The Medical Basis for
Radiation Accident Preparedness

The Medical Basis for Radiation Accident Preparedness

Proceedings of the REAC/TS International Conference:
The Medical Basis for Radiation Accident Preparedness,
October 18–20, 1979, Oak Ridge, Tennessee, U.S.A.

Editors:

Karl F. Hübner, M.D. and
Shirley A. Fry, M.B., Ch.B.
Oak Ridge Associated Universities

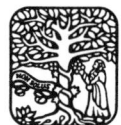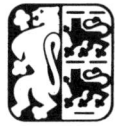

Elsevier/North-Holland
New York • Amsterdam • Oxford

In the interest of a rapid publication, this book has not received the standard attention of the Desk Editorial Department and thus, Elsevier North Holland, Inc. bears no editorial responsibility for this volume.

Published by:

Elsevier North Holland, Inc.
52 Vanderbilt Avenue, New York, New York 10017

Sole distributors outside U.S.A. and Canada:

Elsevier/North-Holland Biomedical Press
335 Jan van Galenstraat, P.O. Box 211
Amsterdam, The Netherlands

Library of Congress Cataloging in Publication Data

REAC/TS International Conference: The Medical Basis for Radiation Accident
     Preparedness, Oak Ridge, Tenn., 1979.
The medical basis for radiation accident preparedness.

Includes bibliographical references and index.
1. Radiation—Toxicology—Congresses. 2. Radiation workers—Diseases and
     hygiene—Congresses. 3. Nuclear facilities—Accidents—
     Congresses. I. Hübner, Karl F. II. Fry, Shirley A. III. Radiation
     Emergency Assistance Center/Training Site
     (U.S.) IV. Title. [DNLM: 1. Radiation injuries—Prevention and
     control—Congresses. WN650 R106m 1979]
RA1231.R2R23   1979   616.9'89707   80-16567
ISBN 0-444-00431-9

Manufactured in the United States of America

Contents

Preface

The International Conference on The Medical Basis for Radiation Accident Preparedness was organized by the staff of the Radiation Emergency Assistance Center/Training Site (REAC/TS) of the Medical and Health Sciences Division of Oak Ridge Associated Universities (ORAU). The philosophical importance of relating, through investigation and education, the intellectual resources of higher education to the important social problems associated with energy, health, and the environment was the foundation of the meeting.

The symposium, held under the auspices of the U.S. Department of Energy, was the ninth (a list is provided on p. xiii) since 1960 of a series of international conferences addressing the various aspects of radiation accidents. The approach of this most recent conference differed somewhat from that of those preceding it, in that it sought an international review of the gamut of the medical aspects of radiation injury, not only for the experts in the field, but also for other physicians and scientists who, in view of current events, have had the need to know thrust upon them.

To widen the circle of the enlightened is, as its name implies, one of the charges of REAC/TS. REAC/TS also shares in a responsibility with other scientists to interpret contemporary problems to society and, as Dr. Philip L. Johnson, executive director of ORAU stated, to put the challenge of expectation into perspective with the possibility of attainment. The importance placed on these responsibilities in the United States was attested to by the participation in the conference of Dr. Shields Warren, the first director of the Atomic Energy Commission's

Division of Biology and Medicine, and two of his successors, Dr. John R. Totter and Dr. William W. Burr, Jr., the present director of the Office of Health and Environmental Research of the U.S. Department of Energy. Under their guidance, the knowledge and appreciation of the health effects of radiation have developed to the benefit of man.

Karl F. Hübner
Shirley A. Fry

Conferences and Symposia
on Radiation Accidents

1. Scientific Meeting on the Diagnosis and Treatment of Acute Radiation Injury (WHO), Geneva, October, 1960, New York, International Documents Service, 1961.
2. Symposium on Radiation Accidents and Emergencies in Medicine, Research and Industry. Mid-West Chapter Health Physics Society, Medical Physics Society of Illinois and American Industrial Hygiene Association, Chicago, 1963, Springfield, Illinois, Thomas, 1965.
3. Risk Evaluation for Protection of the Public in the Event of Radiation Accidents; A Report Published on Behalf of IAEA and WHO, Vienna, International Atomic Energy Agency, 1967 (IAEA Safety Series No. 21).
4. Accidental Irradiation at Place of Work; Proceedings of the International Symposium, Nice, 1966, Liege, EURATOM, 1967.
5. Symposium on the Handling of Radiation Accidents. (IAEA, WHO), Vienna, 1969, Vienna, International Atomic Energy Agency, 1969.
6. International Workshop on Recent Advances in Medical Management in Radiation Accidents, U.S. Atomic Energy Commission/Pan American Health Organization, Washington, September 16–19, 1973 (Unpublished).
7. International Seminar on Diagnosis and Treatment of Incorporated Radionuclides. (IAEA and WHO) Vienna, 1975, International Atomic Energy Agency, 1976.
8. Symposium on Handling Radiation Accidents 1977, Proceedings of a Symposium (IAEA, WHO), Vienna, 1977, International Atomic Energy Agency, Vienna, 1977.

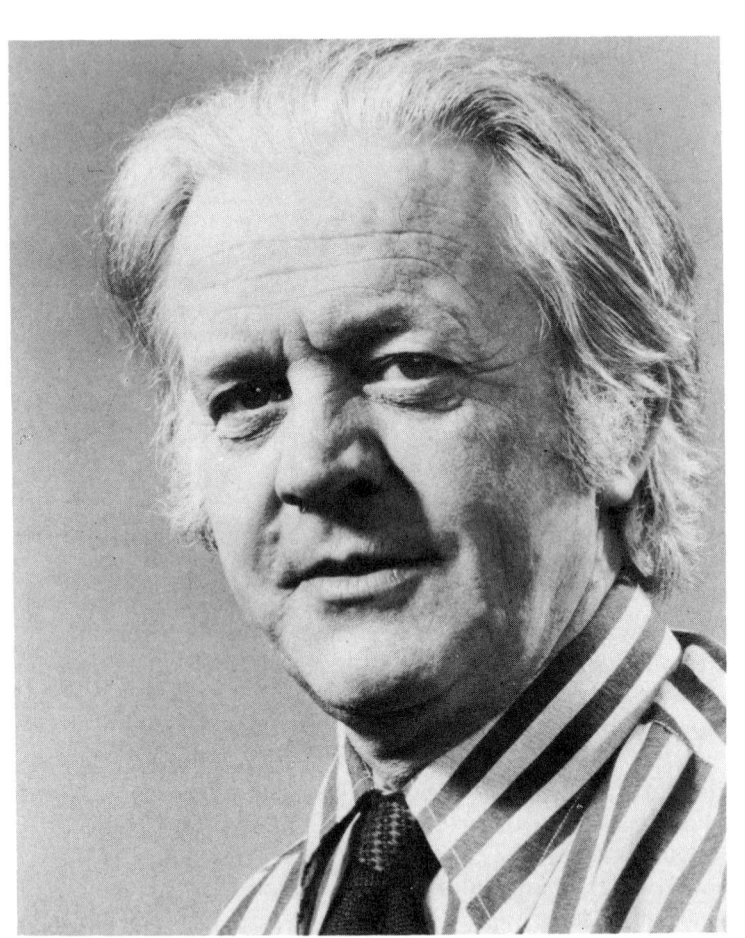

Dedication

During the initial planning for this Conference, we had hoped to be able to invite Dr. Geoffrey Dolphin of the National Radiological Protection Board in the United Kingdom to participate in this meeting and present one of the presentations in the section on Cytogenetic Dosimetry. It was in our preliminary communications with various persons from Great Britain that we first learned that Dr. Dolphin was seriously ill, and late this summer we were very saddened to learn of his untimely death.

For those of us in the field of radiation cytogenetics this is indeed a great loss. Dr. Dolphin's scientific contributions in the use of cytogenetic methodology in human dose assessment had been numerous, particularly during the last decade, and all of us who had the opportunity to know him, to talk with him regarding mutual scientific problems and interests, benefited greatly from the association with him. His enthusiasm for his work, his willingness to share his thoughts and ideas, his work and his wit, were his trademarks, and the lack of his presence at assemblies such as this is truly unfortunate.

It seems appropriate we formally recognize his numerous contributions in radiation biology by dedicating the proceedings of this conference to his memory. We have asked Dr. Geoffrey Schofield, who is the Chief Medical Director of the British Nuclear Fuels Limited, to speak briefly at this dedication. Dr. Schofield, in addition to collaborating on several scientific projects with Dr. Dolphin, was also a close personal friend for many years.

L. G. Littlefield

It is with very mixed feelings that I take on this duty. I'm very honored to be able to speak for Geoff Dolphin, who has been a very close friend and colleague for over 20 years. I think this is a great loss to this Conference and to the world of radiobiology in general.

Geoff started out his career as a pure physicist. He qualified at Reading University, and, following that, he went into the Royal Air Force where he worked with radar. After coming out of the Royal Air Force, he got his Ph.D. in pure physics at Reading University, and, as a matter of interest for those of you who knew the sort of work that he did, his Ph.D. was on the viscosity of air. Now you can't get more physical than that, can you? He had an excellent mind and was very capable in dealing with people, understanding what made people think, being able to bridge the gap between doctors and physicists. He developed an interest in medical physics and went to St. Bartholomew's Hospital in London as a researcher in medical physics. During the course of this particular activity, he came to the United States for the first time with his wife, Yvonne, and the children where he worked at Yale for a year; and, of course, we know of his daughter Annette, following in father's footsteps, who is at present working at Yale. Very nice, I think.

While Geoff was in the States, he made an awful lot of friends, of course, and these stayed with him. That says an awful lot for his totality. Eventually, he drifted away from physics, and he became a man of parts. The occasion arose when he had to get a new passport, and he spoke to his friend Ken Dunkin and asked how he should describe himself on his passport. They scratched their heads, and Ken, being a Scotsman, said "Well, in Scotland professors of physics are called professors of natural philosophy. Why don't you call yourself a natural philosopher?" And Geoff called himself a natural philosopher. I don't think you can have a better term for a man of his stature. He joined the Authority Health and Safety Branch, as it was in 1959, and he was one of the senior members of that organization from the word go. Eventually, this changed hands, like all the organizations do, and the National Radiological Protection Board was formed in 1971. Geoff became one of its Assistant Directors with particular reference to research. It was during this time that he became so interested in cytogenetics, of course.

Originally, in the United Kingdom, we had picked out all the people who were overexposed at Windscale, and the medical research council had looked at them. Geoff became extremely interested in this, and he set up an excellent cytogenetics section at the NRCB. Another side of his activities, of course, was concerned with the ICRP, and here he was a well-known member for many, many years. He started with the ICRP in 1964 as a member of the task group from ICRP Committee 4, on the evaluation of radiation doses to body tissues from internal contamination. From 1966 to 1968, he was a member of the task group of Committee

Mark, Committee 1 on spatial distribution of radiation dose. In 1969, he became a member of ICRP Committee 2, and since that time until his death, he was a member of ICRP Committee 2 and also its secretary. I'm told the secretarial duties have never been done so well as they were done when Geoff was doing this.

He reached the peak of his scientific career in 1978 when he was awarded the Doctor of Science from Reading University. The degree of Doctor of Science in the United Kingdom is one that is given to very, very few. You really must be the absolute tops in your field to be awarded this particular degree. Now those of you who knew Geoff, knew that he was very unassuming; never assumed that he was good at anything. But on one occasion, just after he got his DSc, he whispered it to me over a noggin one evening, "You know, I'm really rather pleased about this DSc." Now for Geoff to say that would be equivalent to the rest of us standing on the housetops and shouting it to the country.

One of the other important aspects about Geoff Dolphin was his ability to teach, to lecture, and to explain—to explain things in a simplified manner that even the rather less intelligent people like myself could actually understand. His lectures were superb, and he always stuck by the maxim of lecturers that you must never, ever put too much on a slide because no one would read it. Geoff's slides were known everywhere. They were beautiful; they were simple. He was a great man for the model, and his ability to make things clear was really quite profound. The only snag was that having made things clear, by the time you got down the corridor you'd have forgotten what he'd said.

I've said that his wit was extraordinary, quick as a flash, and there is a rather nice little tale that some of you may have heard. When Geoff was in conversation with an extremely earnest young man, and they were talking about the fission product deposition in humans with particular reference to zinc 65, the earnest young man said to Geoff, "Well, you realize, of course, that zinc 65 is deposited in the testes, and furthermore, it's deposited in the sperm. What do you think about that?" And Geoff quick as a flash said "It must have galvanized them." Such was this man of many parts. I think really that this is the moat on which I ought to formally dedicate this conference to Dr. Geoffrey Dolphin and at the same time extend the condolences and sympathies of everybody here, to his wife Yvonne and to his daughters Annette and Phillipa. Thank you very much.

G. B. Schofield

Introduction

Ruth C. Clusen

Assistant Secretary for Environment, U.S. Department of Energy

Environmental concerns don't stop at borders or at waters' edge, they are worldwide. I always knew that. But the presence at this symposium of distinguished scientists, physicians, and engineers from 17 other countries is proof of the international character of those concerns.

This symposium focuses on nuclear energy. Environmental concerns related to nonnuclear energy sources are receiving equal attention. Just a scant 50 miles from Oak Ridge, my office is supporting, simultaneously with this meeting, an international symposium on the potential environmental and health effects of atmospheric sulfur deposition.

Observation is the classic method of training physicians. Doctors, however, don't see many radiation-accident victims. Because professors in teaching hospitals do not encounter many such cases in their rounds, no medical school, I am told, teaches care of radiation-accident victims; that, of course, is one of the reasons for this meeting. This symposium is a way each of the participants can help colleagues, by imparting this hard-to-find knowledge. We are fortunate such accidents are rare—as a human concern.

Since 1960, there have been eight conferences or symposia on radiation accidents in Europe or the United States. This, the ninth, is the first sponsored by the Department of Energy, but the second sponsored by the office I now head. That seeming paradox can be explained by the fact that, despite several changes in name and in home agency, my office is a lineal descendant of the former Atomic Energy Commission's Division of Biological-Environmental Research. The 1973 International Workshop on Recent Advances in Medical Management in Radiation Accidents had two other sponsors. One was the Division of Operational

Safety—now called the Operational and Environmental Safety Division. The other was the Pan American Health Organization. Since the World Health Organization held the first symposium in Geneva 19 years ago this month, Euratom and the International Atomic Energy Agency have also sponsored meetings. I am impressed by the company we keep. My pride in being part of such history is great, I assure you.

There are at least two other "firsts" connected with this symposium. It is the first to be directed toward those outside or on the fringes of the nuclear industry along with, of course, those of you who have been involved directly for years. I speak of the emergency room physician at a hospital that happens to be near a road used by trucks carrying such hazardous substances as radioactive waste, of the occupational physician of a power and light company that is building or soon will put into operation a reactor, of the physician or scientist from one of the many laboratories or hospitals dealing with radioactive materials. Each has to be prepared to act in the event of an accident involving one or a few persons, or an accident compounded by an uncontrolled release of radiation or radioactive materials that could adversely affect a large population.

Another first: this symposium encourages the reporting of the current status of the survivors of earlier accidents. That is necessary if diagnosis and treatment of radiation injuries are to be improved and the knowledge of long-term radiation effects extended. In these presentations and discussions the last 35 years are reviewed by the very physicians who participated in developing knowledge in this field.

Detailed review of past accidents and of their survivors forms a broad medical basis to enable physicians to react intelligently to the unique needs of the moment and to modify or extend therapy protocols. "Unique" is the proper word because victims of various types of radiation accidents have been so few, that experts have found every case differs from others enough to prevent using fixed procedures.

There are increasing applications of radiation and radioactive materials in diagnostic and therapeutic medicine, in medical and scientific research. There are nuclear fuels being used as energy sources, although new starts on nuclear power plants have slowed or nearly stopped. That slowdown occurred before Three Mile Island, which has added to the speculation about the future of the nuclear power industry.

National and international public worry over most things nuclear contrasts, almost in a contradictory fashion, with the rarity of radiation accidents. Since that awesome dawn of the nuclear age at Hiroshima in 1945 there have been 45 known, serious radiation accidents. Thirty of them have been in the United States. Approximately 800 persons were involved, of whom 14 (four in this country) died of acute effects of radiation. About 50 others were seriously injured by radiation in those accidents.

No known radiation injuries were recorded outside the Three Mile Island Plant. More than 50,000 traffic deaths occurred in the United States again last year. Fires in houses, hotels, and other buildings caused 8,700 deaths and 280,000 injuries in 1978. To say, therefore, that radiation accidents and resultant casualties are rare is no misstatement of fact. To say that there will be a few in the future may be prophetic, but also it could prove to be untrue. We dare not make such predictions. It is imprudent.

Prudence has been demonstrated in the past, however. It continues to be, as witnessed in this symposium. All radiation accidents are documented in the Registry System established under the Atomic Energy Commission and continued today, right here in Oak Ridge by the Radiation Emergency Assistance Center/Training Site—usually called REAC/TS. The staff also maintains other registries of past and present employees of the Department of Energy and its predecessors, whose exposures exceeded the annual occupational limits, and of accidents in other countries. The registries are an integral part of the research and educational program of the assistance center.

Prudence, too, was behind the establishment in 1962 of annual, national medical symposia at various government laboratories, including what was then called the Oak Ridge Institute of Nuclear Studies—now the Oak Ridge Associated Universities (ORAU). Since 1976, ORAU has been conducting these courses for DOE at the Radiation Emergency Assistance Center/Training Site. Seminar-like courses are offered regularly. Experts from this country—most of them here—have lectured about their experiences, diagnostic and therapeutic methods. Just since November of 1976, eighteen courses have trained 300 persons. There have been three course titles: Medical Planning and Care in Radiation Accidents, Health Physics in Radiation Accidents, and Handling of Radiation Accidents by Emergency Personnel. The registries provide the documentation for the courses.

Among those trained have been hospital administrators, state and local health and energy disaster officials, fire rescue officers, policemen, and others. Also among them were 14 physicians, health physicists, scientists, and registered nurses from five other countries. All of this training comes under a heading of preparedness. How well are we prepared?

Excellent safety practices are the best prevention of radiation accidents. That is one of my functions as head of the Office of Environment in the Department of Energy. My office oversees safety at the Department's installation and at those operated by its contractors, which have more than 100,000 employees. Those of you attending, however, have the more grim duty—maintaining readiness for what could happen should those safety precautions fail. Human beings do fail, unfortunately.

We in the Office of Environment are part of the National Interagency Radiation Assistance Program, designed to aid in radiation accidents.

This assistance would consist of determining the amount of radiation, monitoring its source and its pathways, helping to clean up any radiation materials that might be spread from the source. REAC/TS provides a different type of response capability. The medical staff at REAC/TS, under the able direction of Dr. Karl Hübner, is instantly available by phone to assist in providing medical advice, consultation, and if necessary to receive and treat accident victims at REAC/TS.

Although these groups are ready at all times to assist, the first line of defense in any radiation accident will be you and your paramedical staff. The more trained people like you that are available around the country and the world, the quicker competent medical assistance can be provided the victims.

Although experiences have proved favorable, the potential for real disaster is great. Peaceful uses of radioactive materials and nuclear energy have been demonstrated to be worthwhile for mankind. But as with anything inherently dangerous—fire, electricity, explosives, transportation vehicles, even drugs—caution must be taken. Things nuclear must be treated even more cautiously. The public seems to have an aversion, a fear, a foreboding about this arcane force. They might even put those who work with radioactive materials in the same class with cultists such as snake handlers. These feelings perhaps emerge from the initial use of nuclear energy, the Bomb. Whatever the reason, it puts you in a class apart.

The mystery—if that's what it is—must be put to rest. The danger, linked with cancer in the minds of so many, must be faced. Not perhaps with the same cavalier attitude we have to such dangers as a slippery bathtub, but perhaps more with the respect we have for a hearth fire. Truth is a great tool. Should you have been involved, when a crisis passes, you might wish to inform the public in a clear and forthright manner of the nature of a victim's plight. Level with the public. The truth might not be pleasant, but certainly it will be less sinister than imaginations will conjure up.

In closing, may I commend each of you for helping to make this symposium a success. It is one of the fine achievements of the Department. I am proud to be part of it.

Ruth C. Clusen
Assistant Secretary for Environment,
U.S. Department of Energy
Oak Ridge, Tennessee

October 18, 1979

List of Participants
International REAC/TS Conference

Baruch Aaron
Aaron Emergency Medical Consultants, Inc., 951 Sherwood Lake Drive, Apartment 1-C, Schereville, Indiana 46375

William Albers
Division of Operational and Environmental Safety, E-201, Department of Energy, Washington, D.C. 20545

Herbert C. Allen
100 Horman Professional Building, Houston, Texas 77030

Bobby R. Adcock
Armed Forces Radiobiology Research Institute (AFRRI), Defense Nuclear Agency, Bethesda, Maryland 20014

Gould A. Andrews*
Professor of Medicine and Radiology, Department of Nuclear Medicine, University of Maryland Hospital, Baltimore, Maryland 21201

John Auxier
Oak Ridge National Laboratory, Building 4500 S, Room G250, P.O. Box X, Oak Ridge, Tennessee 37830

A. J. Barker
General Electric Company, P.O. Box 11508, St. Petersburg, Florida 33733

*Conference speaker.

Flora M. Barlotta*
Department of Internal Medicine, St. Barnabas Medical Center, Livingston, New Jersey 07039

Jerre Batson
Medical and Health Sciences Division, Oak Ridge Associated Universities, P.O. Box 117, Oak Ridge, Tennessee 37830

John A. Beare
Division Director, Health Services Division, Department of Social and Health Services, DSHS Mail Stop OB-44J, Olympia, Washington 98504

John O. Beatty
University of California, Lawrence Livermore Laboratory, 700 East Avenue, Livermore, California 94550

Jay Beaufait
Division of Operational and Environmental Safety, Department of Energy, Mail Stop E-201, Washington, D.C. 20545

Jack Beck*
Professional Training Programs, Oak Ridge Associated Universities, P.O. Box 117, Oak Ridge, Tennessee 37830

Richard E. Benson
Oak Ridge Operations, Department of Energy, P.O. Box E, Oak Ridge, Tennessee 37830

Scott Benson
Department of Energy, Washington, D.C. 20545

Donna Best
Radiation Health, Mare Island Naval Shipyard, Vallejo, California 94592

Mary Ellen Berger
Indian River Community College, 1484 Sunshine Avenue, Port St. Lucie, Florida 33452

Victor P. Bond*
Associate Director, Life Sciences, Chemistry and Safety, Brookhaven National Laboratory, Upton, New York 11973

Antonie Botha
Medical Officer, Atomic Energy Board of South Africa, Office of the Scientific Counsellor, Suite 300, 2555 M Street, NW, Washington, D.C. 20037

Hugh K. Boyd, Jr.
Richland County/City of Columbia Civil Defense, 1401 Hampton Street, Columbia, South Carolina 29201

Bryce D. Breitenstein*
Hanford Environmental Health Foundation, P.O. Box 100, Richland, Washington 99352

James T. Brennan
University of Pennsylvania, 9120 Germantown Avenue, Philadelphia, Pennsylvania 19118

Frank Brooks
Federal Emergency Management Agency, 1725 I Street, NW, Washington, D.C. 20472

Robert E. Brubaker
United Nuclear Corporation, UNC Naval Products, 67 Sandy Desert Road, Uncasville, Connecticut 06382

Austin M. Brues*
Medical Director, Center for Human Radiobiology, Argonne National Laboratory, Argonne, Illinois 60439

Arne O. Bull
Nordic Society of Radiation Protection, University of Oslo, Box 1060, Blindern, Oslo 3, Norway

Elaine M. Bunick
Oak Ridge Hospital of the Methodist Church, 301 Medical Arts Building, Oak Ridge, Tennessee 37830

W. W. Burr, Jr.*
Director, Office of Health and Environmental Research, Department of Energy, Washington, D.C. 20545

Donald Busick
Stanford Linear Accelerator Center, P.O. Box 4349, Stanford, California 94305

Bill Byrd
Medical and Health Sciences Division, Oak Ridge Associated Universities, P.O. Box 117, Oak Ridge, Tennessee 37830

Glyn Caldwell
Chief, Cancer Branch, Bureau of Epidemiology, Center for Disease Control, 1600 Clifton Road, NE, Atlanta, Georgia 30333

Donald P. Cameron
UT-CARL, 1299 Bethel Valley Road, Oak Ridge, Tennessee 37830

Alex G. Carabia
125 West Tennessee Avenue, Oak Ridge, Tennessee 37830

Elbert Carlton
Medical and Health Sciences Division, Oak Ridge Associated Universities, P.O. Box 117, Oak Ridge, Tennessee 37830

W. J. M. Carpay
Netherlands Energy Research Foundation, P.O. Box 1, 1755 ZG Petten (N.H.), The Netherlands

Helen Carpenter
Blount Memorial Hospital, Maryville, Tennessee 37801

K. C. Carstairs
Department of Hematology, Toronto General Hospital, 101 College Street, Toronto, Ontario, Canada M 5 G1L7

Melvin H. Chalfen
Massachusetts Institute of Technology, 77 Massachusetts Avenue, 20B-23B, Cambridge, Massachusetts 02139

Warren A. Christensen
X-Ray Products Corporation, 7829 Industry Avenue, Pico Rivera, California 90660

Roger J. Cloutier
Professional Training Programs, Oak Ridge Associated Universities, P.O. Box 117, Oak Ridge, Tennessee 37830

Ruth Clusen*
Asst. Secretary for Environment, Department of Energy, Washington, D.C. 20545

Jack Coffey
Professional Training Programs, Oak Ridge Associated Universities, P.O. Box 117, Oak Ridge, Tennessee 37830

Vincent P. Collins*
9200 Westheimer, Houston, Texas 77063

Shirley Colyer
Medical and Health Sciences Division, Oak Ridge Associated Universities, P.O. Box 117, Oak Ridge, Tennessee 37830

Robert A. Conard
32 Ivy Lane, Setauket, New York 11733

W. J. D. Cooke
Chalk River Nuclear Laboratories, Atomic Energy of Canada, Ltd. Research Company, Chalk River, Ontario, Canada K0J 1J0

Robert L. Craig
Tennessee Valley Authority, 320 Edney Building, Chattanooga, Tennessee 37401

John Crockett
Medical and Health Sciences Division, Oak Ridge Associated Universities, P.O. Box 117, Oak Ridge, Tennessee 37830

Edgar B. Darden, Jr.
UT-CARL, 1299 Bethel Valley Road, Oak Ridge, Tennessee 37830

Zivan Deanovic
"Ruder Boskovic" Institute, Bijenicka 54, 4100 Zagreb, Yugoslavia

Tede Eston de Eston
Faculdade de Medicina da Universidade de Sao Paulo, Ave. Padre Pereira de Andrade, 545 Apt. 103-E, Sao Paulo, Brazil

Howard Dickson
Health and Safety Research Division, Oak Ridge National Laboratory, P.O. Box Y, Oak Ridge, Tennessee 37830

Weldon D. Dillow
Tennessee Valley Authority, Radiological Hygiene Branch, River Oaks Building, Muscle Shoals, Alabama 35660

Keith H. Dinger
Portsmouth Naval Shipyard, Code 105.5, Portsmouth, New Hampshire 03801

William S. Dingledine
Medical Director, Virginia Electric and Power Company, P.O. Box 26666, Richmond, Virginia 23261

Ronald V. Dorn III
Walter Reed Army Medical Center, OSC Box 172, Washington, D.C. 20012

Thomas J. Doyle
Con Edison, 30 Flatbush Avenue, Brooklyn, New York 11217

Russell DuFrain*
Medical and Health Sciences Division, Oak Ridge Associated Universities, P.O. Box 117, Oak Ridge, Tennessee 37830

Daniel Dupourque
Tennessee Valley Authority, Building 308, Chattanooga, Tennessee 37401

Elizabeth Dupree
Medical and Health Sciences Division, Oak Ridge Associated Universities, P.O. Box 117, Oak Ridge, Tennessee 37830

Robley D. Evans
4621 E. Crystal Lane, Scotsdale, Arizona 85253

Judy W. Ewing
Sandia Laboratories, P.O. Box 5800, Albuquerque, New Mexico 87185

M. H. Faes
Centre d'Etudes de L'Energie Nucleaire, B-2400 MOL, Belgium

James Farmer
Interdevelopment, Inc., 2361 S. Jefferson Davis Highway, Suite 1014, Arlington, Virginia 22202

William E. Felling
Assistant Director, Oak Ridge Associated Universities, P.O. Box 117, Oak Ridge, Tennessee 37830

T. Guy Fortney
Union Carbide Corporation, Nuclear Division, P.O. Box P, Oak Ridge, Tennessee 37830

Robert J. Freedy
Battelle Columbus Laboratories, 505 King Avenue, Columbus, Ohio 43201

Thomas E. Fritz
Argonne National Laboratory, BIM Building 202, 9700 South Cass Avenue, Argonne, Illinois 60437

E. L. Frome
Medical and Health Sciences Division, Oak Ridge Associated Universities, P.O. Box 117, Oak Ridge, Tennessee 37830

Shirley A. Fry*
Medical and Health Sciences Division, Oak Ridge Associated Universities, P.O. Box 117, Oak Ridge, Tennessee 37830

Eleanor M. Garner
2204 Westcliff, Knoxville, Tennessee 37919

Seaton Garrett
Oak Ridge National Laboratory, P.O. Box X, Oak Ridge, Tennessee 37830

Robert M. Gastineau
Medical Director, Westinghouse Bettis Atomic Power Laboratory, Box 79, West Mifflin, Pennsylvania 15122

Mary Esther Gaulden*
Associate Professor and Chief, Radiation Biology, University of Texas Health Science Center at Dallas, 5323 Harry Hines Boulevard, Dallas, Texas 75235

Bill Gerhardt
UT-CARL, 1299 Bethel Valley Road, Oak Ridge, Tennessee 37830

Michael V. Gilberti*
Senior Medical Advisor, Research and Development Laboratory, Gulf Oil Corporation, P.O. Box 1166, Hammarville, Pennsylvania 15230

Carolyn Gooch
Oak Ridge National Laboratory, Building 9207, P.O. Box X, Oak Ridge, Tennessee 37830

John A. Googins
Oregon Health Division, 1400 SW 5th, Portland, Oregon 97201

Douglas Grahn
Argonne National Laboratory, Building 202, 9700 South Cass Avenue, Argonne, Illinois 60439

Rodger W. Granlund
Pennsylvania State University, 228 Academic Projects Building, University Park, Pennsylvania 16802

Robert S. Grier
Los Alamos National Laboratory, Los Alamos, New Mexico 87544

Peter Groer
Institute for Energy Analysis, Oak Ridge Associated Universities, P.O. Box 117, Oak Ridge, Tennessee 37830

Lloyd Hall
Sierra Vista Hospital, 81 Verde Drive, San Luis Obispo, California 93401

Martha Hansard
Medical and Health Sciences Division, Oak Ridge Associated Universities, P.O. Box 117, Oak Ridge, Tennessee 37830

Kent Harding
Department of National Defense, Defense Research Establishment, Ottawa, Ontario, Canada K 1A 0Z4

J. C. Harduin
Cogema–Etablissement de la Hague, BP 270 50107, Cherbourg, France

Robert J. Hart*
Manager, Oak Ridge Operations, Department of Energy, P.O. Box E, Oak Ridge, Tennessee 37830

Ray Hayes
Medical and Health Sciences Division, Oak Ridge Associated Universities, P.O. Box 117, Oak Ridge, Tennessee 37830

Louis H. Hempelmann*
Route 1, P.O. Box 193, Santa Fe, New Mexico 97501

K. Hirashima*
Head, Division of Radiation Health, National Institute of Radiological Sciences, Anagawa, Chiba-shi 260, Japan

Harold Hodges
Medical and Health Sciences Division, Oak Ridge Associated Universities, P.O. Box 117, Oak Ridge, Tennessee 37830

Leo J. Hoge
Knolls Atomic Power Laboratory, Box 1072, Schenectady, New York 12301

F. Eugene Holly*
1622 Van Horne Lane, Redondo Beach, California 90278

Alan Houston
North Sandwich, New Hampshire 03259

Leslie Hovey
St. Francis Memorial Hospital, 900 Hyde Street, San Francisco, California 94109

Christopher D. Hoy
251 West 92nd Street, Apt. 53, New York, New York 10025

K. F. Hübner*
Medical and Health Sciences Division, Oak Ridge Associated Universities, P.O. Box 117, Oak Ridge, Tennessee 37830

Vicki Huff
Medical and Health Sciences Division, Oak Ridge Associated Universities, P.O. Box 117, Oak Ridge, Tennessee 37830

Donna Hudson
Medical and Health Sciences Division, Oak Ridge Associated Universities, P.O. Box 117, Oak Ridge, Tennessee 37830

Shirley Hutton
Blount Memorial Hospital, Maryville, Tennessee 37801

William Jessen*
Swedish State Power Board, Ringhals Nuclear Power Plant, S43022 Vaeroebacka, Sweden

P. Jockey*
Commissariat a L'Energie Atomique, Institute de Protection et de Surete Nucleaire, Department de Protection, 92260 Fontenay-Aux-Roses, France

Philip L. Johnson*
Executive Director, Oak Ridge Associated Universities, P.O. Box 117, Oak Ridge, Tennessee 37830

Gene Joiner
Medical and Health Sciences Division, Oak Ridge Associated Universities, P.O. Box 117, Oak Ridge, Tennessee 37830

Toni Jones
Medical and Health Sciences Division, Oak Ridge Associated Universities, P.O. Box 117, Oak Ridge, Tennessee 37830

Robert J. Kaminski
Walter Reed Army Medical Center, 6 Feather Rock Place, Rockville, Maryland 20850

Anthony J. Keating
Maine Yankee Atomic Power, 767 High Street, Bath, Maine 04530

Charles E. Kent
Professional Training Programs, Oak Ridge Associated Universities, P.O. Box 117, Oak Ridge, Tennessee 37830

Joe Khym
Oak Ridge, Tennessee 37830

S. A. Kingsbury
Florida Power and Light Company, P.O. Box 529100, Miami, Florida 33152

Marion Bart Knight
Tennessee Valley Authority, 315 Edney Building, Chattanooga, Tennessee 37401

Knud Knudsen
34 S. Howells Pt. Road, Bellport, New York 11713

E. Komarov*
World Health Organization, CH-1211 Geneva 27, Switzerland

Leonard Kreisler
Reynolds Electrical and Engineering Company, Inc., P.O. Box 14400, Las Vegas, Nevada 89114

Toshiyuki Kumatori*
Director–General, National Institute of Radiological Sciences, Chiba, Japan

Pierre Lalu
Commissariat a L'Energie Atomique, Centre d'Etudes de Valduc, B.P. 14, 21-120 I.S. Sur-Tille, France

A. W. Lawson
Senior Medical Officer, British Nuclear Fuels, Ltd., Windscale and Calder Works, Seascale, Great Britain

Steve Lawrence
Manager for Administration, Oak Ridge Associated Universities, P.O. Box 117, Oak Ridge, Tennessee 37830

Roland Le Gô*
Service de Protection Sanitaire, Department de Protection, Republic Francaise, Commissariat a L'Energie Atomique, Fontenay-Aux-Roses, France

Howard J. Leitman
Emergency Department, Baptist Hospital of Miami, 8900 SW 88th Street, Miami, Florida 33176

T. A. Lincoln*
Medical Director, Union Carbide Corporation–HSEA, 270 Park Avenue, 22nd Floor, New York, New York 12107

Roger E. Linnemann*
Director, Radiation Management Corporation, University City Science Center, 3508 Market Street, Suite 400, Philadelphia, Pennsylvania 19104

Gayle Littlefield*
Medical and Health Sciences Division, Oak Ridge Associated Universities, P.O. Box 117, Oak Ridge, Tennessee 37830

William Lotz
EPRI, 1800 Massachusetts Avenue, Suite 700, Washington, D.C. 20036

Guido Lozada
St. Francis Memorial Hospital, 900 Hyde Street, San Francisco, California 94109

C. C. Lushbaugh*
Medical and Health Sciences Division, Oak Ridge Associated Universities, P.O. Box 117, Oak Ridge, Tennessee 37830

Sallie McCaskill
Medical and Health Sciences Division, Oak Ridge Associated Universities, P.O. Box 117, Oak Ridge, Tennessee 37830

Janice McConkey
Oak Ridge Hospital of the Methodist Church, 125 W. Tennessee Avenue, Oak Ridge, Tennessee 37830

Donald McNeill
Emergency Department, Good Samaritan Hospital and Medical Center, 1015 NW 22nd, Portland, Oregon 97210

S. Marks*
Environment, Health, and Safety Research Program, Battelle Pacific Northwest Laboratory, Richland, Washington 99352

Samuel O. Massey
Oak Ridge Ear, Nose, and Throat Center, P.O. Box 444, Oak Ridge, Tennessee 37830

Bruce A. Mazat
Armed Forces Radiobiology Research Institute (AFRRI), Defense Nuclear Agency, Bethesda, Maryland 20014

Sam Miller
Clinical Engineering Center, University of New Hampshire, 120 Kingsbury Hospital, Durham, New Hampshire 03824

Dan Morrison
Medical and Health Sciences Division, Oak Ridge Associated Universities, P.O. Box 117, Oak Ridge, Tennessee 37830

Hartman B. Mowery
Defense Nuclear Agency, Washington, D.C. 20305

W. K. Mueller
Gesellschaft fur Reaktorsicherheit (GRS) mbH, Glockengasse 2, 5000 Koln 1, Germany

D.K. Myers*
Head, Radiation Biology Branch, Chalk River Nuclear Laboratories, Chalk River, Ontario, KOJ 1JO Canada

Floyd P. Naugle
Ritenour Health Center, Pennsylvania State University, University Park, Pennsylvania 16802

J. C. Nénot*
Service de Protection Sanitaire, Department de Protection, Republic Francaise, Commissariat a L'Energie Atomique, Fontenay-Aux-Roses, France

Willard S. Osibin
P.O. Box 338, Templeton, California 93465

Bernard M. Olsen
Portsmouth Naval Shipyard, Code 105.2, Portsmouth, New Hampshire 03801

L. M. Outten
Mars Hill College, P.O. Box 722-C, Mars Hill, North Carolina 28754

R. W. Pape
Medical Director, City of Austin Emergency Medical Service, P.O. Box 1088, Austin, Texas 78767

Roy Parker
5061 Abelia Drive, Baton Rouge, Louisiana 70808

Christian Pasquier
Commissariat a L'Energie Atomique, C.E.N. Fontenay-Aux-Roses, DPr D.P.N. 6 92260, France

Frances K. Patterson
University Hospital Pathology Dept., 1924 Alcoa Highway, Knoxville, Tennessee 37920

Clarence H. Peterson
Department of Development, City of Carlsbad, 2404 W. Pierce 4B, EMS NM Med. Sec., Carlsbad, New Mexico 88220

Gary Peterson
Arizona Health Plan, 6524 W. Indian School Road, Phoenix, Arizona 85033

William A. Pillsbury
Baltimore Gas and Electric Company, Room 1511, P.O. Box 1475, Baltimore, Maryland 21203

A. Polednak*
Medical and Health Sciences Division, Oak Ridge Associated Universities, P.O. Box 117, Oak Ridge, Tennessee 37830

George A. Poda*
Medical Superintendent, E. I. du Pont de Nemours and Company, Savannah River Plant, Aiken, South Carolina 29801

Bailey Pullen
P.O. Box 842, University Station, Hammond, Louisiana 70402

S. Rae
National Radiological Protection Board, Harwell, Didcot, Oxon, United Kingdom OX 11 ORO

John Rafter
Medical and Health Sciences Division, Oak Ridge Associated Universities, P.O. Box 117, Oak Ridge, Tennessee 37830

Betty Rakestraw
Blount Memorial Hospital, Maryville, Tennessee 37801

Malcolm Randolph
Health and Safety Research Division, Oak Ridge National Laboratory, Building 7509, P.O. Box X, Oak Ridge, Tennessee 37830

Norman Rasmussen*
Professor of Nuclear Engineering, Massachusetts Institute of Technology, Boston, Massachusetts 02139

Iver S. Ravin
Boston Edison Company, 800 Boylston Street, Boston, Massachusetts 02199

Tang Remsen
Nuclear Regulatory Commission, Office of Inspection and Enforcement, Mail Stop C/W 359, Washington, D.C. 20555

Klaus Renz
Berufsgenossenschaft der Feinmechanik und Electrotechnik, Der Leitende technische Aufichtsbeamte, Postfach 51 05 80, 5000 Koln 51, Germany

Conrad Richter
Medical and Health Sciences Division, Oak Ridge Associated Universities, P.O. Box 117, Oak Ridge, Tennessee 37830

Robert C. Ricks*
Medical and Health Sciences Division, Oak Ridge Associated Universities, P.O. Box 117, Oak Ridge, Tennessee 37830

A. M. Roberts
UK Ministry of Defense, Atomic Weapons Research Establishment, Aldermaston, Reading RG7 4PR, England

D. M. Robie
Medical and Health Sciences Division, Oak Ridge Associated Universities, P.O. Box 117, Oak Ridge, Tennessee 37830

M. J. Robinet
Argonne National Laboratory, Building 14, 9700 S. Cass Avenue, Argonne, Illinois 60439

Robert J. Rodriguez
Union Carbide Corporation, Nuclear Division, Oak Ridge Gaseous Diffusion Plant, P.O. Box P, Oak Ridge, Tennessee 37830

Hans Detlef Roedler
Institute for Radiation Hygiene, Federal Health Office, 8042 Neuherberg, Germany

Genevieve S. Roessler
Department of Nuclear Engineering Sciences, University of Florida, Nuclear Sciences Center, Gainesville, Florida 32611

Kjell Roos
Swedish Board of Health and Welfare, S 162 87 Vollingby, Sweden

Joseph F. Ross*
11246 Cashmere, Los Angeles, California 90049

Mike Ryan
Oak Ridge National Laboratory, P.O. Box X, Oak Ridge, Tennessee 37830

Eugene L. Saenger*
Radioisotope Laboratory, Cincinnati General Hospital, Cincinnati, Ohio 45267

Leonard Sagan
Electric Power Research Institute, 3412 Hillview Avenue, Palo Alto, California 94303

Bruce C. Salo
Loyola University Medical Center, Department of Nuclear Medicine, 2160 South First Avenue, Maywood, Illinois 60153

Anne Sayer
Medical and Health Sciences Division, Oak Ridge Associated Universities, P.O. Box 117, Oak Ridge, Tennessee 37830

William Schecter
St. Francis Memorial Hospital, 900 Hyde Street, San Francisco, California 94109

Audrey Schlaffke
Medical and Health Sciences Division, Oak Ridge Associated Universities, P.O. Box 117, Oak Ridge, Tennessee 37830

Geoffrey B. Schofield*
Company Chief Medical Director, British Nuclear Fuels Limited, Windscale and Calder Works, Seascale, Great Britain

E. Benson Scott*
500 McMillan, West Monroe, Louisiana 71291

Thomas M. Seed
Division of Biological and Medical Research, Argonne National Laboratory, 9700 South Cass Avenue, Argonne, Illinois 60437

Walter Seelentag
Ministry of the Interior, 17-21 st, Bonn, Germany

David H. Sexton
Oak Ridge National Laboratory, P.O. Box X, Oak Ridge, Tennessee 37830

C. J. Schilling
Central Electricity Generating Board, Medical Branch, Courtenay House, Umrwick Lane 1, London, England EC 4

Connell Shearin*
Chief, Plastic Surgery, Bowman Gray School of Medicine, Winston-Salem, North Carolina 27103

K. Shimaoka
New York State Department of Health, Roswell Park Memorial Institute, 666 Elm Street, Buffalo, New York 14263

Charles S. Shoup
80 Outer Drive, Oak Ridge, Tennessee 37830

L. E. Sigmar
Medical Arts Building, Suite 308, Oak Ridge, Tennessee 37830

Warren K. Sinclair
Associate Laboratory Director for Biomedical and Environmental Research, Argonne National Laboratory, 9700 South Cass Avenue, Argonne, Illinois 60439

Ann Sipe
Medical and Health Sciences Division, Oak Ridge Associated Universities, P.O. Box 117, Oak Ridge, Tennessee 37830

John R. Sisk
Oak Ridge National Laboratory, P.O. Box X, Oak Ridge, Tennessee 37830

W. L. Smalley
Division of Safety and Environmental Control, Department of Energy, P.O. Box E, Oak Ridge, Tennessee 37830

R. L. Sphar
U.S. Navy, Bureau of Medicine and Surgery, 2300 E Street, Washington, D.C. 20372

John H. Spickard
EG & G Idaho, Inc., P.O. Box 1625, Idaho Falls, Idaho 83401

Henry H. Stauffer
Medical Services, Lawrence Berkeley Laboratory, University of California, Berkeley, California 94720

Andrew Stehney
Argonne National Laboratory, 9700 South Cass Avenue, Argonne, Illinois 60439

Peter Stern*
Orthopedic Surgery, Cincinnati General Hospital, Cincinnati, Ohio 45267

Ervin Stoll
Nuclear Safety Division, Federal Energy Office, P.O. Box 2649, CH-3001 Berne, Switzerland

John Storer
Biology Division, Oak Ridge National Laboratory, Building 9207, Room 023, P.O. Box X, Oak Ridge, Tennessee 37830

A. N. B. Stott
United Kingdom Atomic Energy Authority, Harwell Laboratory, Didcot, US, Oxford, England

Robert B. Stroube
Virginia Department of Health, Room 701, 109 Governor Street, Richmond, Virginia 23219

Seiji Sudo
Power Reactor annd Nuclear Fuel Development Corporation, Muramatsu, Tokai-mura, Naka-gun, Ibaraki, Japan

Tan Tan Sun
Medical and Health Sciences Division, Oak Ridge Associated Universities, P.O. Box 117, Oak Ridge, Tennessee 37830

Laszlo B. Sztanyik
National Research Institute for Radiobiology and Radiohygiene, P.O. Box 101 H-1775, Budapest, Hungary

John M. Taylor
Sandia Laboratories, Division 1233, Albuquerque, New Mexico 87185

Malcolm Tenney, Jr.
Virginia State Health Department, 609 N. Coalter Street, Box 2708, Staunton, Virginia 24401

John Totter*
Institute for Energy Analysis, Oak Ridge Associated Universities, P.O. Box 117, Oak Ridge, Tennessee 37830

Frank A. Traylor, Jr.
8350 West 38th Avenue, Wheat Ridge, Colorado 80033

Robert A. Trenkle
2226 Matthews Street, SE, Huntsville, Alabama 35801

Klaus R. Trott
Institute of Radiobiology, University of Munich, Osterberg 4 D - 8184 Gmund, West Germany

Nelson Jose de Lima Valverde
Head, Angra Medical Division, Furnas Centrais Eletricas, Rua Real Grandeza 219, Rio de Janeiro, RJ, Brazil

Claude Vigan
Commission of the European Communities, Joint Research Center - 21020 Ispra (VA), Italy

Branko Vitale
"Ruder Boskovic" Institute, Bijenicka 54, 41000, Zagreb, Yugoslavia

Helen Vodopick*
Oak Ridge Medical Clinic, 170 W. Tennessee Avenue, Oak Ridge, Tennessee 37830

George L. Voelz*
Division Leader, Health Research, Los Alamos Scientific Laboratory, Los Alamos, New Mexico 87544

Howard H. Vogel, Jr.
UT Center for the Health Sciences, Department of Radiation Oncology, 800 Madison Avenue, Memphis, Tennessee 38163

Niel Wald*
Department of Industrial Environmental Health Sciences, Graduate School of Public Health, University of Pittsburgh, Pittsburgh, Pennsylvania 15261

Shields Warren*
Cancer Research Institute, New England Deaconess Hospital, 185 Pilgrim Road, Boston, Massachusetts 02215

Ronald Wascom
Louisiana Nuclear Energy Division, P.O. Box 14690, Baton Rouge, Louisiana 70808

W. T. Washam
Goodyear Atomic Corporation, P.O. Box 628, Piketon, Ohio 45661

Lee Washburn
Medical and Health Sciences Division, Oak Ridge Associated Universities, P.O. Box 117, Oak Ridge, Tennessee 37830

John L. Weeks
Atomic Energy of Canada Ltd., Whiteshell Nuclear Research Establishment, Pinawa, Manitoba, Canada R0E 1L0

D. G. Wilson
United Kingdom Atomic Energy Authority, Doun Reay Nuclear Establishment, Thurso, Scotland

Michael C. Wills
Ontario Hydro, Health Services Department, 700 University Avenue, Toronto, Ontario M5G 1X6, Canada

Henry Wolfe
Occupational Health Physician, Operational and Environmental Safety Division, Department of Energy, Mail Stop E-201, Washington, D.C. 20545

Alan Wood
University of Michigan Hospital, 903 Granger, Ann Arbor, Michigan 48104

Sara Wood
Medical and Health Sciences Division, Oak Ridge Associated Universities, P.O. Box 117, Oak Ridge, Tennessee 37830

Henry D. Wyman
E. I. du Pont de Nemours Company, Construction Division, Savannah River Plant, P.O. Box 117, Augusta, Georgia 30903

K. Y. Yeh*
Chinese Academy of Medical Sciences, Beijing, People's Republic of China

Gino Zanolli
Union Carbide Corporation, Nuclear Division, Y-12 Plant, P.O. Box Y, Oak Ridge, Tennessee 37830

The Medical Basis for
Radiation Accident Preparedness

SECTION I:

Radiation Accidents: Total-body Irradiation

Published 1980 by Elsevier North Holland, Inc.
K.F. Hübner and S.A. Fry, eds. The Medical Basis for Radiation Accident Preparedness

Total-body Irradiation:
A Historical Review and Follow-up

C. C. Lushbaugh, Shirley A. Fry,
Karl F. Hübner, and Robert C. Ricks

*Medical and Health Sciences Division, Oak Ridge Associated Universities,
Oak Ridge, Tennessee.*

In order to provide the conference with a quick overview of worldwide radiation accidents that we are about to discuss here, my colleagues, Drs. Shirley Fry and Karl Hübner, and I have prepared for you a handout which historically presents several lists of these accidents by type of exposure. There is appended a second section which acknowledges by name at long last the many physicians and their major support staff who have taken part in these accidents one way or another. We are prepared for you to be quite critical of these lists and hope you will correct our mistakes and omissions. We would be bitterly disappointed if you did not, because updating our knowledge here is what this symposium is all about. It's the first chance in about seven years for all of us internationally to correct our mistaken "facts" and add new information to our radiation accident lore.

The first chart depicts the various symbols used in the subsequent figures. Wherever possible, we have used an open square to indicate an irradiated person; a blackened square depicts a victim who died from one of the radiation syndromes; and in three instances, death by blast injury is shown by cross-hatched squares. Because I once thought that women were not conducive to radiation accidents, I have marked the women involved with the usual symbol. As you will see, the Mexican, Algerian, and recent California accidents destroy this belief.

In the first figure we have depicted the worldwide criticality accidents about which we have information at least sufficient to list them in the REAC/TS Radiation Accident Registry. In the 14 recorded accidents, five persons died from acute radiation effects and three from blast injuries out of the 44 seriously exposed persons. The small asterisks indicate the seven persons who died subsequent to the accidents from various causes. The large asterisks indicate the accidents which will be addressed in this symposium and were added so the participants in this conference can use these figures as though they were score cards and can relate the various papers to come by calendar year. This chart also notes that criticality accidents appear to be a phenomenon of the adolescence of the atomic age.

The next chart depicts the date, place, and numbers of persons involved for accidents where total-body irradiation was from external sources, such as atomic bomb fallout, ^{60}Co irradiators, and radiography sources. In these 20 accidents, 382 persons were involved, 300 of whom were irradiated by fallout from a Bikini test shot and a shifting wind that did not follow predictions. Of these exposees, nine died acutely, and as far as we know, only two persons have died subsequently. As you can see, 19 persons had concomitant local radiation burns, eight of which required surgery. Again the large asterisks indicate the accidents this conference will either "revisit" or learn of anew.

Largely as the result of Dr. Shirley Fry's industry and the cooperation of the U.S. Nuclear Regulatory Commission, our knowledge of the occurrence of local radiation burns has been increased enormously, as the next two lists show. Formerly I was able to follow the format of the two previous charts, but this practice (begun by Dr. Andrews and me in 1969) had to be abandoned in the interest of completeness and accuracy.

An entire section of the conference addresses the problems caused by this type of radiation injury. Obviously this type of accident has become our most common kind. In the 47 recorded ones (there must be many others we have failed to find), 66 persons received serious burns, and 24 required surgery.

The next chart lists by calendar year the incidence of accidents wherein serious levels of internal contamination and radiation exposure occurred. Eight persons were involved in what are euphemistically called medical misadventures; 13 were related to occupational situations; and two are shown as acutely fatal, although we are uncertain about the nature and outcome of the 1961 "Germany" accident.

In the last figure we have classified all 98 of these recorded accidents according to the kind of radiation-producing device or substance involved. One can see from this analysis that accidents occur much more frequently from inadvertent exposure to radioisotopic "sources" or commercial irradiators (^{60}Co, ^{192}Ir, ^{137}Cs, etc.) and to X-ray generators used in laboratory analyses and research than from all other sources of exposure.

Please peruse the list of medical personnel appended to these charts at your leisure during the conference, and let us have your corrections and additions. We are certain that we have omitted many persons whose work and care with these radiation accident victims and survivors should be acknowledged.

ACKNOWLEDGMENTS

This material is based on work performed under Contract No. DE-AC05-76OR00033 between the Department of Energy, Office of Health and Environmental Research, and Oak Ridge Associated Universities.

Overview of Serious Radiation Accidents

TOTAL BODY IRRADIATION (TBI)

- ▣ FATAL TBI c̄ SEVERE INJURY
- ▣ FATAL TBI
- ▨ FATAL BLAST INJURY
- ◸ SURVIVING TBI
- ▲ INTERNAL EXPOSURE

LOCAL EXPOSURE

- ⊡ LOCAL ONLY
- ▣ LOCAL + TBI
- s SURGERY REQUIRED

GENERAL NOTES

- * NATURAL DEATH
- ♀ FEMALE
- p PATIENT
- F FETUS
- R RESCUER
- ○ TOTAL PERSONS INVOLVED IN ACCIDENT
- ☆ REACT/S CONF.-1979

Figure 1. Chart key. This chart is applicable to Figures 2–5 that summarize the major radiation accidents world-wide. In Figures 2–5, each square ☐ represents one individual who received a radiation dose equal to or in excess of the DOE/NRC dose criteria* as recorded in the U.S. and Foreign Radiation Accident Registries (REAC/TS December 1979).

---

*See p. 458, this volume.

Figure 2. Major Radiation Accidents: Criticality Accidents.

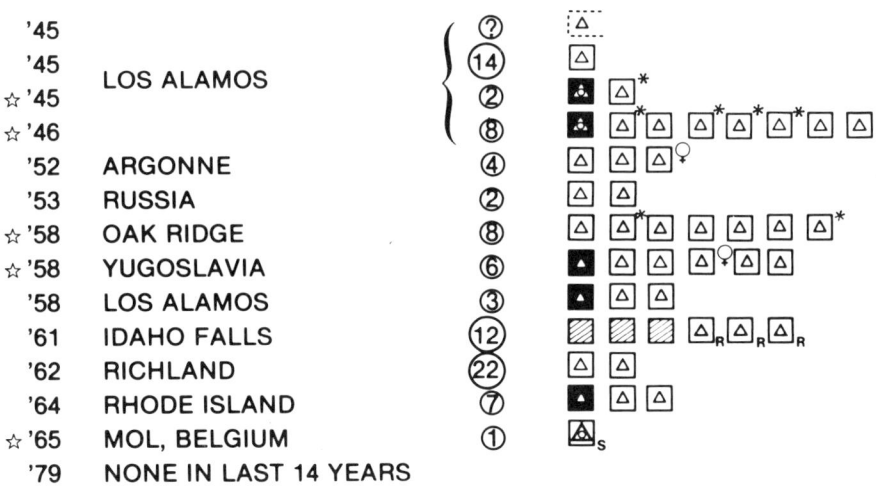

Figure 3. Major Radiation Accidents: Total Body Irradiation from External Sources.

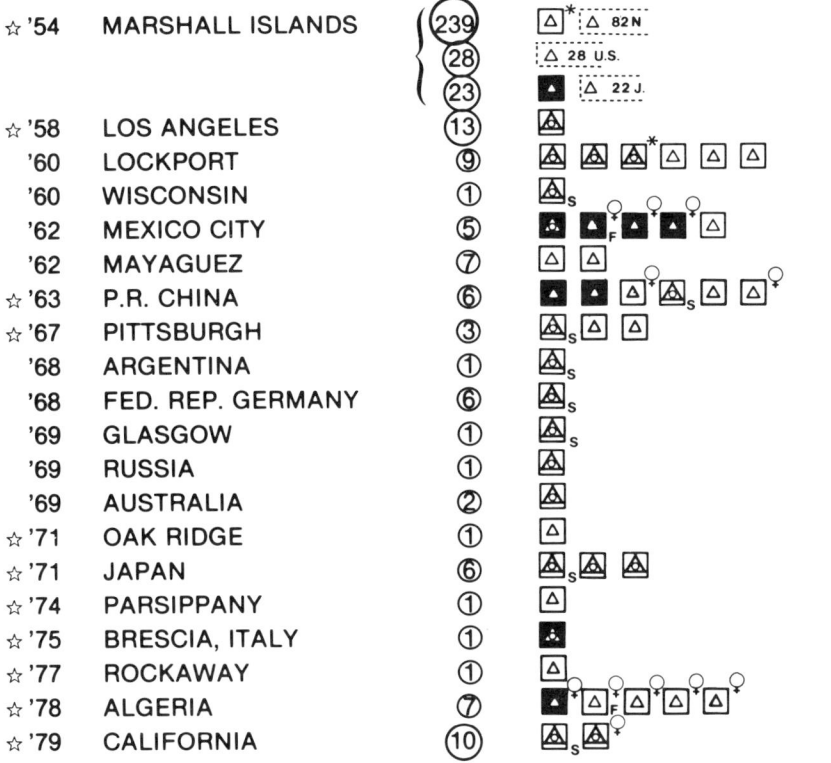

8

'55	HANFORD	^{235}Pu	🄰
'60	RUSSIA	^{226}Ra	🄰
'61	MIAMISBURG	^{238}Pu	🄰 🄰
'61	GERMANY	?	🄰 🄰
'61	MIAMISBURG	^{210}Po	🄰
† '64	NEW YORK	^{241}Am	🄰 🄰
'66	PORTLAND	^{32}P	🄰ᴾ🄰ᴾ🄰ᴾ🄰ᴾ
'66	LEECHBURG	^{235}Pu	🄰
'67	BLOOMSBURG	^{241}Am	🄰
'68	BURBANK	^{238}Pu	🄰 🄰
'68	WISCONSIN	^{198}Au	🄰ᴾ
'69	WISCONSIN	^{35}Sr	🄰ᴾ
'70	DES MOINES	^{32}P	🄰ᴾ
'70	ERWIN	^{235}U	🄰
☆ '76	HANFORD	^{241}Am	🄰
'77	DENVER	^{32}P	🄰ᴾ

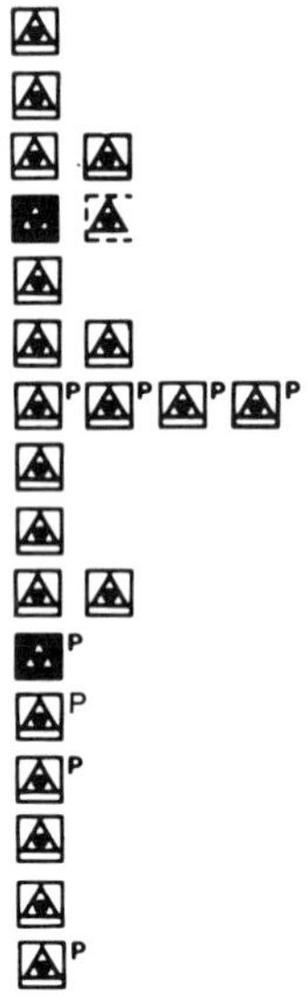

Figure 4. Major Radiation Accidents: Severe Internal Doses.

Classification of Radiation Accidents by "Device"

A. **"Criticalities"**
   1. Critical assemblies — 5
   2. Reactors — 5
   3. Chemical operations — 4
B. **Radiation Devices**
   1. Radioisotope "sources" — 41
   2. X-ray devices — 15
   3. Radar generators — 1
   4. Accelerators — 4
C. **Radioisotopes**
   1. Transuranics — 11
   2. Fission products — 4
   3. Radium spills — 1
   4. Diagnosis and therapy — 7

                                              98

'48	ENIWETOK	β	HAND	④	☐s ☐s ☐s ☐s
	LOS ALAMOS	Ba, La	LEG	①	☐s
'52	LOS ALAMOS	β	HAND	①	☐
'56	LOS ALAMOS	β	HAND	①	☐
'60	SANDIA	ELECTRONS	FACE, TONGUE	①	☐s
'62	ST. PAUL	^{90}Sr	HANDS	②	☐ ☐
'64	BIRMINGHAM	^{60}Co	HANDS	②	☐ ☐
	NEW ORLEANS	^{192}Ir	HAND	①	☐
'65	BURLINGTON	X-RAY	HANDS	③	☐s ☐
	LLL	X-RAY	HAND	①	☐s
	RICHLAND	X-RAY	HAND	①	☐s
	CHICAGO	ELECTRONS	RT. ARM	①	☐s
'66	SALT LAKE CITY	^{192}Ir	HAND	①	☐
'68	W. GERMANY	^{192}Ir	THIGH	⑥	☐s
	INDIA	^{192}Ir	BUTTOCK	①	☐s
	ARGENTINA	^{137}Cs	BOTH LEGS	①	☐s
	SOUTH CAROLINA	^{192}Ir	HAND	①	☐
	HARWELL	?	HAND	①	☐
'69	CHICAGO	^{60}Co	HANDS	⑫	☐ ☐ ☐ ☐ ☐ ☐ ☐ ☐
'70	CAMBRIDGE	REACTOR	HAND	①	☐
'71	NEWPORT NEWS	^{60}Co	HAND	①	☐
	NEW HAVEN	X-RAY	HANDS	②	☐s ☐s
	BIRMINGHAM	^{192}Ir	HAND	①	☐

Figure 5a. Major Radiation Accidents: Local Radiation Burns.

10

Year	Location	Source	Site	Number	
'72	INDIA	X-RAY	HAND	①	▢
'72	CHICAGO	¹⁹²Ir	HAND	①	▢
	PEACH BOTTOM	¹⁹²Ir	HANDS	①	▢ₛ
'74	HASL	X-RAY	HAND	①	▢ₛ
	PEORIA	X-RAY	HANDS	③	▢▢▢
	CHICAGO	⁹⁰Sr	HANDS	②	▢▢
	ALBANY	X-RAY	CHEST	①	▢ₛ
	INDIA	X-RAY	CHEST	①	▢ₚ
	INDIA	X-RAY	ARM	①	▢ᵖ
	AMARILLO	X-RAY	FACE	①	▢
'75	KENTUCKY	¹⁹²Ir	HAND	①	▢ₛ
'76	NEW JERSEY	CYCLOTRON	HAND	①	▢
	BALTIMORE	X-RAY	HAND	①	▢
	PITTSBURGH	¹⁹²Ir	HAND	①	▢
'77	GAINESVILLE	⁶⁰Co	HAND	①	▢
	BERKELEY	X-RAY	HANDS	①	▢ₛ
	SHREVEPORT	⁶⁰Co	HAND	①	▢
☆ '78	MONROE, LA.	¹⁹²Ir	HAND	①	▢ₛ
	E. ALTON	X-RAY	HAND	②	▢▢
☆	ALGERIA	⁶⁰Co	HANDS	②	▢ₛ▢ₛ
☆ '79	NORTH CAROLINA	X-RAY	HAND	①	▢
	NTS	⁶⁰Co	HAND	①	▢
	PARIS, FRANCE	SYNCH'TRON	HAND	①	▢
☆	BATON ROUGE	¹⁹²Ir	HANDS	①	▢

Figure 5b. Major Radiation Accidents: Local Radiation Burns (Continued).

The Which, When, Where and the Physicians of Serious Radiation Accidents

Accident	Date		Medical Staff
Los Alamos 0	6-4-45	LASL	L. H. Hempelmann
		Follow-up:	L. H. Hempelmann, L. G. Littlefield
Los Alamos I* (2 persons)	8-21-45	LASL	L.H. Hempelmann
		Los Alamos Hospital	A.M. Large, J. Brooks, J. DePersio, H. Dwyer
		Consultant	R. S. Stone, L. G. Littlefield
Los Alamos II* (8 persons)	5-21-46	LASL	P. O. Hageman, A. M. Large
		Los Alamos Hospital	J. G. Allen, C. Beller, J. Brooks, L. H. Hempelmann, J. J. Nickson, C. Prosser, H. O. Whipple
		Consultant	S. L. Warren, L. G. Littlefield
Eniwetok (4 persons)	9-7-48	Los Alamos	L. H. Hempelmann, N. P. Knowlton
		Los Alamos Hospital	J. R. Hogness, D. C. Gull, W. R. Oaks, C. L. Schaffer
		St. Louis, Mo. (plastic surgery)	J. B. Brown
		Follow-up:	R. Lapp, H. Andrew, R. Grier, T. Shipman, C. C. Lushbaugh, W. R. Oaks
Kansas City (1 person)	1950's	Kansas City	W. H. Allen
Argonne (4 persons)	6-2-52	Argonne Cancer Research Hospital	R. Hasterlik, A. Finkel, A.M. Brues, L. O. Jacboson
Russia (2 persons)	1953	Moscow	A. Gus'kova, G. D. Baisogolov
Bikini Atoll	3-1-54	Marshall Islands	R. A. Conard, N. R. Schulman, R. S. Farr, W. S. Hall, V. P. Bond, E. Cronkite, J. S. Robertson, G. V. LeRoy, C. L. Dunham, Dr. Weden
		Follow-up:	R. A. Conard, E. P. Cronkite, V. P. Bond, W. W. Sutow, W. C. Maloney, B. Cannon, B. M. Dobyns, A. Lawrey, P. R. Larsen, J. E. Rall, J. Robbins, K. R. Rai, J. Wolff, J. Steele, K. Knudsen, L. M. Meyer, H. S. Pratt
		Japan	M. Tsuzuki, T. Kumatori

The Which, When, Where and the Physicians of Serious Radiation Accidents
(Continued)

Y-12 (Oak Ridge) (8 persons)	6-18-58	Y-12	C. L. Sullivan, C. Congdon, K. S. Lane
		ORINS	M. Brucer, G. A. Andrews, E. B. Andrews, B. Nelson, B. W. Sitterson, A. L. Kretchmar, B. Cooper, M. Perez-Reyes, A. Tsuya
		Consultants:	C. L. Dunham, L. H. Hempelmann
		Follow-up:	G. A. Andrews, B. Nelson, C. L. Edwards, R. M. Kniseley, R. Tanida, K. Goh, K. F. Hübner, H. Vodopick, S. A. Fry, and L. G. Littlefield
Vinca, Yugoslavia (8 persons)	10-15-58	Belgrade	B. Radojicic, M. Antic, S. Hajdukovic
		Curie Foundation, Paris	H. P. Jammet, G. Mathe, J. F. Duplan, G. A. Andrews, B. Pendic, R. Latajet, Dr. Larrieur, D. Kallic, Z. Kjukic, J. Vigne
		Follow-up:	B. Pendic
Los Alamos III (3 persons)	12-30-58	LASL	R. S. Grier, J. S. Benson, C. C. Lushbaugh, P. Harris, T. Shipman, D. Petersen, W. Langham
		Follow-up:	L. H. Hempelmann, G. Voelz, L. G. Littlefield, R. S. Grier
Lockport, N.Y. (9 persons)	3-8-60	Niagara Falls, AFB Hospital	
		U. Rochester SM Hospital	J. Howland, M. Ingram
		Consultant:	C. L. Hansen
		Follow-up:	J. Howland, M. Ingham, G. Casarett
Sandia (1 person)	11-8-60	Albuquerque, N.M.	S. Bliss
Madison, Wisconsin (11 persons)	3-29-60	U. Wisconsin Hospital	E. Rossi
		Follow-up:	E. P. Cronkite, R. A. Love
SL-1 (12 persons)	1-31-61	Idaho Falls	G. Voelz, J. Spickard
		LASL	C. C. Lushbaugh, C. Cavender, P. Harris, D. Petersen
		Follow-up:	J. Spickard

The Which, When, Where and the Physicians of Serious Radiation Accidents
(Continued)

The Mexican Accident (5 persons and fetus)	3-21-62	Oncology Hospital	R. Martinez-Gonzalez, G. Ganem, E. Guttman, M. Lieberman Garcia, G. Cassab
Hanford II (22 persons)	4-7-62	Hanford	P. A. Fuqua, W. R. Norwood, S. Marks
Mayaguez (7 persons)	7-24-62	PRCN Puerto Rico	B. McCandless, A. Contron-Rivera
Peoples Republic of China (6 persons)	1963	?	K.-Y. Yeh, N. Tein, B.-Y. Chiang, F.-W. Chien
Wood River Junction (6 persons)	7-24-64	Rhode Island Hospital	J. S. Karas, M. Albala, T. Forsythe, S. Frater, H. Fanger, M. Bender
Redondo Beach (1 person)	9-24-64	S. Bay Hospital	J. Roberts
New Orleans, LA (2 persons)	1964	Ochsner Clinic	G. H. Porter, W. S. Maxfield
Rockford, IL (1 person)	2-18-64	Argonne Cancer Research Hosp.	A. Tarlov, R. Hasterlik, L. O. Jacobson
Mol, Belgium	12-30-65	Nuclear de Mol U. of Louvain and Curie Foundation, Paris	H. P. Jammet, R. Gongora, R. Le Go, G. Marble, M. Faes, Prof. Morelle
West Indies (1 person)	5-28-66	Antiqua ORINS	— H. Vodopick
Gulf Oil Corp. (3 persons)	10-4-67	U. Pittsburgh Hospital Follow-up:	M. Gilberti, R. R. Schenk, N. Wald M. Gilberti
The Argentinian Accident (1 person)	5-3-63	La Plata	Dr. Paltino, B. Benson, C. C. Lushbaugh
Madison, Wisconsin (1 person)	8-28-68	Argonne Cancer Research Hospital	J. M. Barron, S. Tachin, R. Polycyn, F. W. Fitch, W. A. Sturner
India (1 person)	8-1-68	Stanley Medical Coll. Hosp., Madras	M. Annamalai
New Haven, Conn. (2 persons)	1-71	Yale U. Hospital, Dept. of Surgery	T. Krizek, S. Ariyan, E. V. Kennelly, A. Tarlov
Chiba-Shi, Japan (6 persons)	9-17-71	National Inst. of Radiological Sciences Hospital, Chibashi Follow-up:	T. Kumatori, T. Ishihara, A. Kurisu, H. Sugigana T. Hashizume

14

U. T. Animal Research Lab, Oak Ridge (1 person)	2-4-71	ORINS	G. A. Andrews, H. Vodopick
		Follow-up:	G. Andrews, H. Vodopick, K. F. Hübner, S. A. Fry, N. Gengozian, L. G. Littlefield
Poughkeepsie, N.Y. (1 person)	12-21-72	Gulf Oil Vassar Bros. Hosp. Consultants: ORAU U. Pittsburgh Hosp.	D. Gassaway, M. Gilberti Dr. Tumblety G. A. Andrews, R. Love A. Spritzer, N. Wald
Texas (1 person)	1974	? Follow-up:	T. D. Cronin, V. P. Collins V. P. Collins, M. E. Gaulden
Health and Safety Lab., New York (1 person)	2-4-74	Westwood Pasack Valley Hosp. Consultants:	K. Kalemkeris C. C. Lushbaugh, N. Wald
Peoria, Illinois	3/21-29/74	Caterpillar Tractor Co. Methodist Hospital Follow-up:	C. W. Asbury I. Weigensberg C. W. Asbury, I. Weigensberg
Parsippany, New Jersey (1 person)	6-13-74	St. Barnabas Medical Center Follow-up:	J. A. Hogan, F. Barlotta, M. Olesnicky, Dr. Heins F. Barlotta
Amarillo, Texas (1 person)	9-27-74	On site Consultant:	F. J. Kelly, C. Lang, J. J. Alpar, W. E. Laur, J. Moore C. C. Lushbaugh
The Italian Accident	1-75	Italian AEC Curie Foundation	E. Strambi, H. Jammet, J. C. Nenot, R. Le Go
Louisville, Kentucky	4-16-75	Jewish Hosp. Louisville 5/77	H. Kleinert
ARCO (2 persons)	8-30-76	Hanford Environ. Health Found. Emergency Decon. Facility REAC/TS	B. Breitenstein, P. A. Fuqua, W. R. Norwood L. G. Littlefield
Rockaway, N.J. (1 person)	9-23-77	St. Barnabas Medical Center Consultant:	F. Barlotta, J. Hogan N. Wald
Berkeley, CA (1 person)	1977	Merritt General Hospital LBL REAC/TS	J. Tupper, H. Stauffer, T. Budinger, E. Alpen, S. Wolfe C. C. Lushbaugh, K. Hübner, L. G. Littlefield, R. Ricks

The Which, When, Where and the Physicians of Serious Radiation Accidents
(Continued)

Hanford III (4 persons)	12-16-77	HEHF	B. Breitenstein, D. Norwood, P. Fuqua
		REAC/TS	L. G. Littlefield
W. Monroe, Louisiana (1 person)	5-78	Glenwood Hospital	E. W. Scott, A. Green
		REAC/TS	L. G. Littlefield
Algeria (7 persons)	5-78	Paris	R. Le Go, M. T. Doloy, J. L. Malarbet, M. Veyrat
Winston Salem, N.C. (1 person)	1-4-79	Duke University Medical Center	K. Pickrell
		Bowman Gray Medical Center	J. C. Shearin
		REAC/TS	L. G. Littlefield
San Bernardino, CA (9 persons)	5-22-79	Kaiser Hospital Fontana, CA	W. Gordon, D. DeVor
		UCLA Med. Center	H. Saren, Dr. Ajalat
		Consultants:	M. R. Brown, J. Ross
		REAC/TS	L. G. Littlefield, S. A. Fry, R. Ricks, W. Beck
Baton Rouge, LA (1 person)	8-29-79	Ochsner Foundation New Orleans	D. Busch
		REAC/TS	C. C. Lushbaugh, K. Hübner, S. A. Fry, L. G. Littlefield

*Special assistance in LA I and II was provided by:
Pathology: H. Lisco, F. Inda, C. Eckert
Hematology: L. H. Hempelmann, N. P. Knowlton, C. V. Moore, J. G. Allen
Biochemistry: E. S. G. Barron, S. S. Schwartz
Radiation Physics: H. O. Whipple
Others consulted included: J. C. Aub, H. A. Blair, A. M. Brues, O. Cope, J. Dealy, L. L. Engel, H. L. Hardy, J. W. Howland, L. O. Jacobson, T. R. Noonan, Shields Warren, R. E. Zirkle.
Follow-up examinations and studies: L. Blaney, L. H. Hempelmann, N. P. Knowlton, H. O. Whipple, C. C. Lushbaugh, R. Bakemeier, Dr. Greenberg, and W. R. Oaks.

What Happened to the Survivors of the Early Los Alamos Nuclear Accidents?

Louis H. Hempelmann,* Clarence C. Lushbaugh,+ and George L. Voelz‡

*University of Rochester, Rochester, New York;
+Oak Ridge Associated Universities, Oak Ridge, Tennessee;
‡Los Alamos Scientific Laboratory, Los Alamos, New Mexico.

Within ten months of the end of World War II, two serious nuclear criticality accidents occurred at the Los Alamos Laboratory (Site Y) of the then Manhattan Project. Each accident resulted in the death of the operator, and eight other participants sustained overexposure to ionizing radiations. Both accidents were the result of uncontrolled nuclear chain reactions in so-called critical assembly experiments using metallic plutonium. Because of the nature of the times at the end of World War II, the early published accounts gave little detailed information of the nature of the accidents or of how they occurred. In the present report, we describe the now nonclassified physical aspects of the accidents and bring up to date the medical histories of the survivors, last published in 1951, to show what has happened in the almost 35 years since the exposures occurred.

The criticality experiments were designed to provide information about the fission characteristics of metallic plutonium. The experiments were carried out with a subcritical plutonium sphere exposed to neutrons from a small externally placed neutron source. Because of the size and shape of the sphere, so much neutron leakage occurred from the sphere that in the absence of neutron-reflecting material, a fission chain reaction could not be sustained. By surrounding the sphere with the right amount of tamper (neutron-reflecting) material, it was possible to reflect enough neutrons back into the sphere to achieve a delayed critical state. In this state, a constant rate of self-sustaining nuclear fission chain reactions could be achieved with or without extraneous neutrons. In the prompt critical state, the neutron reflection back into the sphere is great enough to sustain criticality even in the absence of delayed neutrons. When prompt criticality was exceeded, as is believed to have occurred in both accidents, fissioning of plutonium atoms increased exponentially, with the release of a burst of neutrons and gamma rays.

Although the potential danger in this type of experimentation was fully appreciated, the physicists elected to carry out the procedure manually rather than remotely since a reliable remote-control mechanism was not available at the time. The scientists in charge feared that failure of such a mechanism could lead to a minor but still serious nuclear explosion, while manual operators, by meticulous attention to detail, could carry out the experiments with very little radiation exposure even while standing next to the critical assembly. Hundreds of such experiments were carried out properly with negligible exposures of the operators.

In two experiments at Los Alamos after World War II, the critical state was accidentally exceeded. In these two accidents, ten experimenters were seriously irradiated; two of them died within weeks of their exposures. The fatal accidents and a brief description of how they occurred were published in a monograph in 1952.[1] That report focused primarily on the acute illness of the two fatally stricken operators and of seven of the eight survivors, all of whom received substantial doses of neutrons and gamma rays. The eighth survivor refused to consent to the follow-up study. Although all seven survivors have been followed periodically since 1950, their medical courses have not been published in the open literature. In the present report we bring up to date the case histories of seven of the eight survivors of the two Los Alamos accidents.

Description of the Accidents

In both accidents, the uncontrolled chain reactions occurred in a nickel-plated plutonium sphere.[2] The plutonium sphere in both accidents weighed 6.19kg. In the first accident, designated LA-1, the tamper material used to surround the sphere was tungsten carbide (WC) bricks, while that in the second accident, designated LA-2, was beryllium in the form of hemispheres. On both occasions there was a prompt supercritical excursion believed to have been caused by the increased number of neutrons reflected back into the sphere by the tamper material. During the period of the exponentially increasing chain reaction, the assembly was engulfed by a clearly visible blue glow of intensely ionized air caused by electrons and soft X rays. In the LA-1 accident, which occurred at night in a well-illuminated laboratory, the flash lit up a newspaper being read by a security guard 10–12 feet away with his back to the assembly (case 2). In LA-2, in a sunlit room, the glow was seen by five of the seven persons facing the assembly. Data from other published experiments on high-intensity radiation sources suggest that a particle beam does not become visible until the radiation intensity is of the order of 6 × 10⁷ R/sec.[3]

In the LA-1 accident,[4] tungsten carbide (WC) bricks, each weighing 4.4 kg, were stacked around the carefully machined sphere. Two similar but slightly modified experiments with WC bricks had been successfully carried out the day of the accident. The fatal experiment, scheduled for the next morning, called for five bricks of WC on each side. Instead of waiting until the scheduled time, the physicist-operator (case 1) began the experiment on the night of August 21, 1945, at 9:55 P.M. with only a military guard (case 2) in the laboratory. While the guard was seated at a desk 10–12 feet away, the operator added the WC bricks to the assembly. Four layers of bricks were in place and the final brick for the fifth layer was being carried to its place when the operator noted that the neutron flux was increasing rapidly. He attempted to withdraw the final brick (Figure 1), but it slipped out of his hand and fell onto the center of the assembly. The operator immediately pushed the final brick off the assembly with his right hand and dismantled the assembly to the point shown in Figure 2. The operator estimated that he remained in the

Figure 1. Mockup of accident LA-1: assembly before accident.

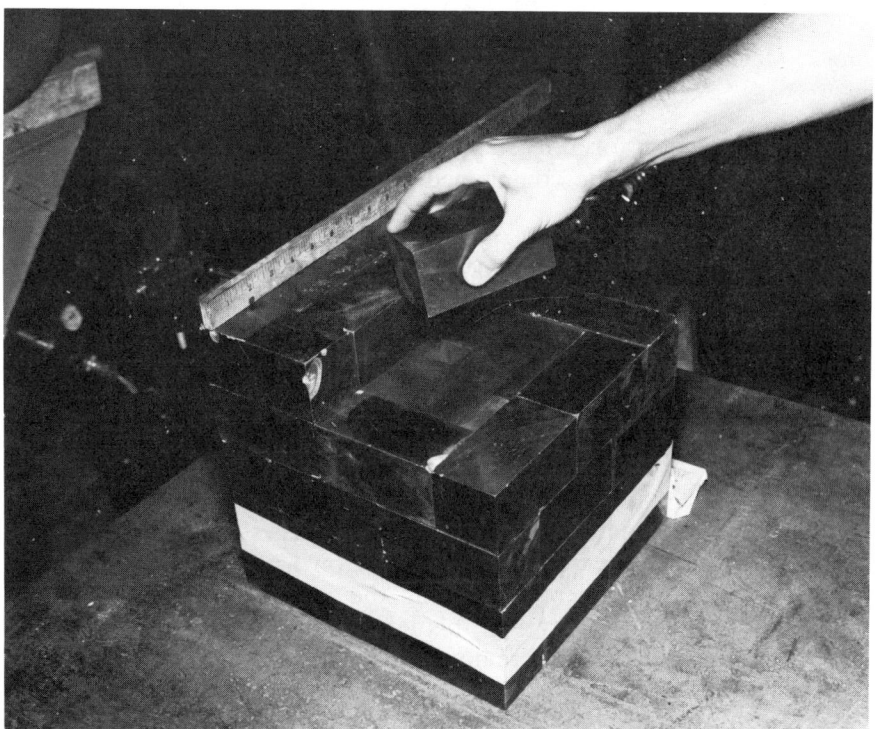

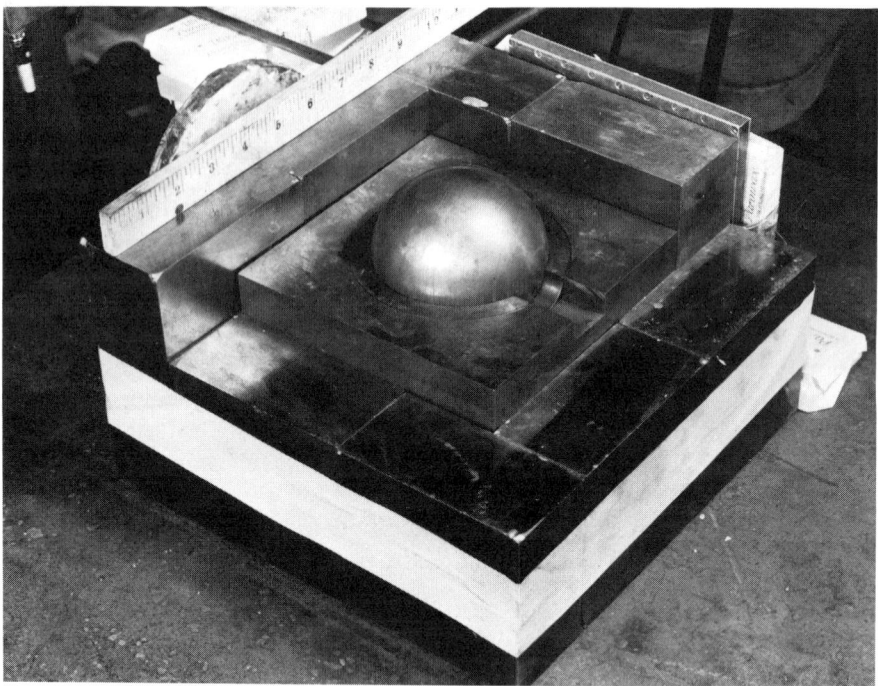

Figure 2. Mockup of accident LA-1: assembly after accident.

vicinity of the reactor for at least 10 min.[3] When seen at the hospital 30 min after the accident, he complained of numbness and tingling of his swollen hands.

In the LA-2 accident on May 21, 1946, [5,6] the physicist in charge (case 3), who was about to leave for the Bikini test, was indoctrinating his successor (case 4) in his new duties. An experiment had not been scheduled, but the physicist decided that the best indoctrination would be an impromptu test, even though six other people were in the laboratory. The tamper material consisted of two concentric hemispherical shells of beryllium, which had been shown to bring the assembly to criticality when the bottom hemisphere measured 13 inches in outside diameter and the upper one 9 inches in diameter[5] (Figure 3). In the presence of a small neutron source (10^6 neutrons/sec), the physicist-operator placed the upper 9-inch hemisphere on 1-inch aluminum shims above the lower hemisphere containing the plutonium sphere. Then, holding the upper hemisphere with his left thumb placed in an opening in the polar point, the operator removed the shims and allowed one edge of the upper hemisphere to be in contact with the lower hemisphere (Figure 3). Still holding the upper hemisphere, he placed a screwdriver under that part of the upper hemisphere not in contact with the lower hemisphere. He was working the screwdriver out from under the hemisphere (Figure 4) when it slipped, with the resultant criticality excursion.[5] The operator threw the shell to the floor immediately, and all personnel left the scene of the accident as rapidly as possible. One of the lesser-exposed experimenters (case 9) returned briefly to the vicinity of the assembly to drop some film badges on the assembly and to make radiation measurements. All subjects were taken to the Los Alamos Hospital for observation.

Radiation Doses

Although 85% of the energy of these chain reactions was dissipated in the form of heat,[7] the biological damage to the exposed subjects was due exclusively to three types of ionizing radiation, namely, neutrons, gamma-rays, and very soft X rays and electrons (in the region of the blue glow). Neutrons, the principal component of the incident radiation, were emitted instantaneously during the fission process. The gamma-ray component was composed of prompt and delayed gamma-rays. The

Figure 3. Mockup of accident LA-2: assembly before accident.

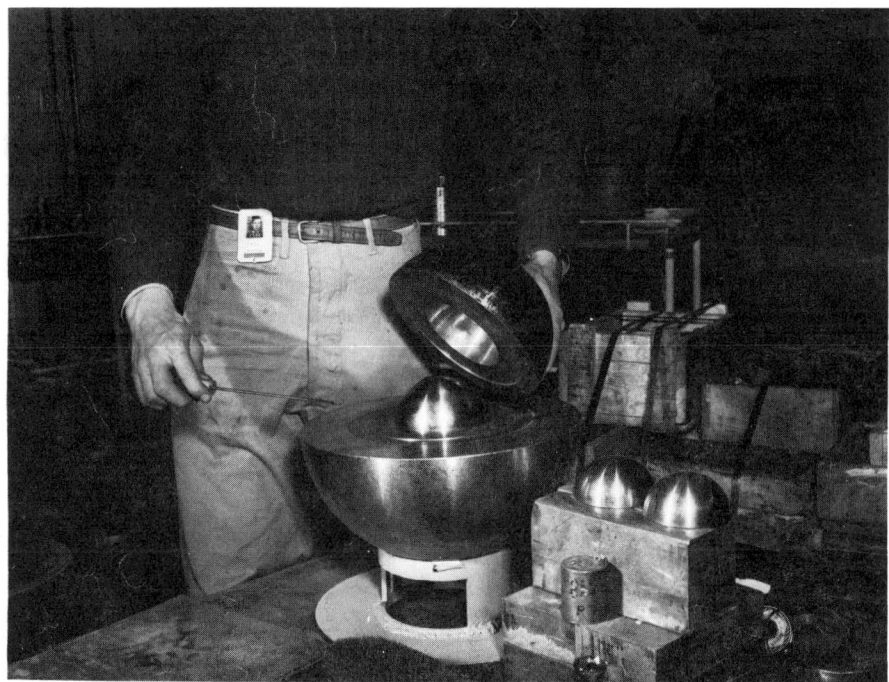

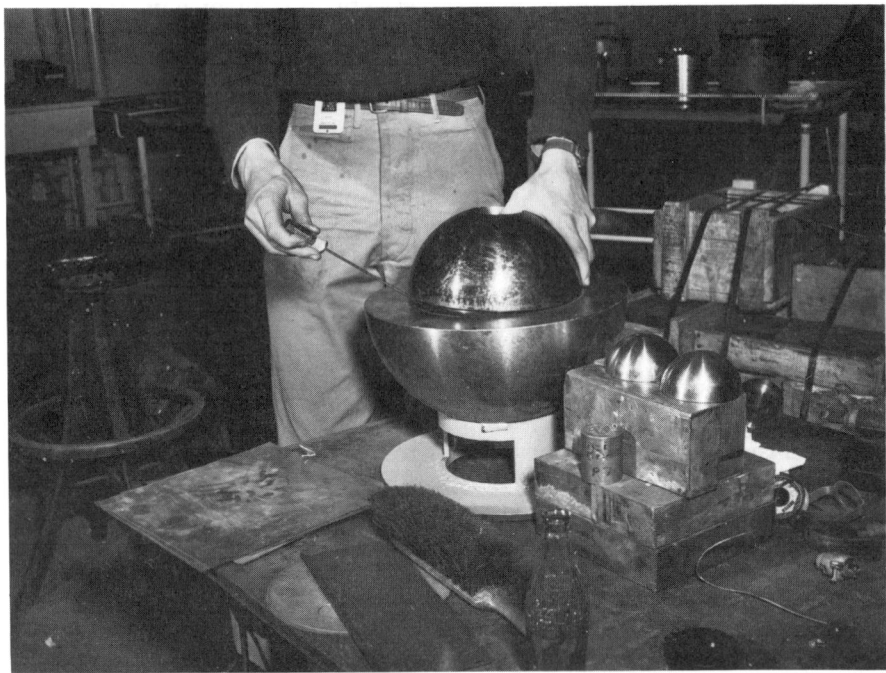

Figure 4. Mockup of accident LA-2: assembly just before accident.

prompt gammas were emitted during the fission process or were given off within the bodies of the subjects as a result of hydrogen capture of neutrons. The delayed gammas were emitted by the fission products and by radioactive elements induced by the incident neutrons. In these cases, the delayed gammas accounted for only a small fraction of the total dose. The radiation in the blue glow was very soft indeed. It is estimated that only 0.1% could have penetrated the tissues of the hands and arms of cases 1 and 3. Although the intensity of these radiations in air was of the order of 7×10^7 R/sec, the tissue doses were probably 3000 to 40,000 rad.[1,3]

Fortunately, it is possible to calculate the neutron doses with reasonable confidence. These doses are based on the sodium 24 (^{24}Na) activity of the serum sodium of the subjects as compared to the studies on human phantoms. At first the energy of the incident neutrons was not known but was assumed to be 0.5 MeV based on information from J.R. Oppenheimer (personal communication). By 1966 the energy spectra of the escaping neutrons had been accurately measured, thereby increasing the accuracy of the latest estimated neutron doses. Since film badges were not worn by the subjects, it is not possible to estimate the gamma doses accurately. The gamma flux with respect to distance from the assembly could be calculated knowing the number of fission reactions. The gamma-ray doses were based on estimates of the time each subject spent in regions of known gamma intensity. In view of the uncertainties of the gamma-ray doses, it is fortunate that they are small compared to the neutron doses. The estimated doses to the hands and arms of cases 1 and 3 are based on studies done elsewhere of beams of charged particles generated by accelerators. For such beams to be visualized, the radiation intensity must be of the order of 7×10^6 R/sec. The estimates of hand doses (3000–40,000 rad) are based on guesses as to how long the hands remained in the blue glow and on knowledge of what fraction of radiation could penetrate the skin.

As more was learned about what happened during a critical excursion, the dose estimates were improved and in the case of neutrons became quite reliable. The evolution of the dose estimates is shown in Table 1.

Table 1. Evolution of Total-Body Radiation Dose (In Rads of Neutrons and Gamma Rays)

	1948 (ref. 6)	1952 (ref. 1)	1957 (ref. 3)	1968 (ref. 8)	1976 (ref. 10)	1978 (ref. 11)
Case 1						
Neutrons	96	96	168		200	200
Gammas	110	110	487		200	110
Case 2						
Neutrons	6	6	9		7-8	8
Gammas	0.1	0.1	3		2	0.1
Case 3						
Neutrons	386	386	407	1000		1000
Gammas	114	114	156	100		114
Case 4						
Neutrons	78	78	82	166		166
Gammas	26	26	41	17		26
Case 6						
Neutrons	37	37	42	51		51
Gammas	11	11	19	5		11
Case 7						
Neutrons	28	28	20	20		33
Gammas	9	9	10	2		9
Case 8						
Neutrons	11	11	11	8-20		12
Gammas	4	4	6	1-2		4
Case 9						
Neutrons	8	8	9	9		9
Gammas	3	3	4	1		3
Case 10						
Neutrons	7	6	6	7		7
Gammas	2	2	3	1		2

The first three dose calculations (in rads) were made by the late Joe Hoffman and were based on studies of ^{24}Na induction by neutrons in phantoms of human bodies. By the time of the 1967 estimates of Hankins and Hansen,[8] of the Los Alamos Scientific Laboratory (LASL), the energy spectra were available for neutrons leaked by several critical assemblies, and data on ^{24}Na induction by neutrons as studied in human phantoms had been extended.[9] The same data were used in the 1976 and 1978 estimates of neutron dose made by James N. P. Lawrence of LASL.[10,11] Refining the neutron dose estimates resulted in an increase in dose for the five most heavily irradiated subjects but did not change much in the rest of the subjects. Comparison of the estimated neutron and gamma-ray doses shows that the radiation was predominantly neutrons (except for case 1, who received a substantial dose of delayed gammas). The composition of the incident radiation was unlike that in the Japanese irradiated by the atomic bombings of 1945. The neutron component of the radiation from the bomb in Hiroshima was only 15–30%, while that in Nagaski was almost nonexistent.[12,13] When organ doses are estimated it must be remembered that the energy of the neutrons was such that they would have penetrated tissue about as well as X rays of less than 100 kV peak.[3]

The relative biological effectiveness (RBE) for neutron exposures in the production of late effects, especially carcinogenesis, is a subject of considerable discussion and interest now. Recent studies of late effects in the irradiated Japanese indicate that the RBE for late effects in man at lower doses may be much higher than for acute radiation effects; for example, the RBE for leukemogenesis is believed to lie between 30 and 50.[12,13] The ICRP in publication 26[14] recommends that an RBE of 10 be used for neutron exposures when the distribution of radiation collision stopping power (kilo-electron volts per micrometer) is not known at all points in the volume of interest. An RBE of 20 is recommended when the collision stopping power (kilo-electron volts per micrometer) in water is known to be 175 or above. This report on a few follow-up cases does not permit a valid statistical evaluation of these RBE values because of the small numbers involved and potential confounding factors, including hereditary influences that cannot be ruled out.

Medical Histories of the Survivors

The estimated exposure doses and main features of the medical histories of the persons irradiated in the two LASL accidents are shown in Table 2. The medical histories of those persons who survived are now discussed, except for that of case 5, who refused to cooperate with this study. The early responses (before 1950) are described elsewhere[1] and will not be repeated here.

Table 2. Summary of Clinical Course of Subjects

Case	Age at exposure (years)	Estimated dose (1978) (rad)		Acute radiation response	Age when last seen or age at death(d)(years)	Diagnosis
		Neutrons	Gamma			
				Accident LA-1		
1	26	200	110	Severe,[a] leading to death in 24 days	26 (d)	Fatal acute radiation syndrome (hematopoetic type)
2	29	8	0.1	None (death in 32 years)	62 (d)	Fatal acute myeloblastic leukemia
				Accident LA-2		
3	32	1000	114	Severe[a] (death in 9 days)	32 (d)	Fatal acute radiation syndrome (gastrointestinal type)
4	34	166	26	Moderate, severe fatigue for 6 months; epilation, aspermia (death in 20 years)	54 (d)	Fatal myocardial infarction (myxedema, compensated, cataracts)
5	Refused consent to follow-up					Alive in 1978
6	54	51	11	None	83 (d)	Clinical aplastic anemia, fatal bacterial endocarditis
7	21	33	9	None	27 (d)	Korean War fatality
8	23	12	4	None (death in 18 years)	42 (d)	Fatal acute myelocytic leukemia
9	36	9	3	Transient nausea	67	Healthy male
10	23	7	2	None	55	Healthy male

[a] See ref. 1.

Cases 1 and 3

These men received the largest doses of radiation and died 24 and 9 days later, respectively, as a result of the exposures. The story of their acute illnesses has been fully documented.[1]

Case 2

This 29-year-old military security guard was exposed to a relatively small dose of neutrons and to a smaller dose of gamma-rays (see Table 2). He returned to civilian life after the war and enjoyed excellent health for 28 years. In 1974 he suffered a heart attack, from which he recovered without complications.

In March, 1976, he was hospitalized for weakness and vertigo. There were no significant physical findings, but the blood picture was distinctly abnormal. There was a pancytopenia with a leukocyte count of 2300 cells per cubic millimeter, a hematocrit of 24%, and a platelet count of 136,000 per cubic millimeter. Although no leukemic cells were seen in the peripheral blood smears, many myeloblastic cells were found in hyperplastic bone marrow. His disease was diagnosed as acute myeloblastic leukemia. During the next six months, the patient responded well to chemotherapy with Purinethol and repeated transfusions. Despite symptomatic improvement, the pancytopenia persisted.

By November, 1976, it had become clear that the disease was no longer being controlled by Purinethol alone. Combined chemotherapy with vincristine, prednisone, and adriamycin was begun, and this induced a satisfactory remission after some initial problems with bleeding and fever. In July, 1977, the patient's condition began to deteriorate. The leukocyte count at this time was 8400 cells per cubic millimeter, the hemoglobin was 10 gm %, and the platelet count was 33,000 per cubic millimeter. Many immature granulocytes, including myeloblasts, were seen in the peripheral blood smear.

The patient improved somewhat after additional chemotherapy, but his clinical course was steadily downhill. His last hospital admission was in December, 1977. At that time he had a platelet count of 3000 cells per cubic millimeter and suffered from combined renal and hepatic failure. He died January 28, 1978, at age 62, 33 years after the accident. At autopsy the diagnosis of acute myelogenous leukemia was confirmed. There was extensive leukemic involvement of all organs and multiple hemorrhages in the heart and lung.

Case 4

This 34-year-old physicist received the highest dose of any of the survivors (see Table 2). He was partly shielded by case 3, as a result of which his head, neck, upper torso, and right arm had a larger dose than the rest of the body.

After recovery from a six-month episode of weakness following exposure, case 4 resumed his scientific duties. Except for mild hypertension, which predated the accident, he appeared to have recovered completely from the effects of the exposure. In December, 1955 (nine years after the accident) he had a moderately severe myocardial infarction, from which he appeared to recover without complications. Although his strength returned gradually, he did not feel normal and had difficulty controlling his weight. These signs and symptoms, together with an elevated blood cholesterol (488 mg) and a low PBI (1.2 mg %), led to a diagnosis of myxedema, which was treated with thyroid hormone. On this replacement therapy, the patient's condition improved, and he returned to normal activity. Although his blood pressure had fallen to normal after the heart attack, his heart gradually increased in size, until in 1964 roentgenographs indicated it to be 17% above the upper limits of normal. In the summer of 1966 (20 years after the accident) he suffered a fatal heart attack at age 54.

At autopsy his heart was greatly enlarged. Severe arteriosclerosis was observed in his coronary arteries as well as in the aorta. There were multiple fresh and healed infarcted areas in the myocardium. The thyroid gland was so atrophied that it was difficult to identify. The normal thyroid tissue had been replaced by dense scar tissue in which there were multiple foci of lymphocytes and plasma cells. There were a few atrophic thyroid follicles scattered throughout the scar tissue and in the lymphoid follicles. The testes were atrophic; microscopically they showed atrophy and hyalinization of the tubular epithelium and a great increase in the interstitial fibrous tissue.

Case 6

This 54-year-old technician received a substantial dose of neutrons and gamma-rays (see Table 2). Considering the magnitude of the dose, it is surprising that this man experienced no acute symptoms and was able to resume his custom of taking 20-mile weekend hikes within two weeks after the accident.

Case 6 enjoyed vigorous good health for 27 years following the accident. In 1973 and again in 1974 (when he was in his 80s) he was hospitalized for acute enteritis (diverticulitis and spastic colitis) and severe secondary anemia (2,500,000 cells per cubic millimeter). On each occasion his condition improved after repeated transfusions.

In the summer of 1975 the patient was hospitalized for severe anemia and congestive heart failure. The anemia was first thought to be hemolytic in nature. He had a marked eosinophilia (up to 2300 cells per cubic millimeter), and his intensely hyperactive bone marrow contained many erythroid precursors. An interesting incidental finding was a monoclonal

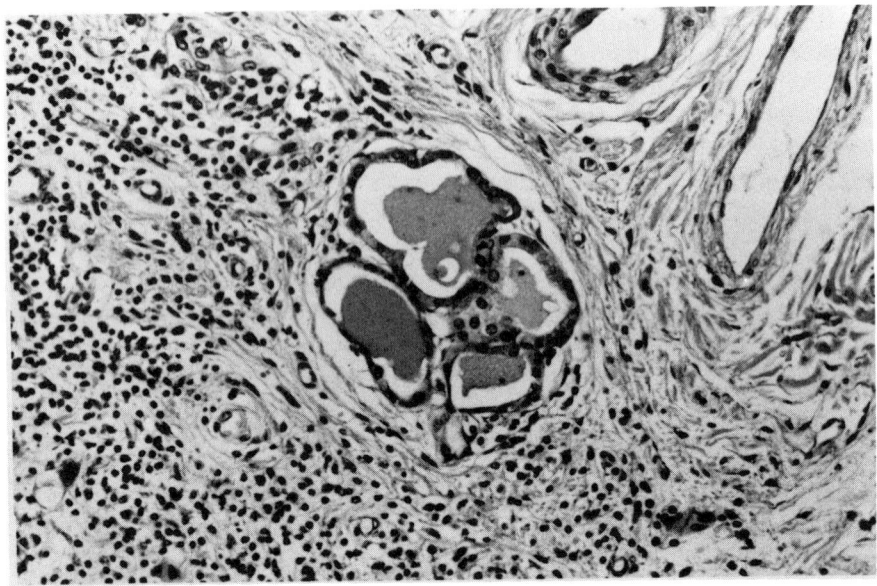

Figure 5A. Photomicrograph (×200) of the thyroid gland of case 4 at autopsy, 20 years post accident; an area showing four surviving thyroid acini in a lymphoid rich stroma.

Figure 5B. Photomicrograph (×200) of the thyroid gland of case 4 at autopsy, 20 years post accident; an area showing highly atypical surviving epithelial remnants failing to form functional acini.

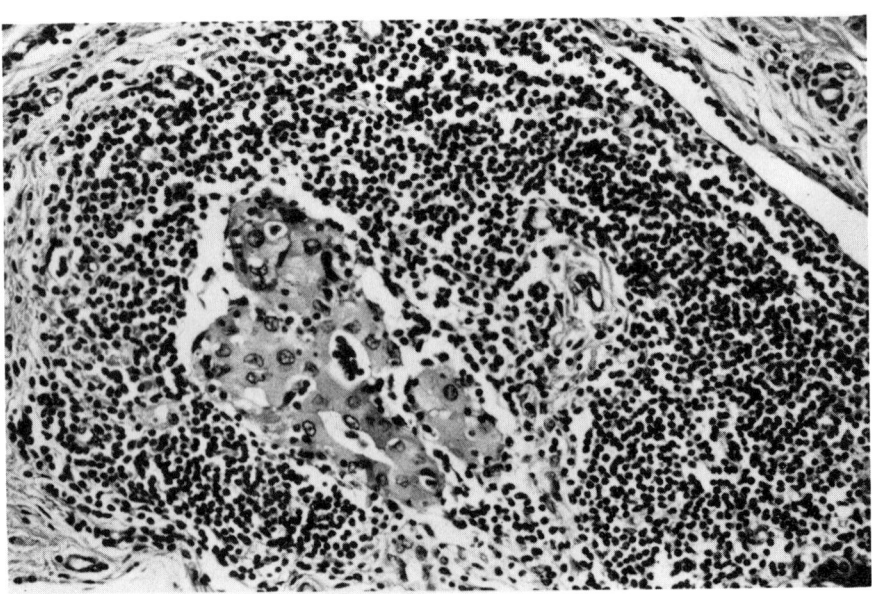

gammapathy with marked increase in the IgG component. At this time it was thought that he might have autoimmune hemolytic anemia about to enter an aplastic crisis. His condition improved after several transfusions.

In the fall of 1975, case 6 was again hospitalized for weakness due to severe anemia (1.7 million cells per cubic millimeter). Physical findings were in keeping with his age, except for enlargement of his heart and liver. His leukocyte count was 17,500 cells per cubic millimeter with a normal differential. His bone marrow was moderately hypercellular with an increase in the myeloblastoid cells showing some shift to the left. There were many immature white cells and orthochromic normoblasts. There was no increase in plasma cells. The megakaryocytes were smaller than normal and increased in number. In addition to the monoclonal gammapathy, Bence Jones proteins were now present in the urine.

Hemolytic anemia was ruled out by appropriate laboratory tests, and multiple myeloma was excluded by the normal appearance of the bones on roentgenograms. It was suggested that the patient had a benign gammapathy sometimes seen in older people, but the exact nature of the refractory anemia was not known. After four transfusions the patient's condition improved, and he was discharged on medication including pyridoxine, folic acid, and prednisone.

In December, 1975, the patient was readmitted to the hospital because of increasing weakness and spiking fever. His condition had deteriorated markedly, and he was found to have heart failure and *Escherichia coli* septicemia. The patient had a heart attack while in the hospital and died just before Christmas, 1975, at age 83 (29 years after the accident).

At autopsy, a vegetative bacterial endocarditis was found as well as *E. coli* septicemia and cardiac and splenic infarcts secondary to emboli. Microscopically, the bone marrow was moderately hyperplastic, with a marked increase in red cell precursors and some increase in plasma cells. The autopsy gave no clues as to the nature of the anemia.

Case 7

This 21-year-old soldier was exposed to an intermediate dose of mixed radiation (see Table 2). When last examined, 28 months after the accident, there were no significant physical or laboratory findings. This man was killed in combat in Korea in 1952 at age 27.

Case 8

This 23-year-old college graduate received a relatively small dose of mixed radiation (see Table 2). After the war he returned to graduate school and became an important executive in industry.

Case 8 enjoyed excellent health until 1964 (18 years after the accident). At this time he developed what was first thought to be acute sinusitis. When antibiotics failed to relieve his symptoms, hemotalogical studies revealed a leukocyte count of 300,000 cells per cubic millimeter, with many blast cells seen in the blood smear. His bone marrow was hypercellular and contained many immature myeloid cells. A diagnosis of acute myelogenous leukemia was made, and he was started on 6-mercaptopurine (6-MP) therapy. He had a satisfactory remission for five months. At this time his medication was changed to methotrexate. At first he seemed to respond, but soon his condition worsened. In March, 1965, his lymph nodes and spleen were palpable, and he developed a superficial ulcer on his palate. His leukocyte count was 22,700 per cubic millimeter; his hematocrit was 21.5%, and his platelet count was 16,000 per cubic millimeter. Many immature granulocytes and an occasional myeloblast were seen in the blood smears. Erythroid elements and megakarocytes were rarely seen in the bone marrow.

After an unsatisfactory trial with prednisone and vincristine, the patient entered the hospital of the Brookhaven National Laboratory in April, 1965, for treatment with extracorporeal irradiation (e.c.i.) of his blood. Shortly after admission he developed a severe headache, with neurological signs which were completely relieved by intrathecal methotrexate. Following daily e.c.i. treatments, the leukocyte count (then 79,000) fell rapidly and stabilized at 30,000 cells per cubic millimeter. His spleen decreased in size, and the patient felt better. In May, 1965, subcutaneous nodules developed, and his spleen and liver became larger. He was given two series of treatments with tritiated thymidine in addition to the e.c.i. His leukocyte count fell to 800 cells per cubic millimeter, and the lymphoid masses shrank in size. His clinical condition went downhill rapidly, and he died after a grand mal seizure on July 18, 1965. Death occurred at age 42, 19 years after the accident.

At autopsy, extensive leukemic infiltration resembling a sarcomatous growth of all organs, soft tissues, and meninges was observed.

Cases 9 and 10

These young men, 36 and 23 years old, respectively, received small doses of mixed radiation (see Table 2). When last examined in 1978 (32 years after the accident), they were found to be in excellent health and spirits. They showed no physical or laboratory evidence of late radiation injury.

Discussion

The accidental total-body exposures of these subjects (nonhomogeneous in the case of the most heavily exposed) were unique in that moderately fast neutrons accounted for almost all of the radiation doses. Although some of the neutron doses are small numerically (in terms of rads), the RBE of at least ten makes the biologically effective dose (rems) high in all cases.

Since ionizing radiations, particularly neutrons, are known to be leukemogenic, it is tempting to attribute the terminal illnesses of cases 2 and 8 to their accidental radiation exposure. Similarly, since the thyroid gland is readily destroyed by radiation,[15] one might suspect that the myxedema of case 4, presumably radiation-induced, may have promoted his coronary disease by elevating the blood cholesterol. This could well have precipitated the first heart attack. By the same line of reasoning, one can imagine that the insult to the hematapoietic tissue of case 6 resulting from the radiation exposure could have been a factor in the development of the terminal refractory anemia.

Our statistician friends assure us that it is dangerous to draw definite conclusions from such small numbers of cases in such limited populations, as there may be etiologic factors other than radiation exposure. For example, a brother of case 2 also died of leukemia (and three other siblings are believed to have had cancer). This makes it likely there is a familial component to the development of the disease. Similarly, the father of case 4 also had a myocardial infarction when he was in his early 40s. This also suggests a genetic factor. And finally, in the case of the refractory anemia of case 6, this disease (in the absence of leukemia) is not usually considered to be a late effect of radiation exposure and is not uncommon in aged patients.

In summary, there have been six persons followed for more than ten years after the criticality accidents, four of whom died 19 or more years after the accident. It seems likely that the two leukemic deaths represent late effects of the radiation exposure, although one may have had a genetic component predisposing to leukemia. The other two deaths could conceivably have been related to the exposures, although one also seems to have a genetic factor. The two survivors were in good health in 1978 and showed no clinical or laboratory evidence of late radiation damage.

References

1. Hempelmann LH, Lisco H, Hoffman JG: The acute radiation syndrome. A study of nine cases and a review of the problem. *Ann Int Med* 36:279, 1952.

2. Stratten WR: *A Review of Criticality Accidents,* unclassified report LA-3611. Los Alamos Scientific Laboratory, Los Alamos, NM, Sept. 22, 1967.

3. Hoffman JG, Hempelmann LH: Estimation of whole body doses in accidental fission bursts. *Amer Journ Roentgenol Rad Therapy & Nuclear Med* 77:144, 1957.

4. Aebersold P, Hempelmann LH, Slotin L: *Report of Accident of August 21, 1945 at Omega Site,* report LAMD-120. Los Alamos Scientific Laboratory, Los Alamos, NM, Sept. 21, 1948.

5. Froman D: *Preliminary Report on the Accident in Parajito Laboratory Los Alamos on May 21, 1946,* memorandum report. Los Alamos Scientific Laboratory, Los Alamos, NM, undated.

6. Hoffman JG: *Radiation Doses in the Parajito Accident of May 21, 1946,* report LA-687. Los Alamos Scientific Laboratory, Los Alamos, NM, May 26, 1948.

7. Kaplan I: *Nuclear Physics.* Wiley Publishing Co., Cambridge, Mass., 1955, p. 505.

8. Hankins DE, Hansen GE: *Revised Dose Estimates for the Criticality Excursion at Los Alamos Scientific Laboratory,* report LA-3861. Los Alamos Scientific Laboratory, Los Alamos, NM, December, 1967.

9. Hankins DF: *A Study of Selected Criticality Dosimetry Methods,* report LA-3910. Los Alamos Scientific Laboratory, Los Alamos, NM, January, 1967.

10. Lawrence JNP: *Reexamination of Exposure of Case 2. LA Accident #1,* internal memorandum to Voelz G, H1-76-320. Los Alamos Scientific Laboratory, Los Alamos, NM, Oct. 4, 1976.

11. Lawrence JNP: *Dosimetry Evaluation Handbook,* internal memorandum on Los Alamos criticality accidents, 1945–1946, personnel exposures, H-1-78. Los Alamos Scientific Laboratory, Los Alamos, NM, Oct. 6, 1978.

12. Rossi HH: Symposium on the radiobiological response relationships at low doses. The effect of small doses of ionizing radiation. Fundamental biological characteristics, *Radiation Res.* 71:1, 1977.

13. Upton AC: Radiobiological effects of low doses: Implications for radiological protection, *Radiation Res.* 71:51, 1977.

14. International Commission on Radiological Protection: ICRP Publication 26. *Ann. ICRP* 1(3):4–5, 1977.

15. Michaelson MS, Quinlan WJ, Casarett G, Mason WB: Radiation induced thyroid dysfunction in the dog. *Radiation Res.* 30:38, 1967.

Follow-up Studies over a 25-Year Period on the Japanese Fishermen Exposed to Radioactive Fallout in 1954

Toshiyuki Kumatori,* Takaaki Ishihara,* Kunitake Hirashima,* Hajime Sugiyama,* Seiji Ishii,+ and Kazuo Miyoshi‡

*National Institute of Radiological Sciences, Anagawa-4, Chiba-shi, Japan, 260;
+Yaizu Municipal Hospital, 1550 Sangamyo, Yaizu-shi, Japan, 425;
‡Tokushima University, School of Medicine, Kuramoto-cho 3, Tokushima-shi, Japan 770.

Introduction

On 1 March 1954 a thermonuclear test explosion was performed at Bikini by U.S. authorities. After the explosion a Japanese fishing vessel in the area, the 5th Fukuryumaru (the Lucky Dragon), with 23 fishermen aboard, was exposed to radioactive fallout produced by the test. On this accidental exposure several medical reports have been published.[1-8] On the same occasion 239 Marshallese and 28 American servicemen were also exposed.

According to a BNL report,[9] "the detonation from a tower of a thermonuclear device, Bravo, in the Castle Series of tests at Bikini resulted in a serious fallout accident. The yield was about 17 megatons, considerably greater than expected, and an unpredicted shift in winds in the upper atmosphere caused the radioactive cloud to drift over and deposit fallout on several inhabited atolls to the east."

The Japanese fishermen, aged 18–39, saw a huge red light in the west at about 3:50 A.M. (Japanese standard time) while they were fishing tuna and heard a few dull sounds several minutes later. The location of the vessel was long. 166°58′ E and lat. 11°53′N, where the distance from the explosion center was about 190 km. At about 7:00 A.M., white ashes began to fall on the vessel, which continued for about 4 1/2 hr. They gave up fishing and returned to their base at Yaizu on 14 March 1954.

After landing, all the fishermen were found to have been injured by the fallout. They were hospitalized by 28 March, 7 of them to the Tokyo University Hospital and the other 16 to the First National Hospital of Tokyo (at present National Hospital Medical Center). They were discharged from both hospitals in May 1955, except one fatal case that died on 23 September 1954. After discharging, the follow-up studies have been performed on an annual basis. The number of persons who accepted the examination has been 10–20 in each year.

The Reproduction of Exposure

A try to reproduce the scene of ashes-fall was performed in cooperation with the fishermen in August 1954. Powders made from the same sort of coral reef were used as white ashes. According to the statements of the fishermen, it was impossible to keep their eyes and mouths open when the intensity of the ashes-fall was most heavy (Figure 1). Their footprints were clearly visible on the deck covered by the ashes (Figure 2). The fishermen wore cotton shirts, rubber aprons, boots, cotton gloves, and hats or caps (Figure 3). The ashes adhered to the bare parts of their bodies, which suggested the cause of skin lesions (Figure 4). In this experiment a quantity of the ashes deposited on the deck was estimated to be 4–8 mg/cm².

Figure 1. The falling ashes (experimentally reproduced).

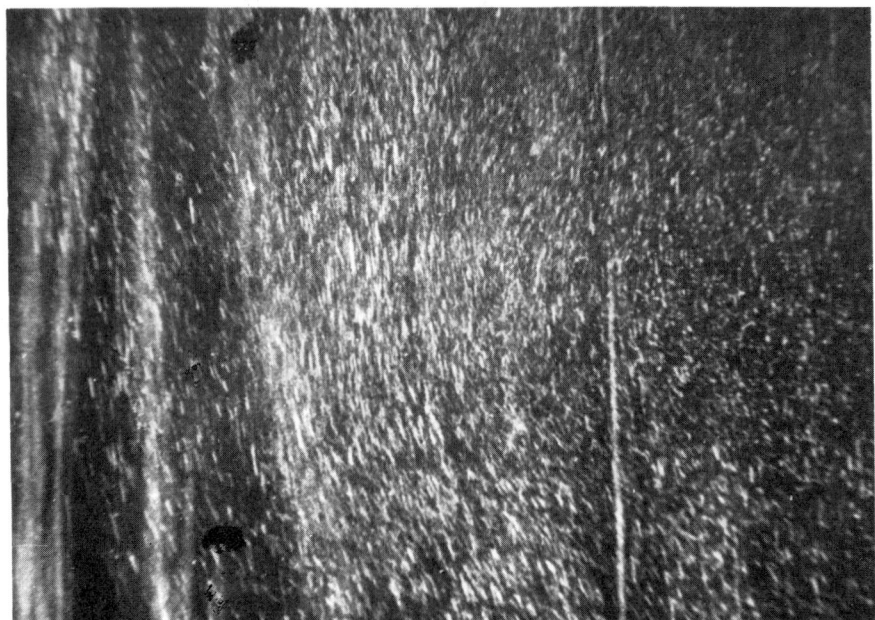

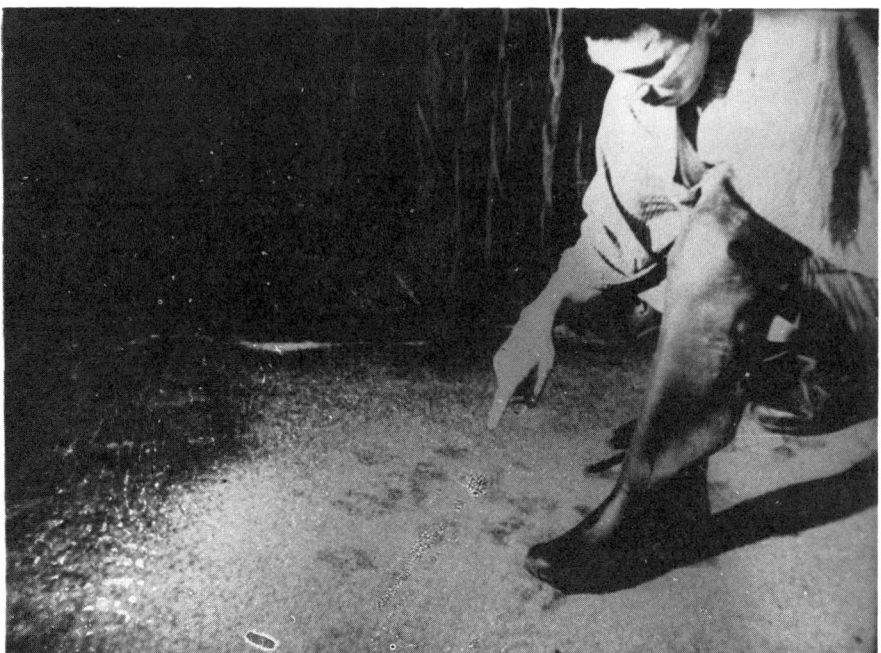

Figure 2. Footprints on the deck (experimentally reproduced).

Analyses of Ashes

Radiochemical analyses of the ashes brought by the crew were performed at Prof. Kimura's laboratory of the University of Tokyo, and by 26 March, 27 nuclides were detected.[10] Rare-earth elements and uranium constituted about 50% and 20% of the gross beta activity respectively.

The specific activity of the ashes was 0.37 millicurie per gram on 23 April. By extrapolation of this data, the specific activity of the ashes at 7:00 A.M. on 1 March was estimated as 1.4 curies per gram.

Estimates of Dose

The fishermen were irradiated in the following ways on the vessel for two weeks:

1. from the radioactive fallout adhered to the body surface,
2. externally from the fallout deposited in the cabins, on the deck, etc.,
3. internally from the incorporated radioactive materials.

The dose estimate in the case of radiological accident is very difficult usually.

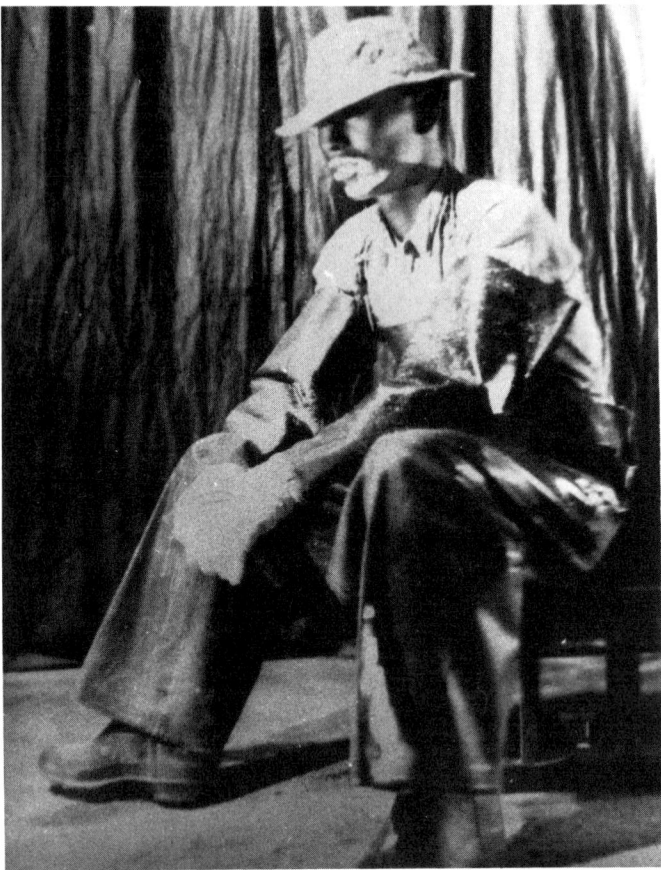

Figure 3. Clothes of the fishermen at the time of the accident.

External Dose (Gamma Radiation)

The external doses were estimated with the following surveys:

1. From the results of a try to reproduce ashes-fall, a rough quantitative estimate of ashes on the deck was made. Then the exposed dose during the time spent on the deck was estimated.
2. The measurements of dose rate at many places of the vessel were done at Yaizu repeatedly. From these data the dose rate during the navigation was calculated.
3. The movements of each fisherman on the vessel were followed every one hour.

Table 1 shows the estimated doses for two weeks. The extrapolated equivalent single dose will be approximately 50% of the total dose, i.e., 80–320 rad.[11]

Internal Exposure

The internal deposition of radioactive materials was proved by the existence of radioactivity in urine, in thyroids, and in several organs of one fatal case.

Radioactivity in Urine

Urine samples of the fishermen were collected and transferred to the Health and Safety Laboratory of U.S. AEC (at present Environmental Research Laboratory) for radiochemical analysis. According to the information from Prof. Eisenbud of the above mentioned laboratory,[12] significant amounts of radioactivity were found in urine samples at about four weeks after the initial exposure (Table 2). This radioactivity decreased rapidly, and about six months later the activity in urine samples became barely detectable. The initial skeletal deposit of ^{89}Sr was estimated as 0.5–5 microcuries.

Radioactivity in the Thyroid

External countings of radioactivity in the thyroid glands were performed on seven fishermen during the fourth to the seventh week. From these observations the effective half-life of ^{131}I on the patients counted two or three times was estimated as 4.8–7.0 days (cases T-2, T-6, T-7, and T-8).

Figure 4. Ashes adhering to the hair; the upper part was protected by a cap (experimentally reproduced).

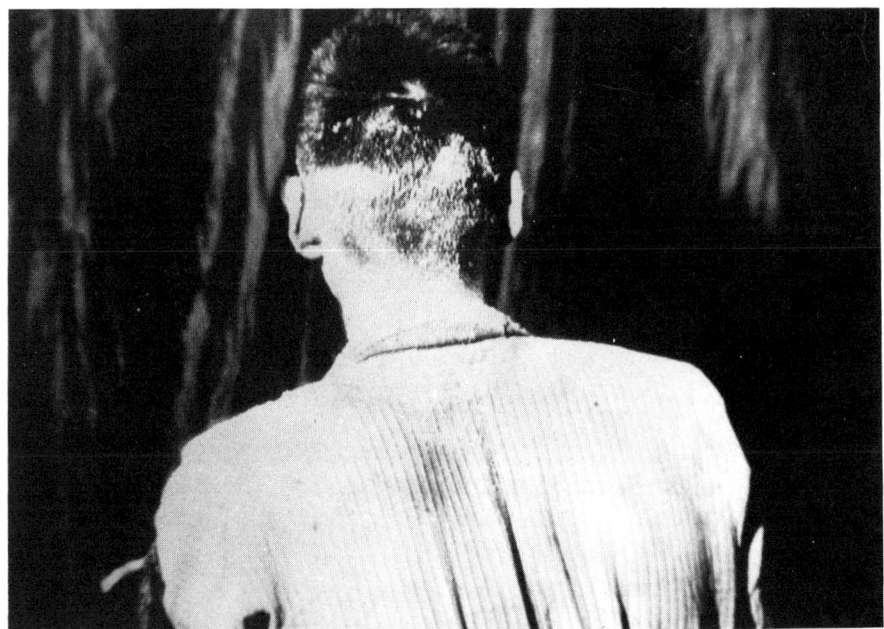

Table 1. Estimated Dose of Whole-Body Gamma Radiation (In Rads)

Subject No.	1st day	Total
T-1	240-290	450-500
T-2	210-260	390-440
T-3	150-200	260-310[a]
T-5	400-430	660-690
T-6	130-180	200-250
T-7	140-190	220-270
T-8	310-360	520-570
K-1	190-220	310-340
K-2	130-180	200-250
K-3	140-190	230-280
K-4	120-170	190-240
K-5	140-190	220-270
K-6	180-230	300-350
K-7	230-280	340-390
K-8	220-270	380-430
K-9	310-360	550-600
K-10	140-190	230-280
K-11	120-170	170-220
K-12	100-150	170-220
K-13	250-300	370-420
K-14	420-500	510-590
K-15	140-190	210-260
K-16	120-170	190-240

[a] T-3 put the fallout material close to his bed. Therefore, about 100 rad should be added, making the total 360-410 rad.

Table 2. Radiochemical Analysis of Urine

Case	Date of Sample	Total Products[a]	Total Activity/24 hr [b]	Percent Sr^{89}	Percent Ba^{140}
T-1	3/29/54	6,100	3,540	5	8.2
T-2	3/29/54	6,000	3,360	0.4	4.0
T-3	3/29/54	8,400	5,380	9	4.6
T-5	3/29/54	54,000	76,680	6.9[c]	
T-6	3/29/54	1,300	1,170		
T-7	3/26/54	550	495	18[c]	
T-8	3/26/54	230	300	21[c]	

[a] Disintegrations per minute per liter.

[b] Disintegrations per minute in 24-hr specimen. Corrected as "per 24h" by Kumatori.

[c] Sr + Ba.

The integrated dose to thyroid glands from incorporated ^{131}I was approximately 20–120 rad. Besides ^{131}I, other iodine isotopes (^{132}I, ^{133}I, and ^{135}I) were absorbed. Among them mainly ^{133}I and ^{135}I contributed to the irradiation of thyroid glands. The dose from ^{133}I was estimated to be twice as much as that from ^{131}I, and the dose from ^{135}I was estimated to be 0.8 times as much as from ^{131}I. Therefore the total thyroid dose from incorporated iodine isotopes seems to be approximately 80–450 rad. These calculations are based on the assumption that the fishermen inhaled each radioiodine isotope at 5 hr after the detonation. Besides the internal exposure the thyroid glands received external irradiation. Table 3 shows the total dose to thyroid glands.

Since the environment of the fishermen on the vessel is considered almost the same, the doses to thyroid glands of other fishermen are probably similar to the doses to these four cases.

Radiochemical Analysis of Organs of the Fatal Cases

1. Radiochemical analysis of organs from the fatal case (K-14) was performed at Prof. K. Kimura's laboratory of Tokyo University.[13] Comparing with controls, the radioactivity of the fatal case was greater but low.

    The estimate of internal dose from these results was very difficult. However, based on these results the dose to liver, kidney, lung, and bone of K-14 are being calculated for trial with MIRD method referring to ICRP Publication 30.[14]

2. Case K-6 died in April 1975. Gamma-emitting nuclides except ^{40}K were not proved in his lung, liver, kidney, spleen, pancreas, and bone. By the radiochemical analyses of vertebral and femoral bones, ^{90}Sr and ^{239}Pu were not detected. From these results it is concluded that there is no significant quantitative difference of long-lived nuclides between the exposed fishermen and normal Japanese at 21 years after the detonation.

Table 3. Dose to Thyroid Gland[a]

| Case | Dose (rad) | | |
	Incorporated Iodine	External	Total
T-7	76	220-270	296- 346
T-2	99	390-440	489- 539
T-6	304	200-250	504- 554
T-8	456	520-570	976-1026

[a] The weight of thyroid gland is assumed as 20 gm.

Whole-body Counting

Whole-body counting was done on 3 persons in September 1962 and 13 persons in January to May 1964. Gamma spectrometric analyses showed no significant difference between the curves of the fishermen and those of the controls.

Progress of Clinical Observations and Laboratory Tests

Signs and Symptoms

Soon after the accident, prodromal syndrome and conjunctivitis were observed, followed by skin lesions and epilations. These are summarized in Figure 5.

Skin Lesions

Skin lesions due to beta radiation occurred in the sequence of erythema, edema, vesicle, erosion, and ulcer or necrosis mainly at the uncovered surface of the bodies. Epilation was observed in 18 fishermen at the occipital area. However, complete epilation was seen in another two persons who did not wear hats at the time of ashes-fall. Figure 6 shows the contaminated and injured area schematically.[15] Wooly hair, eyebrows, eyelashes, beard, axillary hair, and pubic hair were proved to have some radioactivity but were not epilated.

Acute skin lesions recovered in a few months. However, the necrotic area has remained alopecic in one case. Residues of skin lesions are observed in the navel area and on the anterior surface of the ears, where atrophy of epidermis, pigmentation, depigmentation, and capillary dilatation are macroscopically noted in nine cases. However, these findings are becoming not apparent year by year and hard to observe at present in most of them. No sign of malignancy is observed.

Main histological findings are as follows:

1. Acute skin lesions: pigmentation of epidermis, cell infiltration, and capillary dilatation in the corium (fourth week).
2. Necrotic scalp: coagulation necrosis in the whole layer of epidermis, hair follicle, and papilla, demarcated by cell infiltration from the layer of corium (fourth week).
3. Residual beta burn on abdominal wall: atrophy of epidermis with narrowed stratum granulosum and elogation of rete pegs. Fibrosis and collapsed blood capillaries in subepidermis. No evidence of inflammation or neoplasm as well as chronic dermatitis (after ten years).

Hematologic Changes

Hematologic examinations were begun 16 March (16 days after the initial exposure).

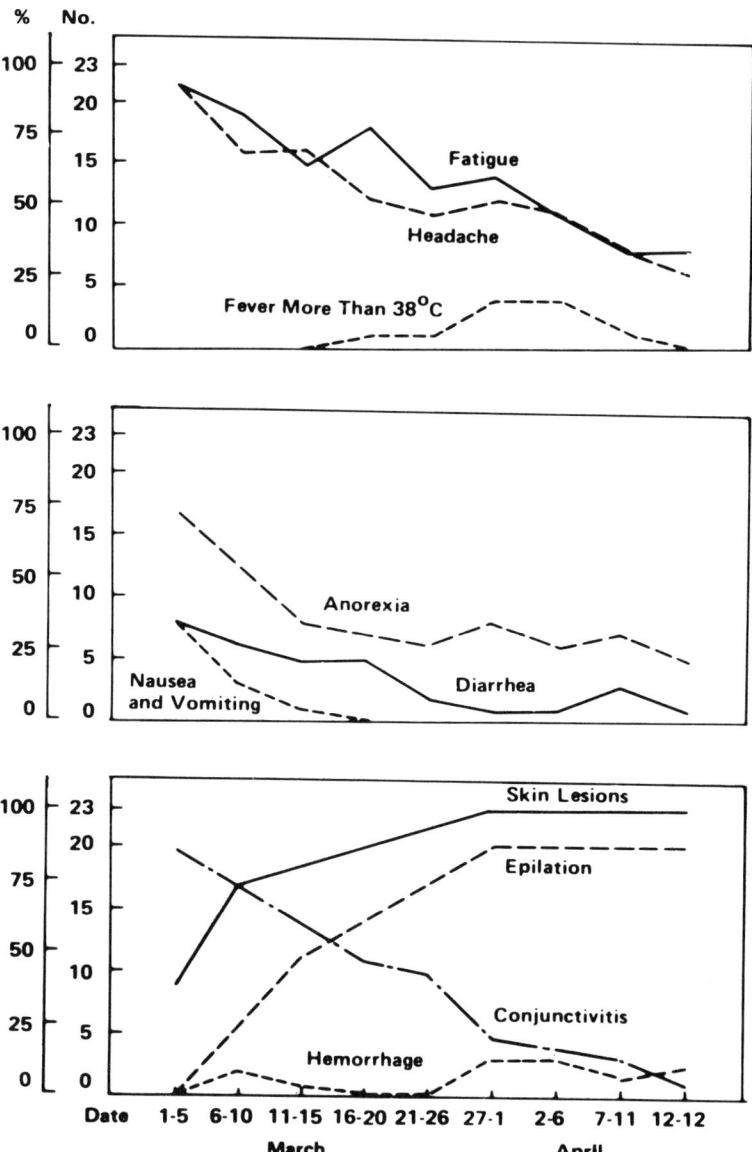

Figure 5. Symptoms and signs in the early stage.

Leukocytes

The total numbers of leukocytes decreased gradually, showing the lowest count at about four to seven weeks after the exposure. In 5 cases the count was less that 2000/mm³, in 13 it was less than 3000, and in 5 it was less than 4000. In one case the number fell to 800. A reverse correlation

42

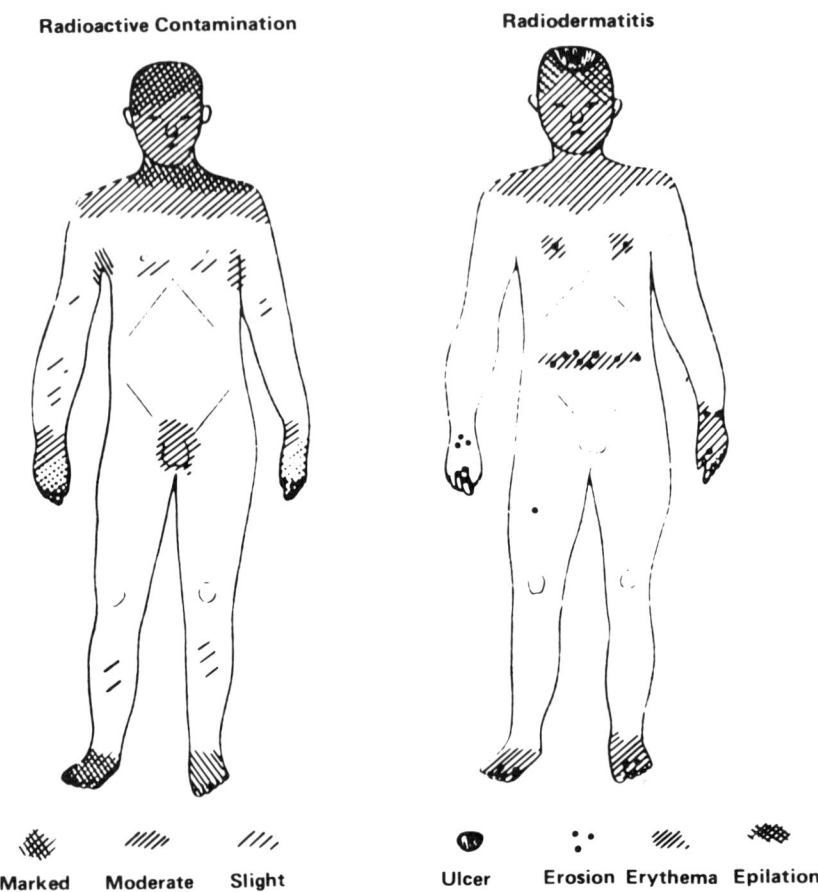

Figure 6. Contamination and lesions of body surface. By courtesy of Dr. K. Ishikawa.

was found between these minimum counts and the doses of individual external radiation.

Lymphopenia was noted at two to eight weeks in all cases. In severe cases, complete recovery was observed after a few years.

Neutropenia was also observed. At four to seven weeks, all cases got minimum values. The relationship between those values and individual radiation doses were similar to that of total leukocyte count (Figure 7).

After eight weeks, recovery was clear, though in some cases immature neutrophils slightly appeared in the peripheral blood. Most cases showed remarkable eosinophilia (maximum more than 40%) at that time, which continued several years in some cases with gradual depression. In a few cases, monocytosis was observed.

Platelets

Platelet counts showed an increasing depression, reaching a minimum at four to seven weeks (15,000–100,000/mm³). Slight coagulation disturbances were observed in several cases. Recovery was observed at eight weeks.

Erythrocytes

A few severe cases showed slight anemia accompanied by remarkable reticulocyte depression. The color indices were over 1.0. The Price-Jones curves were at first displaced to the right of normal but returned almost to normal after one year.

Bone Marrow

In severe cases the bone marrow was highly hypoplastic at the critical stage (Figure 8), but it changed to slightly hypoplastic and then almost normoplastic.

Recovery was not complete even after a year. The coexistence of hypoplastic and hyperplastic areas was observed in histological sections at the recovery stage. This finding was seen even in some sections

Figure 7. Correlation between minimum count of neutrophils and dose.

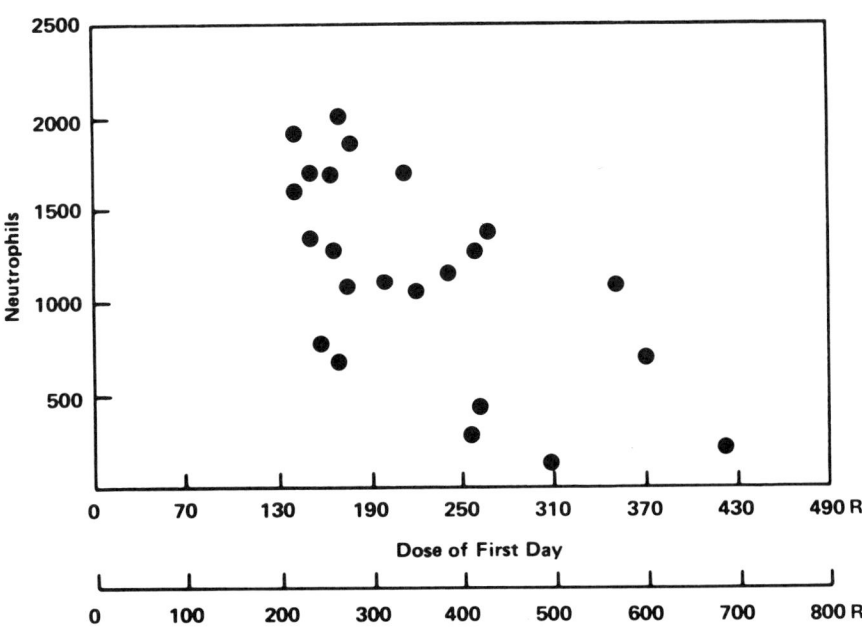

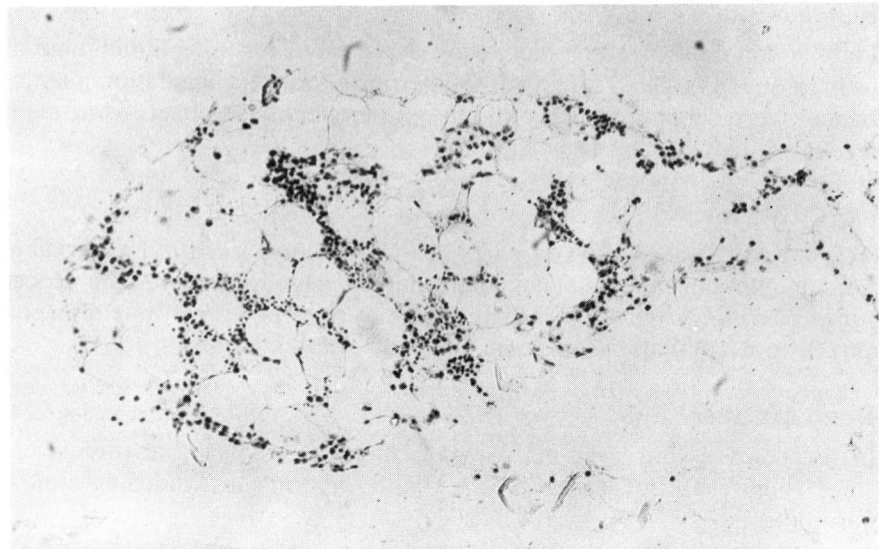

Figure 8. Hypoplastic bone marrow. K-9, 32 days post detonation. 125×.

examined 10–15 years after the exposure (Figure 9). In light cases, only slight depression of bone marrow cells was observed even at the critical stage.

Morphological Abnormalities

Several morphological abnormalities, e.g., abnormal granules in the lymphocytes or neutrophils, vacuoles in various leukocytes and mega-karyocytes, giant nuclei and hypersegmentation of neutrophils, binuclear lymphocytes, abnormal mitosis of erythroblasts, etc., were observed for about one year, especially at the critical and recovery stages. A small increase in "mitotically connected abnormalities" was found in the bone marrow smears of a few cases after 10 years. In T-5 a slight increase of binucleated myelocytes was found at 20 years after exposure.

The bone marrow showed an increased percentage of erythrocytes in some cases even after recovery. In cases T-3 and T-5, slight maturation arrests of neutrophils were observed even at 5 years after the exposure.

Recovering Process of Blood Cells

The cumulative distribution curves of the leukocyte, erythrocyte, and platelet counts were displaced to the left of normal ones at the critical stage. Though the erythrocyte and platelet curves lay on the normal Japanese ones after two years, the leukocyte curve was still displaced slightly to the left of normal after six years (Figures 10 and 11).

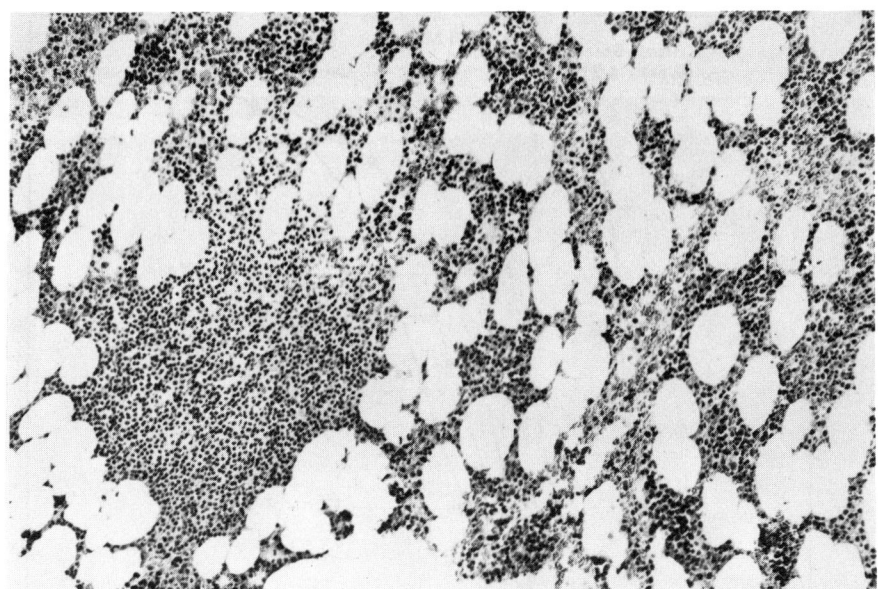

Figure 9. Coexistence of hyperplastic and hypoplastic area. K-9, 14 years post detonation. 125×.

Figure 10. Cumulative distribution curves of erythrocytes count.

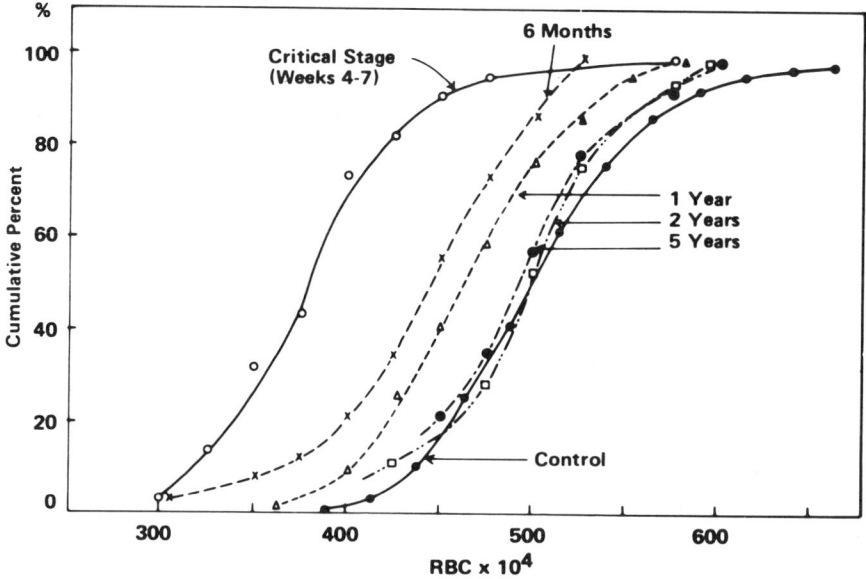

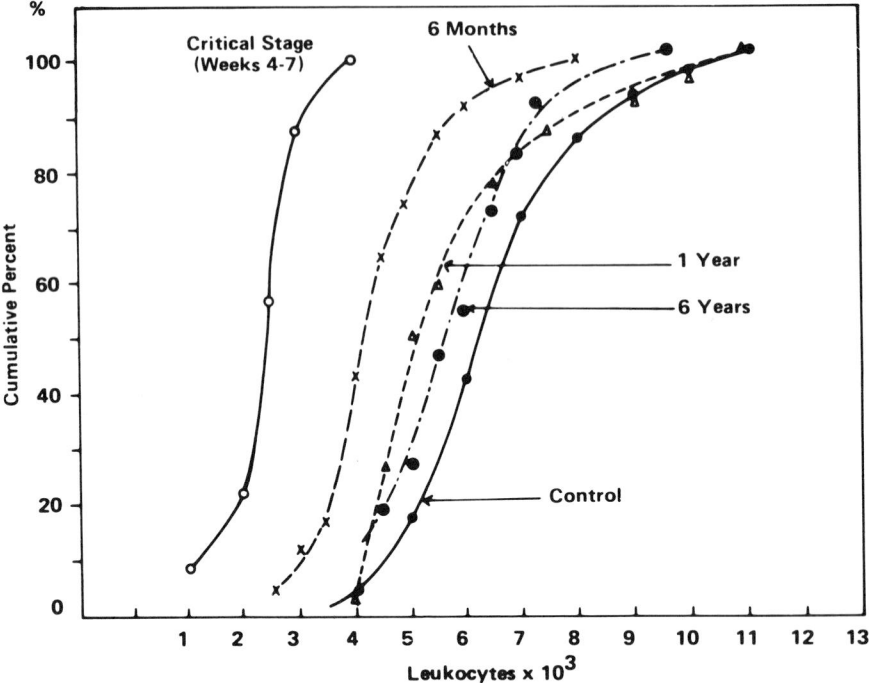

Figure 11. Cumulative distribution curves of leukocyte counts.

The changes of percent depression from average values of leukocytes and platelets are shown in Figure 12, which indicates the general tendency of hematopoietic recovery. The numerical evolution of total leukocytes, neutrophils, and lymphocytes on two severe cases that received annual examination for 25 years is shown in Figure 13. Case T-3 seems to be still leukopenic.

Present hematologic findings are almost normal except T-7, which has been treated as chronic hepatitis and proved thrombopenia.

The assay of CFUc in bone marrow was performed with soft agar culture method at 24 years after exposure. Depressions of CFUc were observed in three cases.

Chromosome Observations

Follow-up of chromosome observations in blood cells has been performed since 1964.[16,17]

In the 1969 examination the close correlation between the percentage of Cs cells and external dose was found.[18]

Table 4 shows the cytogenetic data observed in ten cases that have been examined three to five times since 1964. In comparison with the results obtained in 1967 and 1970 survey the frequency of dicentric plus ring seems to be decreasing. On the other hand, Cs cells remained fairly constant at the frequency of 2 to 3%. In general, both dicentrics plus rings and Cs cells were much more in the peripheral lymphocytes than in the general population; namely, even after 25 years the percentages of dicentric plus rings and Cs cells in the fishermen are about 3 times and 30 times those of normal Japanese in the forties and fifties respectively, which are about 0.1% in both dicentric plus ring and Cs cells (Tonomura; personal communication).

In bone marrow cells, chromosome abnormalities, which were only stable aberrations, were observed. In some cases, clone formation was proved.

Spermatopoiesis

The examinations of spermatopoiesis were performed on 21 cases among 23 cases, including 1 autopsy case.

The number of spermatozoa was depressed by June except five cases, in which the depression was observed at the next examination about four months later. Reduced motility and increased percentages of morpho-

Figure 12. Percentage depression of leukocytes and platelets count.

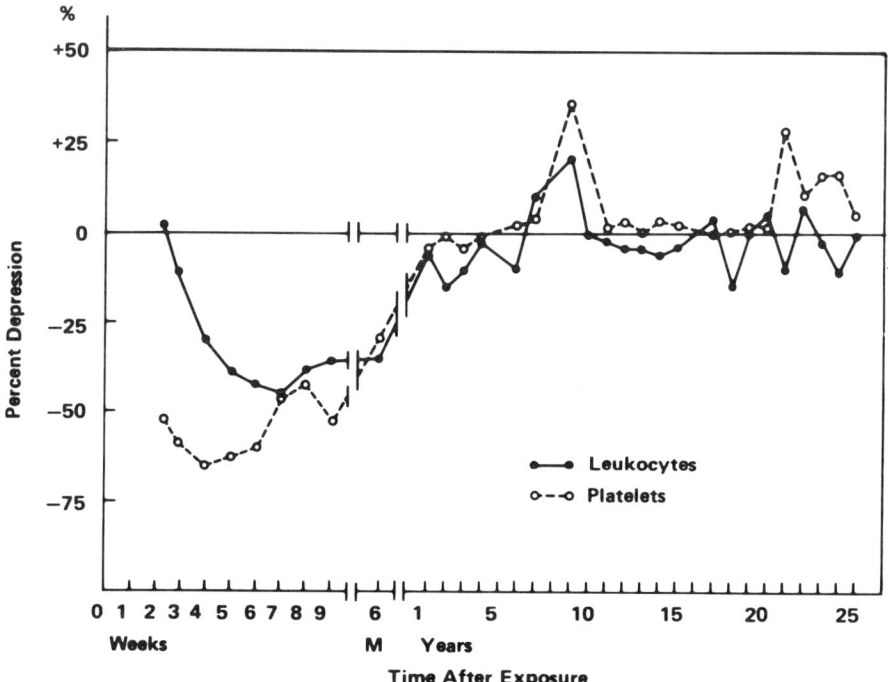

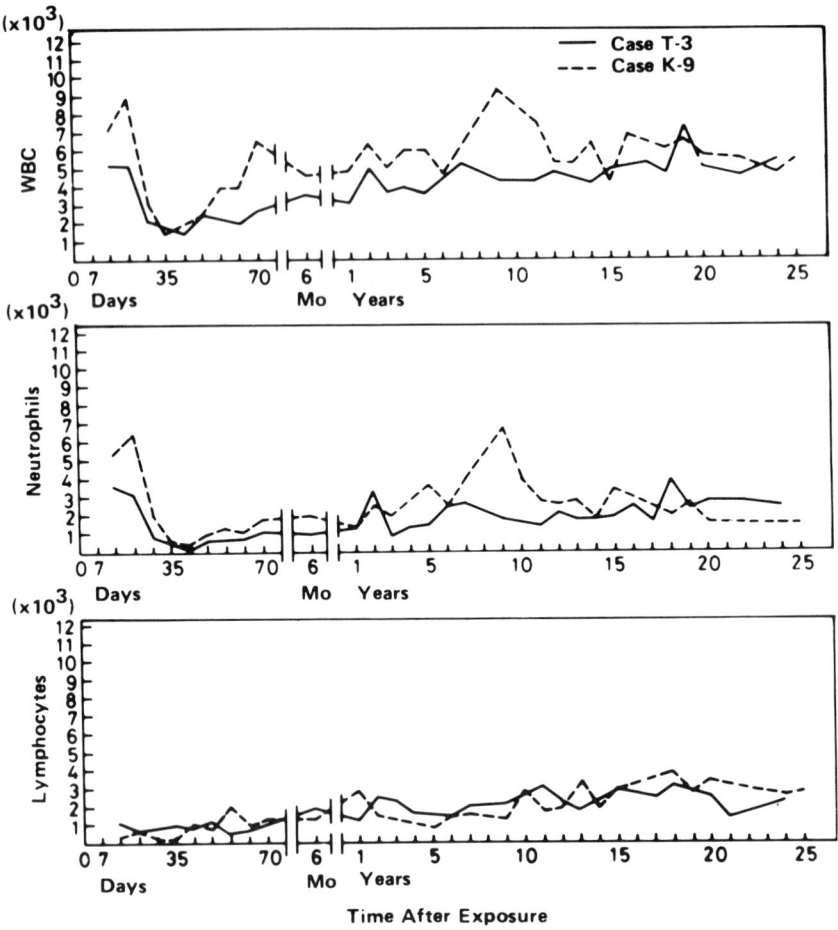

Figure 13. Changes in the number of leukocytes, neutrophils, and lymphocytes of two cases (1954–1979).

Table 4. Incidence of Chromosome Abnormalities in Peripheral Lymphocytes

Years After Exposure	No. of Cases	No. of Cells Examined	Dic + R	Frag	Cs Cells	Aneuploid Cells (Hyper-)
13	9	725	0.83%	0.41%	2.34%	0.14%
15	8	2,912	0.52	0.36	2.10	0.14
20	6	6,000	0.20	0.42		
		973			2.77	0.41
24-25	10	15,000	0.31	0.29		
		2,000			3.15	0.30

ogically abnormal spermatozoa were also noticed.[15] Indications of recovery were seen at approximately two years after the exposure, and most of the patients had healthy children (Figure 14 and Table 5).

The testicle of the fatal case (40 years old) that died 206 days after the exposure "is remarkably atrophic and possesses the interstitial tissue composed of loosely arranged connective tissue. The basement membrane of the seminiferous tubules shows marked thickening. Spermatogonia are extremely decreased in number and in some areas they are completely lacking. No sperma is encountered within the lumen of either seminiferous tubules or epididymis. Sertoli's and Leidig's cells are essentially well preserved."[19]

Ophthalmological Findings

In the evening of the day of exposure, lacrimation, eye wax, and pain in the eyeball annoyed most of them. Two weeks later, severe photophobia, hyperemia, and edema of the conjunctiva were added to the above-mentioned signs. The ophthalmologist diagnosed them as acute kerato-conjunctivitis. Due to the treatment these signs disappeared by the middle of April.

Slight lenticular opacities have been observed in several cases. How-

Figure 14. Changes in the number of spermatozoa.

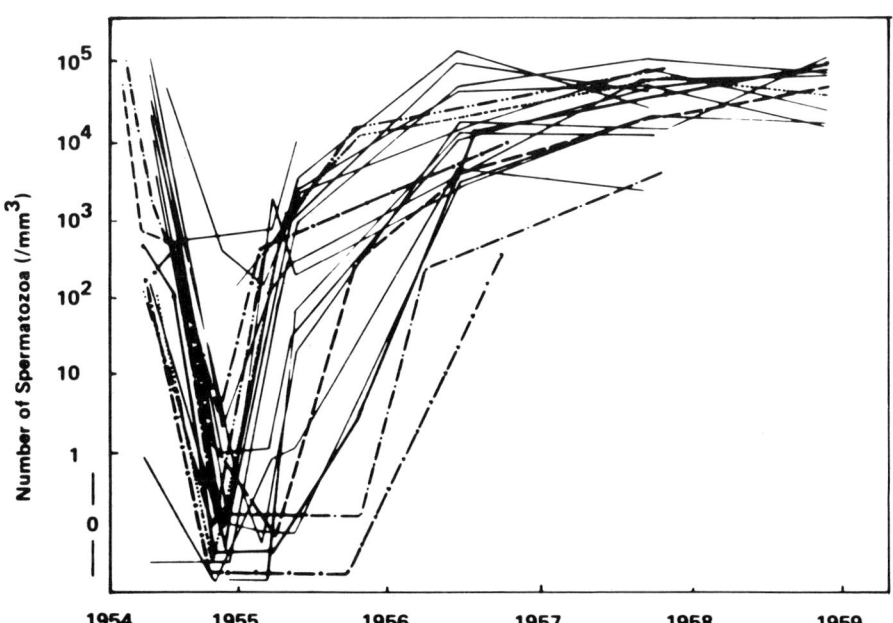

Table 5. Marriage and Children

Case	1954	1955	1956	1957	1958	1959	1960	1961	1962	1963	1964	1965	1966	1967	Age in March 1954
T-1	M(2)[a]		A	f											27
2	M(3)														38
3	M(2)														28
5	M(4)			f											30
6	M(3)														28
7		M						f							27
8						M									26
K-1		M	m		m										22
2				M				f					m		25
3					M	f		m		m	f				25
4		M			m			f				f			24
5						M			m	f			f		22
+6		M		m	A	f		f							26
7									M	m		m	f		18
8				M		f				m					23
9							M	f		m					22
10			M	m								f		m	24
11				M				f	f						23
12							M		f	m					18
13			M			f		f							22
+14	M(3)														39
15	M(2)				f				m						27
16							S	f							20

[a] M, marriage; ( ), no. of children at the time of exposure; m, male; f, female; A, abortion; S, stillbirth; +, fatal case.

ever, these have no characteristics of radiation-induced cataracts as observed in A-bomb survivors.

Thyroid Findings

Dr. Conard et al. report that "in 1963, 9 years after exposure, a 12 year-old girl was found to have an asymptomatic nodule of the thyroid gland. Development of thyroid abnormalities in other subjects continued during subsequent years. At present (1974) 29 to 86 exposed people of Rongelap are affected, including two stunted boys who developed thyroid atrophy without nodularity."

In our cases, in a 1965 examination a nodule of rice corn size was found at left edge of thyroid in K-10. However, it was not observed at next year's examination. Since then it has never appeared. Case K-10 showed the indication of slight depression of T-3. However, any significant clinical change has not been observed in this case. The other cases revealed normal thyroid functions.

Liver Functions

Slight disturbances of liver function were found in a few cases by the laboratory test at the time of hospitalization on 28 March 1954. Since the beginning of May, jaundices were found in 13 cases. A case that revealed remarkable hematologic disturbances (anemia, leukopenia, and thrombopenia) died on 206 days after the exposure. The other cases gradually recovered. However, T-7 and K-6, who had not attended at annual examinations since 1964, were proved to have ascites in 1974. T-7 was also suffering from diabetes mellitus and sepsis. Though T-7 got better, K-6 died in April 1975. Rather fresh liver cirrhosis was observed histologically.

Since these ten years, slight elevation of GOT and GPT has been observed in another four cases.

Concerning these abnormalities, radiation effects should not be ignored. However, it is very difficult to prove the existence of a relationship between the exposure and the liver damage.

Treatment

Skin Lesions

Since the radioactivity of hairs and nails was remarkable, hairs of heads, axillae, and pubes were completely shaved off, and nails were cut off. Necrotized tissue and pus were removed.

The entire surface of the body was cleaned by soap with taking a bath each day. Sodium-EDTA solution was also used for decontamination. At about the middle of April the radioactivity of body surface was no longer detected.

Other treatments such as local administration of ointments and use of antibiotics were done according to the symptoms.

Other Treatments

Since spotlike suppurations were found on the body surface of many cases at the time of hospitalization, antibiotics were used for a few weeks. As in five cases the temperature rose to 38°–39°C in March and April of 1954, a few kinds of antibiotics were used alternately. Blood transfusions were tried for anemic patients.

Other Diseases

Major diseases other than the above-mentioned ones which were observed since 1955 are as follows: r. pulmonary tuberculosis (one in 1955), r. pleuritis (one in 1959), gastric ulcer (one in 1964), diabetes mellitus and sepsis (one in 1974). All of them recovered or improved by medical treatment.

Summary

The follow-up studies on 23 Japanese fishermen exposed to fallout radiation in 1954 were described, including acute effects. In general the current health status of the fishermen is almost normal except slight disturbances of liver function in five cases.

The present conditions which were caused by radiation are residual beta burns in several cases and the increase of chromosome abnormalities in peripheral lymphocytes. Hematologic changes have almost recovered. Radiation-induced cataract has not been proved yet.

However, the further investigation should be continued to detect subtle changes.

ACKNOWLEDGMENTS

We are deeply grateful to many agencies and individuals for valuable assistance to the medical surveys since 1954.

We would like to express our hearty thanks for the good cooperation by the exposed fishermen.

Drs. R. Ichikawa, S. Abe, T. Hashizume, and T. Maruyama of National Institute of Radiological Sciences (NIRS), Dr. T. Tsuchiya of University of Occupational and Environmental Health, and Dr. S. Kimata of Tokyo University School of Medicine were most helpful in the estimate of radiation dose.

We wish to thank Dr. S. Tanaka of the Mitsui Memorial Hospital for his effective advice, and express our gratitude to Dr. R.A. Conard for his excellent information on the exposed Marshallese.

References

1. Miyoshi K, Kumatori T: Clinical and hematological observations on the radiation sickness caused by the ash-fall at Bikini. *Acta Haem Jap* 18:379–406, 1955.

2. Koyama Y, Kumatori T, Shibuya T, Niitani K, Fukuda R, Imamura Y, Sano I, Shigiya R, Koya G, Kono M, Hino Y, Watanabe T, Takemasa Y, Nakamura N, Ozawa Y, Hayashi Y, Hirashima N, Hayafune E, Hamaguchi E, Kimura N, Kanda K, Okamoto S, Hamada M, Ohashi S, Hashimoto K, Kosakai N, Ishii T, Amaki I, Fukazawa Y, Kifune T, Matsumura Y, Nakano I, Taneda K, Hayashi Y, Murata M: Clinical course of the radiation sickness caused by Bikini ashes (intermediate report). *Iryo* 9:1–45, 1955.

3. Mikamo Y, Miyoshi K, Shimizu K, Ishikawa K, Kuriyama S, Koyama Y, Kumatori T: Clinical and haematological studies on Bikini patients, in: *Research in the Effects and Influences of the Nuclear Bomb Test Explosions II.* Tokyo, Japan Society for the Promotion of Science, 1956, pp. 1313–1331.

4. Kumatori T, Miyoshi K: Clinical studies on persons injured by radioactive materials, in: *Diagnosis and Treatment of Radioactive Poisoning.* Vienna, International Atomic Energy Agency, 1963, pp. 253–272.

5. Kumatori T, Ishihara T, Ueda T, Miyoshi K: *Medical survey of Japanese exposed to fallout radiation in 1954.* Chiba, National Institute of Radiological Sciences, 1965.

6. Kumatori T: Hematological effects on heavily irradiated Japanese fishermen, in Sugahara T, Hug O (eds.): *Biological Aspects of Radiation Protection.* Tokyo, Igaku Shoin, 1971, pp. 64–73.

7. Kumatori T: Clinical, especially hematological observations over the 20-year period on the Japanese fishermen exposed to fallout in 1954. *Acta Haem Jap* 38:635–645, 1975.

8. Kumatori T: Clinical aspects of the effects of ionizing radiation, in Finckh ES (ed.): *The Effects of Environment on Cells and Tissues.* Amsterdam-Oxford, Excerpta Medica, 1976, pp. 123–135.

9. Conard RA, Knudsen KD, Dobyns BM, Meyer LM, Sutow WW, Lowrey A, Larsen PR, Rall JE, Robbins J, Rai KR, Wolff J, Steele J, Cohn SH, Oh YH, Greenhouse NA, Eicher M, Motoro F, Riklon E, Anjain J: *A Twenty-year Review of Medical Findings in a Marshallese Population Accidentally Exposed to Radioactive Fallout,* BNL 50424. Upton, New York, Brookhaven National Laboratory, 1975.

10. Kimura K, Minami E, Honda M, Yokohama Y, Ikeda N, Fuwa K, Natsume H, Ishimori T, Sasaki Y, Mizumachi K, Asada M, Abe S, Mabuchi H, Suzuki Y, Komatsu K, Nakada K: Radiochemical analysis of falling dust on the fishing boat "Fukuryu Maru" on 1st March, 1954, in: *Research in the Effects and Influences of the Nuclear Bomb Test Explosions I.* Tokyo, Japan Society for the Promotion of Science, 1956, pp. 497–519.

11. *Basic Radiation Protection Criteria,* NCRP Report No. 39. Washington D.C., National Council on Radiation Protection and Measurements, 1971, p. 48.

12. Kobayashi R, Nagai I: Cooperation by the United States in the radiochemical analyses, in: *Research in the Effects and Influences of the Nuclear Bomb Test Explosions II.* Tokyo, Japan Society for the Promotion of Science, 1956, pp. 1435–1445.

13. Kimura K, Ikeda N, Kimura K, Kawanishi H, Kimura M: Radiochemical analysis of the body of the late Mr. Kuboyama, in: *Research in the Effects and Influences of the Nuclear Bomb Test Explosions I.* Tokyo, Japan Society for the Promotion of Science, 1956, pp. 521–527.

14. International Commission on Radiological Protection: ICRP Publication 30. Part 1, *Limits for Intakes of Radionuclides by Workers.* A report of Committee 2 of the

International Commission on Radiological Protection. Oxford-New York-Frankfurt, Pergamon Press, 1979.

15. Shimizu K, Ishikawa K, Saito Y, Nakamura K, Sato T, Torada S, Sugiyama T, Takayama S, Huruya H, Ono M, Inagaki H: Some observations on the victims of the Bikini H-bomb test, in: *Research in the Effects and Influences of the Nuclear Bomb Test Explosions II.* Tokyo, Japan Society for the Promotion of Science, 1956, pp. 1333–1351.

16. Ishihara T, Kumatori T: Chromosome Studies on Japanese exposed to radiation resulting from nuclear bomb explosions, in Evans HJ, Court Brown WM, McLean AS (eds.): *Human Radiation Cytogenetics.* Amsterdam, North-Holland Publishing Company, 1967, pp. 144–166.

17. Ishihara T, Kumatori T: Cytogenetic studies on fishermen exposed to fallout radiation in 1954. *Japan J Genet* 44:Suppl. 1, 242–251, 1969.

18. Kumatori T, Ishihara T, Kohno S, Inaba M: Chromosome abnormalities of Japanese fishermen exposed to fallout radiation in 1954, in: *NIRS-10, Annual Report 1970–1971.* Chiba, National Institute of Radiological Sciences, 1971, pp. 56–57.

19. Miyake M, Ohashi S: Pathology of the Bikini patients, in: *Research in the Effects and Influences of the Nuclear Bomb Test Explosions, II.* Tokyo, Japan Society for the Promotion of Science, 1956, pp. 1371–1401.

Published 1980 by Elsevier North Holland, Inc.
K.F. Hübner and S.A. Fry, eds. The Medical Basis for Radiation Accident Preparedness

The 1954 Bikini Atoll Incident: An Update of the Findings in the Marshallese People

Robert A. Conard

Consultant and former Head of the Marshall Island Medical Program at Brookhaven National Laboratory.

The thyroid findings in the Marshallese people accidentally exposed to radioactive fallout following the detonation of a nuclear device at Bikini in 1954 are reported in detail in a 20-year review[1] and other reports.[2,3] A 25-year review is being written. A brief updating is presented here.

The Marshallese populations with exposure data are listed in Table 1. The early effects of exposure on the Rongelap group were similar to those reported by Dr. Kumatori for the fishermen on the *Lucky Dragon.* Transient nausea and vomiting occurred in that group and to a lesser degree in the Ailingnae group but were not reported in the Utirik group.

The major findings in the Rongelap group were depression of blood leukocytes and platelets to about one-half normal levels for 4 to 6 weeks, widespread "beta" burns of the skin with epilation, and significant internal absorption of radionuclides. These findings were less pronounced in the Ailingnae group and were not documented in the Utirik population. These observations are described in detail in earlier reports. During the first decade there were few findings that could definitely be associated with radiation exposure; although there did appear to be a lag in complete recovery of leukocytes in the Rongelap group. During the second decade, however, there were serious developments in the exposed Rongelap group—a death from acute myelogenous leukemia and numerous thyroid abnormalities along with growth retardation in some of the children.

Development of Thyroid Abnormalities

Radiochemical urine analyses shortly after the accident revealed measurable amounts of radionuclides, particularly isotopes of strontium,

Table 1. Exposures of Marshallese Populations

Atoll	Distance from Bikini	No. of people	Amount of fallout	Estimated gamma dose
Rongelap	~100 miles	67	Heavy (snow-like)	175 rad
Ailingae	~110 miles	19	Moderate (mist-like)	69 rad
Utirik	~300 miles	158	Not visible	14 rad

barium, and iodine. The significance of the radioiodine exposure was not fully appreciated at that time. When thyroid abnormalities began to appear, a re-evaluation of thyroid dose indicated an estimated dose of 335 rad to Rongelap adults and doses ranging from 700 to 1400 rad in the children exposed at less than 10 years of age. Lower doses were calculated for the other populations. The higher doses in the children were related to the smaller sizes of their thyroid glands. The largest component was ^{131}I, but shorter-lived isotopes of iodine, particularly ^{132}I, ^{133}I, and ^{135}I, contributed more than half the dose.

The first indication of thyroid trouble was the finding of growth retardation in a number of exposed Rongelap children, and later correlation with decreasing thyroid hormone levels indicated decreased function of the gland. Two boys developed frank myxedema. It was about this time (1964) that thyroid nodules began appearing, particularly in the exposed children. In subsequent years, the nodules continued to appear in the Rongelap and Ailingnae group and, beginning about 1967, in the Utirik groups. Table 2 shows the numbers of subjects who have had thyroid nodules up to the present.

The Rongelap and Ailingnae people are seen to have greatly increased numbers of nodules, both benign and malignant, and the Utirik group also appears to have increased numbers compared with the unexposed

Table 2. Thyroid Nodules Appearing from 1964 to 1979.

Group	Total nodules	Cancer[a]
Rongelap and Ailingnae (135-1150 rads)	36.0% (31/86)	4.7% (4/86)
Utirik (30-95 rads)	9.5% (15/158)	1.9% (3/158)
Unexposed	6.6% (29/437)	0.9% (4/437)

[a] The number of cancer cases is tentative since final diagnoses on some recent cases are pending.

people. In the Rongelap-Ailingnae group, 65% of those exposed as children had nodules compared with 27% of those exposed as adults. Paradoxically, in the Utirik population a greater percentage of adults had nodules in spite of a higher dose to the children's glands.

During the past ten years, a disturbing finding has been the further development of thyroid hypofunction, even in some Rongelap people without other detectable abnormalities. Table 3 shows the present status of thyroid hypofunction. The positive category represents individuals who have exhibited two TSH (thyroid-stimulating hormone) levels of 6 μU/ml or greater. The suggestive category represents individuals who have two TSH levels of 4 to 6.

The association of radiation exposure with the development of thyroid abnormalities in the Rongelap population seems apparent though the Utirik findings are less clear-cut. The development of thyroid tumors following radiation exposure is well documented in the Japanese exposed to the atomic bomb and in patients, particularly children, following radiation therapy.

On a risk per rad basis, the induction of thyroid nodules and cancer in the Marshallese appears to be about equal to that following X-ray exposure. Since ^{131}I is believed to be only about one-tenth as effective as X irradiation in producing thyroid abnormalities, it seems likely that in the Marshallese the exposure to the short-lived isotopes of iodine ^{132}I, ^{133}I, and ^{135}I, which have more energetic betas and deliver a faster dose rate than ^{131}I, might account for the high incidence.

The findings in the Marshallese emphasize the importance of thyroid exposure to radioiodines that may result from warfare or accidents in which radioiodines are released. Exposure to penetrating gammas or neutrons is a more serious hazard not only because of their acute effects, but also because of the fatal nature of malignancies such as leukemia which may develop. Deaths due to thyroid abnormalities including cancer

Table 3. Thyroid Hypofunction in Marshallese Populations

Group	Positive	Suggestive	Total[a]
Rongelap + Ailingnae (135-1150 rads)	15% (13/86)	9.3% (8/86)	24.4% (21/86)
Utirik (30-95 rads)	0.8% (1/158)	3.8% (6/158)	4.4% (7/158)
Unexposed	0.6% (1/155)	1.5% (1/67)	3.0% (2/67)

[a] Some of these subjects appear also in the nodule table, i.e., they have both hypofunction and nodularity.

are rare, and such abnormalities are amenable both to preventive measures (such as prophylactic use of stable iodine) and to treatment with hormones and surgery.

References

1. Conard RA: A twenty-year review of medical findings in a Marshallese population accidentally exposed to radioactive fallout. BNL 50424, September, 1975.
2. Conard RA: Summary of thyroid findings in Marshallese 22 years after exposure to radioactive fallout, in De Groot J (ed.): *Radiation Associated Thyroid Carcinoma*. New York, Grune and Stratton, 1977, p. 241.
3. Larsen PR, Conard RA, Knudsen K, Robbins J, Wolff J, Rall JE: Thyroid hypofunction appearing as a delayed manifestation of accidental exposure to radioactive fallout in a Marshallese population, in *Late Biological Effects of Ionizing Radiation,* vol. I, International Atomic Energy Agency, Vienna, 1978, pp. 101–115.

Report of 21-Year Medical Follow-up of Survivors of the Oak Ridge Y-12 Accident

Gould A. Andrews,* Karl F. Hübner,+
Shirley A. Fry,+ Clarence C. Lushbaugh,+
and L. Gayle Littlefield+

*Department of Nuclear Medicine, University of Maryland Hospital,
Baltimore, Maryland;
+Medical and Health Sciences Division, Oak Ridge Associated Universities,
Oak Ridge, Tennessee.

Accidents, industrial and otherwise, involving whole-body exposure of human beings to levels of ionizing radiation sufficient to cause immediate or early harmful effects have occurred only rarely since the first critical excursion at the University of Chicago in 1942. There has been no concomitant increase in the relative incidence of these events despite the increased use of radiation and radioactive materials. Typically, these accidents have involved only a few individuals, and total mortality and morbidity have been low.

Detailed descriptions and analyses of some of these accidents have been widely reported. With the exception of the studies by Conard of the Marshall Islanders exposed to fallout in 1954,[1] however, published reports of the long-term medical follow-up of survivors of this type of event have been infrequent.

This paper reports the medical findings in a 21-year follow-up of the survivors of the serious radiation accident at the Y-12 Plant in Oak Ridge, Tennessee, on June 16, 1958. This group of survivors is unique in that they have continued to live and work, individually and collectively, in the same or a very similar environment as at the time of the accident. The introduction of new variables which frequently compound long-term follow-up studies is therefore less likely. The accident and its early clinical effects and laboratory data have been documented extensively.[2-11] A review of each survivor's status with dose estimates and effects during the first 48 hr after the accident, the clinical course during the period of hospitalization, and subsequent follow-up data are presented in Table 1.

The Accident and its Immediate Effects

Eight Caucasian male workers 25 to 56 years of age were exposed to a mixed neutron–gamma field in a critical excursion triggered by an unplanned transfer of enriched uranium to a 55-gallon drum. Five men received whole-body doses of between 236 and 365 rad, and three others doses below 70 rad. Symptomatic treatment and laboratory studies were begun at the plant site for seven of the eight men. Approximately 11 hr after the accident, the five high-dose victims were transferred to the research hospital of the Oak Ridge Institute of Nuclear Studies, now the Medical and Health Sciences Division of Oak Ridge Associated Universities (ORAU). Two men who had received doses of 68.5 and 22.5 rad, respectively, remained asymptomatic and were released at first. They and the eighth man, who had left the building on hearing the alarm and gone directly home, were recalled and admitted to the hospital on the second postaccident day.

In consultation with national and international experts, the five high-dose survivors (A, B, C, D, and E) were treated conservatively. It was decided not to prepare for bone marrow transplantations because within the estimated dose range the risk of a graft-versus-host reaction was considered to be greater than any potential benefit. Bone marrow transplantation, however, was not ruled out should definite clinical indications develop. Under the circumstances, symptomatic and supportive care was the treatment of choice, with antibiotics being reserved only if definitely indicated. Patients A, B, C, D, and E each developed the characteristic hematological pattern of radiation-induced bone marrow depression, which was most severe in patient A (365 rad). Patient E, with the fifth highest dose (236 rad), ranked second; patients B (270 rad), C (339 rad), and D (327 rad) ranked third, fourth, and fifth, respectively. In the fourth week, mild hemorrhagic phenomena in patients A and C were associated with thrombocytopenia (platelets 10,000 to 20,000/mm^3). Spontaneous recovery of the platelets and granulocytes occurred between the fifth and eighth week. Patients A and B developed mild upper respiratory tract infections not clearly correlated with minimal granulocyte levels and promptly responded to antibiotics. Partial transient epilation, beginning on the 17th day, was noted in patients A, B, C, D, and E. Patients F (68.5 rad), G (68.5 rad), and H (22.5 rad) remained completely asymptomatic and were discharged on the ninth day. They had no hematological changes clearly attributable to radiation exposure; patient G had an unexplained preexisting leukocytosis; patient H had

Table 1. Summary of Immediate and Follow-up Medical Course of All Eight Patients.

Patient Status at Time of Accident	Dose (rad) γ, μ	Hospital Course	Convalescent Course, 12/58	Subsequent History[a] through 3/79
A				
40 yrs., married, 2 children P.H: non-contrib. smoker Chemical operator 6 ft from source	269 γ; 96 μ; dose = 365 rad	0-48 hrs: nausea (persisting 5 days), vomiting 49 hrs.: lymphs 9%: 873 Day 17: epilation began Day 25-28: mild thrombocytopenic signs Day 29: pyrexia, acute tonsillitis Day 44: discharged Wt change: −2 lbs, +8 lbs	Joint stiffness, fatigability, vague visual symptoms, disturbance of balance, decreasing gradually, mild depression	Generally good health with minor complaints. 1962: "about recovered" from weakness, joint and muscle symptoms. 1970: bronchial asthma. 1976: c/o asthma, arthralgia. Hypothyroid, Synthroid prescribed. 1979: Several non-malignant nevi excised in interim. Arthralgia minimal, asthma continues, otherwise in good health. Continues full time employment at Y-12.
B				
32 yrs., married; 2 children P.H: non-contrib. Electrician 15 ft from source	199 γ; 71 μ; dose = 270 rad	0-48 hrs: nausea (persisting 3 days), vomiting, headache 49 hrs: lymphs 9%: 882 Day 10: furuncle Day 13: pyrexia, mild pharyngitis, otitis media Day 17: epilation Day 27: rare RBCs in urine Day 44: discharged Wt change: −2 lbs, +13 lbs	Tendency to tire easily, some muscle soreness, several mild URI's	1965: mild or incipient diabetes, obesity, hyperuricemia. 1968: fasting blood sugar, serum uric acid normal. 1979: good general health continues, no medications. Faint lenticular opacities. Continues full time employment at Y-12.

Table 1. (continued)

C				
39 yrs., married; 4 children P.H: coal miner 12 yrs., smoker Machinist 17 ft from source	250 γ, 89 μ; dose = 339 rad	0-48 hrs: generalized warmth, nausea, vomiting 30 mins day 2 only 49 hrs: lymphs 15%: 1276 Day 10: pyrexia, URI Day 17: epilation Day 25-30: petechiae over trunk, legs; mild fatigue Day 44: discharged Wt change: + 8 lbs	Some weakness in thighs. Headache in sunlight. Some fatigue.	Symptoms decreased with time. 1960: spontaneous bruising. 1967: fatigue, weight loss, infiltrate in apex of right lung: tuberculosis. 1967-69: treatment with tuberculostatica. 1970: infiltrate LUL, lobectomy, invasive multinodular bronchogenic carcinoma; cobalt therapy. Hypercholesterolemia. 1972: metastatic spread. 1973: died 1/13/1973.
D				
50 yrs., married; 1 child P.H: non-contrib. Electrician 16 ft. from source	241 γ, 86 μ; dose = 327 rad	0-72 hrs: intermittent nausea, vomited twice 49 hrs: lymphs 21%: 1827 Day 17: epilation Day 24: discomfort RLQ Day 25: rare RBC in urine Day 44: discharged Wt. change: −2 lbs, +3 lbs	Weakness, forgetfulness, headache, fatigability, abdominal discomfort, nervousness, insomnia, mild depression.	Persistent symptoms, numerous minor complaints, arthralgia and weakness especially in the legs. 1961: hypertrophic degenerative arthritis by X-rays. Continued employment at Y-12 until 1972. 1974: IgA gammopathy, no B-J protein, bone marrow hypocellular, not diagnostic. Medically controlled hypertension.

Table 1. *(continued)*

E 35 yrs., married, 4 children P.H: non-contrib. Machinist 22 ft from source	174 γ, 62 μ; dose = 236 rad	0-48 hrs: asymptomatic for 24 hrs. Nausea, vomiting (X3) day 2 only, malaise, aches in legs 49 hrs: lymphs 21% 945 Day 3: furuncle Day 17: epilation Day 26, 27: Sl. gingival bleeding on brushing Day 44: discharged Wt change: +10 lbs	Fatigability, weakness in legs. Photophobia in sunlight. 8/23/58, nervousness.	1976: IgA level still elevated but decreased. B-J protein negative, bone marrow non-diagnostic. 1979: IgA level still elevated but less than in 1976. No B-J protein, bone scan negative. Prostatic hypertrophy. Physically active.
F 41 yrs., married; 4 children P.H: empyema nephrolithiasis since 1950, smoker, asbestos exposure Welder 20 ft from source	50.5 γ, 18 μ; dose = 68.5 rad	0-48 hrs: weakness 49 hrs: lymphs 25%; 2548 Day 3: nausea 2 hrs. Day 9: discharged Wt change: +5 lbs	Aches, fatigue of thighs, severe "snapping sounds" in many joints. Intermittent fatigability.	Persistent fatigability; minor complaints. 1959: hospitalized for left anterior pain. 1962: hypoglycemia 1965-present: erythroplasia of Queyrat. 1971: renal infection. 1975: prostatitis 1979: good general health; dermatological consultation. Continues employment at Y-12. 1961: right nephrolithiasis, mild hydronephrosis; bleeding peptic ulcer. 1967: mild hypertension, albuminuria. 1972: right nephrolithotomy.

Table 1. *(continued)*

				1973: gastrojejunostomy for acute peptic ulcer. 1974: left nephrolithiasis. 1976: COPD 11/76: hospitalized with pneumonia, medical disability retirement from Y-12. 1979: COPD, little change; physical activity limited; reports past asbestos exposure.
G 56 yrs, married; 5 of 8 children living P.H. 1957: M.I. Maintenance mechanic 20 ft from source	50.5 γ, 18 μ; dose = 68.5 rad	0-48 hrs; asymptomatic 49 hrs: lymphs 15%: 1989 Mild emphysema Day 9: discharged Wt change: +½ lb	Considerable nervousness about late effects of irradiation. Few brief weak spells in mid-July 1958. Some depression. Weakness in legs not prominent.	Few minor complaints. Nervousness about accident persisted. General health good. 1962: Early retirement. 1972: Mild hypertension, RBBB and occasional PVCs. 1976: CVA, fatal in 45 minutes.
H 25 yrs, single P.H: emotional problems F.H: hemoglobinopathy, possible psychoneurosis 50 ft from source	16.8 γ, 6 μ; dose = 22.8 rad	0-48 hrs: asymptomatic 49 hrs: lymphs 33%: 1914 Day 6: URI responded to symptomatic treatment Day 9: discharged Wt change: −1 lb, + 4 lbs	Nervousness, fatigability. Married 2 mos. after accident. Special study of hemoglobin led to incidental discovery of pre-existing familial	Continued psychoneurotic difficulties. Normal, healthy daughters born in 1959 and 1965. Marital problems; separated 1973. 1975: Continued good health

hemoglobinopathy of no clinical significance.

through 8/75. Adenocarcinoma colon in 9/75. No evidence of recurrence or metastates through 3/79.
1976: Ventricular bigeminy.
1977: Auto crash; whiplash injury.
1979: Healthy and more stable. Continues employment in an office job.

[a] Studies in November, 1961, showed sperm counts in six patients who had aspermia or oligospermia 4 months after the accident were consistent with good potential fertility; aspermia persisted in patient C. No radiation-induced dermatological or ophthalmological changes reported in any patient through February, 1979.

transient leukopenia two weeks after the accident. The five high-dose patients were released from the hospital on the 44th day.

The patients were followed at regular intervals after their release. They all complained, to a varying degree, of weakness, fatigue, soreness, and stiffness of joints, the severity and duration of which were not clearly related to radiation dose. These symptoms were quite real, but no organic basis for them was found. They might be explained in part by the abrupt resumption of normal physical activities after a period of deconditioning due to hospital confinement; similar symptoms have been experienced by other radiation accident survivors who have been hospitalized[12] but, as is well known, also accompany extensive courses of radiation therapy. In time these symptoms decreased in severity except in patient D, who continues to complain of stiffness and joint pains, which may now be related to degenerative skeletal changes. Patients A, C, and E complained of disturbances of balance and vision with photophobia and general intolerance of the sun's heat for a few months. Other radiation accident survivors also had similar symptoms. Patient E complained of "dizzy spells" for a period of two years; it is probable that these episodes were all or in part related to hypoglycemia, which was diagnosed in 1962.

During hospitalization and subsequently, special biochemical and hematological studies were done, many of them in collaboration with colleagues from other laboratories.[13-20] Sperm counts showed that the five high-dose patients were aspermic by four months after exposure and hypospermic for at least 21 months; sperm levels adequate for fertility were reached by 41 months after exposure in four of these five patients.[21] Only one of the wives of the seven men participating in the fertility studies later became pregnant; the other six patients had established families prior to the accident; at least one couple chose not to have additional children. Routine and special ophthalmological examinations were done periodically throughout 20 years; several patients have, with time, developed lenticular opacities of various kinds, but none were typical posterior lenticular radiation-induced opacities.

Subsequent Course

Since the initial follow-up during the recovery phase, the eight patients have been recalled at intervals of from one to two years for routine examinations and hematological, biochemical, cytogenetic, and ophthalmological evaluations and special tests if indicated. Two of the survivors are now deceased; the remaining were examined most recently in February, 1979.

Within four months of the accident, all the men had resumed work at the Y-12 Plant, where they were assigned to day-shift jobs with minimal or no radiation exposure. Seven of the men retained their original job classifications. The eighth man (low dose), who had relatively little seniority, was reclassified; his employment was discontinued in a reduction-in-work-force action at the Y-12 Plant in 1965; he has since kept an office job in the Oak Ridge area. One low-dose man (G) was granted early retirement at the age of 62 years in 1964. Patient E, who also had been a hard-rock miner, was granted medical disability retirement in November, 1976, following hospitalization at age 59 for bilateral pneumonia associated with chronic obstructive pulmonary disease.

The previously described symptoms of weakness and fatigability gradually lessened in the months and early years after reconvalescence. It is impossible to define precisely the course of these symptoms or to determine whether they completely in each patient disappeared; in patient D they definitely persisted. The patients, now 71, 61, 60, 56, 53, and 46 years old, respectively, sometimes suggest that they may be simply experiencing the effects of advancing years.

Late in 1961 and early in 1962, a group of nationally known consultants, representing the specialties in neurology, psychiatry, dermatology, orthopedics, male fertility, and ophthalmology, examined the men. Their findings can be summarized as follows:

1. There were no skin changes secondary to irradiation.
2. There was no objective evidence of orthopedic problems that could be related to the radiation exposure.
3. There were no ophthalmological abnormalities attributable to irradiation. Periodic examinations through February, 1979, have resulted in similar conclusions.
4. Sperm studies (one low-dose man was not studied) showed that all but one of the seven had normal or near-normal sperm counts by early 1962. One low-dose man had azoospermia, which may have antedated the accident.[21]
5. Neurological findings and electroencephalograms were normal.
6. Psychologic examination indicated that the accident had had a rather profound effect on the men, and at least two of them evidenced mild depression probably related to it. Sexual activity was decreased in at least half the group, probably because of psychological factors. Only one of the married couples wanted more children; two wives had shown lessened libido, reputedly due to fear of transmitting possible genetic damage induced by the exposure.
7. The patients reported that their weakness was less pronounced.

Long-term Medical Follow-up

Since 1962 the survivors had a variety of not unusual illnesses, and the subsequent medical histories of the survivors are noteworthy only because of their banality.

Patient A

This man, 40 years old at the time of the accident, who had received the highest dose (365 rad), continued to have upper respiratory tract infections for some time after the accident. Episodes of acute prostatitis, which had occurred prior to the accident, continued intermittently since and have responded well to treatment. Symptoms and radiological evidence of calcific tendonitis in the right shoulder were reported in 1965. In the winter of 1970–71, he developed allergic bronchial asthma without a specific antigen being identified. Desensitization with mixed allergens has continued since that time. Dyphylline and potassium iodide were prescribed together with Isuprel. In 1974, a routine physical examination at the plant revealed a "high thyroid count." When seen at ORAU in 1974, a slightly nodular but apparently asymptomatic goiter was found. In 1976, a T_4 of 1.9 μg/dl, a triiodothyronine uptake of 33%, and a FTI of 0.6 were found. He was referred to an endocrinologist, who suspected lymphocytic disease made overt by the potassium iodide therapy; there were few symptoms of thyroid insufficiency. Potassium iodide was discontinued; later Synthroid 75 mg b.i.d. was prescribed and has been continued to the present. In February, 1979, the thyroid gland was not palpable, and the TT_4 was 10.2 μg/dl, T_4I 6.7 μg/dl, T_3 39%, and the FTI 2.6, indicating a euthyroid state. Also, at this examination the hemogram showed a hemoglobin of 13.9 gm%, a hematocrit of 44%, and 6300 leukocytes/mm³, with 59% polys, 31% lymphocytes, 8% eos, and 2% basophils. This patient has continued to work as a chemical operator at the Y-12 Plant since the fourth month after the accident. In recent years he has been engaged in the fabrication of plastics and rubber, involving minimal exposures to solvents and cleaning fluids.

It is concluded 21 years after the accident that this man is in good general health except for mild symptoms of bronchial asthma, to which the slight eosinophilia is probably attributable. Arthralgia, a considerable problem in the past, seemed to be remarkably less at the most recent examination.

Patient B

This patient was 32 years old at the time of the accident. His estimated total-body dose was 270 rad. He has continued to enjoy good general health since the accident, and he is still employed at the Y-12 Plant.

Patient C

This man, 39 years old in 1958, one of the high-dose victims, showed the most profound acute hematologic effects. He had worked as a coal miner from the age of 14 to 33, spending 12 years at underground work, and also was a habitual one-pack-per-day cigarette smoker. In the middle

1960s he developed pulmonary tuberculosis, which responded to tuber-culostatica and finally was considered to be cured in 1969. In April, 1970, a chest radiograph showed focal pulmonary calcifications, bullae, and bilateral apical scarring believed to present healed tuberculosis; however, another roentgenogram later that year showed an infiltrate in the upper lobe of the left lung. A thoracotomy was done, and the left upper lobe was resected for a multinodular bronchogenic carcinoma. The histopath-ologic examination revealed a multicentric origin of the cancer around silicotic nodules and anthracosilicosis with moderate focal fibrosis. After having recovered from postoperative complications he received radiation therapy. He died in 1973 from metastatic spread of the malignancy. No autopsy was done.

Patient D

This man was 50 years old at the time of exposure. He had many symptoms, especially muscle and joint pains, not substantiated by objective findings and changing significantly through the years. Serum protein studies, which had been normal in 1958 and 1965, began to show a progressive globulin increase starting in 1968 and reaching a level of 4.7 gm% in 1974; albumin levels decreased slowly to 3.4 gm% in 1976. Serum immunoglobulins, which had not been measured earlier, were abnormal in 1974 (Table 2 and Figure 1). The abnormality has continued, with fluctuating values but without Bence-Jones proteinuria. In early 1974, 6% plasma cells, with some young forms, were found in the bone marrow; a radiographic bone survey and a technetium 99m diphosphonate bone scan revealed no lesions. In October, 1976, the symptoms and physical findings were unchanged, although IgA was further elevated. Some osteoporosis without focal lesions was noted on X-ray examination, and there were 9% plasma cells and many smudge cells in the bone marrow. At the most recent examination (February, 1979), this patient's general condition was essentially unchanged; elevation of IgA continued but was reduced from the 1976 level, while the other gamma-globulin levels were in the normal range; a bone survey showed generalized degenerative changes and hypertrophic infractions of T-11 and T-12, but there was no evidence of focal lytic lesions. Tests for Bence-Jones

Table 2. Immunoglobulins in Patient D

	2/4/74	4/18/74	6/9/75	10/25/79	3/5/79
Total protein	7.6 gm %	7.9 gm %	7.5 gm %	8 gm %	8 gm %
IgG	1400 mg %	1000 mg %	590 mg %	1000 mg %	740 mg %
IgA	2800 mg %	900 mg %	1200 mg %	3950 mg %	2400 mg %
IgM	32 mg %	25 mg %	30 mg %	36.5 mg %	25.0 mg %

(−)   (+)

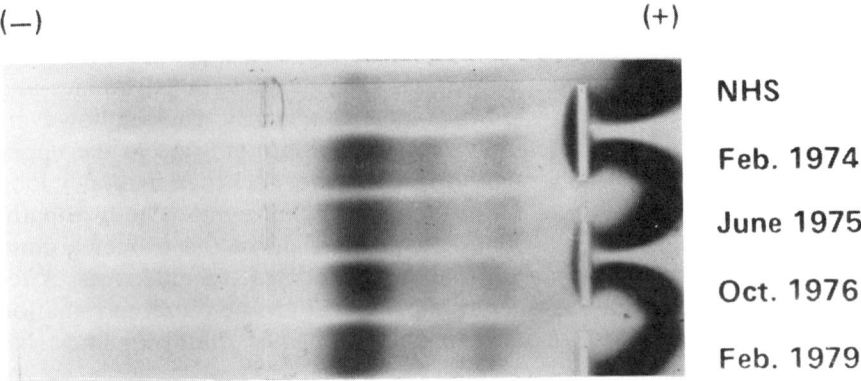

NHS

Feb. 1974

June 1975

Oct. 1976

Feb. 1979

Figure 1. Electrophoretograms on Na-acetate demonstrating increased and changing Ig^A levels in patient D. NHS, normal human serum. This figure was provided by and is shown here with the permission of Dr. A. Solomon, University of Tennessee Memorial Research Center, Knoxville, Tennessee.

protein have been consistently negative. Hematological findings were also unremarkable, and it was felt that a bone marrow examination was not indicated at this time. The patient, now 71 years old, was advised to consult a urologist for evaluation of symptoms of prostatic hypertrophy which have developed recently.

Patient E

This man was 35 years old at the time of the accident; he has had an unremarkable medical history since then. In 1965, he developed a skin condition diagnosed as lichen planus et atrophicus. The problem continued; a revised diagnosis of erythroplasia of Queyrat has been made; the patient remains in the care of a dermatologist.

Patient F

This man's whole-body dose was 68.5 rad. He was 41 years old when the Y-12 accident occurred. Since then he has undergone surgery for nephrolithiasis and for the treatment of an acute peptic ulcer and a hiatal hernia. In November, 1976, he was hospitalized for a pneumonia. Earlier in 1976, the diagnosis of COPD had been established, and he received a medical disability retirement later that year. There has been little change in his somewhat limited physical activity during the past three years.

Patient G

Having been 56 years of age in 1958 made this man the oldest individual involved in the accident. His radiation dose was 68.5 rad. His general health was good throughout the 1960s. In 1972, mild hypertension and a right bundle branch block with occasional premature ventricular systoles were diagnosed. He remained well and active until his death from an acute cerebral vascular accident in March, 1976, at the age of 74. No autopsy was done.

Patient H

This man was 25 years old when he received a 22.5-rad whole-body dose. He was doing quite well on July 14, 1975, and physical and routine laboratory examinations were unremarkable. Hemoglobin was 15 gm%. However, within two months he developed severe abdominal symptoms preceded by the rapid weight loss of 35 pounds. On September 22, 1975, he had a right colectomy for an extensive adenocarcinoma of the colon. There was also a periappendiceal abscess. There was no gross evidence of metastases, and five lymph nodes showed hyperplasia but no histologic evidence of neoplasm. He had an uncomplicated postoperative course, and in November, 1975, his CEA titer was 0. In October, 1976, he had returned to a normal weight and had no evidence of recurrence of the malignancy. An irregular cardiac rhythm was reported by the patient in 1976; ventricular bigeminy was diagnosed by a cardiologist. In January, 1977, this patient sustained a whiplash injury in a serious automobile accident; the injury responded to traction therapy. In April, 1978, and February, 1979, the patient's progress had been maintained, and he appeared to be in good condition; the CEA titer continued to be within the normal range.

Hematologic Follow-up of the Whole Group

Complete blood counts are shown in Figure 2. The hemograms returned essentially to normal and remained without much variation over the years. The averages may be altered somewhat by inclusion, up until 1973, of patient C, who had tuberculosis and also developed lung cancer. As shown in Figure 2, lymphocyte counts, and less consistently granulocyte counts, have been slightly lower than before the accident. In 1979 the average blood values for the five high-dose men showed little change for platelets and hemoglobin over the 1976 values. However, neutrophil and lymphocyte counts were increased over the 1976 values. In 1976, neutrophil and lymphocyte counts reflect the transient leukopenia in patient E (3045 neutrophils and 826 lymphocytes); in 1979 this patient's leukocyte count was within the normal range; this situation is reflected in the steep rise of the average absolute neutrophil and lymphocyte counts from the 1976 levels. Only time and future follow-up examinations will tell whether or not the rise is real and sustained.

Repeated bone marrow examinations over the years have usually shown no significant abnormalities. No effort has been made to repeat

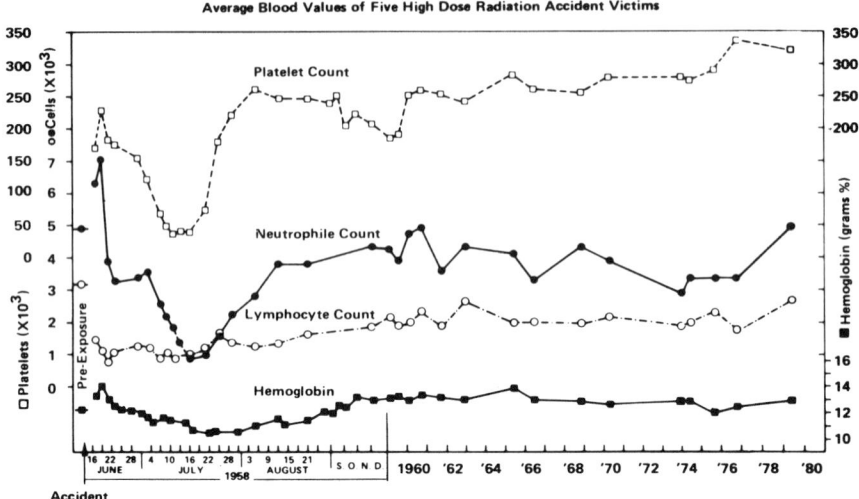

Figure 2. Average blood values of the five "high-dose" men. The preaccident values present the averages of from four to nine counts for each employee, all taken from preemployment or annual physical examinations, not during known illness.

the detailed quantitative morphologic studies made earlier.[17] In one patient, E, the marrow has sometimes been described as hypocellular in the presence of normal blood values; and in patient D a bone marrow examination in 1976 showed an increase in plasma cells, including some immature forms.

Biochemical Tests

After the initial hospital stay, biochemical studies were not carried out as systematically as the hematological studies except in patient D. Repeated assessments of thyroid function have been within the normal range; the thyroid dysfunction of patient A was diagnosed and was treated by an endocrinologist. Maturity onset diabetes mellitus associated with obesity was diagnosed together with hyperuricemia in patient B in 1965 and has been controlled by diet and dietary restrictions.

Cytogenetic Studies

The nature and persistence of radiation-induced chromosome abnormalities in these patients have been studied on seven occasions since the accident. Initially, two and one-half years after the accident, Bender and Gooch[22] found approximately 3% lymphocyte metaphases with ring or dicentric chromosomes, and the frequency of chromosome aberrations in the various men showed "a rough correlation with dose." One year later,[23] dicentrics were still observed, and the authors noted 4.1% translocations, inversions, or deletions (abnormal monocentrics), which are considered "stable" aberrations. Seven,[24] eight, and ten years[25] after the accident, Goh still noted dicentrics, rings, and translocations in an abnormally high number of metaphases and approximately 2% of the metaphases with a small G chromosome. In more recent studies, karyotypic analyses and chromosome banding techniques have been used to assess more critically the frequency of "stable" aberrations persisting in lymphocytes 16 and 17 years after exposure. The results, reported in detail elsewhere,[26] showed only 14 dicentrics in 1142 metaphases from patients A, B, D, E, F, and H, whereas 100 translocations, inversions, and deletions were found. Eighty-five of the abnormal monocentrics were observed in the three men with the highest exposures (A, B, and C). In addition, five possible clones of cells (two or more metaphases having apparently identical karyotypic abnormalities) were detected in preparations from these six men. Only one small G chromosome was noted.

Discussion

With the increasing use of nuclear energy, there is a continuing need for, and interest in, knowledge of effects of accidental radiation exposures. Although most serious radiation accidents have been reported, there are gaps in our knowledge of human radiation effects because (1) the number of severe accidents has been small, (2) low-exposure accidents or those involving only a small part of the body are not usually reported, and (3) late follow-up reports have seldom been made. The experience of this accident emphasized the following to those present:

1. Excessive reaction and apprehension are generated by such events.
2. The medical resources available even 20 years ago could be marshaled effectively in time to deal with this type of exposure involving only external irradiation.
3. Recovery from most of the initial manifestations of organic injury is spontaneous and complete.
4. Cytogenetically identifiable stigmata persist but are of unknown significance.

Today we would be better equipped to protect these patients from infection and hemorrhage; fortunately in this accident the injury did not produce lethal granulocytopenia and thrombocytopenia. There were only minor infections and no serious hemorrhage manifestations. Preparations for bone marrow transplantation were based on little experience in human beings at that time, and adequate tissue typing procedures were not available; it is believed now that the decision not to attempt bone marrow grafts was right.

The mechanism for the mild but persistent reduction in blood lymphocytes is now known; however, the inherent potential for spontaneous and lasting recovery from hematologic injury was demonstrated. (This pattern of prompt recovery is not seen in patients who have received chronic or protracted irradiation at doses high enough to produce clinical symptoms.)

All persons accidentally exposed to high levels of radiation should have a lifetime follow-up for early diagnosis and treatment of neoplasms. It is also desirable to build a background of knowledge on this topic. If carefully managed, by considerate physicians, this follow-up can be reassuring instead of causing apprehension. The results of such a study will be useful in determining whether the expectations based on animal models and previous human experience are valid. The study may be particularly helpful in revealing unexpected results, if any, and in determining the time intervals between exposure and the onset of delayed somatic effects. Routine examinations will give physicians an opportunity to encourage exposed persons to avoid factors such as smoking that might enhance the risk of later malignancy. Data from accidents can be compared with some from the atomic bomb casualties, which are difficult to evaluate because of indefinite doses, associated malnutrition, trauma, thermal burns, and extended exposure to fallout.

The problem of thyroid disease deserves special mention. It is well established that radiation to the neck region, especially early in life, increases the incidence of thyroid cancer.[27–29] Thyroid cancer has not been reported following occupational exposures. One employee exposed in the 1946 Los Alamos accident developed myxedema ten years later and at his death in 1966 was found to have complete thyroid atrophy. There is no way of knowing whether this thyroid atrophy was directly related to the exposure or spontaneous or radiation-induced autoimmune disease, but since this patient received a significant dose of fission neutrons to the head and neck (Hempelmann, personal communication, 1978), the thyroid destruction must be attributed to the accident. However, with therapeutic radiation to the neck, myxedema is not a frequent occurrence. In another unrelated accident a man who survived an external dose of 1200 rad to the head and neck continues to be without symptoms of thyroid dysfunction 18 years after the accident. At each follow-up visit any radiation accident victim should have the thyroid palpated for nodules. (Incorporation of radioactive iodine, as occurred in the Marshall Islanders, produces a heightened risk of thyroid cancer. Internal contamination with radionuclides presents different risk problems, beyond the scope of this paper.) In the present study an asymptomatic nodular goiter was discovered in 1974 in the man who received the highest dose in the accident 16 years earlier. The situation was compounded by the daily administration of potassium iodide as an expectorant for about three years prior to the detection of the goiter. Since the development of thyroid adenoma is a recognized adverse effect of potassium iodide therapy, it is difficult to be absolutely certain about the role of radiation in the development of hypothyroidism in this case.

The delayed carcinogenic effect of radiation alone in animal models and in groups of accidentally and therapeutically irradiated humans is also well documented; the role of radiation in the presence of other carcinogens is as yet less well defined, although a study of uranium miners has shown that the incidence of respiratory tract cancer in smokers was ten times greater than in those who did not smoke (17:1.7/10,000 per year) and that miners who smoked more than one package of cigarettes daily had a shorter tumor latency period than nonsmokers.[30] A multinodular bronchogenic carcinoma was diagnosed 12 years after the accidental exposure of one of the Y-12 group to 339 rad. This patient had a history of exposure to silicon and anthracotic underground before entering employment at Y-12, as well as a long history of cigarette smoking. Anthracotic and silicotic changes were found in his subsequently resected lung. Radiation may have contributed to the development of neoplasia in this case, but in view of the relatively short latent period and a history of chronic exposure to other carcinogens, its role cannot be considered primary.

The incidence of carcinoma in the ileocecal region of the colon in the general male population below the age of 41 years in the absence of familial polyposis is quite low (less than 8% of large intestine carcinomata in the general population of females and males, with a peak incidence in the seventh decade); an adenocarcinoma did occur, however, at the age of 41 years in the man who received the lowest dose in the accident. An increased incidence of carcinoma of the large intestine has been reported in two groups of patients treated with radiation for metropathia hemorrhagica, the mean doses being 190 rad (99.4% of the study population) and 800 rad, respectively;[31,32] these doses are significantly higher and more localized than in this accident case. Similarly, patients with ankylosing spondylitis who received a single course of radiotherapy had an increased incidence of carcinoma of the large intestine compared with the incidence in patients who were not treated by radiotherapy. No dose estimates are given in that study, and no dose-response relationship is considered,[33] but in an earlier study which used the same study population, it was stated that few of the over 13,000 patients received a mean spinal bone marrow dose of less than 250 rad, suggesting significantly higher whole-body doses than that received by patient H.[34] The mortality studies of the Hiroshima A-bomb survivors suggest little relationship between radiation exposure and carcinoma of the large intestine; the mortality of the Nagasaki residents is too small to be evidential. The ABCC Tumor Registry data (1950–1974), however, suggest some relation to radiation, although this study is not entirely free of bias.[35] The 17-year latent period, however, conforms to that expected after a small exposure but, of course, also reflects successful survival and consequent aging, making it difficult to associate the occurrence of the carcinoma in this patient to his single whole-body dose of 22.5 rad.

To date, radiation-induced skin dysplasias or neoplasias have not been found as delayed effects of the sublethal whole-body radiation exposures of the early radiation accident survivors except where thermal or beta burns occurred, a probable reason being the radioresistance of the skin at radiation doses within the 200–300 rad dose range and the observation that radiation-induced skin cancers have not been noted in the absence of radiodermatitis.[36] On the other hand, long mean latent periods (25 years for squamous cell carcinoma, 27 years for basal cell carcinoma) have been associated with radiation-induced skin carcinomata. Three skin cancers developed 12–30 years after a series of 13 patients had received a mean dose of 630 R for the treatment of benign conditions.[37] While it is unlikely, therefore, that any of the survivors of the Y-12 accident will develop skin cancer induced by radiation, they must continue to be considered "at risk" for this disease. There is no clinical evidence to suggest that the localized skin changes in patient E, which began seven years after whole-body exposure (236 rad) and are now diagnosed as erythroplasia of Queyrat, are associated with the radiation exposure.

The cytogenetic data suggest that "stable" chromosome abnormalities persist for many years after significant radiation exposures and that in some instances these cells may undergo propagation *in vivo* and give rise to clones with altered karyotypes. Similar findings have been reported in the 25-year follow-up study of older A-bomb survivors[38] and in the 16-year follow-up of the Bikini fishermen exposed to fallout radiation from a nuclear test.[39] Continued cytogenetic evaluations in persons with previous radiation exposure will be required to determine whether the persistence and possible propagation of cytogenetically altered cells can be correlated with later clinical events.

Conclusions

Twenty-one years after a serious radiation accident at the Y-12 Plant in Oak Ridge, Tennessee, all members of the group recovered spontaneously from the acute effects of the radiation. The subsequent course of events indicates that none has developed a medical condition which can be related unequivocally to the acute radiation exposure. In retrospect, the course of treatment adopted for this group of men immediately after the accident can be said to have been adequate and effective and a model for a similar experience in the future.

ACKNOWLEDGMENTS

Oak Ridge Associated Universities operates under Contract Number DE-AC05-76OR00033 with the U.S. Department of Energy.

Space does not permit the acknowledgment of all the staff members and consultants who have participated in the care of these patients. C. R. Sullivan, M.D., Chief Physician at the Y-12 Plant, referred the patients and cooperated in the follow-up. Cooperation in the follow-up by G. Zanolli, M.D., the current Medical Director at the Y-12 Plant, is also gratefully acknowledged. Marshall Brucer, M.D., former Chairman of the Medical Division, took an active part in the management of this accident.[2,3] Much of the early care was given by B. W. Sitterson, M.D. Many of the follow-up clinical observations were made by Ryosaku Tanida, M.D. Other staff physicians participating included Drs. F. Goswitz, A. L. Kretchmar, R. Kniseley, and H. Vodopick, Among ophthalmologists who saw the patients at intervals was K. W. Christenberry, M.D., of Knoxville, and Alan Solomon, M.D., of the University of Tennessee Memorial Research Center and Hospital, Knoxville, provided special serum protein studies on patient D.

The hematological laboratory work was largely done by Ms. Martha Clevenger and more recently by Ms. Shirley Colyer. During the 1960s the cytogenetic studies and analyses were carried out by M. A. Bender, P. C. Gooch, and K-O. Goh; more recently Gayle Littlefield and Eugene Joiner have been responsible for this work. The bibliography includes among its authors a number of outside consultants who were involved.

References

1. Conard RA: *A Twenty-Year Review of Medical Findings in a Marshallese Population Accidentally Exposed to Radioactive Fallout*, U.S. Energy Research and Development Administration report BNL-50424. Brookhaven National Laboratory, 1975.

2. Brucer M (compiler): *The Acute Radiation Syndrome; A Medical Report on the Y-12 Accident, June 16, 1958*, US AEC report ORINS-25. Oak Ridge Institute for Nuclear Studies, 1959.

3. *Accidental Radiation Excursion at the Y-12 Plant, June 16, 1958*, US AEC report Y-1234. Union Carbide Nuclear Company, Y-12 Plant, 1958.

4. Callihan D, Thomas JT: Accidental radiation excursion at the Oak Ridge Y-12 Plant. I. Description and physics of the accident. *Health Phys* 1:363–372, 1959.

5. McLendon JD: Accidental radiation excursion at the Oak Ridge Y-12 Plant. II. Health physics aspects of the accident. *Health Phys* 2:21–29, 1959.

6. Hurst GS, Ritchie RH, Emerson LC: Accidental radiation excursion at the Oak Ridge Y-12 Plant. III. Determination of radiation doses. *Health Phys* 2:121–133, 1959.

7. Dosimetry of the Y-12 accident, in *Health Physics Division Annual Progress Report for Period Ending July 31, 1959*, US AEC report ORNL-2806. Oak Ridge National Laboratory, 1959, pp. 127–132.

8. Hurst GA, Ritchie RH (eds.): *Radiation Accidents: Dosimetric Aspects of Neutron and Gamma-Ray Exposures*, US AEC report ORNL-2748 (pt. A). Oak Ridge National Laboratory, 1959.

9. Andrews GA, Sitterson BW, Kretchmar AL, Brucer M: Accidental radiation excursion at the Oak Ridge Y-12 Plant. IV. Preliminary report on clinical and laboratory effects in the irradiated employees. *Health Phys* 2:134–138, 1959.

10. Andrews GA, Sitterson BW, Kretchmar AL, Brucer M: Criticality accident at the Y-

12 plant, in *Diagnosis and Treatment of Acute Radiation Injury.* Geneva, World Health Organization, 1961, pp. 27–48.

11. Andrews GA: Criticality accidents in Vinca, Yugoslavia, and Oak Ridge. Comparison of radiation injuries and results of therapy. *JAMA* 179:191–197, 1962.

12. Vodopick H, Andrews GA: Accidental radiation exposure. *Arch Environ Health* 28:53–56, 1974.

13. Kretchmar AL: An alteration in the excretion of free serine in urine from irradiated humans. *Nature* 183:1809–1810, 1959.

14. Rubini JR, Cronkite EP, Bond VP, Fliedner TM: Urinary excretion of beta aminoiso-butyric acid (BAIBA) in irradiated human beings. *Proc Soc Exp Biol Med* 100:130–133, 1959.

15. Bond VP, Fliedner TM, Cronkite EP, Andrews G: Deoxyribonucleic acid synthesizing cells in the blood of man and dog exposed to total body radiation. *J Lab Clin Med* 57:711–717, 1961.

16. Fliedner TM, Cronkite EP, Bond VP, Rubini JR, Andrews G: Mitotic index of human bone marrow in healthy individuals and irradiated human beings. *Acta Haematol* 22:65–78, 1959.

17. Fliedner TM, Cronkite EP, Bond VP, Andrews G: Mitotic activity and cytology of human bone marrow after accidental exposure to ionizing radiation, in *Proceedings of the Seventh Congress, European Society of Haematology, London, 1959* [vol. II, pt. 1]. Karger, Basel, 1960, pp. 458–467.

18. Fliedner TM: Zur Hämatologie des akuten Strahlensyndroms. *Strahlentherapie* 112:543–560, 1960.

19. Sise HE, Gauthier J, Becker R, Bolger J: Blood coagulation factors in total body irradiation. *Blood* 18:702–709, 1961.

20. Fliedner TM, Andrews GA, Cronkite EP, Bond VP: Early and late cytologic effects of whole body irradiation on human marrow. *Blood* 23:471–487, 1964.

21. MacLeod J, Hotchkiss RS, Sitterson BW: Recovery of male fertility after sterilization by nuclear radiation. *JAMA* 187:637–641, 1964.

22. Bender MA, Gooch PC: Persistent chromosome aberrations in irradiated human subjects. *Radiat Res* 16:44–53, 1962.

23. Bender MA, Gooch PC: Persistent chromosome aberrations in irradiated human subjects. II. Three and one-half year investigation. *Radiat Res* 18:389–396, 1963.

24. Goh K-O: Total-body irradiation and human chromosomes: cytogenetic studies of the peripheral blood and bone marrow leukocytes seven years after total-body irradiation. *Radiat Res* 35:155–170, 1968.

25. Goh K-O: Total-body irradiation and human chromosomes. IV. Cytogenetic follow-up studies eight and ten and one-half years after total-body irradiation. *Radiat Res* 62:364–373, 1975.

26. Littlefield LG, Joiner EE: *Cytogenic follow-up studies in six radiation accident victims* (16 and 17 years postexposure), in *Late Biological Effects of Ionizing Radiation.* Vienna, International Atomic Energy Agency, 1978, vol. I, pp. 297–308.

27. Modan B, Baidatz B, Mart H, Steinitz R, Levin SG: Radiation-induced head and neck tumors. *Lancet* 1:277–279, 1974.

28. Hemplemann LH, Hall WJ, Phillips M, Cooper RA, Ames WR: Neoplasms in persons treated with X-ray in infancy: fourth survey in 20 years. *J Natl Cancer Inst* 55:519–530, 1975.

29. Saenger EL, Silverman, FN, Sterling TD, Turner ME: Neoplasia following therapeutic irradiation for benign conditions in childhood. *Radiology* 74:889–904, 1960.

30. Schutterman W: The combined effects of ionizing radiation and smoking in the development of bronchial carcinoma. *Z Erkr Atmungsorgane* 150:243–249, 1978.

31. Brinkley D, Haybittle JL: The late effects of artificial menopause by X-radiation. *Brit J Radiol* 42:519–521, 1969.

32. Smith PG, Doll R: Late effects of X-irradiation in patients treated for metropathia hemorrhagica. *Brit J Radiol* 49:224–236, 1976.

33. Court Brown WM, Doll R: Mortality from cancer and other causes after radiotherapy for ankylosing spondylitis. *Brit Med J* 2:1327–1332, 1965.

34. Court Brown WM, Doll R: Leukemia-aplastic anaemia in patients irradiated for ankylosing spondylitis. *Medical Research Council, Special Report Series* (London), 295, 1957.

35. Beebe GW, Kato, H, Land CE: Studies of mortality of A-bomb survivors. 6. Mortality and radiation dose, 1950–1974. *Rad Res* 75:138–201, 1978.

36. National Academy of Sciences–National Research Council: The effects on populations of exposure to low levels of ionizing radiation. A report of the Advisory Committee on the Biological Effects of Ionizing Radiations. Division of Medical Sciences, November, 1972.

37. Andrews P: Rodent ulcers induced by X-rays and radium. Univ. of London, Thesis for M.D., 1957.

38. Awa AA: Chromosome aberrations in somatic cells. *J Radiat Res* 16 (Suppl.):122, 1975.

39. Ishihara T, Kumatori T: Chromosomes studies on Japanese exposed to radiation resulting from nuclear bomb explosions, in Evans HJ, Court Brown WM, McLean AS (eds.): *Human Radiation Cytogenetics*. New York, John Wiley & Sons, 1967, pp. 144–166.

The People's Republic of China Accident in 1963

Ye Gen-yao, Liu Yong, Tien Nue, Chiang Ben-yun, Chien Feng-wei, and Xiae Chien-ling

Chinese Academy of Medical Sciences, Beijing, China.

On January 11, 1963, a ^{60}Co gamma-ray source of about 10 curies used for irradiation of seeds was taken by a rural child to his home. Six persons were exposed to an accidental nonuniform gamma-ray irradiation for a period of five to nine days in five of them (child's mother, two brothers, a sister, and himself) and 9 hr in another one, who was the child's uncle and happened to stay at their home overnight. The gamma-ray irradiation from the ^{60}Co source resulted in acute radiation sickness of all six persons accompanied by different degrees of localized radiation injury. The radiation doses estimated by physics dosimetrists in the six patients are listed in Table 1. The estimated whole-body average doses, essential clinical findings, and therapeutic outcomes of the six patients are presented in Table 2.

In the early stage after irradiation, most of the patients showed general malaise, lassitude, anorexia, nausea, and vomiting, and some of them also experienced dull pain in the abdomen. There was a striking depletion of bone marrow nucleated cells, which was closely correlated in degree with the radiation doses. The erythroid precursors were somewhat more sensitive to radiation than those of the granuloid system. The decrease in number of leukocytes per day in these patients was in parallel with the doses of radiation. During the early convalescent period, the monocytes recovered rather earlier in the peripheral blood than did the granulocytes and reticulocytes.

Systemic infections and high fever occurred in five patients (A, B, C, E, and F). The time of onset of these symptoms depends upon the severity of the disease (refer to Table 2). We obtained positive blood

Table 1. Estimated Radiation Dose in Six Patients (In Rads)

Patient	Scalp	Cranium Center	Neck	Chest Center	Abdomen Center	Symphysis Pubis	Knee	Ankle	Whole Body Average Dose
E	3.8×10^3	2.1×10^3	1.7×10^3	2.4×10^3	1.9×10^4	9.5×10^3	3.5×10^2	4.6×10	8×10^3
F	7.5×10	1.1×10^2	1.7×10^2	4.3×10^2	3.8×10^3	7.8×10^3	2.5×10^3	3.8×10^2	4×10^3
A	4.3×10	6.2×10	1.1×10^2	2.7×10^2	1.8×10^3	1.3×10^3	4.0×10^2	6.7×10^2	8×10^2
B	1.7×10^2	2.4×10^2	2.8×10^2	3.7×10^2	7.6×10^2	7.3×10^2	4.4×10^2	3.6×10^2	6×10^2
C	1.7×10^3	9.7×10^2	5.9×10^2	5.5×10^2	1.8×10^2	1.6×10^2	– – –	– – –	4×10^2
D	1.1×10	1.5×10	2.1×10	3.7×10	1.1×10^2	2.1×10^2	– – –	– – –	2×10

cultures in three severe cases, viz., patient E, *Escherichia coli;* patient F, *Staphylococcus sp.;* patient A, *Clostridium perfringens*. At the climax of the disease, the blood pressure of patient A dropped to 80/60 mm Hg, and the number of blood cells further decreased during the febrile period. As soon as the high fever subsided the number of granulocytes began to recover almost instantaneously.

Loss of hair was observed in all the cases except the one who received the least dose of radiation.

The principles of therapy and the essential therapeutic measures were: complete rest and adequate nutrition, the ward and all nursing services being strictly controlled to avoid contamination. During the latent period of radiation sickness, preventive treatment of anti-infection drugs and transfusions of blood were given as indicated. When infection and fever emerged, antibiotics were administered on account of positive blood cultures or the existence of infection foci (Figures 1–4). Transplantations of homologous bone marrow were prescribed to those patients who presumably received lethal doses of radiation and suffered a serious degree of immunosuppression. Others were treated with fresh leukocytes and platelets (Table 3). After appropriate therapy, the patients eventually were tided over the crisis and entered the period of convalescence at about one month post irradiation. There were neither evidences of graft-versus-host reaction nor permanent graft in those who had received bone marrow transplantation. Thus the acute radiation sickness within certain degrees of severity was essentially cured within a period of about two months.

Among these cases, four were followed up for a period of 14 years. The general conditions of the patients are apparently good as judged from the results of examinations of certain endocrine functions, sensory

Table 2. Estimated Whole-body Average Dose, Essential Clinical Findings, Diagnosis, and Therapeutic Outcomes in Six Patients

Patient	Whole-body average dose (rad)	Nadir value of W.B.C. No/mm^3	Nadir value of W.B.C. Time (day)	Commencement of fever (day)	Commencement of bleeding (day)	Diagnosis (type of acute radiation sickness)	Therapeutic outcome
E	8×10^3	100	10	8	10	Intestinal type	Died, at 12th day
F	4×10^3	55	10	8	8	Intestinal type	Died, at 11th day
A	8×10^2	55	25	8	8	Severe bone marrow injury	Survived
B	6×10^2	297	17	20	15	Severe bone marrow injury	Survived
C	4×10^2	213	28	26	8	Moderate bone marrow injury	Survived
D	2×10^2	6000				Mild bone marrow depression	Survived

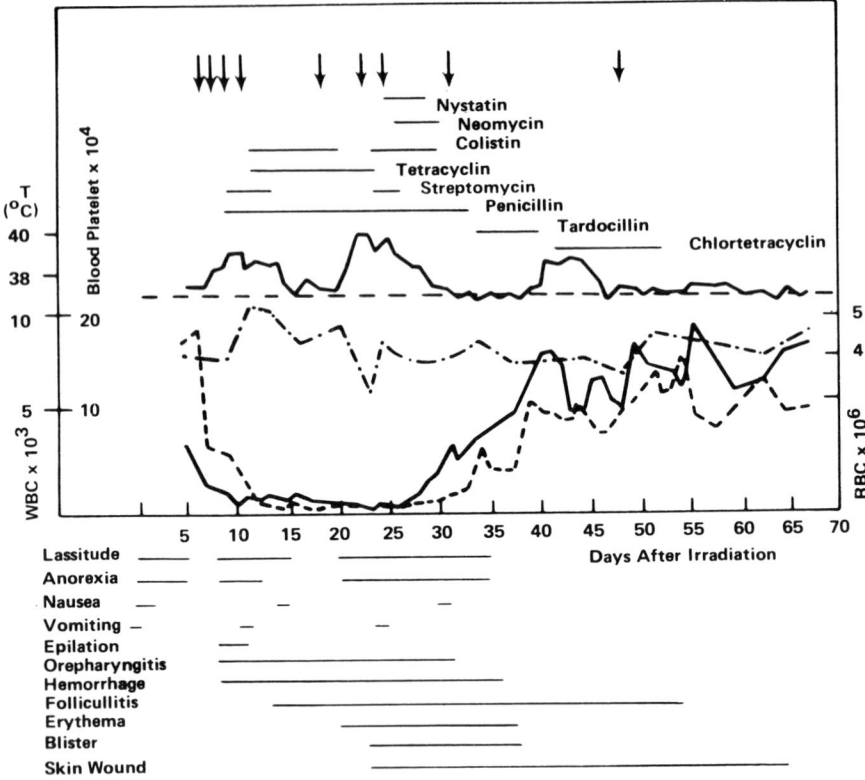

Figure 1. Clinical course and treatment of patient A.

organs, and others, but in three of them the adrenocortical response to ACTH was subnormal. The accidental doses of radiation over the region of sexual glands in a woman patient aged 44 and a boy patient aged 20 were rather high, estimated about 1800 rad and 730 rad, respectively, leading to immediate onset of amenorrhea and permanent sterility. In view of the fact that the sterile boy patient remained normal in sexual activity, it is likely that the testicular hormone secretory cells are more radioresistant than the germinal cells. Another girl patient, then 13 years old, received about 180 rad over the ovarian region. Subsequent development and function of the sexual organs were not affected. She gave birth to a daughter and a son after marriage. The physical and the intellectual development of the offspring were apparently normal. The karyotype analysis and chromosome examination of the children revealed nothing deviated from their parents. Another man patient of 39 years of age showed transient aspermia after exposure to 210 rad of irradiation over the testicular region but recovered uneventfully afterwards.

Immunological tests of the patients showed normal rate of lymphocyte transformation and E-rosette formation. Serum contents of IgA, IgG, IgE, and IgM were within the range of normal variations except one whose IgG level was obviously subnormal.

Up to 14 years since the radiation accident, chromosome aberrations in the peripheral lymphocytes were observed in all the cases. The recovery of the hemopoietic system is worthy of mention: the slow recovery of peripheral lymphocytes, the persistence of aberrant mitotic cells in the bone marrow, and a delayed eosinophilia in some of the patients.

Changes in electroencephalograms occurred only in those who received high cranial doses. In these cases, paroxysmal median and high θ waves were observed in frontal, parietal, and temporal regions. Local irradiation

Figure 2. Clinical course and treatment of patient B.

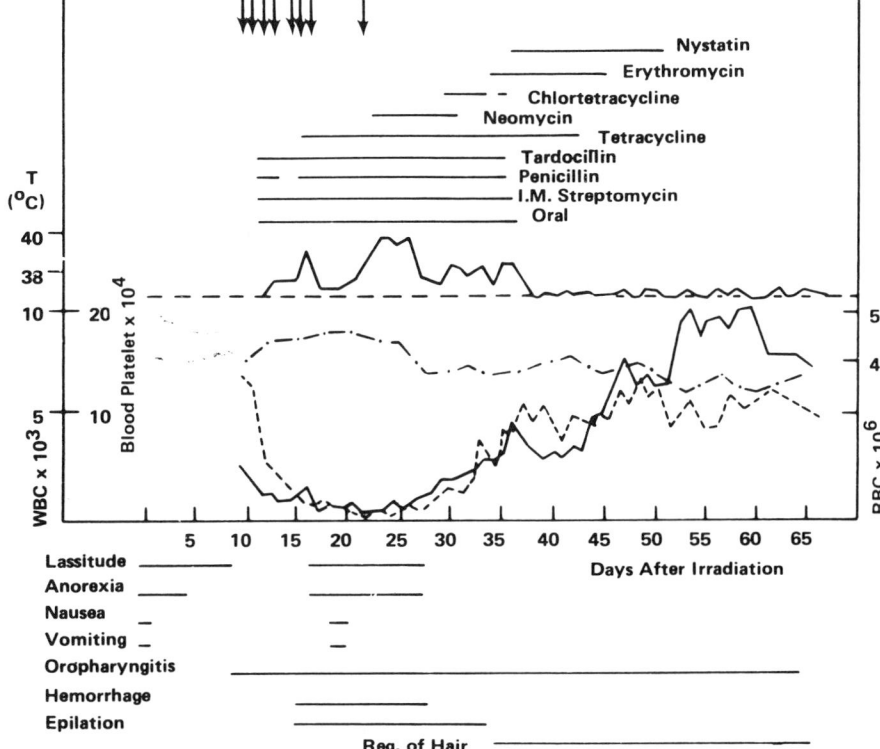

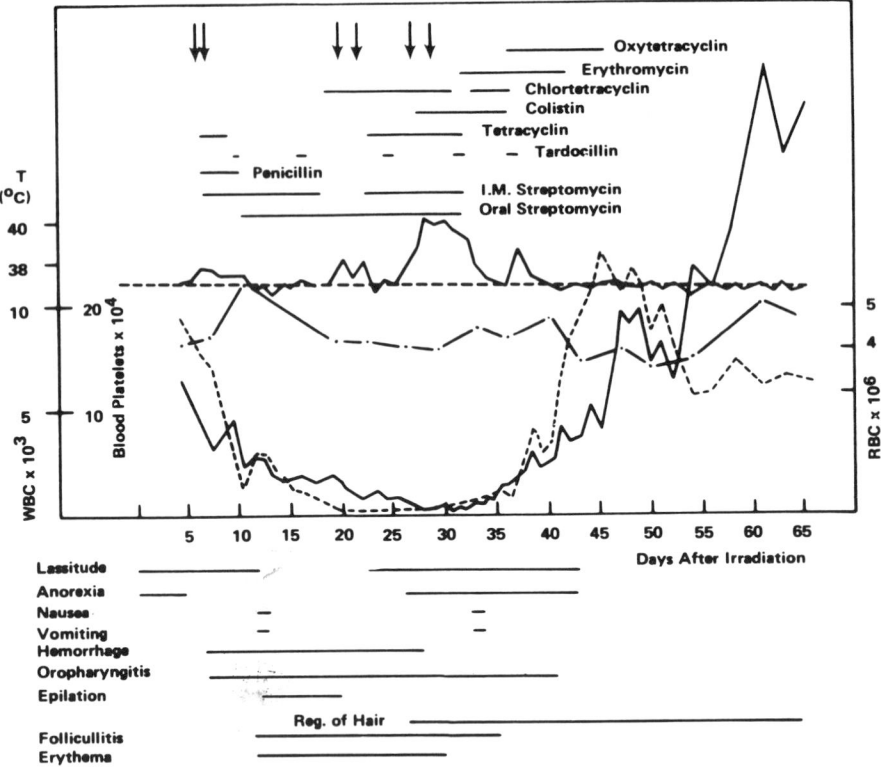

Figure 3. Clinical course and treatment of patient C.

of high doses, occasionally up to 20,000 rad, caused severe burns of the skin and damage to the skeleton. As a result the left leg of a man patient was amputated for necrosis of tibia and fibia. Another woman patient remained to have an unhealed small skin ulcer treated and suffered from a pathological fracture of the femur of the same leg. The latter was reunited after surgical intervention.

In our cases of radiation accident, we have not yet seen any neoplastic changes nor any genetic abnormalities of the offspring within the limited observation period.

Summary

In 1963, we treated six cases of acute radiation sickness (200–8000 rad) that resulted from an accidental nonuniform ^{60}Co gamma-ray irradiation of about 10 curies; two of them died of intestinal-type radiation sickness within two weeks. Four cases survived, and one of them recovered from septicemic shock. Loss of hair, systemic infection, high fever, and bleeding occurred in five patients. The essential therapeutic measures were strict isolation, preventive treatment with anti-infection drugs, fresh blood transfusion, and sometimes infusion of blood formed elements. Among the survivors, two received homologous bone marrow transplantation. There were neither evidences of graft-versus-host reaction nor permanent graft in those who had received bone marrow transplantation.

The general conditions of four patients followed up for a period of 14 years are apparently good with transparent lens, normal thyroid function, and normal immunological reactions, except one who had a low serum IgG level. Three of them showed subnormal adrenocortical activity and impairment of sex gland function. However, a girl patient (400 rad) gave birth to two children with apparently normal genetical constitutions.

Figure 4. Clinical course and treatment of patient D.

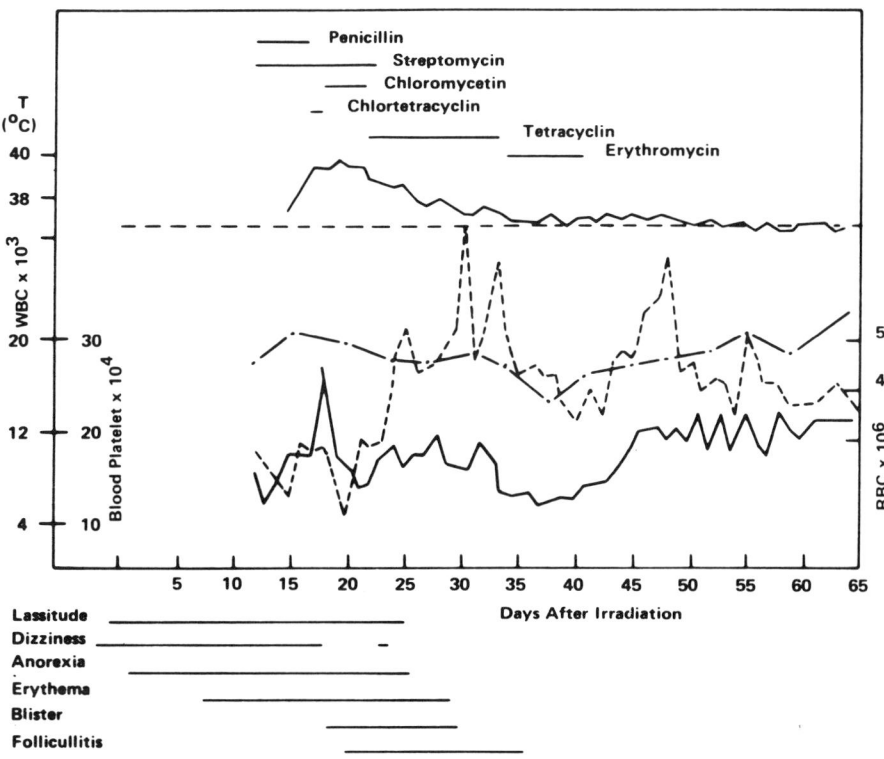

Table 3. Treatment with Blood, Blood Constituents, and Bone Marrow

Patient	Whole blood		Bl. platelets conc.			Bl. platelets, WBC conc.				Homolog. bone marrow		
	Vol. (c.c.)	Date	Vol. (c.c)	No. of bl. platelets	Date	Vol. (c.c)	No. of bl. platelets	No. of WBC	Date	Vol. (c.c.)	No. of nucleated cells	Date
E	400	10				25		2.67×10^9	12			
	1100	11										
	200	12										
F	600	7								250	4.5×10^9	9
	400	8										
	400	10										
A	400	7	52	74.7×10^9	19	100	26.7×10^9	2.0×10^9	11, 3A.M.			
	400	8	43.5	65×10^9	21	101	70×10^9	2.5×10^9	11, 11P.M.			
	400	10	182	95.5×10^9	24	87	0.9×10^9	0.5×10^9	18			
	400	23					47.3×10^9	2.7×10^9	25			
	400	32										
	400	48										
B	200	10				66	2.2×10^9	1.2×10^9	15	240	4.9×10^9	13
	400	11				120	31.5×10^9	5.6×10^9	22	230	7.7×10^9	16
	400	12								200	5.2×10^9	17
C	400	6	60	53.2×10^9	19							
	400	7										
	400	22										
	400	27										
	400	29										
D	0	0	0			0				0		

Serial electroencephalographic changes occurred only in those who received high cranial doses. In all the cases, persistence of chromosome aberration in peripheral lymphocytes was observed. With high doses, the remote regional effects led to amputation of one leg in one patient and pathological fracture of the femur in another.

Clinical and Biological Comparison of Two Acute Accidental Irradiations: Mol (1965) and Brescia (1975)

H. Jammet,[*] R. Gongora,[*] R. Le Gô,[+] and M. T. Doloy[+]

[*]Institut Curie, Service de Radiopathologie, 26 rue d'Ulm, 75005, Paris, France;
[+]Institut de Protection et de Sûreté Nucléaire, Département de Protection, B. P. No. 6, 92260 Fontenay-aux-Roses, France.

Introduction

The two accidental irradiations at Mol (Belgium) in 1965 (M) and Brescia (Italy) in 1975 (B) have been shown to be of great interest because they can be considered as typical examples of very acute irradiation cases in the lethal range. One of the persons is still alive, the Mol case. The other one had only a short survival of 12 days.

Clinical Evolution

From the clinical point of view, the two cases demonstrated the classical phases of the acute irradiation syndrome, namely,[1-4] the prodromal phase, the latent period, and the critical phase.

The Prodromal Phase

This phase was marked for the two persons by nausea and vomiting, respectively, 30 min (B) and 2 hr (M) after the accident.

In both cases these symptoms lasted only a few hours.

In the Mol case, an early erythema was observed during the first days.

The Latent Period

This period was latent only from the clinical point of view. As will be shown later, the hematological syndrome was patent at that time.

The duration of this period was three weeks for M, nine days for B. We should note here that the dose estimates were 550 rad for M and 1200 rad for B, expressed as mean homogeneous equivalent dose.

The Critical Phase

The critical phase was inaugurated by rise in fever to around 40°C for M and which reached 41.3° once for B, with progressive alteration of the general condition (Figure 1).

From this point the subsequent evolutions of M and B were different.

For M, the critical period lasted four weeks and was also marked by some infectious manifestations:

(1) locally: evolution of a typical radionecrotic lesion of the foot which had been on the top of the reactor;
(2) development of mouth mycosis caused by *Candida albicans*;
(3) some intercurrent bacteremia was observed;

Figure 1. Temperature curves in the Mol (M) and Brescia (B) accidents.

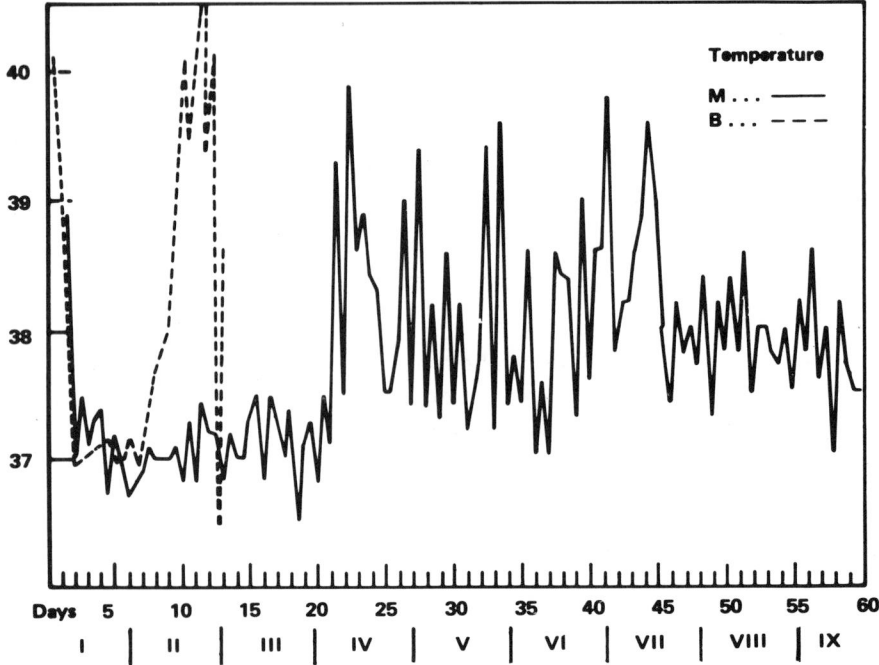

(4) neither an important hemorrhagic syndrome nor a septicemic infection developed, probably because sterile conditions for housing were observed, together with the use of multiple antibiotic and mycostatic therapy.

Nevertheless, all the conditions for a possible bone marrow graft had been prepared, and three potential donors from his family had been grouped as suitable.

Despite the progressive hematological restoration in progress since the fifth week, the clinical critical phase lasted two weeks longer until the real beginning of the restoration phase for M.

For case B, who was more heavily irradiated, the critical phase was in fact abortive, leading in a few days to the fatal issue.

The last hours were marked by a dramatic deregulation of the cardiac rhythm with extreme tachycardia, the respiration rhythm with Cheyne-Stokes rhythm, and thermal regulation, with very high oscillations of central temperature from one hour to the other.

This complete vegetative deregulation was certainly linked to the microscopic hemorrhagic focus observed post-mortem in the central trunk substance.

The Hematological Syndrome

The hematological syndrome in the Mol case was really typical, in the sense of the manifestation of each of the described characteristics of the hematological curves in experimental irradiation.

For this reason, we can now consider this case as a real reference for comparison with any other irradiation cases in the human being.

Another important aspect of these curves that should be noted is the fact that the counts and differential counts of cells were carried out daily during a period of 50 days and three times a week until the third month. This permitted a very precise estimation of the amplitudes and slopes of variation of the blood cell populations.

In all these curves, the absolute numbers of cells per cubic millimeter are plotted on semilogarithmic coordinates, which allows a very simple estimation of the slopes.

The two cases, M and B, are plotted on the same diagram, for each cell line.

Polymorphonuclear Features

The observed features of this curve (Figure 2) for Mol were: (1) early peak, spanned over the first 24 hr, whose amplitude reached 16,500 (such peaks were observed in the Los Alamos accidents at 4500 and 1500 rad, giving peaks of 25,000 and 28,000); (2) a general slope of falling

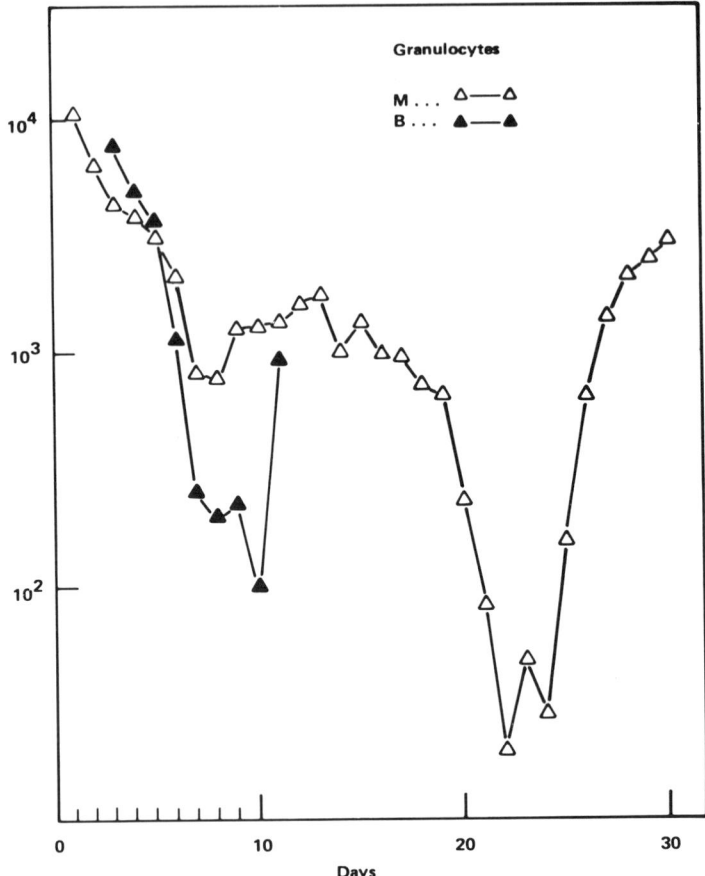

Figure 2. Polymorphonuclear curves in the M and B accidents.

neutrophils leads to a minimum of 20 per microliter at day 25; and (3) an intermediate rebound wave spanning over the second week.

For Brescia the first hematological points were obtained from the hospitals of Pontevico for days 1 and 2 and Tortona for day 3; the rest of the results were obtained in Paris. The granulocyte count reached the level of 100 at the tenth day, the day before the death. The depopulation was still more severe, partially masked by a perfusion of fresh leukocytes (2×10^{11} cells). No rebound can be seen on this slope.

The existence of an early peak could not be determined for the first three days. The comparison between the slopes of disappearance of granulocytes for the Vinca, Mol, and Brescia accidents showed that B was even more injured than M (Figure 3).

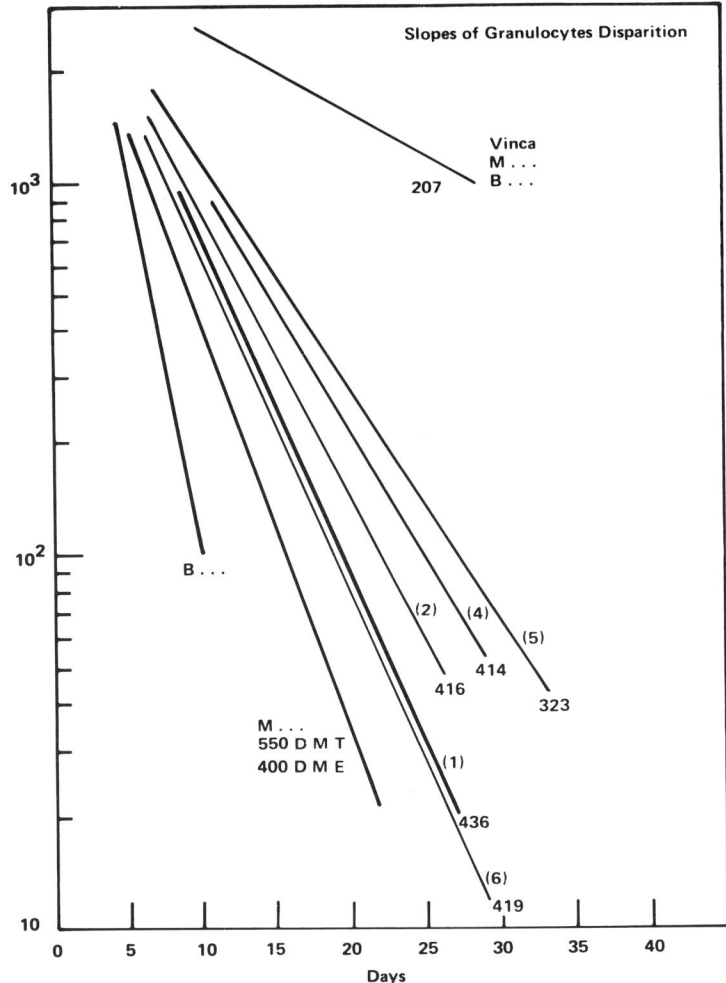

Figure 3. Comparison between the polymorph slopes of different accidents.

Lymphocytes

In both cases the lymphocyte curve (Figure 4) showed a very rapid decreasing slope. This feature is known to be a good index of the severity of the hematological damage and it was the case for these two persons.

In case M, the lymphocyte count decreased to the minimum of 140 cells/μl after four days, then presented regular oscillations around a level of about 250. The initial slope of this curve showed that it was more pronounced than that of the equivalent curve for the three Vinca victims irradiated at 436, 426, and 414 rad.

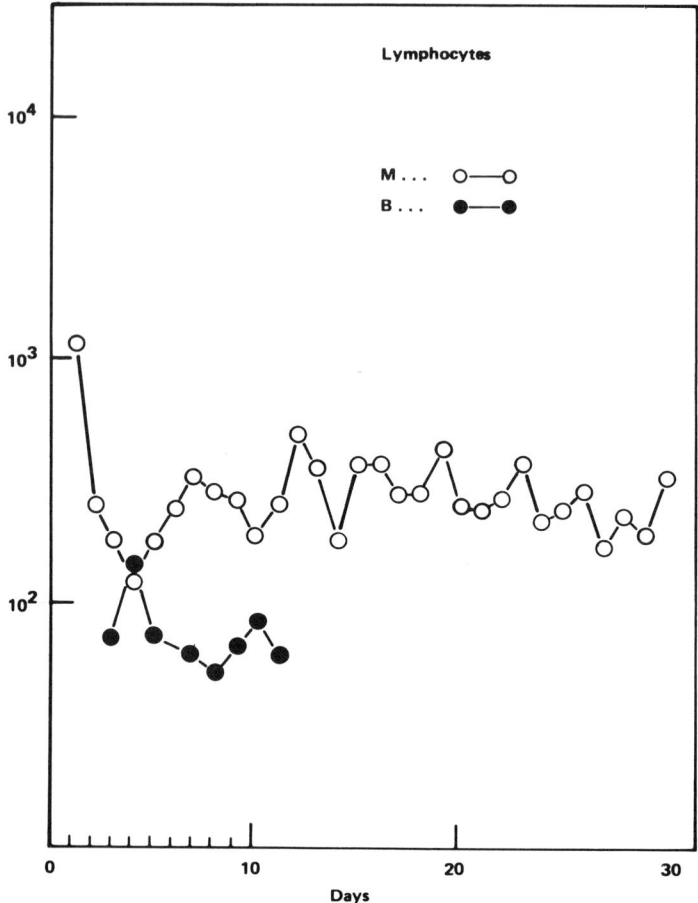

Figure 4. Lymphocyte curves in the M and B accidents.

In case B, the slope was still more pronounced on day J plus 7, at which time we obtained the first blood sample: the absolute number of lymphocytes was 60 per microliter, and it remained low subsequently, under the level of 100.

This figure of 60 per microliter, together with the other hematological parameters from the first sample (230 polymorph, zero reticulocytes), allowed us to infer that the severity of this case was in the lethal range.

The binucleated lymphocytes showed a first wave at a level of 38 per 10,000 on day 15 and another slight increase after day 30, for case M.

Thrombocytes

For case M the thrombocyte curve (Figure 5) showed a very clear steady depressive evolution, falling to the level of 25,000 platelets per microliter on day 20. This level persisted for one week more, indicating a permanent

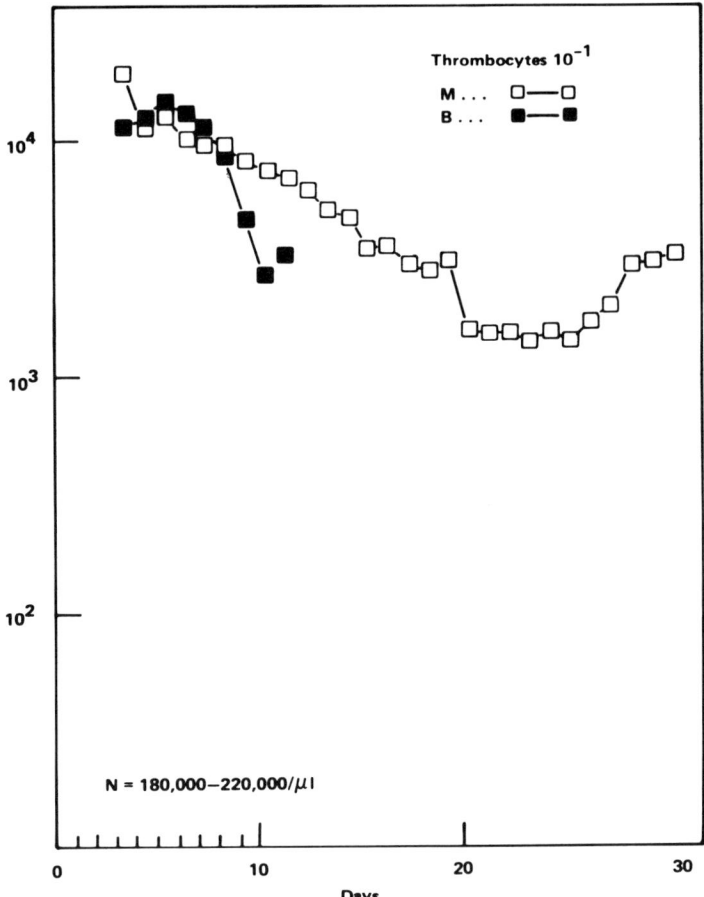

Figure 5. Thrombocyte curves in the M and B accidents.

hemorrhagic risk, as is observed for such a platelet level in the cases of toxic thrombocytopenia.

A comparison with other irradiation cases was difficult due to the differences in laboratory techniques for the platelet count.

However, comparison with case M was possible for case B. It showed a sharper and earlier decrease in the platelet curve, already at the level of 26,000 on day 10 (during the same period it was about 85,000 for Mol), and a perfusion of five units of platelets (one unit is 50 billions) hardly modified the slope for the last 24 hr.

Red Cell Line

The red cell line (RBC) (Figure 6) was also affected by the bone marrow depopulation, but the very large size of this compartment and its subsequent inertia explain the slow decrease in the RBC count observed for case M.

We note that the daily subtraction of some 10 to 15 cc of blood for biological purposes should be taken into account both as a slight accentuation in the decrease of the RBC curve and perhaps as a positive feedback effect on the bone marrow stimulation to regenerate.

Inversely the reticulocyte count was a crucial indicator for cases M and B (Figure 6). For M's curve the features were very similar to those of the polymorph curve, showing a drop to near zero with an intermediate rebound. For B the only figures observed were zero counts of reticulocytes, and these results reinforced the early impression of a desperate case.

Figure 6. Red cell line in the M accident.

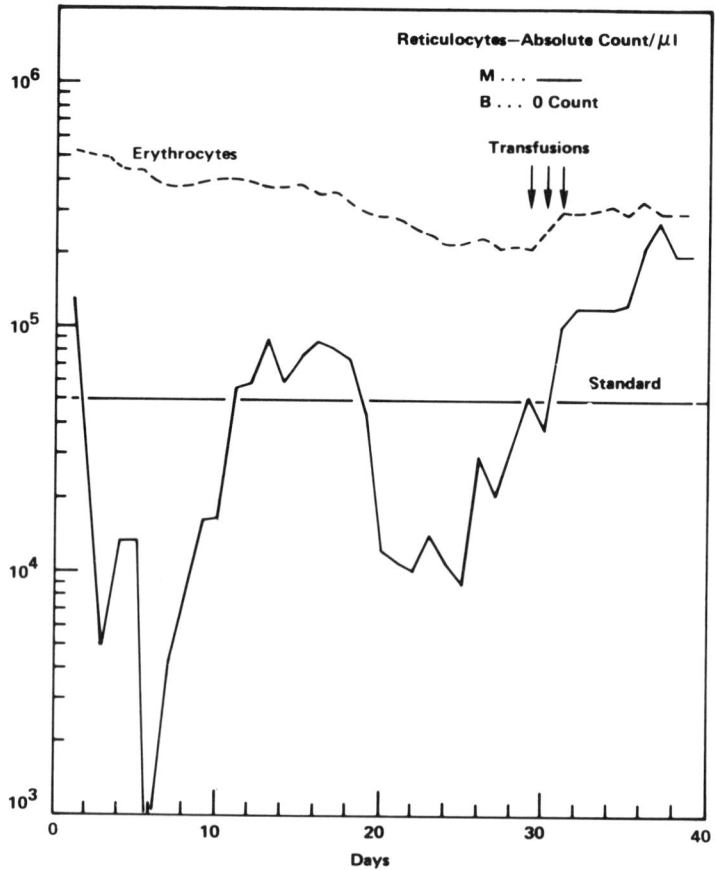

Hematological Evolution

This aspect of the curves (Figure 7) can be described only for M. For B, death occurred on day 11, during the course of decreases in the different blood cell counts. Despite the very low figures reached in the blood, the real mechanism of death was not primarily the bone marrow aplasia. The signs observed were typically due to the lesions of the central nervous system, which had received probably more than 3500 rad at one time.

For M, after a period of critical aplasia that lasted from days 18 to 26, a very sharp restoration of the hematological curves was observed,

Figure 7. Hematological evolution in the M and B accidents.

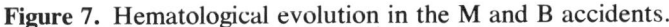

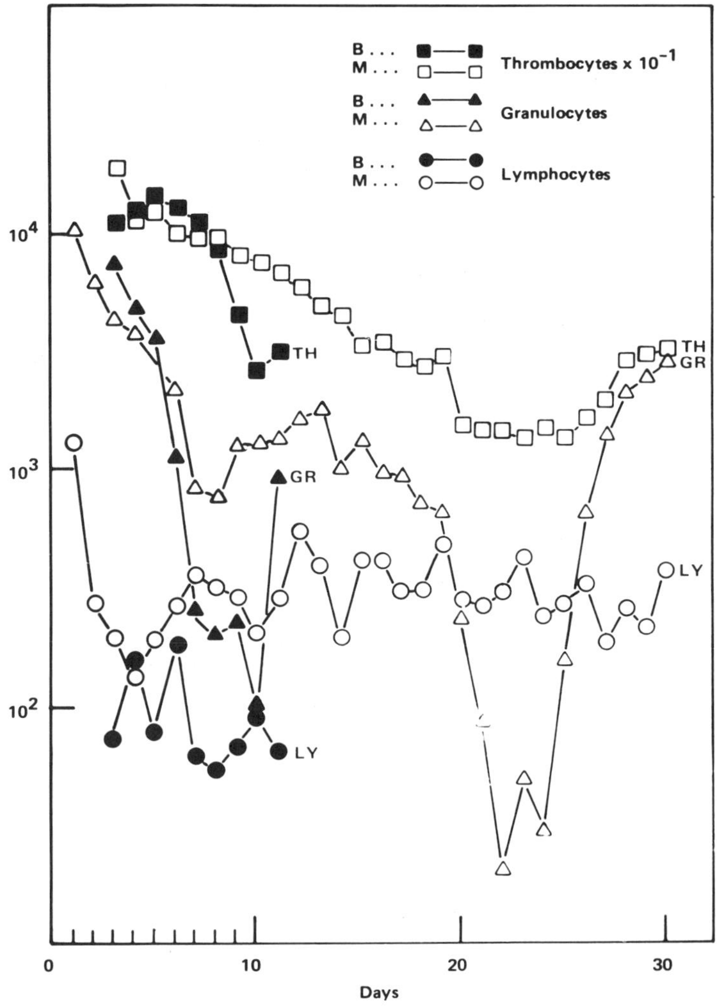

which was especially striking on the two most sensitive, the polymorph and reticulocyte curves. The normal levels were restored in six to eight days. The platelets were restored more slowly but regularly.

The lymphocyte count did not obey the same rule. It remained low (mean level of 300) for one week more during the sharp ascendance of polymorphs. Then within two days it reached a new plateau at a mean level of 900.

Myelemia

In the beginning and during the course of the restoration period an important wave of myelemia was observed with cells as young as promyelocytes and numerous myelo- and metamyelocytes and some plasmocytes passing into the peripheral blood, many of them with mitotic figures.

This evolution was consistent with the results of the incorporation of radioactive iron injected on day 7 (1 microcurie). Instead of the normally observed 80% activity passing into the blood in 6–7 days, the curve showed about 15% of the injected activity. No fecal elimination of iron in relation with intestinal microhemorrhage could be detected.

Bone Marrow Examinations

A number of medullograms were studied in the Mol case.[4] The bone marrow was completely desertic in the sternal puncture for Brescia.

For Mol, the same observation was made in the bone marrow from the sternum, from iliac spines anterior and posterior, even from the calcaneum of the foot which was protected on the concrete rim of the reactor.

As soon as the dosimetry results from the reconstruction of the accident were available, we constructed a transparent mannikin to represent the dose distribution in three dimensions.[4,5]

It appeared that the entire trunk had received doses between 1000 and 300 rad (500 R at the breast pocket).

So the only pieces of skeleton which were at levels near or under 200 were the cervical vertebrae. Therefore, after some hesitation, we decided to perform a bone marrow aspiration from the posterior apophysis of the C-6 vertebra. This smear contained rich marrow on day 15.

This finding made in the middle of the critical period was one of the strongest arguments for the therapeutic abstention with respect to bone marrow graft.

Late Evolution of Case M

After three months of medical care in Paris, the M case was moved to a hospital in Louvain (Belgium). The hematological restoration was at that time complete. The patient still presented epilation of the side of the head and a complete azoospermia.

Moreover, the radiodermatitis lesions of the leg were so severe as to require leg amputation some months later. This person is now in good health and is regularly sent to Paris for chromosome examinations.

Chromosome Analyses

The results of chromosome analyses on M and B produced some important data to estimate the level of irradiation.[6,7]

For M the very low level of blood lymphocytes in culture permitted us to examine only 24 good mitoses in the first sampling. In these 24 caryograms, all types of lesion have been observed: deletions, translocations, dicentrics, rings. Some of the cells showed two or even three dicentrics. At that time (1965) the only available reference curves for chromosome dosimetry were the results of Bender and Kelly, based upon a 72-hr culture time. Plotting our results on these curves gave the figures of 500 rad for the dicentric curve and 470 rad for the break curve (Figure 8).

Figure 8. Dose/dicentrics relationship (results of Bender and Kelly) and plot of M score.

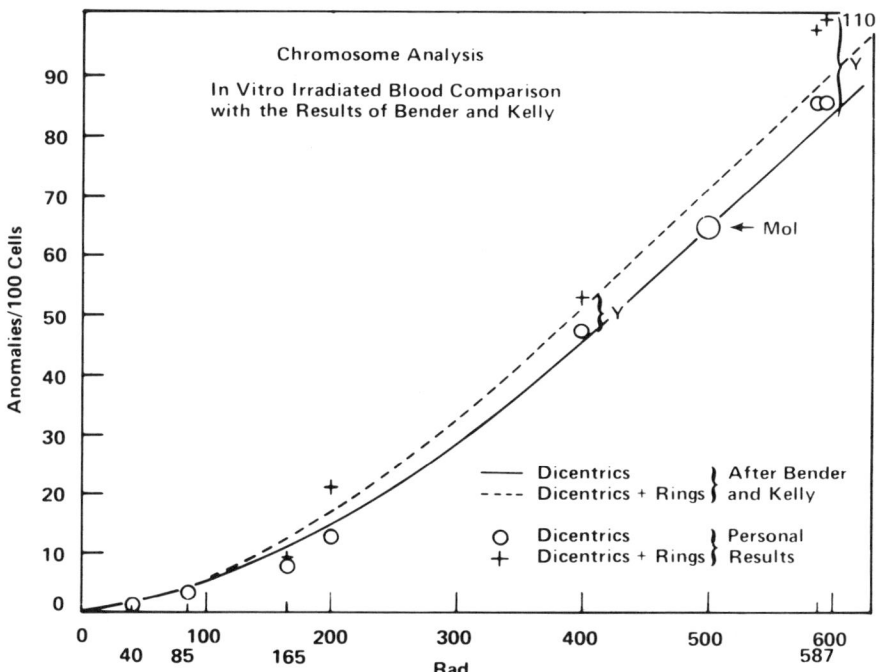

These results are expressed in the form of mean homogeneous equivalent dose. They were in good agreement with the results of the physical dosimetry (Table 1).

For Brescia, the reconstruction of the accident could give only a relative estimate, due to the fact that the exact duration of the exposure was not known.

Therefore the chromosome analysis was of prime importance. It was performed on the basis of a 48-hr culture time to allow the plot on our ^{60}Co reference curve *in vitro*: 230 cells were examined. The mean value of dicentrics led to the estimate of a homogeneous equivalent of 1200 rad of ^{60}Co, that is, 4.95 dicentrics per cell (Table 2).

Moreover, the frequency distribution histogram of the dicentrics did not follow a normal Poisson distribution (Figure 9).

Instead, this frequency distribution showed a bimodal aspect, with one of the modes giving an estimated dose of 870 rad and the other an estimated dose over the level of 3000. (Some of the observed cells presented 13, 14, and 15 dicentrics and were probably subjected to the highest dose level in the cervicocephalic region.)

This observation underlines the importance of the frequency distribution of the chromosome lesions, in relation to the inhomogeneity of the dose distribution within the body.

Conclusions

These two observations allow us to underline the importance of a number of steps to be taken in handling an irradiation accident. The blood sampling should be done as soon as possible to determine the "normal" figures before the beginning of the hematological depression and also to detect an eventual early granulocyte peak. The hematological curves should be plotted daily. This allows useful comparisons between the slopes of these curves from different irradiated persons whose evolution is known.

Table 1. Chromosome Analysis in Case M

Time of sampling	J + 3
Culture time	72 hr
Total cells analyzed	66
Aberrations per 100 cells	
Dicentrics	71
Dicentrics plus rings	75
Acentric fragments	75
Dose estimate (rad)	
Based upon dicentrics	534
Based upon dicentrics plus rings	526

Table 2. Chromosome Analysis in Case B

Time of sampling	J + 7
Culture time	48 hr
Total cells examined	238
Aberrations per 100 cells	
Dicentrics	477
Dicentrics plus rings	543
Accentric fragments	381
Dose estimate (rad)	
Based upon dicentrics	1155
Based upon dicentrics plus rings	1145
Based upon accentrics	1260

The reconstruction of the accident, when possible, can allow the construction a transparent mannikin to show the dose distribution to the different critical organs and especially to the bone marrow. In other cases, doses to the brain (Brescia), to the heart (Los Alamos), or to a main arterial trunk (Argentina Republic accident) can be determined.

The chromosome analysis represents a major tool for the estimation of one of the aspects of the dose, the mean homogeneous equivalent dose. In some cases it can also allow an estimate of an inhomogeneity in the dose distribution if the very high doses received can produce more than one dicentric per cell.

Figure 9. Frequency distribution of the dicentric number per cell in the B accident.

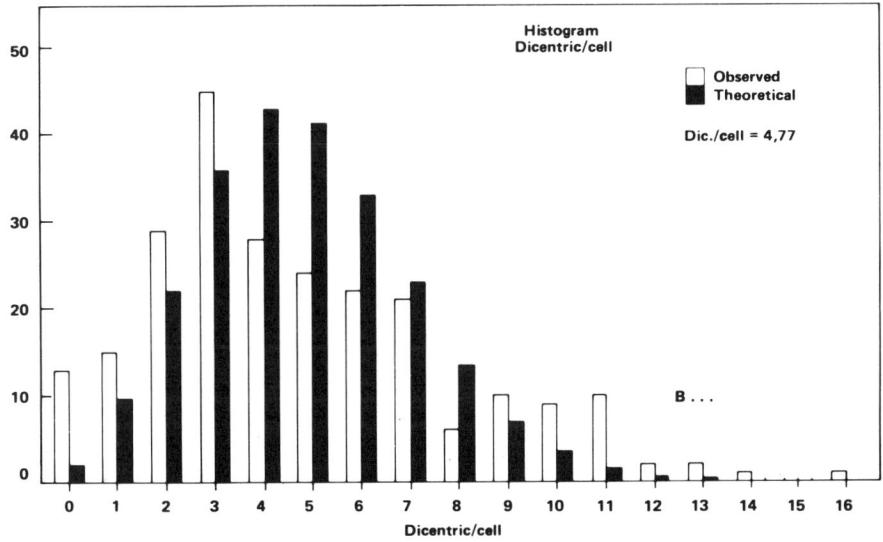

The results of these tests should be compared with the hematological curves—the early lymphocyte slope, the decrease in polymorph counts, the reticulocyte curve, and the platelet curve. These are the most sensitive and precise indicators. These alone are the real proof of bone marrow damage, and regardless of the rad dose estimates it is the extent of the lesions, the bone marrow aplasia, that must be dealt with.

ACKNOWLEDGMENTS
We thank particularly for their contribution to this study Mr. J. L. Malarbet, Miss Veyrat, and Mrs. Roy and the personnel and laboratories at Institut Curie and Commissariat à l'Energie Atomique.

References

1. Diagnostic et traitement des radiolésions aigues, *C.R. Symposium IAEA/OMS Genève 1964*. OMS Genève, 1964.

2. Biola MT: Utilisation des effets cytogénétiques en tant que dosimètre biologique. *Radioprotection* 1:67–88, 1966.

3. Le Gô RJP: Aspects quantitatifs des effets hématologiques des radiations ionisantes. *Radioprotection* 1:89–106, 1966.

4. Le Gô RJP: Description and analysis of the criticality accident at the Venus reactor, Mol on 30th December 1965. Biological aspects, in *Accidental Irradiation at Place of Work*. Euratom, Dec. 1967, Proc. Intern. Symp., Nice, France, 26–29 April 1966, pp. 671–683.

5. Jammet H, Gongora R, Le Gô R: Observation clinique et traitement d'un cas d'irradiation globale accidentelle. *Proc. 1st Int. Congress of Radiation Protection, Rome, Italy, Sept. 5–10, 1966*. Pergamon Press, 1968, pp. 1249–1290.

6. Doloy MT, Le Gô R, Ducatez G, Lepetit J, Bourguignon M: Utilisation des analyses chromosomiques pour l'estimation d'une dose d'irradiation accidentelle chez l'homme, *IRPA IV° Congrès International Paris 1977*. IRPA 1977, vol. 4, No. 435, pp. 1199–1202.

7. Jammet H, Strambi E, Gongora R, Nenot JC: Intérêt de l'association des méthodes physiques et biologiques pour l'évaluation de la dose et de sa répartition dans les cas d'irradiation globale aigue accidentelle, *C.R. IRPA Symposium, Paris, 1978*, No. 457.

A Dosimetric Study of the Belgian (1965) and Italian (1975) Accidents

N. C. Parmentier,* J. C. Nénot,* and H. J. Jammet+

Institut de Protection et de Sûreté Nucléaire, Départment de Protection, Centre d'Etudes Nucléaires, B. P. No. 6, 92260 Fontenay-aux-Roses, France; +Institut Curie, Service de Radiopathologie, 26 rue d'Ulm, 75005 Paris, France.

Introduction

When a competent team of physicians is faced with an acute case of whole-body irradiation, the first question concerns the level of the dose delivered to the patient and subsequently its space and time distributions. The physical and bioclinical approaches are complementary and give their first results after delays of the same order of magnitude. The limit of the dosimetric reconstitution is often the appreciation of the irradiation duration, as the only parameter which can be appreciated with accuracy is the value of the dose rates. On the other hand, only the dosimetric study can appreciate whether the exposure is uniform or not; this an important, if not the most important, factor in order to establish a prognosis and consequently the therapy procedures.[1-3]

A good illustration can be given by the comparison of two acute cases of whole-body irradiation. The first one occurred in Mol, Belgium, on 30 December 1965.[4] The patient was irradiated by neutrons and photons because of a criticality excursion from a small experimental reactor. The second one occurred in northern Italy, on 13 May 1975, in a small installation for cereal irradiation.[5] The subject was irradiated during a few minutes by a source of cobalt 60. In Mol, the accident was immediately known and the patient was admitted to a hospital within 7 hr. At that time, the chest dosimeter indicated a 550-rad gamma and 50-rad neutron dose, evaluated by the measurement of radioinduced sodium 24 (315 microcurie measured in the whole-body counter). In Italy, the nuclear nature of the accident was not evident in the first hours after the accident; the patient landed in Paris on 17 May, four days after the irradiation, when the severity of his case had been recognized in local hospitals. At that time, it was evident, from the evolution of the clinical syndrome, that the irradiation level was very high, probably over the lethal dose.

First Approximation of the Magnitude of the Exposure

In the Mol case, the order of magnitude was known from the chest dosimeter and ^{24}Na measurements, whereas dosimetric information was missing in the Italian case. In both cases, it was soon established that the irradiation was nonuniform. In the Belgian case, the irradiation was distributed from bottom to top, and the position of the subject was quickly known with accuracy after different photographs of a worker simulating the conditions of the accident had been shown to the patient; the induced radioactivity measured in the hairs and nails showed great discrepancies, resulting in corresponding neutron absorbed doses ranging from 40 rad to nearly 500 rad on the leg which was the nearest to the source. In the Italian case, the position of the subject as he described it, the small size of the irradiation chamber, and the relative positions of the patient and the responsible source (Figure 1) ascertained whole-body but not uniform exposure. The most exposed portions were the left shoulder and arm, the front and lateral parts of the neck, the top of the skull, and the face. Because of the high level of the dose suspected, the

Figure 1. Position of workers during exposure. The Belgian is on the right, the Italian on the left.

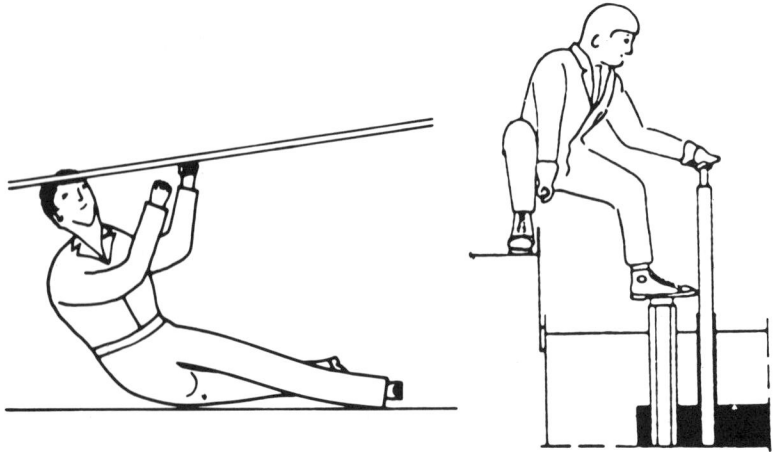

prognosis was mainly dependent on the existence or not of a relatively radiation-shielded area, possibly the left foot and ankle.

Reconstitution of the Accidents

In both accidents, the reconstitution was carried out as soon as possible, seven days after the accident in Belgium, four days in Italy. The phantoms used were Rando-type phantoms (soft-tissue equivalent), with a real skeleton and lungs made of tissue-equivalent material. The phantoms have over 30 horizontal sections, each of them being 1 inch thick, in which the dosimeters were placed. Different types of dosimeters were used: film badges like those used for routine monitoring, different types of lithium fluoride thermoluminescent dosimeters for gamma rays, and S, Au, and Au–Cd detectors for neutron irradiation. Over 300 dosimeters were set inside the phantom and ten on its surface.

Nonuniform distribution of the dose was quickly established after reading of the surface dosimeters. In Mol, the dose was the highest for the left foot, decreasing from bottom to top, from forward to backward, and from left to right. The doses were about 4000 rad at the foot surface, 1200 rad on the pubis, and 500 rad at the top of the head. In the Italian accident only dose rates could be measured (Figure 2), as the duration of the irradiation (2–4 min) could not be evaluated with any accuracy at that time; the dose rates were about 1200 rad/min on the left shoulder, 800 on the anterior left side of the neck, and 600 at the top of the skull. It was then certain that high doses had been delivered to this patient, since the brain dose, for instance, ranged from 1200 to 2400 rad.

From the results of the dosimeters set inside the phantom, it was possible to evaluate with great accuracy the dose distribution within the body. The position and the number of dosimeters had been chosen in relation with anatomical and physiological parameters, such as the percentage of bone marrow present in a given section. Compilation of all these data allowed us to draw isodose curves, giving a clear and synthetic view of the dose distributions. These isodoses on a sagittal median plane and on a frontal median plane are shown in Figures 3 and 4, respectively. In the Italian case, only dose rates were appreciated through this method; for a better comparison, irradiation levels are expressed in terms of total doses; the determination of the absolute dose in the Italian case was made possible by the comparison of the estimated duration of the irradiation and the biological and clinical findings. The important points that can be derived from the isodose curves are for the Belgian patient, doses in the trunk from 300 rad in the upper part to 1000 in the lower part, whereas the Italian patient presented doses above 1000 rad in the whole trunk and up to 2400 rad in the left anterior part of the neck (Figure 3). A first estimate of the prognosis could be derived from doses

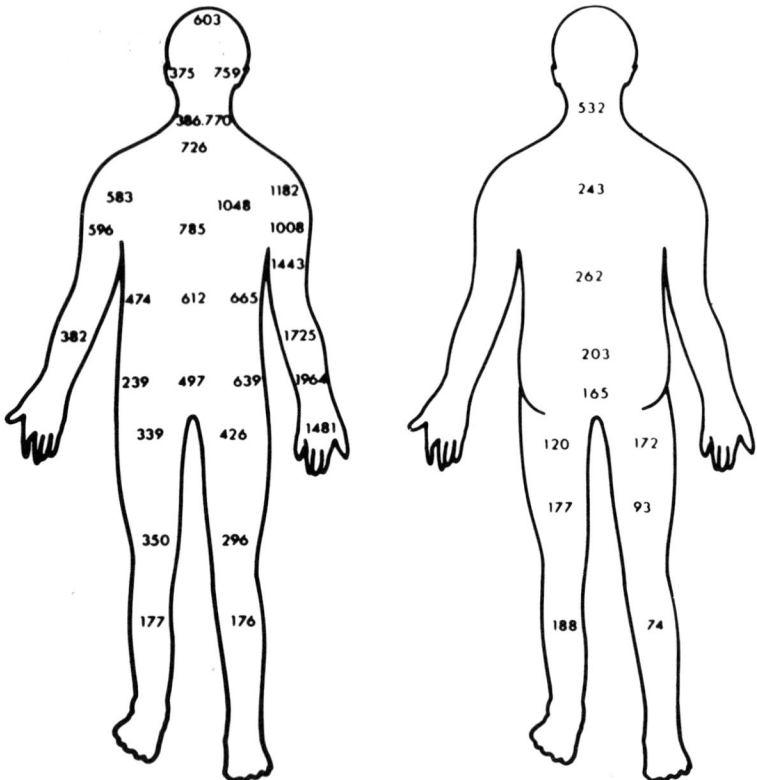

Figure 2. Skin doses measured on the phantom, Italian case (1975).

delivered to the Belgian's dorsal rachis, which received a dose below 300 rad, allowing survival in spite of a mean whole-body dose of about 500 rad; in opposition, the very high dose delivered to the Italian patient's neck explained the early necrosis of the pharynx (Figure 4).

Evaluation of Doses Delivered to Organs and to Bone Marrow

The doses delivered to various organs were calculated, but, except for the bone marrow, the results were approximate, as each organ could not be localized exactly in the phantom. Most doses were between 200 and 500 rad for almost all the organs of the Belgian patient (Table 1), giving good survival chances to this worker, whereas they exceeded 1000 rad for the organs of the Italian patient, which could be considered as a desperate case, in spite of the nonuniform distribution of the dose (Table

1). Bone marrow doses were established with great accuracy. In the Belgian case, the calculation of bone marrow doses gave about 200–300 rad for skull, humerus, and cervical vertebrae, between 500 and 1000 rad for the six lower ribs, lumbar vertebrae, sacrum, and false pelvis. The percentage of bone marrow irradiated at doses between 200 and 300 rad was evaluated at 16% (Table 2); the mean bone marrow dose, calculated by summation of all the doses delivered to the different medullary territories, was estimated at about 500 rad. Though this level is higher than the estimated LD 50 in humans,[6,7] the fact that 16% of the bone marrow received less than 300 rad was in favor of a relatively optimistic prognosis. In the Italian case, 87% of the bone marrow absorbed doses over 800 rad, and 13% absorbed doses between 400 and 800 rad; the levels of these doses were responsible for the very early and complete medullary aplasia.[8] The mean bone marrow dose was estimated at about 1200 rad.

Figure 3. Comparison of isodoses in the sagittal median plane. The Belgian case is on the right, the Italian case on the left.

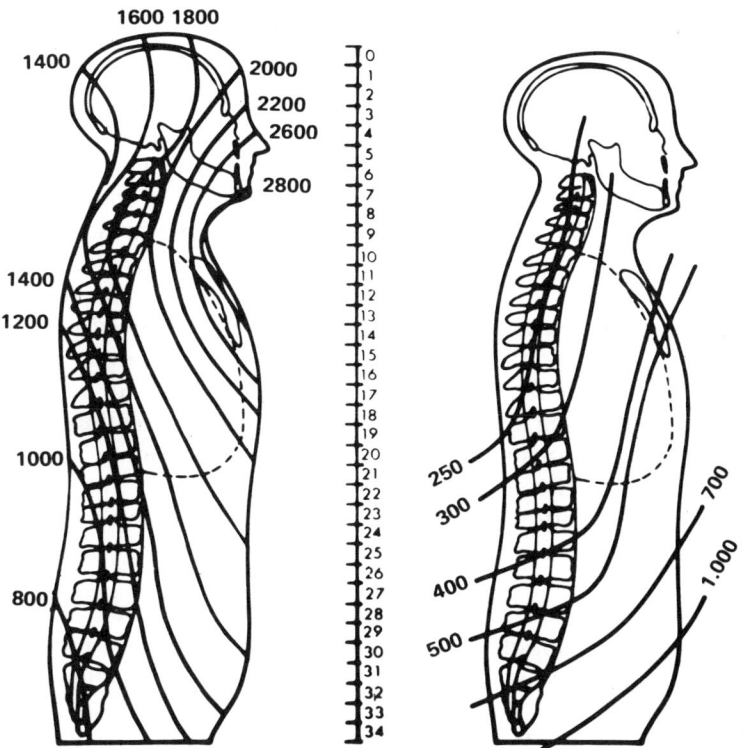

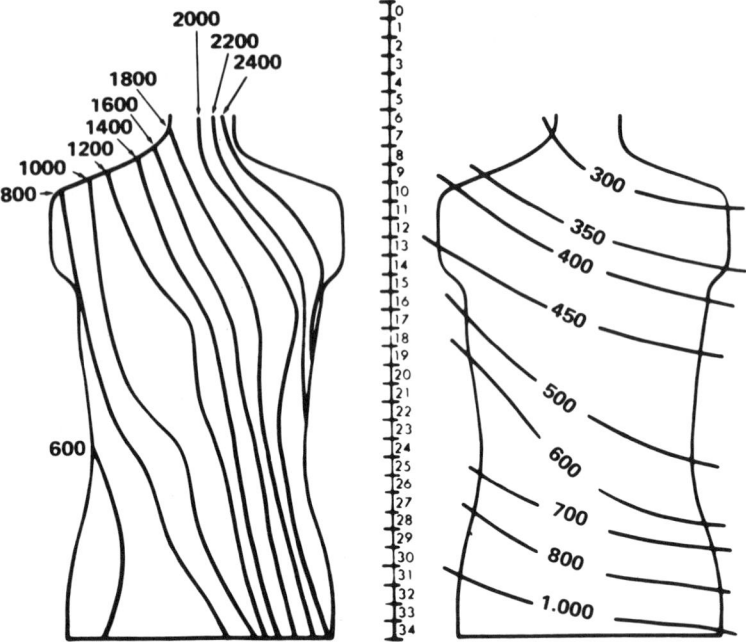

Figure 4. Comparison of isodoses in the frontal median plane. The Belgian case is on the right, the Italian case on the left.

Besides the vital prognosis, it was essential in the Belgian case to evaluate the functional prognosis, as the left foot was heavily irradiated, at doses reaching almost 5000 rad. The dosimetric study, performed with a foot phantom, made of mix D, with a real skeleton, showed doses to bone of 2500 rad at the ankle, 4000 rad at the toe joints. It was evident that amputation could not be avoided, but the question was raised where it had to be done, as it was not reasonable to think of amputation in an area that had absorbed doses ranging from 2000 to 3000 rad. It was shown that the dose to the thigh was 1500 rad; the amputation was carried out in good conditions six months after the irradiation.

The doses delivered to the gonads were about 1000 rad. At this level, prognosis was clear: sterility was certain, total, and permanent.

Conclusions

In both cases, it has been possible, step by step, to obtain a good picture of the dose distribution, giving invaluable help to the physicians clinically in charge of the patients.

One should notice that the Italian case was a typical gamma-irradiation

Table 1. Comparison of Doses Delivered to Various Organs (Rads)

Organs	Belgium, 1965	Italy, 1975
Brain		
Right	} 200-300	1600-2000
Left		1200-1600
Hypophysis	330	1800
Pharynx-esophagus		} 2000-2200
Thyroid	300	
Heart	400-450	1400-2000
Spleen	400	2000
Liver	400-500	1200-1400
Large intestine (transverse colon)	450-500	1000-1800
Adrenals		
Right	} 350-400	{ 800
Left		1600
Kidneys		
Right	} 400-500	{ 800
Left		1600
Gonads	>1100	1600

case. The Belgian case was also considered in 1965 as a gamma-irradiation case, because the neutron contribution to the absorbed dose was considered as negligible. But, in view of the most recent results in neutron radiobiology, namely, variation of RBE with the absorbed dose, it is now necessary to reconsider the neutron absorbed dose contribution. For example, the mean marrow dose may be estimated as follows: 500

Table 2. Comparison of Doses Delivered to the Bone Marrow

Dose range (rads)	Percent of irradiated bone marrow	
	Belgium, 1965	Italy, 1975
200-300	16	
300-400	28	
400-500	8	
400-800		13
500-1000	48	
800-1200		33.3
1200-1600		33.7
1600-2000		4.5
2000-2400		13.5
2400-3000		2

rad gamma dose and 50 rad neutron dose, which should be affected by an RBE of about 3.

ACKNOWLEDGMENTS
The author wishes to express his gratitude to all the physicians and scientists who did not spare their time and care in these circumstances, whether in Belgium, Italy, or France.

References

1. IAEA-WHO-ILO: *Manual on Early Medical Treatment of Possible Radiation Injury*, Safety Series No. 47. Vienna, IAEA, 1978.

2. ICRP Publication 28: *The Principles and General Procedures for Handling Emergency and Accidental Exposures of Workers*. Oxford, Pergamon Press, 1979.

3. Jammet H, Le Gô R, Lafuma J: *Accidents radiologiques. Conduite à tenir en cas d'irradiation externe accidentelle ou de contamination radioactive accidentelle*, Note CEA-N-1365. Paris, Commissariat à l'Energie Atomique, 1970.

4. Parmentier NC, Boulenger R, Portal G: Problèmes de dosimétrie lors de l'accident de criticité survenu au réacteur Vénus à MOL, en date du 30 décembre 1965, in *Proceedings of the First International Congress of Radiation Protection, Roma, Italy, Sept. 5–10, 1966*. Oxford, Pergamon Press, 1968, pp. 1231–1248.

5. Jammet H, Strambi E, Gongora R, Nénot JC: Intérêt de l'association des méthodes physiques et biologiques pour l'évaluation de la dose et de sa répartition dans les cas d'irradiation globale aiguë accidentelle, in *Proceedings of the Fourth International Congress of the International Radiation Protection Association, Paris, France, April 24–30, 1977*. 1977, vol. 3, pp. 961–968.

6. Sub-Committee on the Treatment of Radiation of Injury: *The Treatment of Radiation Injury*, Washington, Committee on Pathological Effects of Atomic Radiation, National Academy of Sciences, National Research Council, 1963.

7. Langham W (ed.): *Radiobiological Factors in Manned Space Flight*, Washington, National Academy of Sciences, 1967.

8. Norwood WD: *Health Protection of Radiation Workers*. Springfield, Ill., C. Thomas, 1975.

The 1978 Algerian Accident: Four Cases of Protracted Whole-body Irradiation

H. Jammet,* R. Gongora,* P. Pouillard,* R. Le Gô,+ and N. Parmentier+

*Institut Curie, Service de Radiopathologie, Service de Médecine Oncologique, 26 rue d'Ulm, 75005, Paris, France;
+Institut de Protection et de Sûreté Nucléire, Département de Protection, B. P. No. 6, 92260 Fontenay-aux-Roses, France.

A Case History

On May 5th, 1978, an iridium 192 source of 25 curies for gammagraphy fell from a truck on the road from Algiers to Setif. It was found within one or two days by two young boys, three and seven years old, who handled this bright metallic pencil-like object for some hours.

Later their grandmother (47 years old) took the source away from them and hid it in their kitchen. The source remained about five or six weeks in this room, where several persons were irradiated under various conditions. Among them, four young female patients, 14 to 20 years old, received a daily and protracted irradiation. They stayed between 0.80 and 1.50 m from the source, which delivered a dose rate in the range of 8 R/hr at 1 m. The exposure time was estimated to be 6 to 8 hr daily.

The Algerian authorities looked actively for the missing source and finally located it on June 12th, 38 days after it had been lost. During the two following days these patients were successively treated in the hospitals of Setif and Algiers. Then, after various delays from 2 to 20 days, they were evacuated from Algiers to Paris, where they were taken to the Curie Foundation Hospital.

Early Clinical Findings

It is worthy of note here that during the four or five weeks that the source was irradiating the four patients the clinical and biological evolution remained completely unknown. Therefore at the outset of the observations the course of the evolution had reached the level of an acute radiation syndrome at its critical period.

DJ (19 years old), the first patient to be evacuated, had shown severe mucous bleeding (from mouth and digestive tract) during her stay in Algiers. She presented ecchymotic suffusion on the eyelid and purpura of the abdominal wall. The general state was poor, with prostration, anorexia, nausea.

Four days later, NG (20 years old), pregnant eight weeks, arrived in Paris with a similar hemorrhagic and digestive syndrome. She had been given a transfusion (total blood) in Algeria some days before.

Two weeks later, at intervals of three days, two other patients arrived in Paris: FA (17 years old) and NO (14 years old), their hematological state having been judged critical by the medical staff in Algiers. They also presented a digestive syndrome plus purpura.

Faced primarily with these four patients, in addition to others whose story will not be presented in this paper, a number of questions had to be answered as soon as possible: (1) estimation of the probable irradiation dose and distribution; (2) estimation of the level of severity of the cellular damage based upon biological results (chromosome analysis and hematological curves); (3) how the sterile housing conditions were to be managed; (4) which therapeutic rules were to be adopted.

The Dosimetry Problems

Physical Dosimetry

The dosimetry problems were difficult to solve, as there was uncertainty about each of the irradiation parameters: (1) the precise day the source arrived in the house; (2) the exact patient-source distances according to the different occupational activities of the women (cooking, washing, grooming) and of the girls doing their homework; (3) uncertainties as to the postures (standing or squatting) and orientation (front, back, or profile) toward the source; (4) uncertainties about the duration of presence in the kitchen throughout the day, estimated between 6 and 8 hr; and (5) uncertainties about the shadowing of different persons by one another.

Therefore a simulation of the accident was set up on the spot in Algeria by the Dosimetry Laboratory of our institute. This simulation allowed us to get a map of the distribution of doses for a given position at a mean distance and to calculate the isodoses for other positions. Then the isodoses could be determined according to the different positions, attitudes, and length of presence in the proximity of the source (Figures 1–2; Table 1).

Figure 1 shows the map of the kitchen, with the working area in front of a table and between it and a small piece of furniture on which the source was hidden in a wooden basket. Figures 2A and 2B show isodose maps after the reconstruction in a human phantom for two hypothetic positions: standing and squatting. They show that for a mean source distance of 1.24 m the calculated dose could be about 2500 rad at the skin with a transmission of about 45% to the vertebrae in a vertical position and 30% in a squatting position. In this last position the head received a very high dose whatever the orientation: front or profile. It could be noted that the medullary mean cumulated dose could have been as high as about 1100–1350 rad.

Figure 1. Map of the kitchen where the four patients were irradiated during cooking activities.

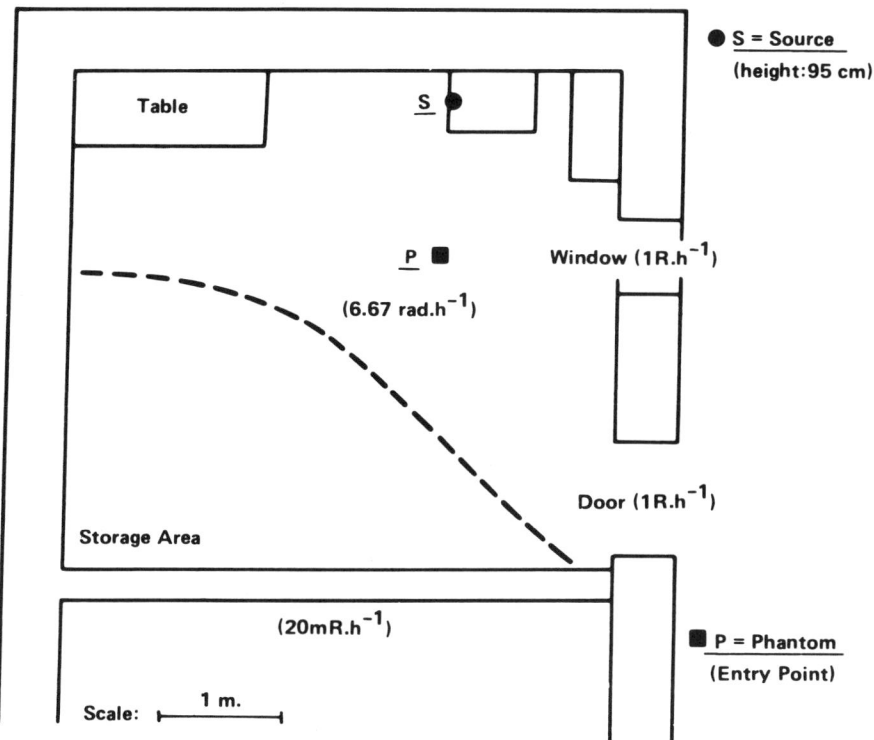

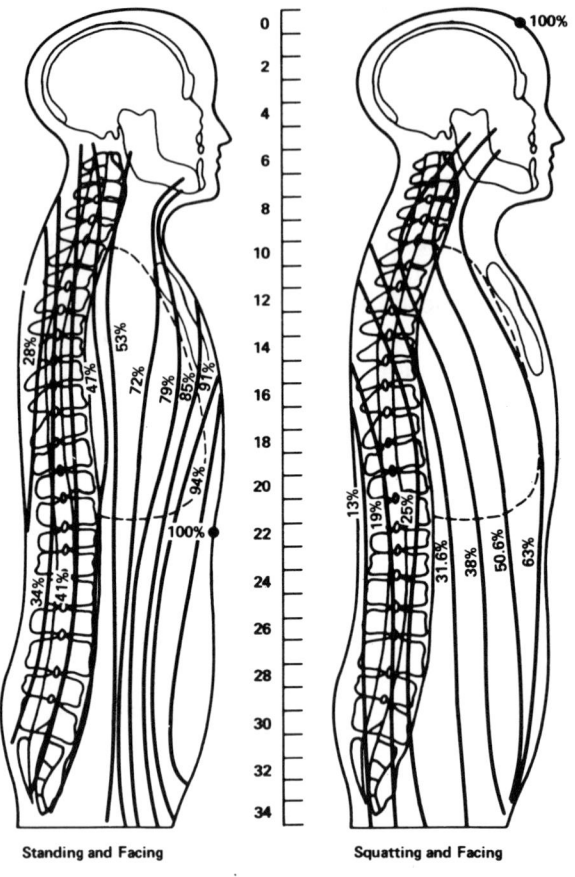

Standing and Facing   Squatting and Facing

Source: 16 Ci—Distance: 1.24 m

Figure 2A. Isodose map from reconstruction in a human phantom for the standing position. **2B.** Isodose map from reconstruction in a human phantom for the squatting position.

Chromosome Analyses

The chromosome analyses in these peculiar cases yielded results which appeared to be in large discrepancy with the real clinical and biological states observed in the four patients.

Thus their results could not be taken into consideration in the sense of a tool of biological dosimetry, as can be done in cases of acute single exposure.

This failure of chromosome analyses to allow dose estimates yielded some special problems which can be summarized as follows.

First, as will be shown later, the hematological findings indicated damage to the hemopoietic tissues far higher than that which the chromosome-based dose estimates yielded.

Second, these estimations are based on an experimental curve whose conditions of irradiation were different: single, acute, homogeneous.

Third, the patients exhibited evidence that the majority (50–100%) of the lymphocytes had completed one or several mitoses at the time of the observation. This estimation was based upon the loss of the fragment which normally stays with the dicentrics.

Fourth, the "normal" lymphocytes from the transfused blood could have been in competition with the heavily damaged patient lymphocytes in the blood cultures, thus eliminating those cells suffering from a heavier burden of aberrations (some of the lymphocytes in culture contained the Y chromosome, necessarily introduced by the transfusions).

However, some attempts to correct the distortion of the observed dicentric frequency introduced by mitotic activity and by transfused lymphocytes were made.

The rule of dicentric disappearance not being precisely known, two different hypotheses were used to approximate the dicentric loss in the course of a mitosis. The first hypothesis was that the dicentric frequency is divided by a factor of two. The second hypothesis was that each dicentric present in the cell reduces the chances of that cell surviving by a factor by two.

These two corrective factors yield two values for the induced abnormality frequencies, which are rather close. Another type of correction took into account the introduction of normal cells by transfusions. It was based on the ratio between the number of cells in the class with one and in the class with two dicentrics. From this ratio a theoretical Poisson distribution could be drawn, which gave a theoretical frequency for the class with zero dicentric, that is, the class of normal cells. However, this correction does not take into account the relative heterogeneity of the dose distribution. In any case the new results are still in discrepancy with the severity of the hematological syndrome.

Table 1. Calculated Doses from Reconstruction in a Phantom (Estimated Exposure in Rads)

Patient	Max skin dose	Mean medullary dose
DJ	2800	1200-1400
NG	2800	1250-1400
FA	2600	1100-1300
NO	2300	1000-1200

Early Hematological Findings

The early blood cell counts already showed the severity of the situation for the four patients. The lymphocytes (norm: 2000–2500 per microliter) (Figure 3) were at the levels of 150–200 per microliter (less than 10% of the norm) for NG and NO. The polymorphs (norm: 4000–6000 per microliter) (Figure 4) were 100 to zero for DJ, NG, and FA; 30 for NO. The reticulocytes (norm: 100,000–150,000) (Figure 5) were 100–200 for NG and NO; zero for DJ and FA. The thrombocytes (norm: 250,000–300,000) (Figure 6) were 20,000–30,000 for DJ, NG, and NO; 7000 for FA.

These initial observations showed hematological damage in the critical period whose level was in the range of the damage observed in the most severe accidents known, such as Mol 1965, or even more severe. Moreover, the bone marrow examinations from various points (sternum, iliac spines) showed a zero cellularity.

Electroencephalograms

For the four patients, very similar abnormalities were found on the electroencephalograms (Dr. Court). They can be summarized as follows: (1) a general disorganization of the cerebral electric activity, particularly of the alpha rhythm, whose modulations disappeared; (2) spindles of diffusely scattered waves (frequency 1–4 Hz) with durations of between 200 and 1000 msec; (3) predominance of these abnormalities in the right parieto-occipital regions for the two older patients, DJ and NG; (4) graphoparoxystic abnormalities (spikes or waves and spikes) for patient NO.

Compared with experimental data on *Macaca mulatta,* these electro-encephalogram modifications favored the hypothesis of a global cumu-lated irradiation between 600 and 1000 rad, combined with a heteroge-neous irradiation of the head more intense on the right side, where the doses could have been higher than 1000 rad.

Clinical Survey

The first observed clinical manifestations were insidious: loss of appetite, progressive asthenia leading to a true prostration within three weeks. Then a typical acute radiation syndrome with its digestive manifestations (nausea, vomiting, diarrhea), hemorrhagia (purpura, epistaxis, bleeding gingiva, hemoptysis, hematuria, melena, metrorrhagia) was observed. These symptoms occurred at different times after arrival in Paris and according to the dose received and the time factor. Moreover, the four patients presented fever that exceeded 39°C. Partial or total loss of hair was also observed.

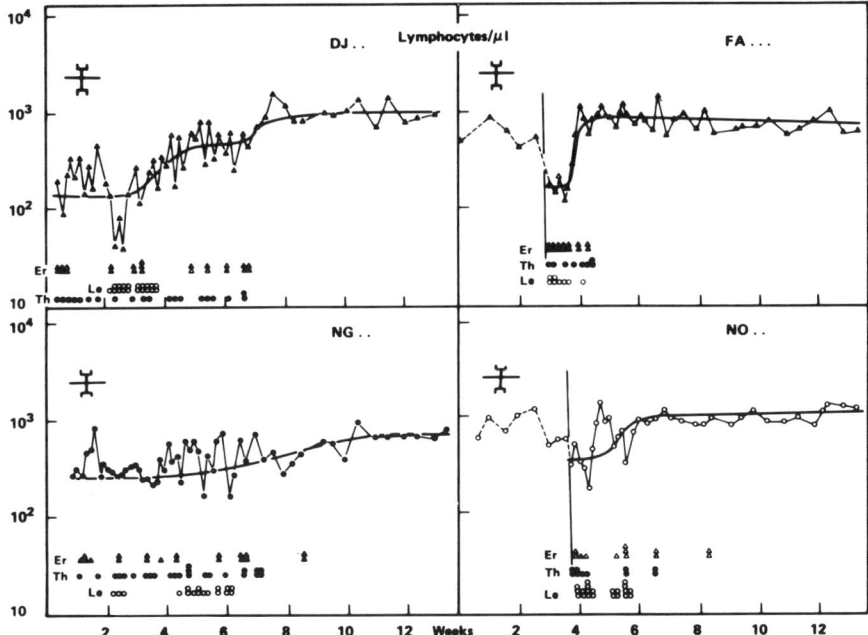

Figure 3. Lymphocyte evolution for the four patients. Exact daily plots, plus corrected (for transfusions) smoothed curve. $\triangle$ = red blood cell unit; $\circ$ = white blood cell units; $\bullet$ = platelet units.

This very severe evolution, dominated by the infectious and hemorrhagic manifestations, lasted eight weeks, despite the establishment of an intensive care, vigorous anti-infectious treatment, and daily balance of the hematological deficiency. During this period the patients presented aphthoid or ulceronecrotic lesions of mouth and lips, leading in one case to severe feeding difficulties and inability to speak.

The bacteriologic and mycologic monitoring of the patients needed several hundred analyses of blood, skin, mucosae, urine, and feces, and several hundred antibiograms.

During the course of the hemorrhagic syndrome, one of the patients had retinal hemorrhage. Another presented a cataclysmic buccal bleeding of about 800 cc due to a vessel ulceration.

Hematological Evolution

The hematological evolution is presented in Figures 3 to 6. Each cell line evolution is shown for the four patients simultaneously: lymphocytes (Figure 3), granulocytes (Figure 4), reticulocytes (Figure 5), and throm-

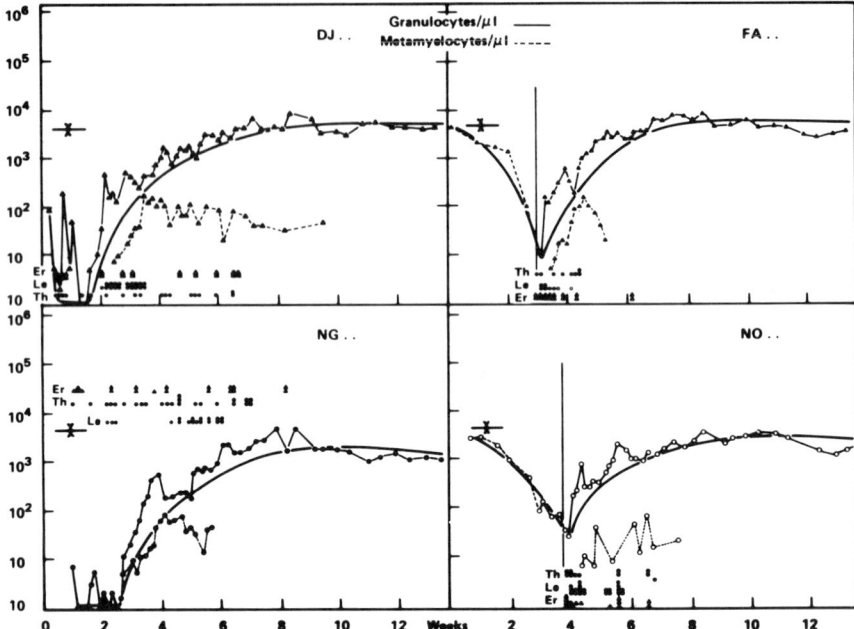

Figure 4. Polymorphonuclear evolution for the four patients. Exact daily plots, plus corrected (for transfusions) smoothed curve. (See legend to Figure 3.)

bocytes (Figure 6). In each of these figures the exact plots of the daily results are represented. The number of perfusions of each variety of packed cells was based on the daily hematological results and by the clinical events such as hemorrhagia, fever, or bacteremia as well. Therefore the plotted points of these curves do not reflect the patient's blood image but the modified image caused by the perfusions.

Thus we had to estimate the increment of cell numeration that each bag of fresh cells yielded. On this basis a computer correction with smoothing yielded the second curve which is drawn on each of the hematological curves. This corrected curve did reflect more accurately the real hematological evolution of the patients.

As can be seen from Figures 3–6, the evolution was very severe for the four patients. The blood cell counts remained during three weeks at levels as low as the following:

0–200 polymorphs	0–4% of norm
0–100 reticulocytes	0–0.1% of norm
25–50,000 thrombocytes	8–15% of norm
200–300 lymphocytes	10–15% of norm

But as far as lymphocytes were concerned, the minimum values they reached in an earlier period, during weeks 1–5, were not known. An important difference between the evolution of these cases of protracted irradiation and known cases of acute irradiation lies in the fact that the critical period was also protracted and necessitated a constant therapeutic effort. Despite the fact that each of the patients was given several (one to three) bags of freshly isolated cells of each line (red, white, platelets) daily, the blood count levels remained very low, at the limit of the infectious and hemorrhagic risks, for a critical period which lasted between 30 and 60 days after the end of the irradiation period.

Restoration Period

The restoration period started late and progressed very slowly, spanning four to five weeks before reaching a stabilization level. This again is in opposition to the fast restoration observed in acute irradiation cases. The first positive index of the bone marrow refunctioning was the progressive appearance of myeloid young cells (myelocytes, metamyelocytes) in the

Figure 5. Reticulocyte evolution for the four patients. Exact daily plots, plus corrected (for transfusions) smoothed curve. (See legend to Figure 3.)

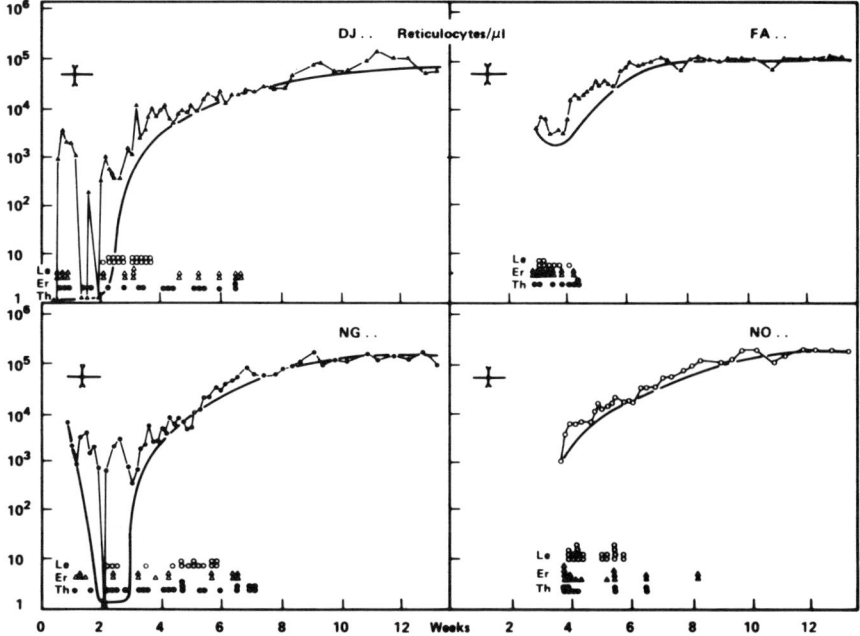

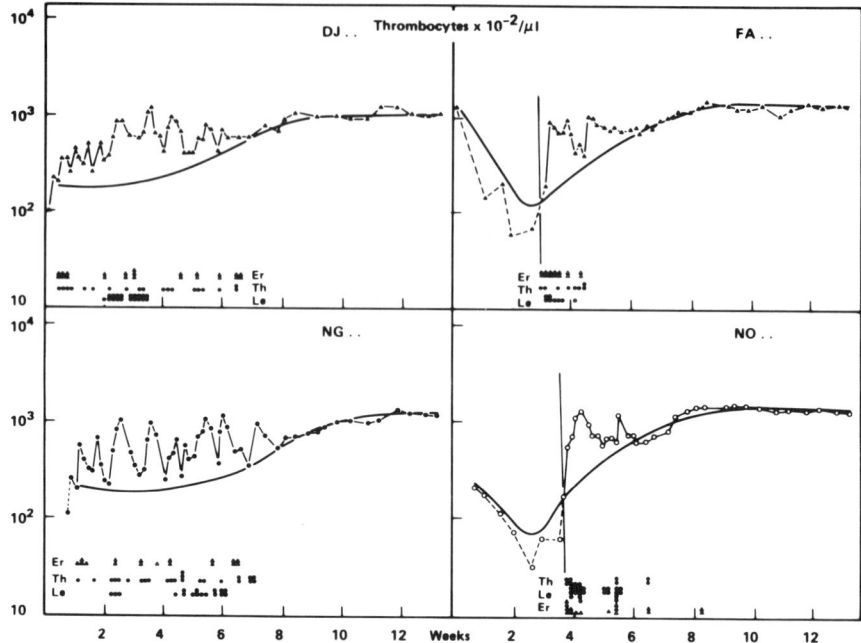

Figure 6. Thrombocyte evolution for the four patients, plus corrected (for transfusions) smoothed curve. (See legend to Figure 3.)

peripheral blood. Also, some monocytes were seen at this time. The presence of both cell types was considered as a proof of spontaneous regeneration because these two cytologic elements could not have been introduced from therapeutic transfusions.

Shortly after, the totality of cell lines began to rise slowly. Concomitantly, the restoration of the general state was observed, and the patients could be removed from sterile conditions; the anti-infectious treatment was also stopped.

Figure 7 shows a panoramic view of the hematological evolution for the four patients. Each of the cell lines is represented by its corrected smoothed curve.

The very slow restoration process can be seen for each family of curves. The special shape of the lymphocyte curve can be noted with its successive steps in plateau.

An important feature of this hematological evolution also lies in the fact that the different stabilization levels reached by the cell lines remain under the physiological level, indicating the persistence of a sequela of the hematological function and tissues, probably linked with a persistent loss of a noticeable part of the hematopoietic "nests" of bone marrow.

Thus the stabilization levels remain steady under the normal values (Table 2). The polymorph plateau remained between 35 and 60% of norm for two patients, NG and NO. The lymphocyte plateau was between 35 and 60% for the four patients. The thrombocyte plateau was between 55 and 60% for the four patients. Inversely, the reticulocyte curves showed a wave of rebound reaching 140–280% for the four patients.

Biochemical Findings

A number of biochemical modifications were noted. Some of them covered a long period and were observed on the four patients: hypoproteinemia, hypouricemia, hypokalemia, and hypocholesterolemia (Figure 8).

Other modifications were episodic: for instance, L.D.H. was increased for three patients during the fifth week. One patient presented an episodic increase of S.G.O.T., another an increase of P.K. It is to be noted that these modifications were dissociated, and their significance is still not established.

Figure 7. Panoramic view of the hematological evolution for the four patients. Each cell line is represented by its corrected smoothed curve.

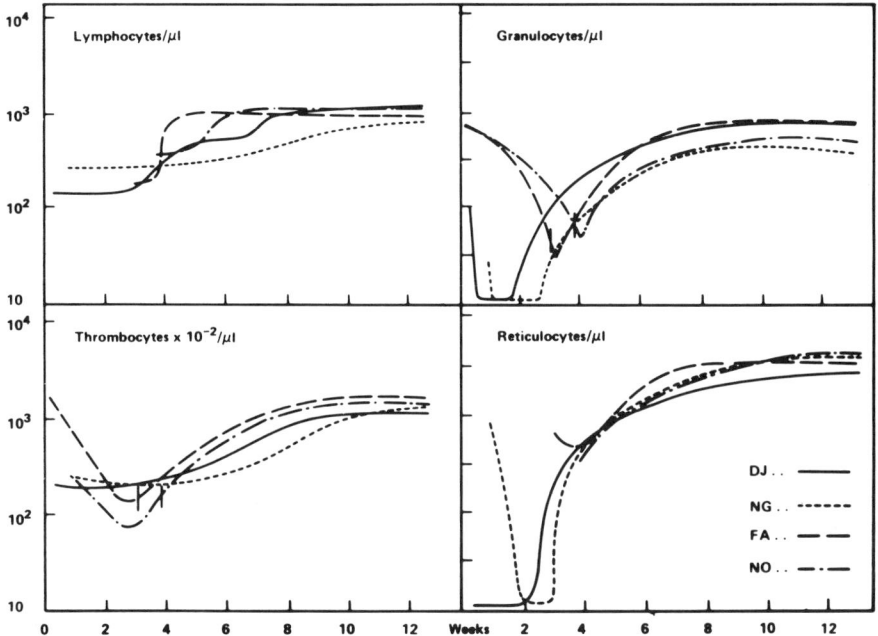

Table 2. Stabilization Levels of the Cell Lines as Percentages of the Normal Levels Five Months After the End of the Irradiation Period

Cell line	Patient DJ	Patient NG	Patient FA	Patient NO
Granulocytes	100%	37%	100%	50%
Lymphocytes	40%	40%	36%	60%
Reticulocytes	140%	240%	200%	280%
Thrombocytes	55%	55%	60%	60%

Endocrinology

The results of hormonal explorations can be summarized as follows: (1) slight adrenal deficiency for the androgenic secretion (perhaps in relation with corticotherapy), (2) cessation of ovarian activity (therapeutic inhibition); (3) normal activity of gonadotropic functions (normal prolactin); (4) normal thyroid activity; (5) normal parathormone levels.

Because NG was pregnant during the irradiation period, special attention should be paid to this patient. The death of the fetus was evident on 10 July at the age of 9.5 weeks. A spontaneous abortion occurred on 6 August. The fetus was 48 mm long. The thymus was present. The liver showed hematopoietic cell islets. All organs were present and histologically normal. The young woman was pregnant again in the course of 1979.

Therapeutic Management

The four patients posed very special therapeutic problems due to the long duration of the critical period of the bone marrow aplasia and its infectious and hemorrhagic consequences. Moreover, oral feeding was not possible, which led to parenteral alimentation, and the perturbation of the main metabolic functions needed intensive care.

First, the patients were isolated for seven weeks in plastic sterile chambers that received sterile air and were air-conditioned. The asepsis was controlled daily, and the dust quantity and granulometry were registered continuously.

Despite the precautions against external contamination, endogeneous bacteria and mycoorganisms were present, and the four patients developed local infections or septicemia, which necessitated major antibiotic and antimycotic treatment based upon repeated antibiograms. One of the patients, for instance, was given flucytosine, 150 gm; amphotericin B, 408 gm; cephalotin, 297 gm (Table 3).

Second, given the hematologic syndrome, the possibility of a bone marrow transplantation was considered during the critical period because of the difficulty in controlling infectious and hemorrhagic syndromes. However, uncertainty about a possible graft-versus-host syndrome in case of transplantation led to the decision to undertake hematologic compensatory therapy. This required repeated transfusions of multiple bags of RBC, WBC, and platelets in order to maintain a minimum level of the circulating cells. The quantities administered were considerable. One of the patients, for example, received 12 packed RBC transfusions (4125×10^{10} cells) and 10 transfusions of leukocytes (42×10^{10} cells) (Figure 9). Such a demand necessitated a cooperation of several trans-fusion centers and activation of efficient supply routes. In addition, this therapy required a strict surveillance of tolerance and systematic detec-tion of antierythrocytic irregular agglutinins. These were always negative. Nevertheless, transfusion shocks were observed.

Third, reanimation also included the maintenance of hydroelectrolytic balance. Thus the liquid compensation by both intravenous and oral administration exceeded 5 liters a day. One of the patients, for example,

Figure 8. Evolution of chlolesterol in case DJ.

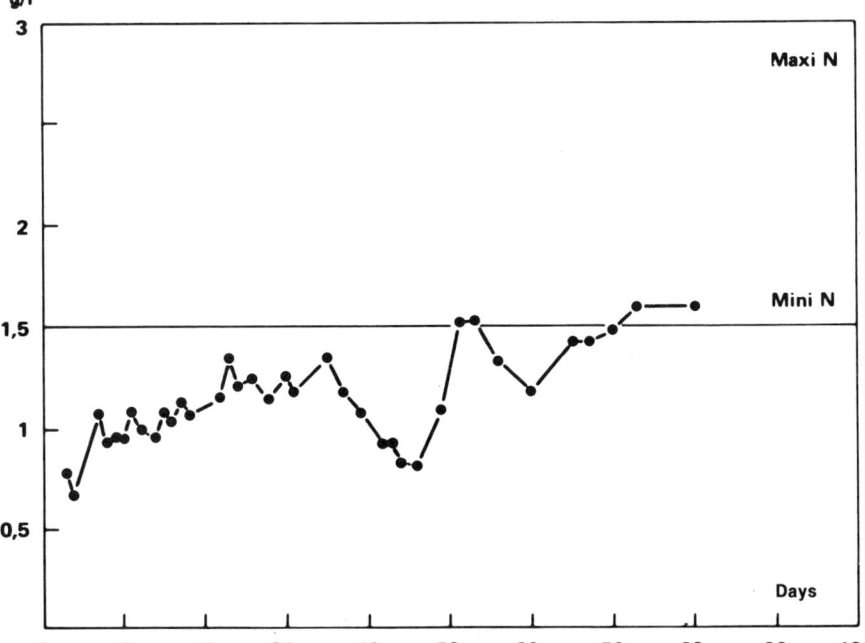

Table 3. Antibiotic and Antimycotic Therapy

	Patient DJ	Patient NG	Patient FA	Patient NO
Antimycotics:				
Flucytosin	150 gm/42 days	105 gm/21 days	80 gm/32 days	65 gm/26 days
Amphotericin B	408 gm/51 days	360 gm/46 days	280 gm/35 days	280 gm/35 days
Antibiotics:				
Ampicillin		192 gm/16 days	72 gm/12 days	
Cephalotin	297 gm/33 days	12 gm/ 2 days	96 gm/16 days	168 gm/28 days
Colimycin			18 M UI/9 days	12 M UI/6 days
Gentamicin	6.40 gm/34 days	6.72 gm/42 days	2.88 gm/18 days	4.48 gm/28 days
Kanamicin	3.75 gm/5 days			
Penicillin G			75 UI/5 days	
Polymyxin B	5.40 gm/27 days	2.80 gm/14 days		
Spiramycetin		16 gm/8 days		
Sulfamethoxazol			17.6 gm/11 days	
+Trimethoprime			3.52 gm/11 days	

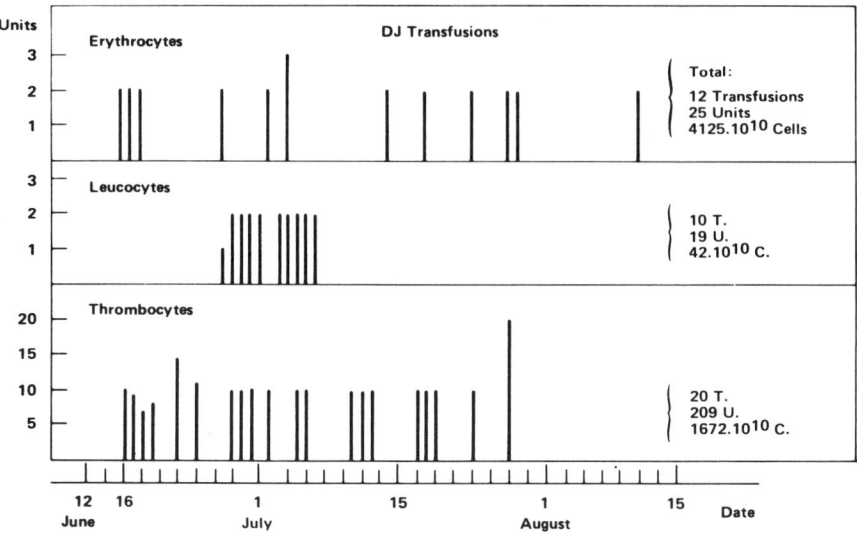

Figure 9. Map of different transfusions in case DJ.

received 222 liters of different sera (Figure 10). Another patient received a daily dose of 498 mEq of Na^+, 121 mEq of K^+, and 635 mEq of Cl^-. In general, it was difficult to maintain K^+ at a normal level.

Nutritive requirements were satisfied by intravenous administration of proteins, lipides, and glucides for a daily total of 2000 calories, with all essential vitamins.

Figure 10. Map of liquid administration in case DJ.

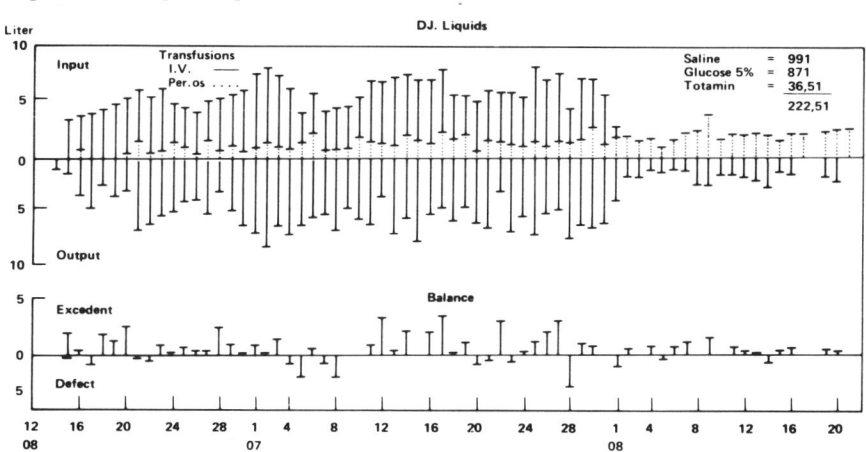

128

Fourth, the main objective of hormonal therapy was to compensate for adrenal deficiency, to block ovarian function in order to inhibit uncontrollable menstrual flux likely to trigger cataclysmic hemorrhages. It was essential to avoid spontaneous abortion for the pregnant patient during the critical phase. This patient was given progesterone and chlormadinone acetate. The other three were given ethinyl-estradiol, lynestrenol, and norethisterone acetate. All received corticoids.

Conclusion

These cases are of particular interest from several viewpoints. It is the first observation of accidental irradiation that spanned so long a period (five or six weeks) and for which the daily data could be collected during several months.[1-8] The dosimetry problems arose from uncertainties of time, position, and posture during the irradiation period.

Chromosome analysis could not at first be referred to an appropriate reference curve, and the dose estimates were biased by the introduction of transfused cells and by intercurrent mitoses. The hematological curves led to the most precise estimation of the bone marrow damage level. They were the solid reference points on which to base therapeutic management, Given the uncertainty of bone marrow reactions to grafts, the restoration therapy based on fresh cell transfusions was the only reasonable action.

The duration of the critical period was much longer than in the acute accidents and required enormous quantities of fresh cells to treat the four patients simultaneously. Intensive anti-infectious and hydroelectrolytic therapy was necessary. The restoration levels of the different cell lines remained below the norm except for the reticulocytes, thus indicating a permanent defect in the hematopoietic nests.

A periodic survey of the patients could be useful, especially with respect to chromosome examinations to detect an eventual malignant clone formation. The long-term prognosis remains uncertain for both stochastic and nonstochastic effects.

ACKNOWLEDGMENTS
We thank particularly all the persons who have given their time and assistance for these patients, among them Drs. Pasquier, Court, Menoux, and Jockey, Mrs. Doloy, Valle, and Roy, Mr. Malarbet, Miss Veyrat, the personnel of laboratories in Institut Curie and C.E.A., and the staff and personnel of transfusion centers in Paris.

References

1. Gonzalez R, Berumen L: Etude de cinq sujets soumis à une irradiation totale subaiguë accidentelle. *Rev Franç Etudes Clin Biol* 8:1009–1011, 1963.
2. Andrews G: Mexican Co[60] radiation accident. *Isotopes Radiat Technol* 1:1963–1964.
3. Sugiyama H, Kurisu A, Hirashima K, Kumatori T: Clinical studies on radiation injuries resulting from accidental exposure to an iridium-192 radiographic source. *J Radiat Res* 14:275–286, 1974.

4. Hirashima K, Ishihara T, Kumatori T, Sugiyama H, Kurisu A: Hematological studies of six cases of accidental exposure to an iridium radiographic source. *J Radiat Res* 14:287–296, 1973.

5. Wakabayashi K, Isurugi K, Tamaoki B, Akaboshi S: Serum levels of luteinizing hormone (LH) and follicle-stimulating hormone (FSH) in subjects accidentally exposed to ^{192}Ir gamma rays. *J Radiat Res* 14:297–303, 1973.

6. Nakamura W, Mizobuchi K, Sawada F, and coll: Biochemical analyses of some metabolites in urine and blood in persons exposed accidentally to a source of [192]Ir. *J Radiat Res* 14:304–320, 1973.

7. Hashizume T, Kato Y, Nakajima T, Yamaguchi H, Fujimoto K: Dose estimation of non-occupational persons accidentally exposed to ^{192}Ir gamma-rays. *J Radiat Res* 14:320–327, 1973.

8. Ishihara T, Kohno S, Hirashima K, Kumatori T, Sugiyama H, Kurisu A: Chromosome aberrations in persons accidentally exposed to ^{192}Ir gamma-rays. *J Radiat Res* 14:328–335, 1973.

Published 1980 by Elsevier North Holland, Inc.
K.F. Hübner and S.A. Fry, eds. The Medical Basis for Radiation Accident Preparedness

The 1967 Radiation Accident Near Pittsburgh, Pennsylvania, and a Follow-up Report

Michael V. Gilberti

Research and Development Laboratory, Hammarville, Pennsylvania.

Introduction

With the current increased use of nuclear energy, the chances of radiation accidents occurring as a result of human error are much more probable. Even previously unreported exposures are now being brought to our attention. Acceptable treatment can only be rendered by using the knowledge and experience gained from previous accidents.

Since the chance of any one type of accident being repeated may be small, it would seem appropriate to report the unusual and interesting clinical features of three patients who were accidentally exposed to high doses of ionizing radiation. These men exhibited features of the acute radiation syndrome and required the astute clinical judgment and applied skills of many experts in the field of nuclear medicine for successful treatment of the critical stages. I have been following these three men for the past 12 years and have had the opportunity to observe some of the long-term effects of severe radiation exposure. Their clinical course, treatment of the acute and chronic changes, and their current health status serve as the basis of this report.

Review of Previous Accidents

There have been increasing numbers of total-body radiation accidents involving either (1) uncontrolled criticality excursions with the victims exposed to fission neutrons as well as gamma and particulate radiation; (2) photon and electron exposures from high-energy accelerators; (3) X-ray exposure from machines; (4) radioisotopes freed accidentally into the environment; or (5) encapsulated but unrecognized radiation sources.[1] Lushbaugh[2] tabulated 25 accidents that occurred between 1945 and 1968 and involved 94 persons, 29 with serious injuries, and 12 fatalities.

An industrial worker in Rockford, Illinois, in 1965 received the very high exposure of 29,000 rad to the right ankle and 42,000 rad to the right hand, with less than 5 rad to the interior of the body.[3] No acute radiation sickness followed, but within six months after the accident, above-the-knee and above-the-elbow amputations were necessary for the two extremities. Gangrenous extremities occurred in three of the earlier criticality accident victims. Two of them died early, however, 30 and 9 days after exposure, and no definitive management for the local injury could be undertaken.[1]

The victims of two most recent American criticality accidents (in Los Alamos and Rhode Island) succumbed within 33 and 49 hr with extravascular edema and impaired cardiac function after severe total-body irradiation.[1]

From this review it becomes apparent that in most of the accidents either local or systemic injury clearly predominated, but one of our patients exhibited not only symptoms of the acute radiation syndrome but also severe local injury to the arms and legs bilaterally.

Description of Accident

On 4 October 1967, three technicians were simultaneously accidentally exposed to whole-body radiation from a Van de Graaff linear accelerator. This three-story accelerator was shielded by a concrete wall and generated electrons down a tube at a target of gold, where a steady stream of X-rays was produced. These X-rays were beamed to a secondary beryllium target and converted to neutrons, which irradiated petroleum samples for various analyses.

The water cooling system failed on this Van de Graaff, and the men were called to repair the cooling system. They unlatched the control panel, removed a key from the private vault, unlocked the safety tunnel door, and finally opened the inside door to the target room. Each and every one of the four maneuvers was designed to automatically shut down the accelerator. These men were not aware that the safety interlock system had failed.

Patient C worked to replace the coil for 20 min. His hands and feet were in line of the X-ray beam. Worker B handed him tools from about 1 foot behind. Man A had excused himself after a few minutes to make a trip to the men's room while C and B finished the work. Fortunately for these men, the beryllium target was rotated away from the line of the

X-ray beam, and so they were not exposed to any significant neutron exposure.

When the patients presented their early symptoms to the medical department, the assessment of the magnitude of the problem required two immediate evaluations: (1) as precise confirmation as possible about the physical facts of the radiation exposure, i.e., measurement of the dose received by the patients, and (2) the clinical evaluation of the magnitude and extent of the injury as promptly and completely as possible in order to render the appropriate clinical management.

To make the first evaluation, Dr. Neil Wald,[4] who at that time was director of the University of Pittsburgh's Radiological Health Division, conducted dosimetry tests in the target room with a tissue-equivalent plastic phantom loaded with film badges and thermoluminescent dosimeters. These tests indicated that patient A, age 31, received in the neighborhood of 100 rad; patient B, age 29, 300 rad; and patient C, age 40, 600 rad to the whole body. In addition, patient C sustained exposure of about 5900 rad to the hands and 2700 rad to the feet for approximately 20 min.

Clinical Observations and Treatment

The accident occurred at approximately 9:00 A.M., and 45 min later, C reported to the medical department complaining of nausea, vomiting, and generalized muscular aches. The nurse in the medical department was not particularly disturbed at first, since there was a mild flu epidemic at that time and she had seen several other people presenting similar symptoms that morning. She gave him Compazine with improvement in symptoms. However, when B also became nauseated and presented himself with similar symptoms, there was an immediate suspicion of radiation exposure in view of the knowledge that they were working on the accelerator. Their film badges were immediately checked, and the reports indicated that they had been exposed to large doses of radiation.

They were admitted to The Western Pennsylvania Hospital in Pittsburgh, Pennsylvania, and placed in reverse isolation in an area with laminar-flow filters to reduce the environmental contamination. Our concern was the prevention and treatment of infections and/or hemorrhages as sequelae of agranulocytosis and thrombocytopenia resulting from damage to the hemopoietic system and bone marrow suppression.

Numerous experts in the field of radiation were consulted as the need dictated. Dr. Gould Andrews, who at the time was chairman of the Medical and Health Sciences Division, Oak Ridge Associated Universities, at Oak Ridge, Tennessee, took an active part in the care and treatment of these cases. Drs. Abraham Broude and Kenneth Brown, from the Infectious Disease Department of the University of Pittsburgh, worked diligently in the management of the antibiotic therapy. Studies of the microbial flora of the nose, throat, skin, urine, and stool specimens were done by Drs. Ed Balish and Ted A. Pearson.

Heavy antibiotic therapy was used in the two high-dose patients consisting of Oxacillin, Neomycin, Streptomycin, and Mystatin orally and triple antibiotic ointment (Polymyxin, Neomycin, and Bacitracin) locally in the nares.[5] All urine cultures were negative for a 90-day period post exposure. In the entire period, not one of the three men developed septicemia. The only serious infection was in gangrenous tissue in patient C.

Patient A, with the least amount of exposure, had very few clinical symptoms. He developed diarrhea the day after exposure. His bowels moved three times and were loose, but no blood was noted, and he felt as if he had the flu. The third day he felt as though he had a hangover without a headache, and on the fourth day he was completely asymptomatic. His clinical course was rather uneventful. He had two episodes of mild pharyngitis, and throat cultures revealed alpha streptococci and diphtheroids. His hemopoietic picture did not change very much and reverted back to normal much sooner than the other two men. His hemopoietic profile revealed the lowest WBC count of his clinical course to be 4400/cc with 75% polymorphonuclear leukocytes, 17% lymphocytes, 4% monocytes, 2% eosinophils, and 2% metamyelocytes on 14 October 1967. From then on his white count gradually rose to normal levels. The platelet count was 270,000/cc, and the reticulocyte count was 0.5%. He was released from reverse isolation on 21 October 1967. His bone marrow showed very little suppression.

Patient B, with roughly 300 rad exposure, felt nauseated, continued to vomit, and required intravenous feedings for several days. His hemopoietic picture changed more dramatically. His WBC started to drop rapidly about the fifth day and reached the nadir on 4 November 1967, with an absolute count of 520 WBC/cc. The platelet count lagged a little behind to about the tenth day and reached bottom on 1 November 1967, with a reading of 3000/cc.

We felt that we were faced with a critical situation, and after considerable discussion with the consultants, he was given a platelet transfusion on 4 November 1967. His bone marrow began to show evidence of improvement the next day and continued on the upgrade. He was removed from isolation on 16 November 1967. Since this patient did not have an identical twin, we were considering the possibility of giving him an allogenic bone marrow graft. His siblings were typed by Dr. Bernard Amos in the event that we had to do so. Other considerations were administering an infusion of leukocytes from a chronic myelogenous leukemia donor and the possibility of a cross circulation as a last resort to provide him with a large number of granulocytes.

In patient C, the clinical course was much more complicated and was unique in that he had an identical twin brother. He had suffered not only much more severe general-body radiation, but also extensive local exposure to the hands and feet, since he had his hands directly under the radiation beam for approximately 20 min. He developed hematological evidence of severe hemopoietic injury. The nadir was reached about the 20th postaccident day with absolute counts of 870 WBC/mm³ and 24,000 platelets/mm³. His bone marrow was completely depleted, and he developed a pancytopenia.

Dr. E. Donnal Thomas was consulted early, and he and his team performed an isogenic bone-marrow transplant on the eighth postirradiation day; the patient's twin brother served as the donor. The marrow ordinarily regenerates between 10 and 15 days after the transplant.[6] On the 15th day, we were getting a little concerned because there was no peripheral evidence of regeneration, and debated whether another graft should be attempted. However, we waited a few days longer on the recommendation of Dr. Thomas, and eventually there was evidence of repopulation of the marrow. He was removed from reverse isolation on 16 November 1967.

About the 17th day after exposure, epilation started in the patient and progressed to complete loss of hair from extremities, scalp, and beard. In January 1968, hair was beginning to grow back on the scalp. However, hair on the arms and legs never regrew.

The dermatological and local changes were difficult to resolve, and the main surgical concern was the treatment of the local effects of the radiation exposure to all four extremities. Mild erythema of the fingers and hands developed one day after the accident and subsided over the next five days, to recur on the tenth postaccident day. The erythema was associated with tenderness, warmth, and slight edema. A febrile course began and continued over the next two months. During this time there was a steady progression from erythema to bullae formation (day 10), to complete superficial desquamation of the fingers (day 32), ending in *Pseudomonas* and *Pyocyaneus* infections and gangrene. At a somewhat slower progression, petechiae in the dorsum of the feet and legs progressed to bullae and again extensive loss of epidermis.

The management of the local injury was one of optimism. We were following the recommendation and procedures advocated by many reports in the surgical literature, which basically were conservative treatment, avoidance of amputation, subsequent removal of the involved skin, and eventually resurfacing the areas with free skin grafts.[7] Most of the reports in the literature dealt with accidents involving lower dose levels and with a somewhat less penetrating field to the extremities, and information which might have been helpful in this situation was not available.

We expected ultimate healing under thorough, successive topical regimens of Burow's solution, lanolin cream, silver nitrate soaks, and antibiotic and corticosteroid ointments under the direction of the dermatologists. Four months after the injury, it became evident that standard dermatological therapy was ineffective and that surgical removal of the dead tissue was necessary.

Following each of the early procedures, the amputation sites manifested lack of healing and further necrosis. Eleven separate operative sessions, some combining revisions of more than one extremity, were performed throughout a 22-month period following the injury. The four-month delay in instituting the first of many operative procedures was partly because of the insidious onset and progression of the pathological condition or radiation necrosis. We also wanted to keep surgical treatment at a minimum until hemopoietic recovery had occurred.

Some of the delay was because of other factors: optimism about topical therapy in treating the superficial, visible epidermal changes while hoping for revascularization; obeying standard surgical rules to amputate only when accurate demarcation of nonviable tissue has occurred and preserve as much length as possible for better function; and the patient was unwilling to accept amputation at that time.[7] This conservatism might have been justified in dealing with trauma cases where one digit and portion of a thumb might have provided good opposition and function. In this severe injury, however, the underlying pathological process[8,9] of diffuse obliterative endarteritis, with resultant ischemia, necrosis, and infection, certainly could not have been reversed by any amount of or duration of topical therapy, despite clean granulation tissue in the early stages, because the accident involved high-energy X-rays in a large dose and a highly penetrating exposure in a short period of time.

Although obedience to the standard rules was desirable in order to try to preserve useful digits and two legs intact to below the knee, the multiple procedures necessary at a gradually ascending level, coupled with poor healing and prolonged morbidity, speak for themselves.

In retrospect we would recommend much earlier amputation at a definitive level, within two or three months after exposure. Earlier operation would have had several advantages: a decrease in infection, probably a shorter period of severe pain and reduction in pain medication, possibly a reduction in hospital stay, and earlier rehabilitation.

Correlation of dosimetry information with clinical observation aids in determining the correct level for amputation. It should be pointed out that the time of onset of tissue injury is directly related to the dose. In general, the higher the dose, the sooner the signs of injury will occur.

The early erythema and especially the bleb formation did give a demarcation of nonviable tissue corresponding to areas of later skin discoloration and final ulceration. Epilation occurred over the entire body and therefore was not a satisfactory guideline.[7] This man eventually was sent to Rusk Institute in New York for rehabilitation and was fitted with prostheses on all extremities.

The gonadal changes on all of the men were monitored by Dr. C. Alvin Paulsen, from the University of Washington, who did both sperm counts and testosterone monitoring. There was no change in testosterone production, but there was complete azoospermia in all three patients. These studies indicated that it took 400 days before patient A fully recovered, patient B approximately 600 days, and patient C 700 days (C. A. Paulsen, personal communication). There is a linear relationship between the degree of exposure and duration of azoospermia.

Follow-up Clinical Picture

These men have been followed carefully since the accident. Patients A and B returned to work at the Research Center in jobs that do not expose them to any form of radiation. Periodic laboratory studies to check on their hematological profile have been done.

Patient A has been back to work at the Gulf Research Laboratories since 9 January 1968, doing chemical analyses, and has not been in areas where radiation is present as far as his work is concerned. He has been feeling well except for occasional gastric distress, which he attributes to a peptic ulcer that he claims was present before his radiation exposure. He takes antacids with immediate relief of the slight gastric symptoms. He has refused G.I. series fearing additional radiation exposure, since the gastric symptoms are not severe.

He has a history of having had eye trouble with his left eye, and a small epidermal inclusion cyst of the left conjunctiva was removed on 23 June 1976. He was examined by an ophthalmologist on 30 August 1979, and it was reported that he has dryness of his tear ducts that would require chemical assistance.

His entire physical examination on 4 September 1979 was entirely negative. There were no palpable nodes. The thyroid was normal to palpation. The spleen and liver were normal to palpation. His heart revealed no abnormalities. Chest, abdomen, extremities, and neurological examination were entirely negative. The laboratory studies, which included SMA 12, were normal. Thyroid uptake and scan performed on 23 and 24 August 1979 were normal. Sperm count done on 21 August 1979 was normal. His CBC has been done every three months and has been normal with a normal white count and differential and normal platelet count. The latest bone marrow study, done on 21 August 1979, revealed a normal marrow with normal cellular elements. An X-ray of the chest, taken on 21 August 1979, was normal.

One interesting feature regarding this man is that his wife gave birth to a female child on 28 December 1970. The child is entirely normal and healthy except that she had an ocular muscular defect, which required corrective surgery. The ophthalmologist stated that this is a rather common birth defect and probably was not genetically related to the father's radiation exposure.

Patient B, exposed to 300 rad, returned to work on 4 March 1968. He was doing well until about the middle of November in 1969, when he started to complain of weakness and fatigue, tremulousness, and slight weight loss. He was followed by an internist, and all lab work, including thyroid and adrenocortical tests, was normal. The internist at first felt the symptoms were because of apprehension and anxiety, and placed him on Librium, with no improvement in four to six weeks. Lab studies were repeated on 8 January 1970, and there was a slight elevation of the PBI (8.6 mg %).

On 8 January 1970, a repeat PBI was 11 mg %, and MPI was also elevated. He was seen by an endocrinologist and after serious consideration was placed on propylthiouracil and Luminal and was followed with weekly blood studies. He was continued on propylthiouracil until 10 March 1971, at which time the medication was stopped, and was symptom-free from the thyroid problems and in euthyroid state.

In May 1974, he first suffered an epileptic seizure one morning about 6:00 A.M., which was observed by his wife. He had gone to bed feeling well the night before, and as far as could be determined there were no contributing circumstances. He does not drink alcoholic beverages and had not been on any medication. All laboratory studies at this time were normal.

On 16 August 1974, he was admitted to The Western Pennsylvania Hospital because of a grand mal seizure with tonic and clonic movements but no incontinence. His electroencephalogram on that admission was abnormal with diffuse dysarrhythmia. A diagnosis of seizure disorder, "probably idiopathic epilepsy," was made by the neurologist who has been following him. He was placed on Dilantin 100 mg daily and has been well controlled on this regimen.

All other laboratory studies were normal. His blood counts, including WBC and differential, were normal. A 5-hr glucose tolerance curve was normal. His electrocardiogram was normal. He was examined on 4 September 1979, and he stated that he feels fine. He has lost very little time from work. He also had no palpable nodes. The liver and spleen were not enlarged.

The neurological examination was also negative. His laboratory studies, which included SMA 12, were all within normal limits. His CBC and differential and WBC and differential were normal. His bone marrow studies were normal. Thyroid scan and uptake were normal. His sperm count was normal. The electroencephalogram at this time revealed abnormal spike waves and poly spike discharges occurring randomly on either side, consistent with interseizure electroencephalogram tracing. It did not reveal any features suggesting localization or focus. His brain scan was reported as normal dynamic and static brain scan. His eyes were examined in June 1979, and there were no significant findings.

Patient C, the man with the greatest whole-body exposure and severe local burns to the hands and feet, is still alive. Soon after his discharge from the hospital he showed signs of diabetes mellitus. His fasting blood sugars were persistently elevated, and he was placed on a dietary regimen and 40 units of NPH insulin daily.

He has been the most difficult of the three to treat because of his mental attitude. He seems to be more difficult to reason with and understandably so—I'm sure that it's because of the mental trauma resulting from his handicap. (The other two patients have not displayed the personality changes that this man has shown. I have suggested psychological evaluation, but they have not seemed receptive to the idea.)

In April 1974, patient C developed a bilateral chronic suppurative otitis media with active drainage in the right ear. Cultures from the ears revealed *Pseudomonas* organisms, and he was treated by an otologist with appropriate antibiotics. Audiological examination at that time revealed a mild to moderately severe mid- and high-frequency mixed hearing loss.

On 22 March 1976, he was readmitted to The Western Pennsylvania Hospital with chest pains, which developed in the middle of the afternoon before admission. Enzyme levels were abnormal, and electrocardiograms showed gradual evolution of an anterior wall myocardial infarction. He was treated and discharged on 9 April 1976. Since that time he has been doing relatively well. He is still on 40 units of NPH insulin daily. However, it has been very difficult to control his highly elevated triglycerides (379 mg %) and type IV hyperlipoproteinemia. His wife stated that he does not follow his dietary regimen.

His most recent laboratory studies revealed a normal CBC, WBC, and differential. His platelet count was normal. His bone marrow studies revealed a normal marrow. His thyroid uptake with iodine 123 was normal; however, the scan revealed uneven distribution of activity throughout the gland and both lobes irregular in contour. No discrete nodules were evident. His triglycerides were 360 mg % and fasting blood sugar 75 mg %. His electrocardiogram on 31 August 1979 revealed changes consistent with an old inferior wall myocardial infarction. An X-ray of the chest, taken on 28 August 1979, was within normal limits.

Ophthalmological examination on September 1, 1979, revealed bilateral mild lens opacity, not interfering with vision.

Evaluation of his physical capabilities shows that he is using his prostheses rather well. He has hooks on both upper extremities and is able to feed himself, shave, and maneuver a wheelchair. He has become involved in local politics and has served as commissioner of his township and shown considerable interest in the local civic problems.

References

1. Andrews GA, Balish E, Edwards CL: Possibilities for improved treatment of persons exposed in radiation accidents, read before the Symposium on Handling of Radiation Accidents, Vienna, International Atomic Energy Agency, World Health Organization, 1969.

2. Lushbaugh CC: Reflections on some recent progress in human radiobiology, in Augenstein LG, Mason R, Zelle M (eds.): *Advances in Radiation Biology.* New York, Academic Press Inc., 1969, vol. 3, pp. 277–310.

3. Lanzl LH, Rozenfeld ML: Injury due to accidental high-dose exposure to 10 MeV electrons. *Health Phys* 13:241–251, 1967.

4. Wald N: Dosimetry and management planning, read before the Symposium on Acute Radiation Syndrome, Western Pennsylvania Hospital, Pittsburgh, Pennsylvania, 1968.

5. Balish E, Pearson TA: Studies on the microflora of three men accidentally exposed to total-body irradiation.

6. Thomas ED: Bone marrow transplant and administration of selected blood products, read before the Symposium on Acute Radiation Syndrome, Western Pennsylvania Hospital, Pittsburgh, Pennsylvania, 1968.

7. Schenck R, Gilberti MV: Four extremity radiation necroses. *Arch Surg,* 100:1970.

8. Rubin P, Casarett GW: *Clinical Radiation Pathology.* Philadelphia, W. B. Saunders Company, 1968, vol. 1, pp. 62–119.

9. Wohlbach SB: The pathological histology of chronic X-ray dermatitis and early carcinoma. *J Med Res* 21:415–449, 1909.

The University of Tennessee Comparative Animal Research Laboratory Accident in 1971

Helen Vodopick* and Gould A. Andrews[+]

*Oak Ridge Medical Clinic, P.C., Oak Ridge, Tennessee;
[+]Department of Nuclear Medicine, University of Maryland Hospital,
Baltimore, Maryland.

The nuclear industry, although in its infancy of development, is one of the safest and most regulated industries today. In spite of these many checks and balances, accidents still occur. One such accident involving an essentially whole-body exposure at a high dose rate was previously reported,[1] and now 8.5 years post exposure, follow-up data are given.

Radiation Accident in 1971

On 4 February 1971, a 32-year-old research technologist and a senior control operator were performing seed irradiation experiments in the Variable Dose Rate Irradiation Facility (VDRIF) at the University of Tennessee Comparative Animal Research Laboratory (CARL). Description of this facility is given elsewhere.[2] A series of experiments had been completed earlier that morning. At approximately 11:30 A.M. the research technologist and the control operator discussed the sequence in which further samples would be irradiated. At the end of this discussion, the technologist, who presumed the previous irradiation had ended, proceeded to the irradiation room to remove the set of seeds and replace them with another. He was positioned 50 cm in front of an unshielded 7700-curie cobalt 60 source for an estimated 40 sec. During this time he positioned the sample vials in a holder located 17 cm in front of the source, where the exposure rate was 2500 R/min. He did not notice the source was out of its shield. As the technologist left the radiation room and entered the control room, the operator, who had been unaware of the technologist's movements, looked at the control panel and realized the ^{60}Co source had been exposed while the technologist was in the room. The exact amount of radiation exposure was not known until the thermoluminescent personnel dosimeter worn at the technologist's waist was returned 28 hr later and indicated his whole-body exposure was 260 R, with the right hand receiving an estimated 1200 R. Studies later carried out with an Anderson Rando phantom gave more information on the dose distribution. More detail on this study can be found in a previous publication.[3] This dosimeter worn by the technologist was used as the most accurate measure of his exposure. When the dose distribution studies were carried out on the phantom, these values were normalized to the dosimeter value (Table 1). The radiation distribution was uneven because of the position of the source and the patient (Figure 1). Average midline dose to the torso was estimated to be 127 rad, and to the marrow, 118 rad.

The exposed man was brought by car to the Oak Ridge Associated Universities (ORAU) Medical Division 1 hr after his exposure. When first examined, 2 hr after the accident, the patient appeared apprehensive but not acutely ill. Physical examination revealed no abnormality. His hand showed no redness, swelling, or tenderness. However, episodes of sudden vomiting not preceded by nausea occurred 2.25 hr post exposure and recurred ten times during the next 24 hr. Diarrhea and fever were not present.

After 24 hr, he complained of burning and itching of his eyes. Some conjunctival redness, not present on admission, remained for 24 hr but cleared spontaneously. Later examination by an ophthalmologist revealed no pathologic changes. To avoid nosocomial infection he was allowed to go home on the seventh day. He returned daily for blood counts and exercise test. When his blood counts began to fall, he was readmitted to

Table 1. Estimates of Dose to Organ Based on Reconstruction of Accident and Phantom Dosimetry

Organ	Average dose rate (rad/min)	Dose in 40 sec [a] (rad)	Dose normalized to patient's badge (rad)
Bone marrow	157	105	118
Intestines	220	147	166
Kidneys	137	91	103
Lenses of eyes	206	137	155
Spleen	153	102	115
Stomach	217	145	163
Midline	169	113	127

[a] Patient's exposure time estimated as 40 sec.

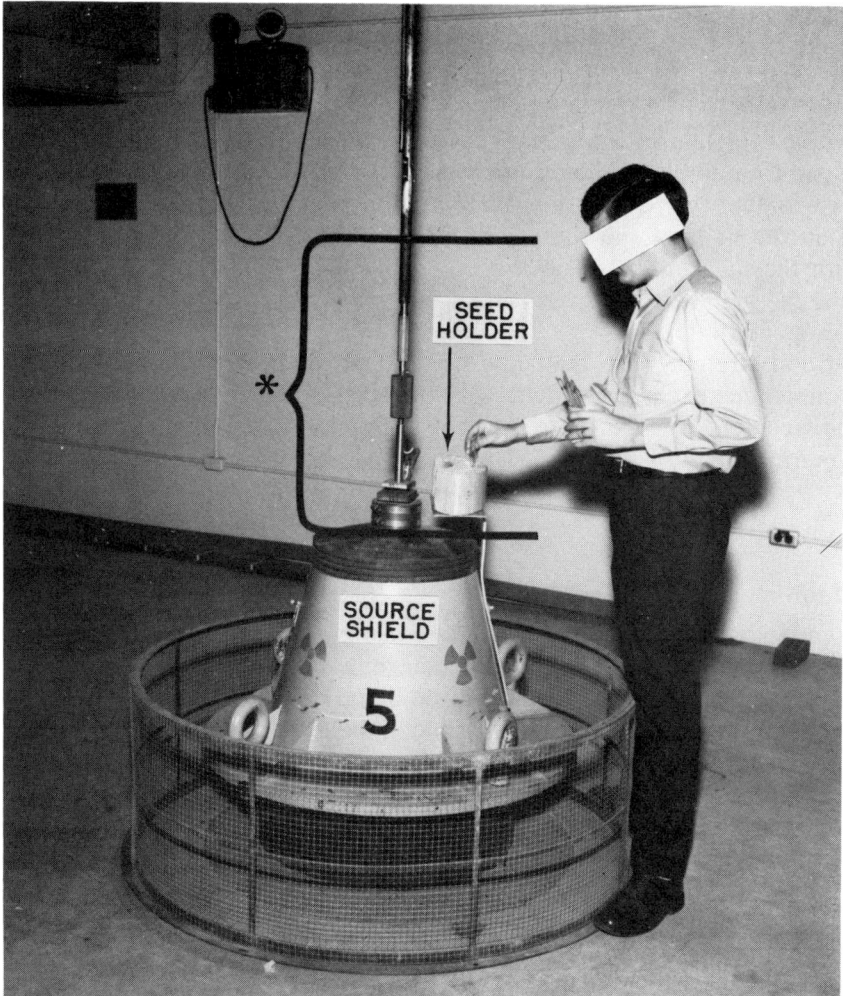

Figure 1. Illustration showing position of unshielded source in relation to the accident victim (simulated picture). The area bracketed * in the picture indicates the ⁶⁰Co source when it is out of its shield.

the laminar air-flow unit to reduce his exposure to infection. No prophylactic antibiotics or transfusions were given.

During maximum hematological depression, from day 24 to 34 post exposure, the patient remained well. On day 36 a mouth infection diagnosed as Vincent's angina was treated with orally administered penicillin and hydrogen peroxide mouth washes. On day 48, all his blood counts had returned to normal. He was then discharged to be followed as an outpatient.

Three days after his exposure, his right hand, which received more irradiation than any other part of his body, began to hurt intermittently, especially after use. Occasionally the pain would awaken him from sleep. There were no objective findings of radiation damage, such as hair loss, swelling, or temperature change. Radial pulses were easily palpable and of good quality. No ulcerations developed. However, four months after the accident the patient noted a faint white horizontal line in the midpart of all the nails of the right hand only. These lines eventually grew out with the nail and were no longer visible after six more weeks. At this time the pain subsided, but it recurred some months later and eventually disappeared.

Soon after the accident, and continuing for four months, the patient experienced excessive fatigue with the least exertion. Eleven weeks after the accident he was able to return to work in an area free of any abnormal level of radiation.

Laboratory Values

Methods

Hematologic studies were performed using these technics: cyanmethemoglobin method for hemoglobin determination;[4] Wintrobe hematocrit tubes for measurement of packed red blood cell volume;[5] electronic cell counting in triplicate for white blood cell number, Brecher-Cronkite method for platelet enumeration.[6] Two hundred white blood cells were counted on each Wright stained blood smear. Oliver's method was used for creatine phosphokinase[7] and Goodwin's method for iron determination.[8]

Results

The initial white blood cell (WBC) changes were consistent with a recent radiation exposure (Figure 2). When the patient's blood count 2 hr post exposure was compared to his preemployment blood count, no difference was found. By 4 hr a definite change had occurred. The total WBC count had risen to $15,800/mm^3$, and the absolute lymphocyte count had dropped from $2840/mm^3$ to $948/mm^3$. At 12 hr the total WBC count had returned to the value found at admission. The absolute lymphocyte count, except for a slight rise at 16.5 hr, remained about $1000/mm^3$ for four weeks following his exposure. Nadir of the WBC count occurred on day 36 and was followed by spontaneous recovery.

Platelet count depression beginning on day 14 reached nadir on day 29, with the lowest platelet count being $37,000/mm^3$. Spontaneous bleeding did not develop. Recovery of platelet count followed a pattern expected after such an irradiation exposure.

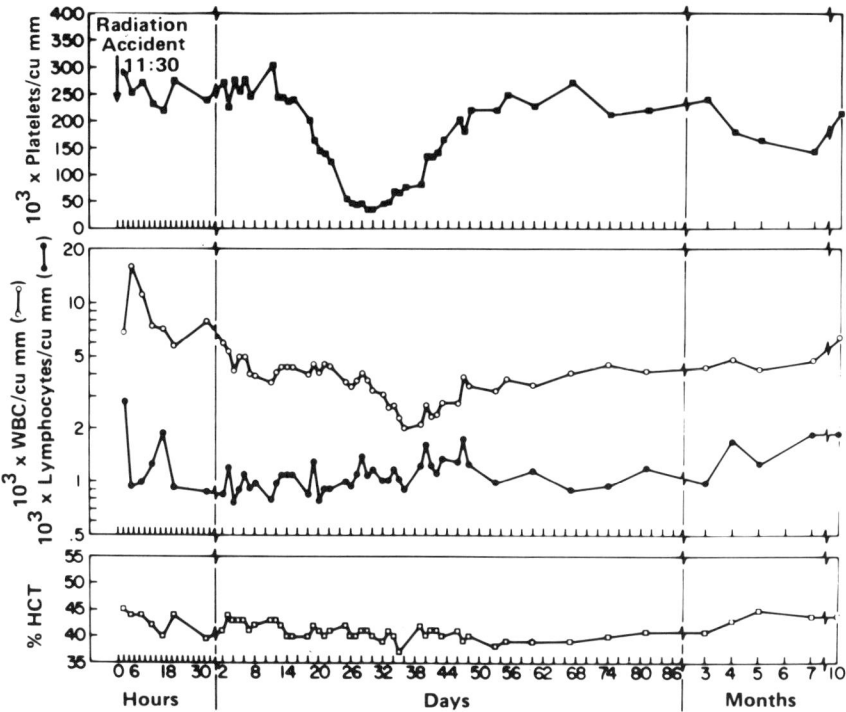

Figure 2. Hematologic changes of patient accidentally irradiated with 250 R at a high dose rate.

Sternal marrow aspirates were performed at 29 hr, 5 days, and 19 days post exposure. Initial marrow revealed normocellularity with some me-galoblastic changes of the erythroid series and with a myeloid:erythroid (M:E) ratio of 4.8. The second marrow was hypocellular with an M:E ratio of 5. Mature granulocytes were hypersegmented. The last marrow examined, on day 19, was moderately hypercellular with slight erythroid hyperplasia (M:E ratio of 1.1).

Cytogenetic analysis of the marrow was done on each of the specimens obtained.[9] On the first aspirate, abnormalities in 70% of the metaphases were noted; chromatid breaks were the most frequent finding. Because of hypocellularity on the second aspirate (day 5), cytogenetic analysis was not possible. The last cytogenetic preparation, on day 19, showed only one dicentric chromosome in the 100 metaphases counted.

Serum iron on admission was slightly above normal range, 180 μg/dl, and rose to 310 μg/dl on day 5. By day 12, serum iron had fallen to 170 μg/dl (Figure 3). These changes were felt to be due to decreased utilization of iron by erythroid precursors in the marrow damaged or

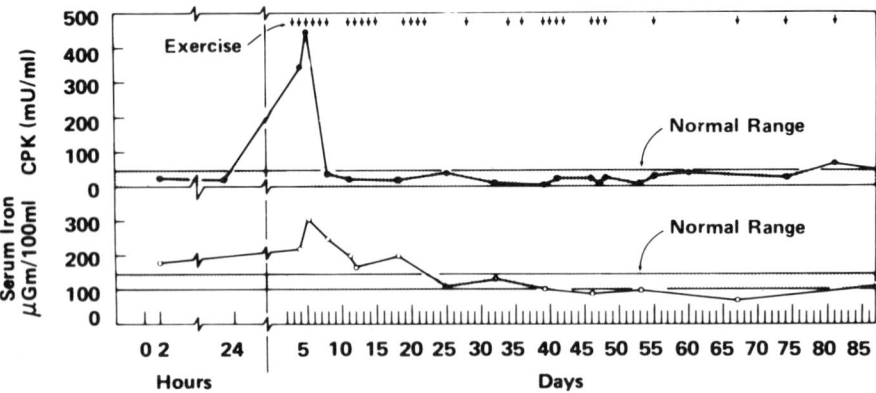

Figure 3. The serum CPK value rose to nine times normal values and serum iron doubled on the fifth day post irradiation. The possible meaning of these abnormalities is discussed in the text.

arrested by the radiation. With restoration of marrow production the serum iron returned to normal.

Semen examination was done 6 and 14 months post exposure. Low concentration of sperm (2.3 million/mm³) on the first specimen and normal concentration (77 million/mm³) on the second specimen were found. Slight morphological abnormality was detected only in the first specimen.

Exercise tolerance was measured by means of an ergometer on a stationary bicycle with varying work loads. Exercising was begun on day 3 and was measured periodically well beyond his recovery. Definite changes in his serum creatine phosphokinase (CPK) level occurred (Figure 3). At the time of admission his CPK was normal, 25 milliunits/ml, but on days 4 and 5, the CPK level rose to 343 and 455 milliunits/ml respectively. In three more days, the CPK had returned to normal. In humans, abnormal elevation of CPK, an enzyme found in skeletal muscle, cardiac muscle, liver, and red blood cells, occurs only after some damage to these tissues. Injury permits the enzyme to leak out of the cell. With increased stress produced by the exercise, the release of CPK may have been accelerated. Whether this elevated enzyme level produced any symptoms is uncertain, but it may have some bearing on excessive fatigue experienced by this patient and other radiation accident victims.

Cause of the Accident

Once it was established that a radiation accident had occurred, investigation was immediately begun to determine its cause.[10] The irradiation facility consisted of a control room separated from the irradiation room by a maze, this passageway having an entrance door from the control room and an exit doorway into the irradiation room. Red warning lights activated by initiation of an irradiation program were positioned over each of these doors, one within the irradiation room itself. Three sodium iodide radiation detectors were located in the control room. Measures had been taken to ensure that no one could enter the irradiation room when any of the sources were out of their shields. An electric lock system on the door of the maze was activated when any of the radiation sources were unshielded. If the door was opened during an irradiation, the sources automatically returned to their shielded container. In the irradiation room was a television camera equipped with scan and zoom controls which allowed visual monitoring in the control room. An audible warning horn sounded in the irradiation room for 75 sec before initiating a program.

Several malfunctions in equipment were discovered by the investigating team: (1) the red warning light in the irradiation room was inoperable, but the other red flashing light was operating properly; (2) incomplete closing of the maze door resulted in failure of the electric lock to prevent entry; (3) the door limit switch had been tied in a closed position several days before the accident; (4) the maze door limit switch did not automatically cause the source to be lowered when the door was opened. Operational errors were also found: established procedures were not followed, and the technologist did not observe the radiation monitors, which were functioning properly in the control room, the flashing red light over the control room maze door, and the raised source in the irradiation room.

Modifications were made after the accident to prevent a repeat occurrence. Most important was the formal training and testing procedure for the facility operators and technologists. More stringent radiation safety and maintenance checks were made. All limit switches were bolted firmly in place. Electric door locks were replaced with a prison-type lock, which could not be opened unless all sources were in their shielded position and an "open" button on the console had been pushed. Additional red warning lights were installed in the control room and maze. A new indicator of source position replaced the old digital indicator on the control panel.

Follow-up Data

The patient, now 40 years old, has been in good health. He has required no medical care or routine medications. He experienced what he described as "weak spells," rarely more than twice monthly. These feelings of generalized weakness lasted for 2 to 3 hr and subsided with rest. They have caused no incapacitation nor any work loss. In spite of good physical strength, he still has intermittent problems with his right hand.

He felt that occasionally his dexterity with fine movement was impaired. Some intermittent pain in the middle and ring fingers was not relieved by cracking his knuckles. Firmly grasping objects occasionally produced pain in the index finger. Objective signs of any abnormality were absent. All nails were healthy and without abnormal marks.

Although he wears glasses, he has had no visual problems. Recent examination by an ophthalmologist revealed some presbyopia and far-sightedness but no cataract formation. No change in thyroid size or contour was detected on recent physical examination.

Primarily because of the patient's and his wife's fear of radiation-induced congenital defects, conception was intentionally delayed for seven years. A second healthy daughter without any physical defects was born in April 1979. An older daughter had been conceived one month prior to the 1971 accident.

The laboratory studies done in July 1979 were all normal, including a complete blood cell count, WBC differential count, urinalysis, multi-chemistry profile, and thyroid profile. The patient has made a good adjustment and exhibits no preoccupation regarding his accident.

Comments

The long-term sequelae following high-dose irradiation are partially known. Experience has been obtained from chronic or repeated exposure to local areas as well as from single high-dose total-body exposures. The induction of leukemia or cancer is the most serious result. The high incidence of leukemia in patients irradiated for ankylosing spondylitis, in radiologists of decades ago, and in the Hiroshima-Nagasaki survivors is well documented. But still unknown is the smallest dose necessary to induce the changes that lead to leukemia or cancer. Even small doses of superficial irradiation given for acne or for thymic enlargement have been linked to the induction of thyroid carcinoma. But only a small portion of the patients so irradiated develop cancer. Changes such as cataract formation, chronic ulcerations, and permanent sterility are not fatal but certainly can lead to various degrees of physical or psychological impairment.

In 8.5 years post irradiation this patient has exhibited no permanent adverse sequelae. The recent birth of a healthy, normal daughter negates the problem of permanent sterility or spermatic abnormality. He remains gainfully employed and is physically active. No psychological trauma is evident.

The nuclear industry is one of the safest industries in the United States. If human error and mechanical failure could be eliminated, it would become the safest industry in the world. Until these flaws are completely corrected, there will continue to be periodic accidents of varying magnitude. Ability to handle such accidents well depends on the continued training of qualified persons. With better training of personnel working with radiation and with better technology and more safeguards, the accident rate could be reduced to zero.

ACKNOWLEDGMENTS
The reproduction of the figures and Table 1 used in this article has been permitted by the American Medical Association, copyright 1974.

Kathryn Lore and Shirley Colyer performed the hematology determinations; R. Ricks, Ph.D., the physiological studies; L. Gayle Littlefield, Ph.D., the cytogenetic studies; Allen Webb, the chemistry determinations; J. MacLeod, Ph.D., the microscopic examination of the sperm morphology; and W. L. Beck, M.S., the phantom radiation dosimetry studies.

References

1. Vodopick H, Andrews GA: Accidental radiation exposure. *Arch Environ Health* 28:53–56, 1974.

2. Cheka JS, Robinson EM, Wade L, Jr. Gramly WA: The UT-AEC Agriculture Research Laboratory Variable Gamma Dose Rate Facility. *Health Phys* 20:339–343, 1971.

3. Beck WL, Stokes TR, Wade L, Jr: Dosimetry for a total-body irradiation accident (abstract). *Health Phys* 23:419, 1972.

4. Cartwright GE: *Diagnostic Laboratory Hematology*, ed. 3. New York, Grune & Stratton Inc., 1973, pp. 49–50.

5. Wintrobe MM: A simple and accurate hematocrit. *J Lab Clin Med* 15:287–289, 1929.

6 Brecher G, Cronkite EP: Morphology and enumeration of human blood platelets. *J Appl Physiol* 3:365–377, 1950.

7. Oliver IT: A spectrophotometric method for the determination of creatine phosphokinase and myokinase. *Biochem J* 61:116–122, 1955.

8. Goodwin JF, Murphy B, Buillemette M: Direct measurement of serum iron and binding capacity. *Clin Chem* 12:47–57, 1966.

9. Brewen JG, Preston RJ, Littlefield LG: Radiation-induced human chromosome aberration yields following an accidental whole-body exposure to ^{60}Co X-rays. *Radiat Res* 49:647–656, 1972.

10. Wade L, Jr: Accidental ^{60}Co exposure at the University of Tennessee–Atomic Energy Commission Agricultural Research Laboratory. *Nucl Safety* 13:304–308, 1972.

The New Jersey Radiation Accidents of 1974 and 1977

Flora M. Barlotta

St. Barnabas Medical Center, Livingston, New Jersey.

As our knowledge about pancytopenic patients with leukemia and aplastic anemia grows and as we advance our expertise in the component therapy of blood banking, the care of the radiation accident victim with severe bone marrow depression becomes less chaotic and, in most instances, can be carried out in a community hospital by clinical hematologists.

In 1974 and 1977, industrial radiation accidents occurred in plants using cobalt 60 sources for product sterilization. Both of these victims were admitted to the Saint Barnabas Medical Center in Livingston, New Jersey. I was responsible for the care of the 1977 case. Dr. James Hogan attended the first man, and he reported the case at Oak Ridge in 1975. Being clinical hematologists, we employed the principles of supportive care used with leukemia patients. Of course, both of the men presented here were healthy, nonimmunosuppressed individuals. What they had in common with a leukemic patient was a depressed bone marrow and pancytopenia. There was no associated organ failure or ongoing chemotherapy with which to contend.

Once their initial gastrointestinal symptoms subsided, there were few therapeutic efforts required until the severe granulocytopenia appeared. The predictable effect of external radiation on the bone marrow is well known, and the curves of our patients' serial blood counts match those of other reported cases.[1] The summaries of the two cases follow.

Case 1

A 61-year-old man was brought to the Saint Barnabas Medical Center emergency room on 13 June 1974, at 6:30 P.M., one-half hour after having had a 5–10 sec accidental exposure to a 120,000-curie cobalt 60 industrial source. The patient failed to use the survey meter and, thinking the cobalt source was "down," entered the hot cell. When he realized that the source was "up," he turned, exposing his left side, and walked out of the room. The exposure was not uniform, since part of the patient's body was shielded by two Teflon-filled fiber drums.

One hour after exposure the patient experienced nausea and headache and then vomited several times. Nausea remained for the next 18 hr. At the time of admission to the hospital (about 6 hr after the patient was brought to the emergency room), the physical examination revealed some scleral injection. The patient was alert and nontoxic. The vital signs were normal. The past medical history was that of a healthy man.

The blood count (5 hr after exposure) showed a white blood count (WBC) of 11,200/cc, an absolute lymphocyte count of 1568/cc, a platelet count of 177,000/cc, and a hemoglobin of 13.1 gm %. The serum electrolytes, total protein, hepatic and renal function tests, and urinalysis were normal. The absolute lymphocyte counts at 12 hr and 36 hr were 1027/cc and 500/cc, respectively. Figure 1 demonstrates the serial blood counts.

The patient was placed in a private room. Visitors were not allowed, and hospital personnel wore gowns, caps, masks, and gloves in the room. For 17 days the patient showed no untoward signs. He was apprehensive at times but functioned normally. Then, on day 18, epilation began on the head and then the trunk, arms, and left leg. Petechiae appeared on the trunk on day 25. On day 26, the WBC was 800/cc and the platelet count 8000/cc. Because the patient complained of dizziness and headache (hemoglobin 10.1 gm %), ten units of platelet concentrates were transfused. This was done again on postexposure days 28, 29, 30, 31, and 34. No sign of hemorrhage was noted. Bowel sterilization was begun on day 26.

The next day the patient had a temperature of 38.7°C and was toxic. Cultures of the blood, sputum, nose, throat, and urine were sterile. Intravenous methicillin and gentamicin were given. Ten units of leukocyte concentrates were transfused on days 29, 30, and 31. During this time the patient was extremely toxic and remained febrile. On day 29, methicillin was stopped, and carbenicillin and cephalothin were given. No elevation of the WBC occurred after the granulocyte transfusions.

A septic course prevailed until the 32nd postexposure day. Monocytes appeared in the peripheral blood smear. On day 28, the patient was afebrile, and the antibiotics were discontinued. Improvement continued, and on 27 July 1974 (day 45) the patient was discharged with a hemoglobin of 10.3 gm %, a platelet count of 370,000/cc, and a WBC of 5100/cc. His chief complaint at that time was weakness.

The patient was followed in the office. His blood count was totally normal by 24 October 1974. By November, he felt well enough to return

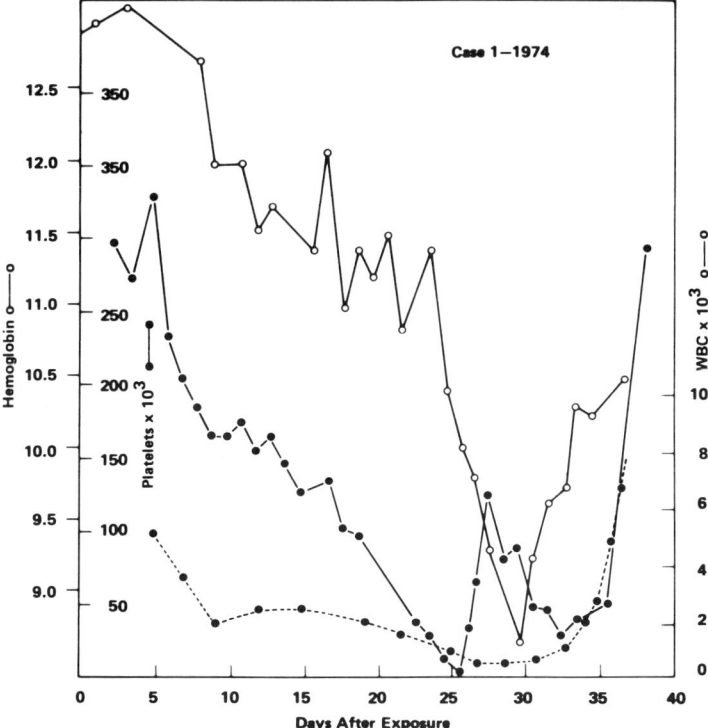

Figure 1. Serial blood counts, case 1.

to work. Jaundice was seen early in January, 1975, and liver function tests were indicative of hepatocellular dysfunction. The hepatitis associated antigen test was negative, but the liver biopsy was consistent with viral hepatitis. Recovery was uneventful. The patient has moved from New Jersey and has not responded to requests for follow-up information.

Case 2

A 32-year-old man was admitted to Saint Barnabas Medical Center 15 hr after having had an estimated ten seconds of exposure to a 500,000-curie cobalt 60 source. The accident occurred around midnight on 23 September 1977 at a New Jersey plant that uses radiation to sterilize medical and chemical products. The patient felt a tingling sensation on his arms as he began to work at a conveyor belt about 9 ft from the source. He left the area immediately after seeing that the source was out of its storage pool. Construction at the facility caused alterations of the hot-cell entry, the source-up warning sign was obscured from view, and the electrical interlock on the door was not in order. He was taken to a nearby emergency room but was discharged. About 2 hr after exposure, he went to the emergency room of another community hospital, where antiemetics were given because of nausea and vomiting. He was observed for an hour and a half, and when the gastrointestinal symptoms subsided, he was sent home. Neither facility performed any blood tests. Fifteen hours after the accident, he was admitted to our hospital at the suggestion of the plant supervisor.

A poor diet was the only remarkable feature of his medical history. The physical examination revealed scleral injection and mild facial erythema. The patient was afebrile and alert.

The admission hemoglobin was 16.1 gm %, the hematocrit 46.1%, and the WBC 5700/cc, with 83% polymorphs, 3% bands, 10% lymphocytes, and 4% monocytes. The platelet count was 299,000/cc, the reticulocyte count 0.8%, and the red blood cell morphology normal. Figure 2 demonstrates the serial blood counts.

The following determinations were normal at the time of admission: chemical profile, serum protein electrophoresis, immunoglobulin quantitation, B and T cell quantitation, T3 and T4, chest X-ray, and serum folic acid level. A bone marrow aspiration was performed on the day of

Figure 2. Serial blood counts, case 2. Supplied by the Metpath Laboratories, New Jersey.

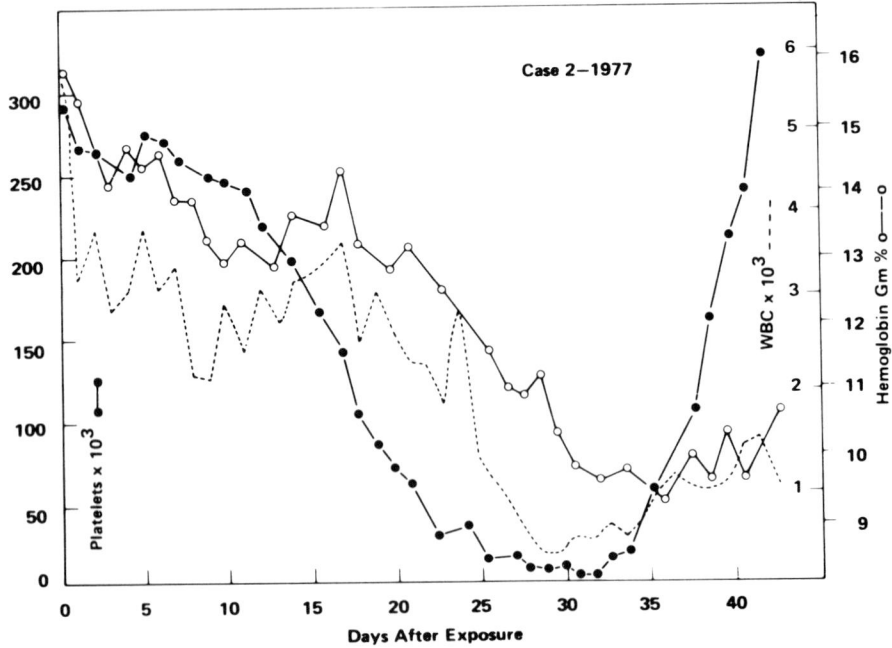

admission and, except for some nuclear cytoplasmic dissociation of the erythroid series, was normal. Since the physical dosimetry measurements had not yet been made, HLA typing was done in preparation for possible bone marrow transplantation.

The patient was placed in a private room, and modified reverse isolation was carried out. Hospital personnel and visitors (limited to the patient's parents) wore mask and gown when in the room and washed their hands before touching the patient. Daily skin cleaning with a "pre-op" plastic scrub brush was performed by the patient.

By reconstructing the event at the scene of the accident and with the use of chromosome aberration dosimetry, the radiation exposure estimate was between 200 and 225 rad, later adjusted to 200 rad. Film-badge dosimetry was calculated at 125 rad. This was lower because the badge was worn on the patient's right back hip pocket and his orientation toward the source was anterior. The exposure was not uniform, since the lower half of the body was shielded by metal drums in the work area.

The absolute lymphocyte count at 16 hr was 570/cc and at 47 hr, 790/cc. On the twelfth hospital day, bowel sterilization was attempted with oral cloxacillin and neomycin. On postexposure day 22, mild epilation from the head and beard occurred. (The patient had shoulder-length hair and a full beard, and the hair loss was not readily apparent.) The patient remained asymptomatic even though the white blood count fell to 400/cc with an absolute neutrophil count of 60/cc.

On day 32 (when the WBC was 600 and the absolute neutrophil count 54/cc), the patient developed chills and a temperature of 38.3°C. Physical examination revealed a hyperemic pharynx. Cultures of the throat, blood, and urine were obtained, and intravenous gentamicin, cephalothin, and carbenicillin were given. The platelet count was 7000/cc, having fallen below 100,000/cc on the 20th day. A few petechiae were seen on the legs, but no other bleeding was noted. All cultures were sterile, and the patient was afebrile in two days and remained so.

On day 37 a bone marrow aspiration showed hypocellularity with depressed granulopoiesis and megakaryocytes but good erythroid activity. The hemoglobin was at its nadir of 9.4 gm %, and the WBC was 1100/cc with 12% monocytes. On the 43rd postexposure day the patient continued to be asymptomatic and afebrile. Antibiotic therapy was discontinued. On day 44 the patient was discharged with a hemoglobin of 10.8 gm %, a WBC of 1200/cc, and a platelet count of 402,000/cc. No support with packed red blood cells, granulocytes, or platelet concentrates was necessary. A sperm count performed on day 24 was 17 million/cc (normal: 60–150 million/cc); the test was not repeated.

At the time of discharge the absolute granulocyte count was not yet considered adequate, but the patient would no longer remain confined in the hospital. He was seen in the outpatient department, and he demonstrated no untoward signs. The return of the WBC to normal levels took longer than is usual in radiation accidents. Since the patient's diet had been poor, folic acid supplements were given during the hospitalization, but this vitamin seemed to have had no effect. The prolonged leukopenia remains unexplained. Two months after the accident, his bone marrow was normal, and the hemoglobin was 13.8 gm %, the hematocrit 41.2%, the WBC 4500/cc with a normal differential count, and the platelet count 331,000/cc. He was last seen on 27 April 1978 and was well. There is no further information, since the patient has not responded to requests for a follow-up visit.

Discussion

Accurate dosimetry should be performed as quickly as possible, because if there is good evidence that the dose exceeded 400 rad and severe hemopoietic toxicity will result, a bone marrow transplant should be considered. Preparations for this procedure should take place early and not during the phase of the severe pancytopenia which occurs in the fourth week.

The dose estimates varied widely in the first case. The plant personnel and our physicist made estimates by reconstructing the events at the accident sites. Estimates by the film badge vendor were not accurate because of light contamination (case 1), the location of the badge on the victim (case 2), and uneven exposure (both cases). Chromosome aberration studies were done on both patients, and the results indicated severe damage. Dr. Wald estimated an exposure of about 410 rad for case 1 and between 200 and 225 rad for case 2. Figure 3 shows some of the chromosome abnormalities detected in case 2. All of the studies demonstrated significant numbers of rings, dicentrics, breaks, fragments, and translocations. Observation of the absolute lymphocyte count (total WBC times percent lymphocytes) during the first 48 hr gave a good estimate and indicated severe injury in both patients.

If a patient is a bone marrow transplant candidate, an appropriate facility is contacted and a suitable donor sought.[2] A patient who is not a transplant candidate should be sent to a hospital where adequate hematologic support can be given. Table 1 compares the clinical events of our cases. As you can see, nothing of significance happened during the first three weeks. One wonders if it is essential to have the radiation accident victim hospitalized for the first 15 days. Careful outpatient management would be of some economic importance if many people were injured in an accident.

Neither of our patients required red blood cell transfusions. No gross blood loss was noted. The bone marrows were severely depressed, but the decline of the red cell mass was gradual due to the relatively long life

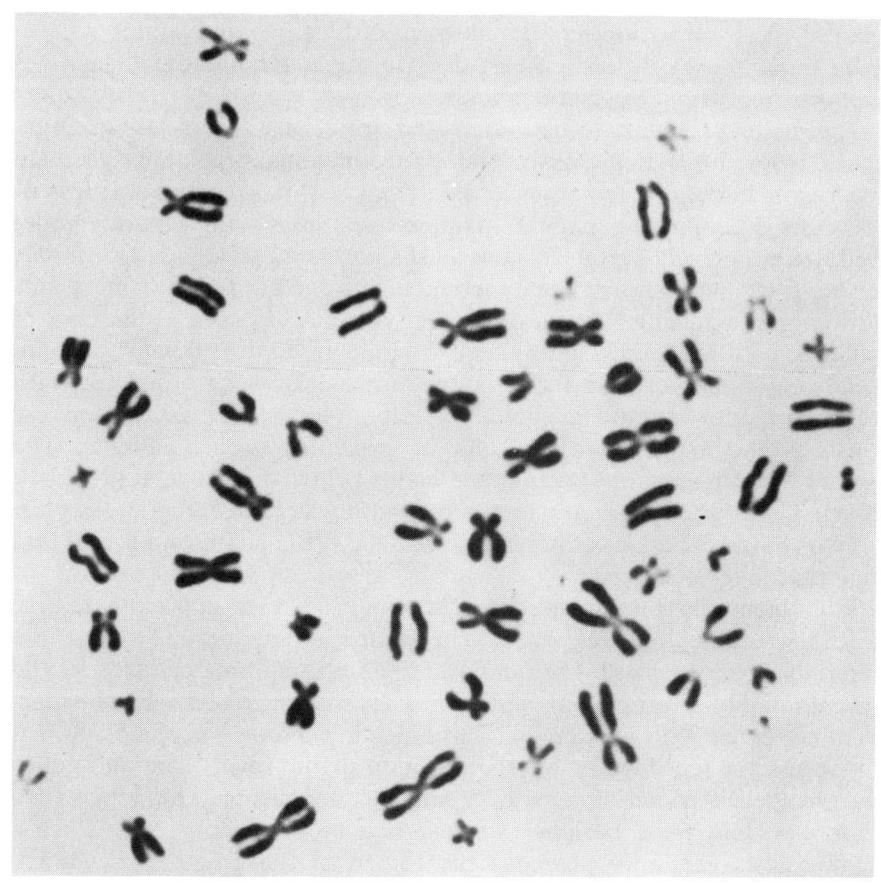

Figure 3. Chromosome aberrations, case 2.

Table 1. Postexposure Clinical Events

Case 1	Event	Case 2
Day 18	Epilation	Day 22
Day 20 <100,000	Thrombocytopenia	Day 20 <100,000
Day 26 (8000/mm^3)	Platelet nadir	Day 33 (7000/mm^3)
Day 25	Petechiae	Day 20
Day 28 (300/mm^3)	WBC nadir	Day 30 (400/mm^3)
Day 28 (for 7 days)	Fever	Day 32 (for 2 days)
Day 31	Initial monocytosis	Day 35
Day 30 (8.7 gm %)	Hemoglobin nadir	Day 37 (9.4 gm %)
9	No. of days WBC below 1000/mm^3	10

span of the erythrocyte and the absence of bleeding and hemolysis. An older patient with ischemic heart disease might require transfusions to support myocardial oxygen demands.

The major problems to be anticipated are sepsis and bleeding. Organisms from the patient's skin and gastrointestinal tract are the main sources of infection, and transmission from hospital personnel is less of a factor. Keeping the patient in a private room with separate toilet facilities is helpful. Certainly, face masks and hand washing are in order for the staff and visitors. The experience with the life island, laminar airflow rooms, and other forms of protective isolation used in the care of patients with leukemia and aplastic anemia is controversial.[3] Careful cleansing of the scalp and skin is encouraged. Bowel sterilization with nonabsorbable antibiotics should be attempted, since Gram-negative sepsis is the main cause of death in granulocytopenic patients. The patient with an absolute granulocyte count below 1000/cc is at great risk of sepsis, but the risk is greatest in one with less than 500 granulocytes/cc. Our patients had less than 100/cc at their WBC nadir, and it is at that time that fever occurred.

In the acute radiation syndrome, one can predict the approximate time of the granulocytopenic phase. The patient's temperature should be carefully observed, and when it starts to climb, multiple cultures should be obtained and intravenous antibiotics given immediately. Broad-spectrum coverage with gentamicin, carbenicillin, and/or a cephalosporin is continued for ten days or for the duration of the fever. The antibiotics are changed if bacterial sensitivity studies so indicate. The appearance of monocytes in the peripheral smear is a most welcome sign since a monocytosis generally precedes the return of the granulocytic leukocytes.[4]

The administration of billions of granulocytes with leukocyte concentrates will help reduce infection. Sensitization occurs, however, and the antibodies formed negate the effects of the transfusions. No substantial increase of the white blood count is seen after the transfusion.[5] The patient can experience fever, shaking chills, and respiratory distress after granulocyte transfusion;[6] therefore many clinicians use this product only in the severely septic granulocytopenic patient who loses ground despite adequate antibiotic therapy. The first case had an extremely toxic course around the time of his leukocyte transfusions. We do not know if he survived because of the WBC transfusions or in spite of them. Fortunately, the second patient did not require any replacement therapy.

The other potential problem in a myelosuppressed patient is bleeding secondary to thrombocytopenia. When the first patient complained of dizziness, his platelet count was 8000/cc. Because of his age (61 years) and the possibility of central nervous system bleeding, platelet concentrates were given. Bleeding can occur at platelet counts below 100,000/

cc, often occurs below 50,000/cc, but usually does not present in a dangerous fashion until the count is below 10,000/cc. Giving platelet concentrates is a matter of clinical judgment; the platelet count alone does not form one's decision. If the clinician aims for a platelet count around 20,000/cc,[7] the risk of bleeding decreases. A normal platelet count is rarely achieved, especially in the presence of infection. When platelets from random donors are used in leukemic patients, antibodies to platelet and lymphocyte antigens can develop by six weeks.[8] Since the severe thrombocytopenia of the radiation accident victim lasts about ten days, antibody formation should not pose a great problem.

Seven months after having received platelet and granulocyte concentrates, the first patient developed antigen-negative hepatitis, demonstrating another risk of such therapy. By increasing the use of voluntary donors, the incidence of transmissible diseases from human blood products has diminished.[9]

Radiation accident victims are the object of radio, television, and newspaper bulletins. I am sure we cannot know the extent of their anxiety during those early postexposure days while they wait for "the ax to fall." These patients are isolated, greeted by masked visitors, and subjected to numerous procedures. They read and watch television to relieve the boredom of their isolation. Some news items are alarming, and I would recommend that the patients be spared the exposure to such reading material, and that the physicians and other hospital representatives be honest but discreet in their communications with the press. I do not believe the patient is well served by hearing about his case on a television broadcast; his progress reports should be given by his doctor. Radiation accidents are of public interest because they concern the public safety, but a patient's right to privacy must be respected, and I make a plea that we give consideration to the psychological aspects of the patient's care.

ACKNOWLEDGMENTS
Dr. Louis Sanfilippo, the Director of Radiotherapy, and Dr. David Steidley, the radiotherapy physicist, gave valuable assistance with their dosimetry estimates and their generous contributions of knowledge and time. Dr. Neil Wald, consultant to the Nuclear Regulatory Commission, performed the chromosome aberration dosimetries. Mrs. Genevieve Collins assisted with the manuscript preparation.

References

1. Andrews GA, Haywood FF: Clinical and biological consequences of nuclear explosions. *The Practitioner* 207:331–342, 1971.
2. Thomas ED, Fefer A, Buckner CD, Storb R: Current status of bone marrow transplantation for aplastic anemia and acute leukemia. *Blood* 49:671–681, 1977.

3. Jameson B, Gamble DR, Lynch J, Key HEM: Five year analysis of protective isolation. *Lancet* 1:1034–1036, 1971.

4. Erslev AJ, Gabuzda TG: *Pathophysiology of Blood*. Philadelphia, W. B. Saunders Company, 1975, p. 107.

5. Graw RG Jr, Herzig G, Perry S, Henderson ES: Normal granulocyte transfusion therapy. *NEJM* 287:367–371, 1972.

6. Clift RA, Sanders I, Thomas ED, Williams B, Buckner CD: A study of prophylactic granulocyte transfusions. *NEJM* 298:1052–1057, 1978.

7. Clift RA, Buckner CD: Supportive measures for patients with aplastic anemia, in Thomas ED (ed.): *Clinics in Haematology*. London, W. B. Saunders Company Limited, October 1978, 7(3):623–637.

8. Hoak JC, Koepke JA: Platelet transfusions, in Cash JD (ed.): *Clinics in Haematology*. London, W. B. Saunders Company Limited, February 1976, 5(1):69–79.

9. Wallace J: Blood transfusion and transmissible disease, in Cash JD (ed.): *Clinics in Haematology*. London, W. B. Saunders Company Limited, February 1976, 5(1):183–200.

Discussion for Section I

A. O. BULL: No one so far in this conference is using the new SI units. There is a factor of 100 in between the old rad and the new Gy, and between the rem and the new Sv. Our students are now familiar with the new unit, but not with the old one, so we can foresee some confusion and probably some serious errors if we are not very careful.

E. L. SAENGER: Thank you. We will all stand corrected on not using the SI units, and we will hope that SI units may end up in parentheses.

R. D. EVANS: The ratio of 100, which relates the familiar rad unit to the SI Gray unit, has impeded usage of SI units for a variety of reasons. There is a simple remedy. Recall that the SI meter is simply 100 centimeters. Similarly, the SI Gray is simply 100 rad. Thus, the familiar rad unit may equally well be read as one centigray (cGy). Likewise, 1 rem may be read as one centisievert.

A. O. BULL: I have a question to Dr. Karl Hübner. In his lecture on the Y-12 accident he gave the gamma and neutron doses in rads. What QF factor for the neutrons should be considered to give the dose in rems?

K. F. HÜBNER: Let me refer the answer to this question to Dr. Auxier, who has done the dosimetry for the Y-12 accident victims based on sodium activation and special RBE considerations.

J. A. AUXIER: The quality factor is not defined for high-dose levels but is intended for routine occupational conditions. At the dose levels reported for the Y-12 accident, some estimate of Relative Biological Effectiveness (RBE) can be made for the neutrons and gamma rays. For short-term (40-day) hematological effects, the RBE for the neutrons relative to the gammas was probably between 1.5 and 2, based on data from all criticality accidents. For long-term effects, i.e., cancer and leukemia, the RBE is highly dose dependent, increasing inversely with dose, such that in the range of 100 to 400 rads total dose, the RBE decreases from about 3 at 100 rads to near unity at 400 rads. For doses as low as a few rads to red bone marrow, the RBE for leukemia is 10 or greater; this is because the effectiveness of gamma rays for producing leukemia is or approaches zero at doses of up to a few tens of rads. This can be stated, generally, as follows: the incidence of leukemia increases approximately linearly with neutron dose, but as the square of the gamma dose, to doses approaching the mid-lethal dose for hematopoietic death, at which point the curves are nearly the same.

G. L. VOELZ: The doses to the Y-12 persons seem to have been calculated differently for cases A-D than the E-H cases. I refer to the total rads that are divided into gamma and neutrons. It is listed as rads, but the total suggests some modifier (RBE?) was used.

K. F. HÜBNER: The discrepancy in the total doses and gamma and neutron doses is not due to applying a special "RBE-modifier," but rather an error in transferring the dose information from one table to another. The printed table should have the correct gamma and neutron doses, with the sum of the two representing the total dose in rad.

H. H. VOGEL, JR.: Was there significant evidence of increased thyroid abnormalities among the Utirik children and adults exposed to low doses of radiation in the 1954 Marshallese accident? How reliable was the dosimetry at Utirik?

R. A. CONARD: The children of both Rongelap and Utirik had increased doses to their thyroid glands compared with the adults because of the smaller sizes of their glands. There was an increase in thyroid abnormalities in the Utirik children, but paradoxically the percentage of abnormalities in their group was lower than in the adults, in contrast to the Rongelap children who had a much higher percentage than the adults. Because of the importance of low-dose effects, the dosimetry of the Utirik people is being reinvestigated.

N. WALD: To what was the fatal outcome of one of the fishermen patients due? Do you consider it a result of direct radiation damage?

T. KUMATORI: Since the radiation dose to the liver is not known because of unknown movement of incorporated short-lived isotopes, it is difficult to relate the liver damage to radiation directly, although radiation played an important role.

K. SHIMAOKA: I should like to make a comment in regard to radiation-induced thyroid disease. The thyroid tissue had been considered to be radioresistant. However, late effects of low-dose radiation therapy to the thyroid have been found to be responsible for various thyroid diseases, including carcinoma of this gland. We have recently studied thyroid function of malignant lymphoma patients who underwent radiation therapy; 30 patients received radiation therapy that included the neck in its field, with a tumor dose of 2500-4000 rad (median 3600 rad), and 52 had radiation therapy that did not include the neck in its field and/or chemotherapy. The average interval between therapy and evaluation of thyroid function was 3.6 years. Among 30 patients with neck irradiation, 19 (63%) were found to have TSH elevation, 16 (53%) positive titers of antithyroglobulin and/or antimicrosomal antibody, and 5 (17%) clinical hypothyroidism. While among 52 patients whose neck was not irradiated, 8 (15%) were found to have TSH elevation, 11 (21%) positive antibody titers, and 1 (2%) clinical hypothyroidism. These results are on statistical analyses $p < .001$ for TSH, $p < .01$ for antibody, and $p < .05$ for clinical hypothyroidism.

These results indicate that derangement of thyroid function does occur following a moderate dose of therapeutic irradiation of the gland. Reduced thyroid reserve and elevation of antithyroid antibody titers, which in many cases are associated with the development of chronic thyroiditis, occur. These are most commonly seen conditions in patients whose thyroid was irradiated. As in the case of Graves' disease treated by radioiodine, the prevalence of reduced thyroid reserve and hypothyroidism increases, as more time elapses. We have not yet observed the occurrence of thyroid malignancy in these patients.

M. E. GAULDEN: Dr. Barlotta or Dr. Wald, how many hours after radiation exposure was the blood from the two patients taken for chromosome studies and for how long were the lymphocytes cultured?

N. WALD: In the first New Jersey accident the blood was taken between 24 and 48 hours. In the second accident, the sample was obtained somewhere around day 3. There was a second sample in the first New Jersey accident on day 8 and a second sample in the second accident that came out with virtually identical results, which gives some feeling for the amount of time one has for this kind of sampling. The cultures were 48 to 50 hours in both cases.

G. CALDWELL: I would like to ask Dr. Le Gô what abnormalities were found in the spontaneously aborted fetus?

M. E. GAULDEN: At what stage after conception was the fetus exposed to radiation, and what was the total estimated dose to the fetus?

R. LE GÔ: The fetus had an estimated age of 9.5 weeks. His death was evident on 10 July. So it can be assumed that the conception occurred immediately before or immediately after the source arrived in the house, with a greater probability for the former case. Specific dosimetric measurements were not devoted to the fetus. But from the theoretical isodose curves, it can be assumed that he received about 25-30% of the entry-point dose. This fetus (45 mm long) had histologically normal organs. No chromosome examinations were made on it because its spontaneous expulsion occurred four weeks after its death.

D. L. MCNEILL: With regard to the Pittsburgh accident, would Dr. Gilberti or Dr. Wald still recommend multiple-level extremity amputations for radiation necrosis or wait for a final level of demarcation? Would infection alter the decision? For patient C with the bone marrow transplant, are the present peripheral blood elements completely from the marrow graft, or are some of the elements from his own marrow?

M. V. GILBERTI: In our approach to this severe radiation injury to all four extremities there was very little information in the literature to give us guidance in the surgical treatment. Most of the reports in the literature dealt with accidents involving lower dose levels and somewhat less penetrating field to the extremities.

We treated this patient with topical therapy, optimism, and by obeying standard surgical rules, to amputate only when accurate demarcation on nonviable tissue had occurred and to preserve as much length as possible for better function. In addition, the patient was unwilling to accept immediate high amputation.

From having had this experience, I would now recommend much earlier amputation at a definitive level, within two to three months after exposure. Earlier amputation would decrease the incidence of infection, shorten the period of severe pain, afford a reduction of hospital stay, and obtain much earlier rehabilitation.

Correlation of the dosimetry information with clinical observation aids in the correct level of amputation. The time of onset of tissue injury is directly related to the doses received. In general, the higher the dose, the sooner the signs of injury will occur. Early erythema with subsequent bleb formation did give a demarcation level of nonviable tissue corresponding to areas of later skin discoloration and final ulceration. Infection was a late sequela in this process and would not alter my decision for earlier definitive amputation.

N. WALD: Now to the second part of Dr. McNeill's question concerning the patient with the bone marrow graft. In isogeneic individuals with the same genetic composition there are no markers by which one can distinguish self from an identical twin donor, and there is no way to recognize the success of the transplant. It was recognized because of the time factor, that is, the fact that 2 weeks after the transplant and only 19 days after the exposure hematologic recovery occurred.

D. L. MCNEILL: Dr. Vodopick, in the case you presented, were the CPK isoenzymes accomplished? Do you feel there may have been an elevation of the myocardial CPK fraction?

H. VODOPICK: No, CPK isoenzymes were not performed. Yes, I would assume the myocardial CPK fraction was elevated. The position of the ^{60}Co source was directly parallel to the anterior chest wall, extending cephalad from the waist. Therefore, the heart certainly received a significant dose. But since no CPK fractionation was done, the myocardial fraction is unknown.

SECTION II:

Radiation Accidents:
Acute Local Irradiation

Clinical Course and Dosimetry of Acute Hand Injuries to Industrial Radiographers from Multicurie Sealed Gamma Sources

Eugene L. Saenger,* James G. Kereiakes,* Niel Wald,+ and George E. Thoma‡

*University of Cincinnati College of Medicine, Cincinnati, Ohio;
+School of Public Health, University of Pittsburgh, Pittsburgh, Pennsylvania;
‡St. Louis University Medical School, St. Louis, Missouri.

Concepts of Local Irradiation Injury

In the last several years there have been a number of incidents in which industrial radiographers and others have received severe radiation injuries to the fingers from inadvertent contact with sealed sources ^{192}Ir, ^{60}Co, and other radiation sources. These injuries are characterized by an initial severe reaction, progressing from erythema and edema to bulla formations at sites of contact, with relatively little reaction at distances of 1–3 cm from the point of contact. Pain is relatively little in the absence of infection. There is often spontaneous resolution of the lesion over a period of 6 to 8 weeks. Plastic surgical repair depends on the severity of the lesion.

Dosimetric measurements and calculations indicate that doses at the surface are in the kilo rad range per curie, and at 1 cm they are 0.1 to 0.01 of these surface doses. In cases involving direct contact with sealed sources the unusually high surface dose is due in part to electron production in the capsule wall. The gamma absorption in tissue is 5–10% per cm. The inverse square law is the principal factor accounting for the relative lack of effect below 2 cm.

In reviewing the topic of acute local radiation a definition is required. In a radiation injury limited to a sufficiently small part of the body, in spite of various local reactions developing within days to a few (~ 3–4) weeks, there may be no clinical manifestations of the acute radiation syndrome. Omitted from this discussion are injuries following any type of radiation therapy. One recognizes immediately reports of acute local radiation injury associated with the acute radiation syndrome involving large volumes of the body.[1,2] The conspicuous characteristic of most of the cases discussed is that clinical symptoms and signs commonly associated with the acute radiation syndrome following "whole-body" irradiation have been in most instances relatively mild or absent. Hematological changes are mild or absent, but frequently characteristic changes in chromosomes of peripheral lymphocytes can be found. If the lower portion of the body is exposed in the male, changes in sperm counts can be observed.

The medical and health physics literature has been followed for many years in order to identify the common characteristics of this type of injury. In addition, experiences of several of the medical consultants to the Nuclear Regulatory Commission (NRC) are included. The frequency of these injuries is very low in relation to the widespread use of industrial radiography using radionuclide sources. When the injuries occur they interfere with or terminate the worker's specific duties as a radiographer.

A few of the incidents have been bizarre. There have been several reports of suicide attempts, one of which successfully used a 5.3 curie source of ^{137}Cs.[3] Political figures have been reported to be apprehensive about being exposed to sources of radioactivity hidden in their living quarters by their hosts.[4] On 1 May 1979 a French executive of a nuclear fuel treatment plant found three radioactive disks under his automobile seat placed there by a dissatisfied employee (personal communication, P. Pellerin).

The largest number of cases in the literature and as reported to the AEC and subsequently to the NRC have occurred because of malfunctions of industrial gamma-ray industrial radiographic units or because of improper operation of the units. The most common radiation source involved in this kind of injury is the gamma camera. It consists of a storage container containing the radioactive source together with a guide tube through which a flexible wire holding the source can be cranked out to the radiographic site. After the exposure is made the source is cranked back to its container for safe storage. The radiographer is responsible for determining the location of the source by the use of a radiation detector usually of the ionization chamber type; the meter is provided with a small source to check that it is operating properly. If the meter does not register, the operator presumes that the source is in its safe. This presumption has led to inadvertent exposure in several ways. In one circumstance the survey meter fails to register because of its own malfunction. The radiographer fails to check the meter with its own test source, and he proceeds to change setups and films while being unwittingly exposed. A second type of error occurs when the radiographer becomes out of phase with the source by not continually using the survey meter. In this instance the source remains in the out position although the radiographer believes he has returned it to the safe position. Another type of exposure occurs when the source capsule is separated from its flexible guide wire. In this situation the source capsule is seen to be free from its guide and often the radiographer or an untrained assistant picks up the capsule and reattaches it. These scenarios account for the largest group of extremity injuries.

Other instances of severe injury result when an uneducated person finds an industrial radiation source lying free and without identification that it is radioactive. These sources are picked up, carried on one's person, and have led to severe injury and in some cases to death.[5,6] Other instances of extremity or severe regional injury have occurred from exposure to electron beams[7,8] and to X-ray spectrometers at 50–60 kV.[9,10]

A simple way to estimate the extent of involvement in these circumstances of partial exposure is to utilize the "Rule of Nines"[11] that has been adopted for the determination of severity of thermal burns (Figure 1). Although this rule is heavily dependent on body surface rather than volume, its use for these kinds of injury is suggested. For example, one hand is considered to represent 1% involvement. A useful classification of skin and extremity injuries from ionizing radiation follows:[12]

Type I. Erythema (only), is equivalent to a first degree thermal burn like mild sunburn. Some time after exposure, a sensation of warmth or itching may occur; the redness, however, can appear as late as 2–3 weeks after exposure, and the length of the symptomless interval depends on the dose. Medical care is not necessary and ability to work is no more impaired than after a similarly severe sunburn. Dry desquamation (scaling) occurs. Brief doses of several hundred rads to skin can cause delayed erythema. In two fatal radiation accidents where skin dose was several thousand rads, erythema developed within 15 to 30 min after exposure.

Type II. Transepidermal injury (wet desquamation), is equivalent to the injury seen in a thermal burn of the second degree. After the erythema develops, blisters form and break open, leaving raw, painful wounds vulnerable to infection. Itching and pain are experienced after exposure. The symptom-free latent period is shorter than in the Type I lesions, and blisters appear within 1–2 weeks, depending on the dose. Recognizable injury of this grade requires a brief skin dose between 1000 and 2000 rad. The need for medical care and the ability to work depend on the size, location, and severity of the lesion. These lesions usually heal with proper care, but the new skin is usually pigmented, thin, and easily injured.

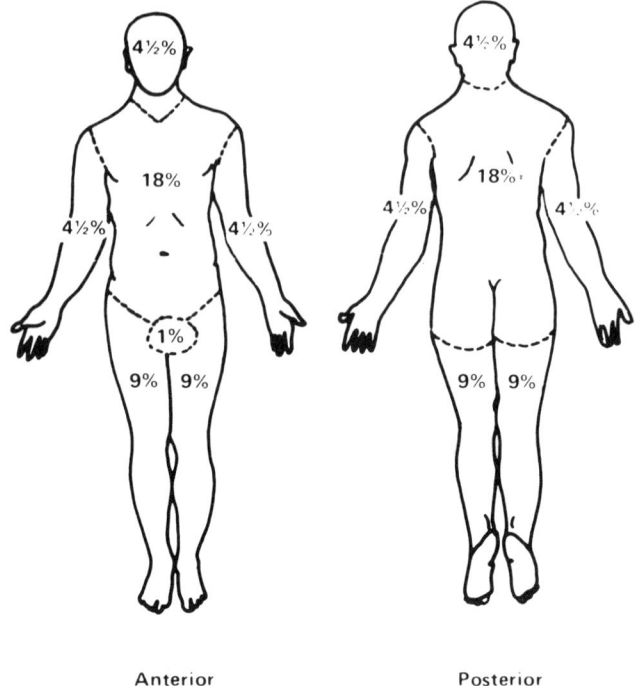

Figure 1. Rule of Nines. A rapid method of estimating the percentage of body surface involved. From Artz and Moncrief.[11]

Type III. Dermal radionecrosis (radiation-induced skin death), is a more serious degree of the Type II lesion, caused by prompt doses of radiation in excess of 2000 rad. Injury of this sort has been observed in persons who handled fresh fission product material or targets in which radioactivity was induced during laboratory experiments by neutron or electron bombardment, and also after accidental exposure of hands to the direct beam of an electron accelerator. The lesions resemble those caused by a severe scalding or chemical burn. Pain occurs promptly and is intense. Medical abatement of pain is urgently needed.

Type IV. Frequently repeated or continuous exposure of the skin to X-rays, gamma rays, or beta rays over a period of months to years causes an eczema-like condition. Once it has developed, it seldom heals completely, and ulceration frequently occurs. Skin cancer occurs in a large (but unknown) proportion of such cases of chronic radiation dermatitis. In the case of persons working with X-rays during a life-time (30+ years), the effective dose levels for skin cancer production are thought to be in the region of several thousand rads when accumulated at rates of about one rad per day.

Radiobiology of the Skin and Underlying Structures

Even in the most severe injuries as defined here, the volumes of tissue are relatively small. In addition there is little or no involvement of major organs or organ systems such as bone marrow, breast, lung, and others where the association of radiation and late development of cancer has been well documented. The usual tissues include skin, muscle, bone, and blood vessels. Early, acute changes are functions of the energy (degree of penetration) of the tissue, dose, and dose rate. Since most accidents involve very high dose rates (500–100,000 rad) delivered in fractions of minutes to several hours, these early changes can be very severe, with the rapid development of tissue necrosis within a period of several weeks. With lower dose rates and doses, changes are protracted and develop only over a period of months or years. The abnormalities are due to a gradual, obliterating endarteritis with resulting fibrosis, atrophy, and eventual tissue death.

Variability in the distribution of radiation, depending on whether it is particulate or electromagnetic, and the energies of these radiations are important considerations in determining the extent of the injury. In general, particulate radiation of less than 10 MeV is of low penetration; producing superficial injuries that involve only the dermis. As the energy and dose rates increase the effects of radiation become more pronounced. These changes can be easily seen by noting the surface and depth dose values in Table 1.[13] For example, ^{192}Ir in a stainless steel capsule has a

Table 1. Approximate Gamma-ray Dose Rates to the Hand for 1 Curie in a Sealed Source[a]

Nuclide	β max (principal) MeV	γ (principal) MeV	Γ R/mCi-h at 1 cm	Surface dose rate[b] R/min	Dose rate at 1 cm tissue depth R/min	Dose rate at 3 cm tissue depth R/min
^{137}Cs	0.51,1.2	0.662	3.26	513	28	3.7
^{60}Co	0.31	1.17, 1.33	13.00	2075	114	16.0
^{192}Ir	0.67	0.468	4.80	813	43	5.5
^{226}Ra	0.4-3.2	0.047-2.4	8.25	1310	72	9.7

[a] Industrial source housings are usually of stainless steel and for the purpose of the calculations, the activity is considered to be a point source. In considering these dose estimates, there is assumed a capsule of outside diameter ¼ inch, with a wall of stainless steel (type 304) which is 1/32 inch thick. Data from National Council on Radiation Protection and Measurements.[13]

[b] The total surface dose rate for the ^{226}Ra source is 1900 R/min based on a 45 percent increase due to electron production in the stainless steel wall. For other nuclides given in the table, the increase in surface dose rate due to electron production in the stainless steel wall is estimated to be 25-45%.

surface dose rate of 813 rad/min/curie, but at 1 cm in tissue the dose rate is 43 rad/min/curie or 5% of that at the surface. At 3 cm the dose rate is 0.7% of the surface dose. Contributing to this peculiar dose distribution is an increase in surface dose rate of about 25–45% due to electron production in the stainless steel capsule wall. Even with exposure to external X-rays of low kilovoltage (<50–60 kV) and industrial or medical X-rays up to 100 kV under circumstances that do not follow good geometry, one should always consider dose distributions within a few millimeters to a few centimeters that do not follow the inverse square law. The surface doses encountered in these cases are in the kilo rad range per curie. The gamma absorption is roughly 5–10% per 1 cm of tissue. Below 2 cm the inverse square law accounts for the relative lack of effect.

The pioneering studies of Strandqvist[14] using X-rays at 250 kV provide an insight into the effect of dosage fractionation, i.e., the effect of recovery (Table 2). Thus erythema can be produced with 1000 rad in one exposure, whereas 1280 rad are required if fractionated over two days or 1490 rad over three days. Necrosis can be produced with a single dose of 3000 rad in a single dose, 3800 rad in two doses in 2 days, or 4400 rad in 3 equal doses in 3 days. Early studies of Low-Beer[15] using ^{32}P beta radiation ($\bar{E}$ max 1.7 MeV, average E ~.57 MeV) show that similar surface doses from protracted beta radiation yield equivalent effects (Table 3).

Clinical Evaluation

An important facet of the great majority of these cases is the absence of systemic manifestations usually found in the acute radiation syndrome. In spite of the intense local injury the clinical and laboratory findings have been minimal. Nevertheless each case requires careful evaluation; the principal steps are listed in Table 4. These studies should provide both a baseline and methods to aid in prognosis, treatment, consideration of possible late effects, and steps directed toward rehabilitation. The use of blood pool imaging and later bone scans of the involved areas should

Table 2. Changes Produced by Fractionation of X-Ray Doses[a]

Effect	Single Dose	Two doses in 2 days	Three doses in 3 days
Erythema	1000	1280	1490
Dry epidermitis	1600	2000	2700
Healing of skin cancer	2450	2800	3250
Necrosis	3000	3800	4400

[a] Data given according to Strandqvist.[14]

Table 3. Effect of [32]P Beta Radiation Produced by 5-cm Diameter Plaques on Human Skin[a]

Effect	Dose rate (microcurie hr/cm^2)	Total dose (R)
Threshold erythema	34	143
Dry desquamation	2000	1700
Bullous epidermitis	4400	7200

[a] Data given according to Low-Beer.[15]

indicate the state of the blood supply and the viability of bone. Comparisons should be made with unirradiated sites if possible. Such studies have not been reported for this type of injury. They have been found useful in other types of trauma and for peripheral vascular disease.

There is some variation in the initial symptoms. The most frequent complaint was a superficial feeling of irritation, tenderness, or itching, often transient and occurring usually within the first 7 to 14 days. Restricted motion or stiffness of the finger was noted early in a few instances. Erythema, edema, and diminished sensation then developed. Bulla formation and ulceration also began. All of these findings occurred from 10 to 30 days in varying degrees. Ulceration was occasionally observed between 10 and 19 days. In the absence of ulceration and infection and with immobilization pain was minimal or absent. The development of vesicles, bullae, and ulceration was associated with increased pain in proportion to the size and depth of the lesions and the presence of secondary infection. These changes developed gradually in 14 to 30 days. The bullae and ulcers are characteristically rather sharply demarcated from adjacent tissue, indicating the confinement of very high doses to limited areas. Depending on the superficiality of the dose these demarcated areas may be the only involved area. Opposing surfaces appear uninvolved. In some instances apparently normal tissues may develop fibrosis and gangrene months to several years later.

Table 4. Useful Steps in Clinical Evaluation of Extremity Injury

History and physical examination
Serial peripheral blood counts
Chromosome analysis of blood lymphocytes
Sperm counts before day 45 and after day 60
Re-enactment of accident
Frequent color photos
Slit lamp exam of eyes
Baseline extremity X-rays
Radionuclide blood pool imaging and bone scan

Epilation is a valuable dosimeter in many radiation accidents. It occurs after doses of 300–1000 rad of beta or gamma radiation but is not as frequently observed in these kinds of injuries. Epilation of hair on the extremities has been less well documented than that of the scalp or face and may require somewhat higher doses for its occurrence than for other parts of the body.

Dry epidermitis or wet epithelitis usually develops 2–3 weeks after exposures of 1000–4000 rad. Restricted motion was an important finding in acute exposure beginning in about 10 to 18 days. It was associated with marked local edema and possibly with some reaction of tendon and synovial surfaces. In some cases this finding persisted and worsened even after recession of the edema.

In the acute phase treatment has been largely symptomatic in order to maintain cleanliness or prevent infection with prophylactic antibiotics and local ointments as are used in thermal burns. Some immobilization is helpful. Grafting of various kinds has often been most important in relieving pain and in restoration of function. Most patients who face the possibility of amputation resist application of this procedure until ulceration or gangrene becomes so severe that there is no likelihood of the success of more conservative methods. It seems best to accede to the patient's wishes in this regard, based on anecdotal experience.

If no grafting procedures or other surgical procedures are performed and there is no necrosis, the extremity heals slowly with a loss of substance of skin, subcutaneous tissues, and muscle. The involved parts are often stiff and tender to pressure, heat, and cold.

Late effects that may be expected are those resulting from insidious but progressive tissue atrophy, fibrosis, and chronic radiodermatitis with tissue breakdown. The hands and fingers may exhibit increased sensitivity to temperature changes and to certain roughened or metallic surfaces. There may be cartilagenous atrophy and other changes of joint spaces and tendon sheaths, leading to progressive limitation of motion.

Finally, the development of skin cancer must always be watched for. Radiation-induced cancer has not been observed in the absence of radiodermatitis.[16] If such dermatitis is severe or progressive, skin grafting should be seriously considered. Amputation is needed only with necrosis and failure of skin grafting.

Since the clinical course of this peculiar type of radiation injury may occasionally be obscure, the evaluation of the patient must be carefully planned. Table 4 presents the studies found to be most useful. Routine hematological tests and chromosome analysis will estimate whole-body doses. The serial ophthalmologic evaluations with a slit lamp are suggested to allay apprehension concerning effects on the lens of the eye. As in all cases of radiation injury, the availability of prompt and continuing medical care and a well-organized plan of rehabilitation will do much to allay the obvious concerns of the injured man and his family during a difficult period.

Prevention of this type of injury can only be attained by continuing education of industrial radiographers. This group of workers usually have only a high-school or technical-school education and no trade journal or society providing national intercommunication. The responsibility for prevention rests almost exclusively with plant management, radiation safety officers, and health physicists who should provide the necessary educational stimulus. In some of cases it would seem that continuing personal contact between the individual radiographer and his supervisors is desirable since there is a tendency for these accidents to occur when the operator becomes excessively preoccupied with his personal emotional problems or interests, at which times his concern for radiation safety may be less than optimal. The diligent use of self-reading pocket dosimeters, film badges or TLD monitors, and portable survey meters are essential for adequate protection.

Equal attention is needed for uninstructed helpers who are usually obtained from unskilled labor pools. Such workers should not participate in radiographic work unless constantly attended and supervised by the qualified radiographer, and wearing appropriate dosimeters.

The frequency of these cases involving industrial radiographers (at least in the experience of licensees of the NRC) has been encouraging in the past 5 years, with a decline in the number of reported cases. In part this change may be attributed to technical design changes of the camera. In great part it has been due to training courses given by employers, the NRC, and local health physicists to technologists who otherwise have not received special instruction in the causes, prevention, and consequences of these kinds of injury.

References

1. Hempelmann LH, Lisco H, Hoffman JG: The acute radiation syndrome. A study of nine cases and a review of the problem. *Ann Int Med* 36:283–465, 1952.

2. Howland JW, Ingram M, Mermagen H, Hansen CL: The Lockport incident: accidental partial body exposure of humans to large doses of X-irradiation, in *Diagnosis and Treatment of Acute Radiation Injury,* proceedings of a scientific meeting jointly sponsored by the International Atomic Energy Agency and the World Health Organization, Geneva, 17–21 October 1960, International Documents Service, New York, 1961.

3. Vassileva B, Kruschkov I: Suizid mit caesium 137. *Psychiat Neurol Med Psych* 30:116–119, 1978.

4. Listening in on the World, *Atlas Magazine,* p. 58, October 1970.

5. Martinez RG, Cassab GH, Ganem GG, Guttman EK, Lieberman ML, Vater LB, Linaires MM, Rodriguez HM: Observations on the accidental exposure of a family to a source of cobalt 60. *Revista Medica Inst Mex Seguro Social* 3(Suppl. 1):14–68, 1964.

6. Beninson D, Placer A, Vander Elst E: Estudio de un case de irradiacion humana accidental, in *Handling of Radiation Accidents,* proceedings of a symposium, Vienna, 19–23 May 1969, International Atomic Energy Agency, SM-119/35, pp. 415–429.

7. Cramer LM, Waite JH, Edgcomb JH, Powell CC, Tuohy JH, Van Scott EJ, Smith RR: Burn following accidental exposure to high-energy radiation. *Ann Surg* 149:286–293, 1959.

8. Fryer MP, Brown JB: Repair of atomic, cathode-ray, cyclotron, and X-ray burns of the hand. *Amer J Surg* 103:688–691, 1962.

9. Report of investigation committee on AEC investigation of accidental X-ray exposure at HASL, New York, on 4 February 1974, U.S. Atomic Energy Commission.

10. Weigensberg IJ, Asbury CW, Feldman A: Injury due to accidental exposure to X-rays from an X-ray fluorescence spectrometer, to be published in *Health Physics.*

11. Artz CP, Moncrief JA: *The Treatment of Burns.* Philadelphia, W.B. Saunders Company, 1969, pp. 90–94.

12. National Council on Radiation Protection and Measurements: Radiological factors affecting decision-making in a nuclear attack, NCRP Report #42, 15 November 1974, Washington, D.C.

13. National Council on Radiation Protection and Measurements: Protection against radiation from brachytherapy sources, NCRP Report #40, 1 March 1972, Washington, D.C.

14. Strandqvist M: Studien über die kumulative Wirkung der Röntgenstrahlen bei Fraktionierung. *Acta Radiol.* 55(Suppl):1–300, 1944.

15. Low-Beer BVA: External therapeutic use of radioactive phosphorus. I. Erythema studies. *Radiology* 47:213–222, 1946.

16. National Academy of Sciences—National Research Council: *The Effects on Populations of Exposure to Low Levels of Ionizing Radiation.* A report of the Advisory Committee on the biological effects of ionizing radiations (BEIR report), Division of Medical Sciences, November, 1972.

The 1971 Chiba, Japan, Accident:
Exposure to Iridium 192

K. Hirashima, H. Sugiyama,
T. Ishihara, A. Kurisu,
T. Hashizume, and T. Kumatori

National Institute of Radiological Sciences, Chiba, Japan.

Onset of the Accident

On Friday, 17 September 1971, an operator was engaged in nondestructive examination with an ^{192}Ir source at a shipyard in Chiba, Japan (Figure 1). The ^{192}Ir source (5.26 curies) was located at the top of a pencil-like stainless steel holder 17 cm long.

After completing the day's work, the operator forgot to confirm that the source-holder had retracted into the shield. The screw which attached the cable to the source-holder was disconnected from the custody box. The loss of the ^{192}Ir holder was not noticed until Monday, 20 September, when the same operator started a radiographic examination. On 23 September, the company reported the loss of ^{192}Ir in the holder to the appropriate authorities. The loss was then reported through the news media.

Meanwhile, in the afternoon of Saturday, 18 September, a construction worker (case YS) employed by a subcontractor of the shipyard found the source-holder on the ground in the shipyard. He picked it up out of curiosity, inserted it between his belt and trousers, and went back to his lodging house by car. While he was en route, the top of the holder was in contact with his right hip for about 10 min and with his left hip for about 30 min.

On the same evening, five of his friends came to his room to watch television. Since they had no knowledge that this metal was radioactive, they in turn fingered the holder for some time. When questioned later, none of them remembered the place where the holder had been left or the period over which the holder had remained in the room. All of them

180

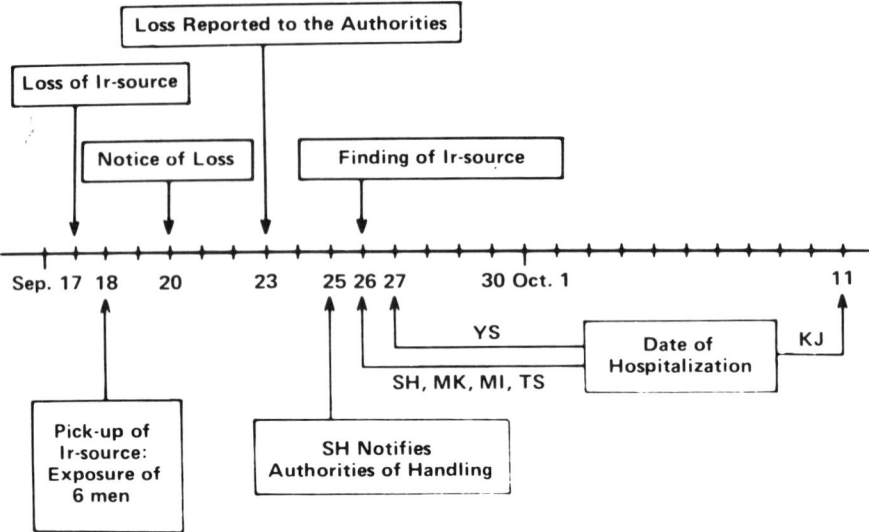

Figure 1. Onset of the accident. From Kumatori et al.[11]

were in the room for at least 1 hour and two of them (cases SH and TS) stayed overnight.

During the next 4 days, five of the men were in and out of the room several times. On 25 September, one of them heard of the loss of the ^{192}Ir source through the news media and notified the authorities that what he had handled at his friend's room might have been the missing holder. On 26 September, the wife of the manager of the lodging house found the source-holder in the garden near the room. All six patients were later hospitalized in the National Institute of Radiological Sciences.

Estimate of Exposed Dose

The management of the six exposed persons was decided on the basis of the individual clinical signs and symptoms as well as their laboratory data, mainly changes in blood cells. Physical dose estimations[1] were derived from measurements of the "mean absorbed dose of the whole body," the "absorbed dose to the skin," and the "gonad dose in one case."

The exposed persons were unable to remember exactly the location of the rod. However, since three of them (cases SH, YS, and MI) wore wrist watches at the time of exposure, we estimated the exposed dose of the jewels (rubies) in their watches by measuring the thermoluminescence intensity of the rubies. The dose rate of 5.26-curie iridium source is 2.17 R/hr at 1 m.

From these data the location of the source could be inferred. The length of the stay and location of the exposed persons within the room were reconstructed by queries. The average whole-body absorbed dose for each person was then estimated (Table 1). In view of the location of the source, the whole-body dose distributions seemed to be uneven.

Since the dose rate on the surface of the ^{192}Ir source was 250 R/min^{-1} curie^{-1}, the absorbed dose rate was 1300 rad/min. As the persons were supposed to have held the rod in their hands for 2 to 7 minutes, the absorbed dose to the fingers was estimated at 2600 to 9100 rad.

Assuming that the ^{192}Ir source had been kept at a distance of 1 cm from the surface of the hips of YS, the absorbed dose rate at the surface of the hips was estimated to be 300 rad/min. Since YS kept the source in contact with his right hip for 10 min and in contact with his left hip for 30 min, the absorbed doses were estimated to be 3000 and 9000 rad, respectively.

The absorbed dose to the testicles of YS was estimated to be 125 rad during this period. Moreover, as he held the source and kept it in his room for about 40 hr, another 50 rad should be added. The total gonad dose was thus approximately 175 rad.

The chromosome aberrations in cultured lymphocytes were examined repeatedly.[2] On the basis of the yields of dicentrics and rings, we made biological estimations of the absorbed dose by using the dose-response relationship for ^{60}Co gamma rays and for Linac X-rays (Table 1). These values were in fairly good agreement with those estimated by physical calculations.

The dose distribution over the whole body in each case was thought to be uneven and did not necessarily agree with the clinical and hematological results. Therefore, we used the technique for more close estimates of localized exposure based on the use of the Qdr value, developed by Sasaki.[3]

One can obtain the Qdr value by calculating the number of dicentrics

Table 1. Estimated Average Whole-Body Absorbed Doses[a]

Patient	Corresponding doses (rad)		Physically estimated doses (rad)
	^{60}Co gamma rays	High energy X-rays	
SH	124	152	133
YS	40	54	50
KJ	26	37	10
MK	12.2	19	25
TS	10.9	17.2	13
MI	9.8	15.6	15

[a] From Kumatori et al.[11]

plus rings in the number of X_1Cu cells in their first division after exposure. The doses estimated from the *Qdr* values were higher than those shown in Table 1, for example 195 rad as compared to 152 rad in case SH (Table 2).

Clinical Findings

The main changes detected clinically are summarized in Table 2.[4,5] They include three instances of skin lesions and one severe, one moderate, and two slight hematopoietic disorders.

Clinical Findings in a Severe Case, Case SH

Patient SH, 25 years of age, was first examined 8 days after the initial exposure. His general condition was quite good, but, when he was hospitalized, he complained of anorexia and nausea without vomiting about three hours after the initial exposure. Hematological data at this time showed only moderate leukopenia (3300 mm³) with lymphopenia (800/mm³). Thereafter he exhibited severe hematopoietic depression between week 3 and week 7 after the exposure. The detailed hematological course in this case is shown in Figure 2.

The hemoglobin level (Hb), the red blood cell (RBC) count, and the hematocrit (Hct) of SH decreased gradually and reached the lowest values at day 39. The depression of reticulocyte production before this period was remarkable. The lowest reticulocyte value was observed at day 23.

An early lymphopenia developed and persisted between day 9 and day 51. The absolute lymphocyte counts in this period ranged from 300/mm³ to 900/mm³. The total white blood cell (WBC) count decreased rapidly until day 11. After the first dip in the WBC count (1600/mm³) at this time, the count increased temporarily and thereafter it reached the lowest value (800/mm³) at day 32. Therefore, the time course of the WBC showed a biphasic pattern, and an abortive rise was remarkably demonstrated in this case. In week 3 to week 7, a severe decrease in neutrophils was observed. The platelet counts dropped very rapidly and reached the lowest value (15,000/mm³) on day 30. A remarkable prolongation of bleeding time (over 10 min) was observed from day 19.

However, the other values of the examination on hemostasis including the coagulation time, one-stage prothrombin time (quick), recalcification time test, fibrinogen concentration, euglobin lysis time, partial thromboplastin time test, and capillary resistance test were almost in the normal range. Clinical symptoms of a hemorrhagic tendency such as petechiae and gingival bleeding were not observed in this period.

The bone marrow of SH was first examined 9 days after the initial exposure. The sample showed remarkable hypocellularity, and a dimi-

Table 2. Main Changes Detected Clinically

Case	Age	Prodromal symptoms	Reduction in the number of blood cells	Skin lesions	Reduction in the number of spermatozoa	Average dose (rad)		
						Physical	Biological	
							From dicentrics +rings	From Q_{dr}
SH	25	+	+++	++	+	133	152	195
YS	20	–	+	+++	+++	50	54	150
KJ	23	–	+	+	+	10	37	55
MK	24	–	+	–	+	25	19	58
TS	30	–	–	–	+	13	17.2	28
MI	24	–	–	–	+	15	15.6	13

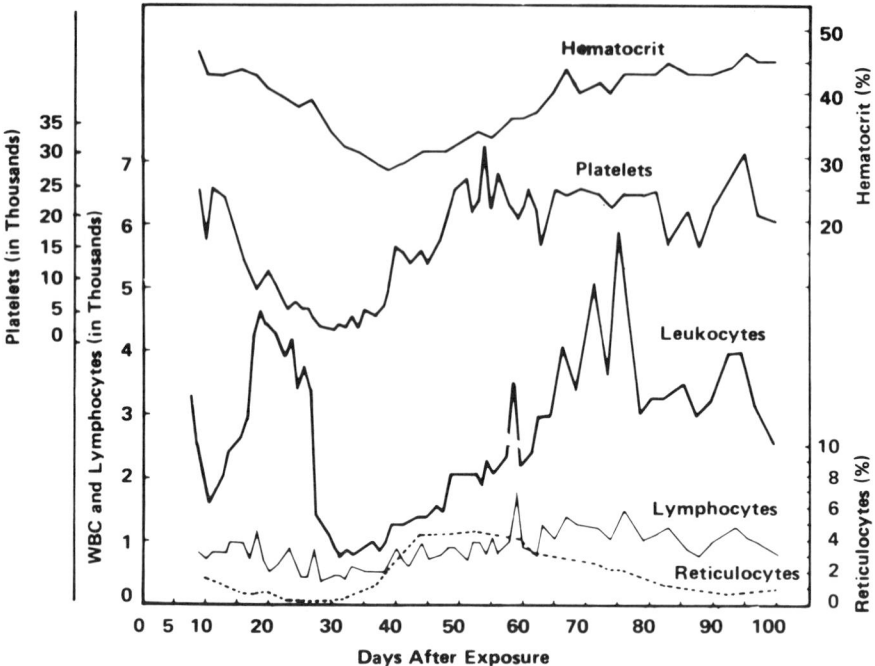

Figure 2. Hematological changes in case SH. From Hirashima et al.[5]

nution in three cell lines was noted while plasma cells and reticulum cells remained. The time course studies on the changes in the sternal myelogram are summarized in Figure 3. The changes in the peripheral blood, such as in the leukocytes and reticulocytes, corresponded to the results of the myelogram.

During the week 3 to week 7, all cell components of hematopoiesis decreased, and the patient exhibited pancytopenia. In this period, we considered it most critical for clinical treatments to know whether the degenerative changes of hematopoiesis were still continuing or not and to detect distinct signs of the initiating recovery process. According to recent theories of hematopoietic injuries caused by ionizing radiation, the depopulation and repopulation of the hematopoietic pluripotential stem cells should play the essential role in the mechanism after irradiation. Therefore, if we can be convinced of the initiation of the recovery process in any hematopoietic cell lines, further potential replacement therapies such as blood transfusion or bone marrow transplantation, which might cause severe side effects, can be avoided.

In case SH (Table 3) the increase in reticulocytes began on day 25, and an increase in the platelets and leukocytes was observed on day 30. However, the changes in these cell counts were too small to ensure the

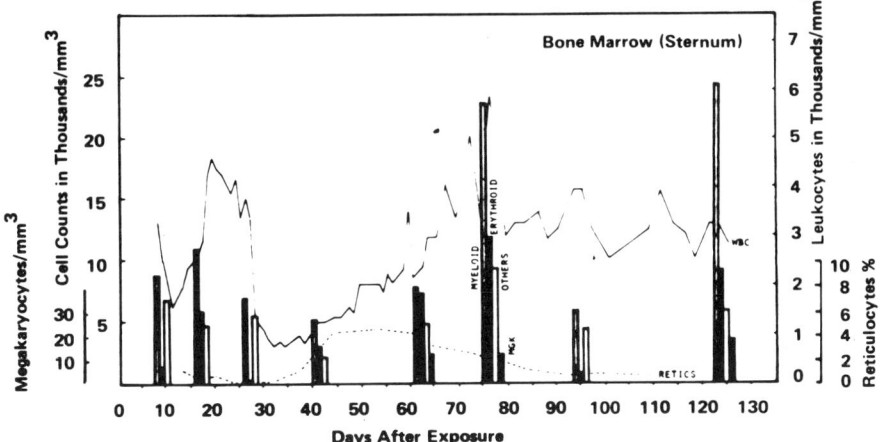

Figure 3. Time-course studies of the sternal myelogram of case SH (MGK, megakaryocytes). From Hirashima et al.[5]

true initiation of hematopoiesis. The most useful method for evaluating the developing recovery is based on the use of the thromboelastograph. The value of the maximum amplitude (m. a.) of the thromboelastogram (Table 3) decreased (34.5 mm) on day 25, but a significant increase in m. a. was observed on day 32 (43.0 mm on day 32, 48.0 mm on day 34). Between day 30 and day 34, although leukocyte and platelet values were the lowest, we were convinced of the initiation of hematopoietic recovery on the basis of thromboelastographic data. Thereafter, the hematopoietic recovery of this patient was rapid.

Patient SH was treated in a bioclean isolator for 34 days with the prophylactic administration of antibiotics (ampicillin, 1500 mg daily, or erythromycin, 900 mg daily, by mouth), and he recovered without either blood or platelet transfusion. During his whole course of treatment, no symptoms of infections were observed.

As shown in Table 2, the average whole-body absorbed dose was estimated as 152 rad on the basis of the yields of dicentrics and rings in the cytogenetic studies. However, the hematopoietic changes were indicative of a greater absorbed dose than this.

According to Wald,[6] the exposure dose in this case, calculated from the drop in the lymphocyte count, is between 200 and 500 rad. Moreover, the hematopoietic depression of this case is in fairly good agreement with the typical case in group II (200–400 rad) of Thoma and Wald's scheme[7] (Figure 4). The main reason for the difference between the hematological results and the exposed doses estimated from cytogenetics we ascribe to the nonuniform exposure in this case. Supposedly, the exposure dose of the trunk including most of active bone marrow and hematopoietic stem

Table 3. Hematological Data in the Critical Stage of Case SH. The Underlined Figures Represent the Lowest Values for Each Category.[a]

Days after Exposure	Hct. (%)	Hb. (gm./dl)	RBC (million/mm³)	WBC (per mm³)	Platelets (thousands/mm³)	Reticulocytes (%)	Thromboelastogram m. a. (mm)
				Hematological Data in the Critical Stage			
20	41	12.0	4.10	4400	110	0.75	
23	40	12.0	4.14	3900	50	<u>0.04</u>	
25	38	11.6	4.08	3400	50	<u>0.10</u>	<u>34.5</u>
27	39	11.4	3.96	3400	35	0.10	
30	34	11.0	3.66	1100	<u>15</u>	0.25	
32	32	9.6	3.45	<u>800</u>	20	0.30	43.0
34	31	9.9	3.31	800	20	0.70	48.0
37	29	9.2	3.14	1000	40	1.15	
39	<u>28</u>	<u>8.6</u>	<u>2.95</u>	1000	80	2.30	47.0
41	29	9.3	3.23	1300	140	1.90	
44	31	10.0	3.20	1400	140	4.40	
48	31	10.2	3.35	1500	200	4.45	

[a] From Hirashima et al.[5]

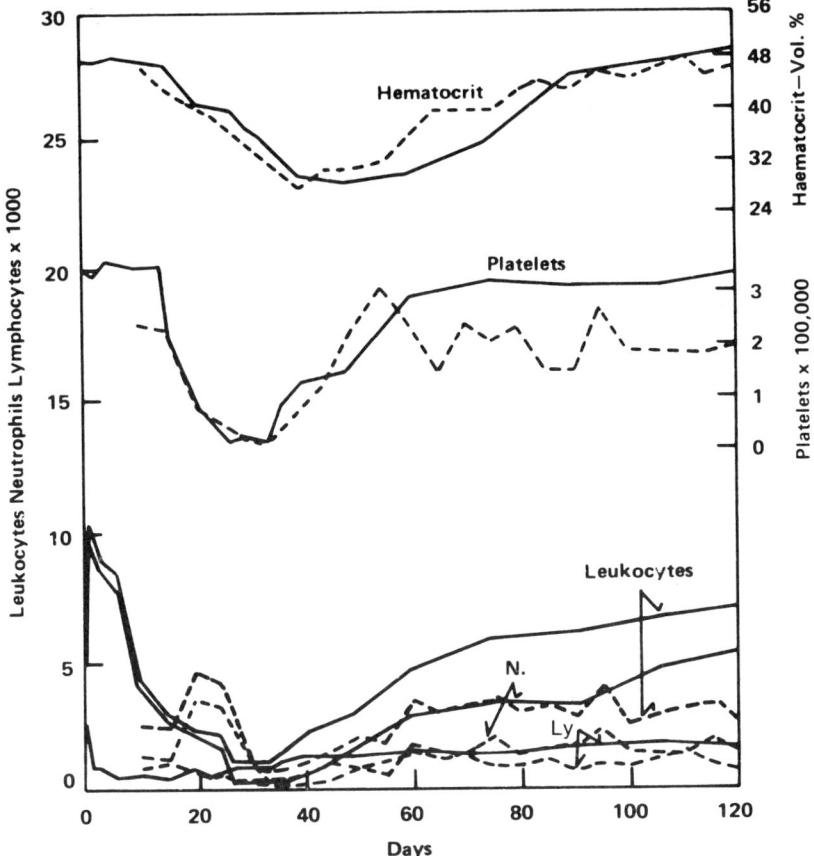

Figure 4. Comparative demonstration of case SH with the typical group II, the hypothetical case of Wald et al. in hematological changes.[6] N, neutrophils, Ly, lymphocytes; —, hypothetical case; ---, case SH. From Hirashima et al.[5]

cells will be much greater than that of the extremities. This conclusion is supported by a value of 500 rad for the maximum absorbed dose on the middle line in the trunk determined as a result of the physical estimates.[1] The doses estimated from the Qdr value seem closer to the hematopoietic depression values. Another reason for this gap must be the difference in the radiosensitivity of peripheral lymphocytes treated with phytohemagglutinin (PHA) according to the method used in our cytogenetic dosimetry and that of the hematopoietic stem cells.

Two weeks after the initial exposure, SH developed painful erythemas associated with swelling of the skin in the palms and fingers of both hands. Within several days, they were accompanied by blisters which ruptured, leaving raw, moist encrusted areas. We were able to alienate the acute symptoms of radiation burns in both hands only by bandaging and treatment with antiseptics.

Toward the end of October 1971, SH noticed the onset of hair loss from the scalp. The epilation stopped soon after, and alopecia was not observed.

On 10 October, the serum glutamic oxaloacetic transaminase (GOT) and glutamic pyruvic transaminase (GPT) activities increased up to 79 and 145 Karmen units, respectively, whereas the serum lactic dehydrogenase (LDH) activity remained normal. Symptoms of hepatitis or coronary artery disease were not evident. The GOT and GPT activities normalized without specific therapy after 6 weeks. The patient was discharged on 28 January 1972, after which time he was followed as an outpatient.

Clinical Findings in Cases YS and KJ

Patient YS, 20 years old, picked the source up and brought it back to the lodging house. He received a biologically estimated dose of 54 rad. He had experienced no prodromal symptoms. He was hospitalized 9 days after the initial exposure. Hematological data at this time revealed only a moderate leukopenia ($3500/mm^3$) with lymphopenia ($840/mm^3$). There was no anemia, and the platelet count was $290,000/mm^3$. The total WBC count decreased until day 11 and the lowest value of the WBC was $2700/mm^3$. Thereafter, the WBC increased with fluctuating waves and reached the normal value at day 25. The sternal bone marrow showed moderate hypoplasia with a relative increase of plasma cells and reticulum cells at day 9.

The bone marrow aspirate from the iliac crest showed more severe hypoplastic changes than the sternal bone marrow on day 17. Furthermore, on day 12 the bone marrow from the iliac crest remained hypoplastic whereas the marrow from the sternum showed evidence of recovery.

Severe radiation dermatitis of the right hand and the hips was noted in case YS. The burns to the hands were less severe than those of case SH and the condition was corrected in November after antiseptic treatment. The skin lesions on the buttocks were formed by contact with the radioactive source. The absorbed dose was estimated at 3000 rad on the right side and 9000 rad on the left. Pain in the buttocks had begun promptly after the initial exposure.

Wet dermatitis was found on both sides after YS was hospitalized, and necrosis of the skin was noted in the center of the lesion in the left hip. Surgical biopsy of the affected skin on the left side was carried out on 25 November, 68 days after the initial exposure. The necrotic ulcer base was underlain by fairly well developed granulation tissue in which the blood vessels had hyalinized, thickened walls. The ulcer margins, sharply demarcated from the necrotic mass, exhibited degeneration, especially the basal layers.

The ulcerous tissue around the necrosis in the left hip was resistant to treatment, and the necrosis was surgically removed on 20 January 1972, 124 days after the initial exposure. The dermatitis had improved without surgery by March 1972. The patient was discharged on 25 March 1972 and thereafter was treated as an outpatient.

Case KJ had no nausea, vomiting, or weakness after exposure, but he noticed an erythematous lesion and pain in the right hand on 29 September. He was hospitalized on 11 October. On admission, a slight leukopenia (3300/mm³) and a blister surrounded by erythema in the right hand were observed. After the radiation dermatitis had improved, he was discharged on 27 November and thereafter was treated as an outpatient. The leukocyte count increased with fluctuating waves and reached a normal value on day 56.

Clinical Findings in Cases MK, MI, and TS

The three other cases did not exhibit prodromal symptoms or radiation dermatitis. They were admitted to the hospital on 26 September. The changes in their blood were minimal, and these three patients were discharged on 16 November.

Other Laboratory Findings

Special biochemical analyses of 11 metabolites in urine and blood, which were regarded as biochemical indicators of radiation effects, were carried out over a long period.[8]

Four metabolites, namely, 5-hydroxyindoleacetic acid, taurine, and Dishe reaction-positive substances (DRPS) in urine and 5-hydroxytryptamine in blood, seemed to reflect the severity of the injuries to some extent. The ratio of one metabolite to another, for example, the ratios of taurine to alanine or DRPS to creatinine, was a better indicator of the injuries than the concentration of any given metabolite itself.

The gonadal effects consisted of impaired spermatogenesis in all cases and elevation of follicle-stimulating hormone concentration in the sera of YS, MK, KJ, and SH; in three of these cases, the elevation became apparent 100 to 150 days after irradiation.[9]

Follow-up Studies

Follow-up studies on the six men have been performed annually since 1972.

The drop in the total lymphocyte count in each case corresponded very well to the exposed doses estimated from the cytogenetic studies during the period of hospitalization (Figure 5). Although no significant hematological disturbances were found in either peripheral blood or bone marrow, long-time observation reveals that the total lymphocyte count of the most severe case (case SH) showed consistently lower values than that of case YS (Figure 6).

In 1976, 5 years after the initial exposure, a quantitative assay of the

Figure 5. Time-course studies of total lymphocyte and neutrophil granulocyte counts in the six cases. From Hirashima et al.[5]

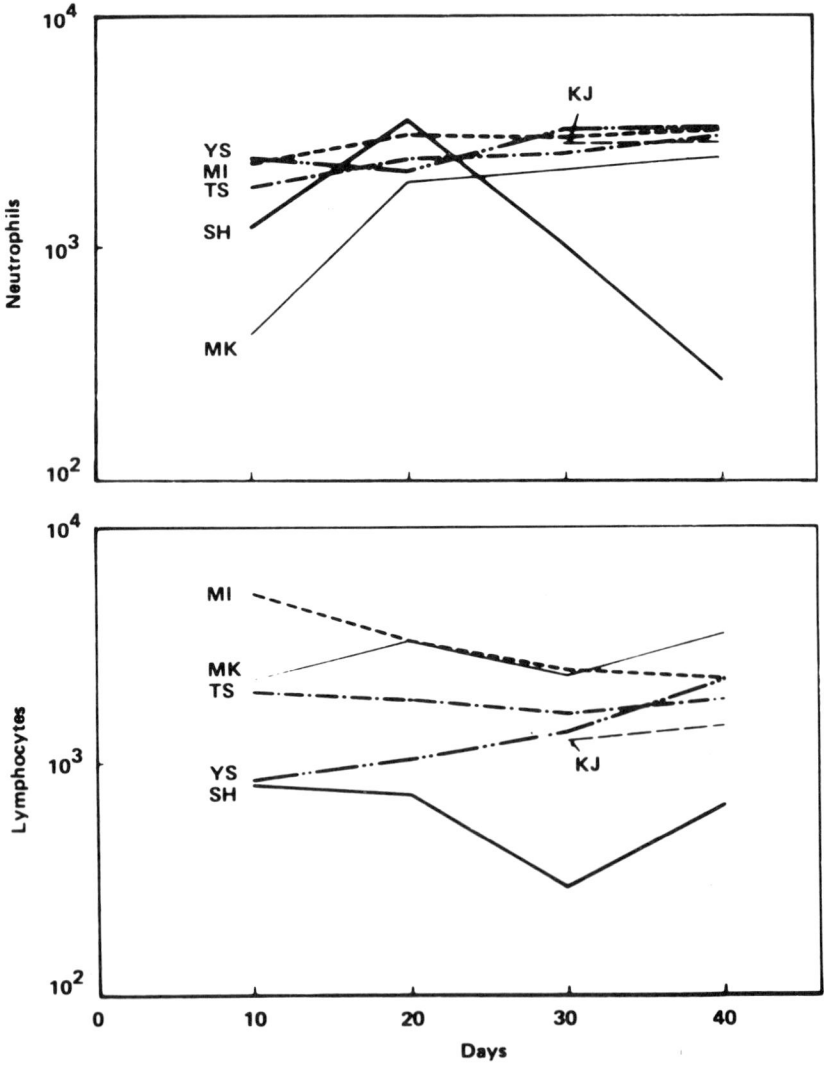

committed (granuloid) stem cells carried out according to the double-layer soft agar cultured method[10] was performed for cases SH and YS. The number of colony-forming units in culture (CFUc) in the marrow of patient SH was very low. In case YS, the CFUc content in the sternal marrow was within normal range while that of the iliac marrow was low (Figure 7).

The PHA-responsiveness of circulating T-lymphocytes which were collected by metrizoate-ficoll solution was also measured in cases SH

Figure 6. Follow-up studies of total leukocytes and neutrophil granulocytes in case SH and YS.

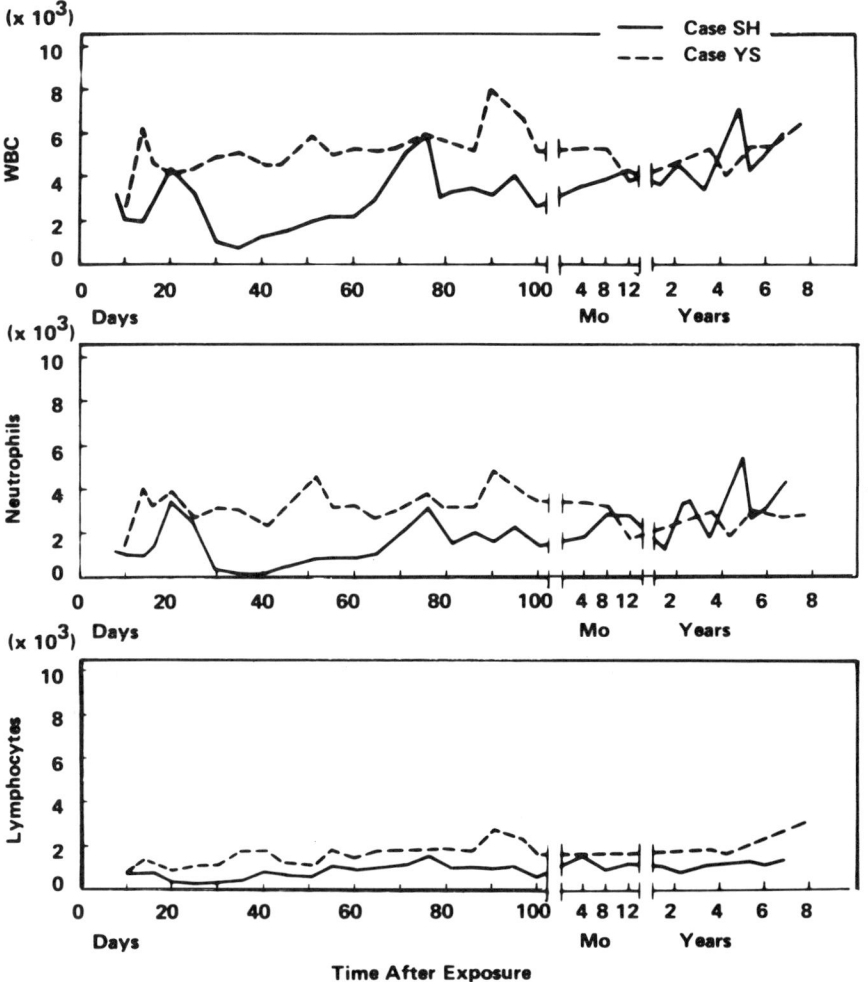

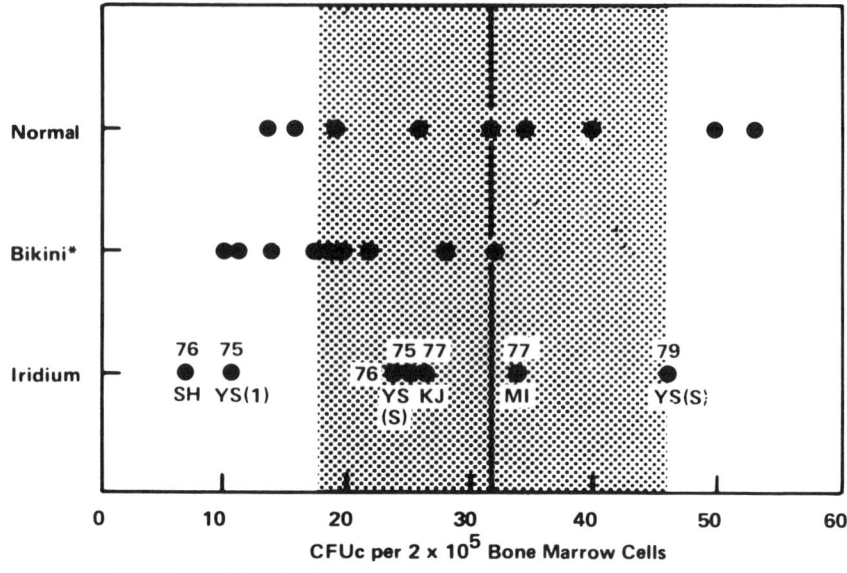

Figure 7. The quantity of committed (granuloid) stem-cells in the marrow of irradiated persons expressed in terms of the colony-forming units in culture (CFUc) per 2×10^5 bone marrow cells. YS(S),79 represents the value of sternal bone marrow in 1979, and YS(I) is the value of iliac bone marrow. No marks in parentheses mean that the data are from the sternal marrow.

and YS. The value for case SH was very low, whereas that of case YS was within normal limits (Figure 8).

Cytogenetic studies of the marrow cells and peripheral lymphocytes have been performed annually. The frequencies of chromosome abnormalities in 1976 were still high, especially in cases SH and YS.

The frequencies of Cu cells (cells with dicentrics plus rings) decreased with time. However, the Qdr values remained almost constant through the years (Figure 9). The number of Cs cells (cells with stable chromosome abnormalities) was fairly constant. The results strongly suggest that the dose estimate from Qdr values is a very useful technique for determining the biological dosimetry; this technique reduces the time lag after exposure and can also detect nonuniformity of exposure.

Nine months after the initial exposure and 5 months after the surgical removal of the necrosis on the right hip of YS, ulceration developed which was excised surgically. Thereafter the wound healed completely. The affected skin of the right hand in case YS was scarred and depigmented. He had flexion contracture of the right ring finger because of the scarring. In 1977, this flexion contracture was treated with skin grafting from a pedicle flap of abdominal skin.

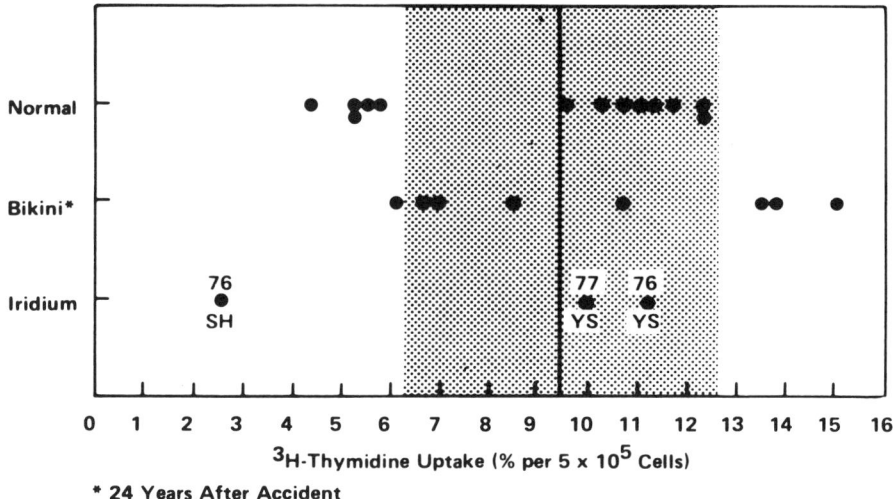

Figure 8. T-lymphocyte function of the irradiated patients expressed in terms of the uptake of ³H-thymidine in PHA-responsive lymphocytes (%/5 × 10⁵ cells). SH 76 represents the value of case SH in 1976.

Figure 9. Shifts with time in the frequency of Cu cells and *Qdr* values in case SH; DIC + R, dicentrics plus rings; Cs, cells with stable chromosome abnormalities.

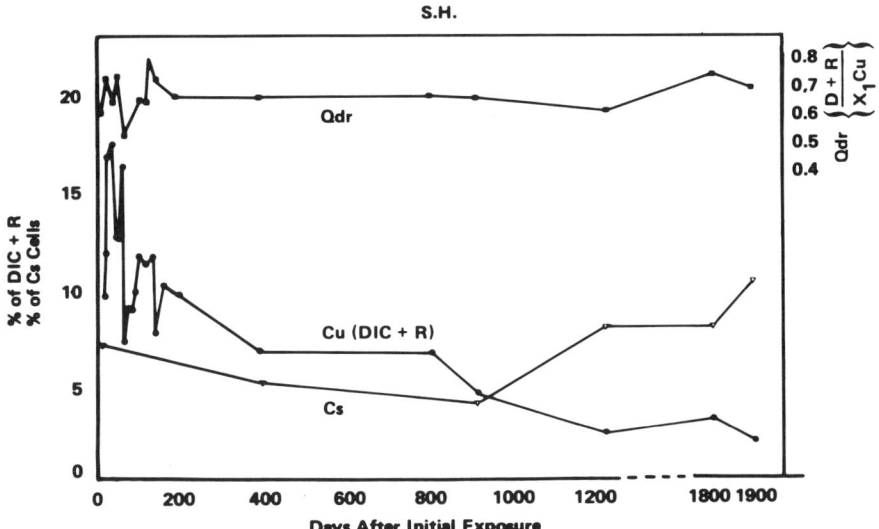

In case SH, the skin lesions in both hands were most remarkable, and there appeared repeatedly erosions of ulcers which healed temporarily with difficulty. However, no sign of skin cancer was observed. In this case, an atrophy of the phalanges, which seems to be due mainly to radiation osteitis, was also observed.

The affected skin of the right hand of case KJ was scarred and inelastic, and also abnormally pigmented or depigmented. However, neither erosion nor ulceration was observed.

A sperm count study was performed by Dr. T. Katayama (Department of Urology, Chiba University, School of Medicine). Five cases showed an almost normal count about 2 months after the accident. The sperm counts 6 months after the exposure showed total azoospermia in case YS; the other five cases had oligospermia (Table 4).

In one case (case YS), a punch biopsy of the testicles was performed in June 1972. Nine months after the exposure, there were marked disturbances of spermatogenesis. Histological findings revealed a decrease in the number of spermatogonia and spermatocytes, a thickening of the basement membrane, hyperplastic Leydig cells, and prominent Sertoli cells. These findings are compatible with atrophy of the testicles. The physically estimated dose to the testicles in this case amounted to about 175 rad. However, YS showed a moderate recovery in the sperm count in January 1973.

Ophthalmologic examinations were done by Dr. S. Kubota (Department of Ophthalmology, Chiba National Hospital). The examinations, carried out in November 1971 and September 1972, revealed quite normal findings in all six cases.

Table 4. Sperm Count.[a]

(millions per ml)

Patient	November 1971	December 1971	March 1972	October 1972	January 1973	March 1973
SH		9	4	1		20
YS	69	10	0		14	
KJ	78		9	15		
MK	27		3			
MI	88		48	15		
TS	84		35	15		

[a] From Sugiyame et al.[4]

Normal count: more than 50 millions per ml (Macleod and Gold).[12]

ACKNOWLEDGMENTS
The authors are much indebted to the International Atomic Energy Agency and the *Journal of Radiation Research* for permitting us to include previously published tables and figures.

References

1. Hashizume T, Kato Y, Nakajima T, Yamaguchi H, Fujimoto K: Dose estimation of nonoccupational persons accidentally exposed to ^{192}Ir gamma-rays. *J Radiat Res* 14:320–327, 1973.

2. Ishihara T, Kohno S, Hirashima K, Kumatori T, Sugiyama H, Kurisu A: Chromosome aberrations in persons accidentally exposed to ^{192}Ir gamma-rays. *J Radiat Res* 14:328–335, 1973.

3. Sasaki MS: Radiation-induced chromosome aberrations in lymphocytes: possible biological dosimeter in man, in Sugahara T, Hug O (eds.): *Biological Aspects of Radiation Protection*. Tokyo, Igaku Shoin Ltd., 1971, pp. 81–90.

4. Sugiyama H, Kurisu A, Hirashima K, Kumatori T: Clinical studies on radiation injuries resulting from accidental exposure to an iridium 192 radiographic source. *J Radiat Res* 14:275–286, 1974.

5. Hirashima K, Ishihara T, Kumatori T, Sugiyama H, Kurisu A: Hematological studies of six cases of accidental exposure to an iridium radiographic source. *J Radiat Res* 14:287–296, 1974.

6. Wald N: Haematological parameters after acute radiation injury, in *Manual on Radiation Haematology,* technical reports series No. 123. Vienna, International Atomic Energy Agency, 1971, pp. 253–264.

7. Thoma GE, Wald N: The diagnosis and management of radiation injury. *J Occupational Med* 1:421–447, 1959.

8. Nakamura W, Mizobuchi K, Sawada F, Kankura T, Kobayashi S, Kojima E, Nishimoto Y, Osawa N, Aoyagi Y, Chiba M: Biochemical analyses of some metabolites in urine and blood in persons exposed accidentally to a source of ^{192}Ir. *J Radiat Res* 14:304–320, 1973.

9. Wakabayashi K, Isurugi K, Tamaoki B, Akaboshi S: Serum levels of luteinizing hormone (LH) and follicle-stimulating hormone (FSH) in subjects accidentally exposed to ^{192}Ir gamma rays. *J Radiat Res* 14:297–303, 1973.

10. Robinson WA, Pike BL: Colony growth of human bone marrow cells *in vitro,* in Stohlman F, Jr. (ed.): *Symposium on Hemopoietic Cellular Differentiation,* New York, Grune and Stratton, pp. 249–259.

11. Kumatori T, Hirashima K, Ishihara T, Kurisu A, Sugiyama H, Hashizume T: Radiation accident caused by an iridium-192 radiographic source, in *Handling of Radiation Accidents, 1977.* Vienna, International Atomic Energy Agency, 1977, pp. 35–44.

12. MacLeod J, Gold RZ: The male factor in fertility and infertility. II. Spermatozoon counts in 1000 men of known fertility and in 1000 cases of infertile marriage. *J Urol* 66:436–449, 1951.

A Case of Child Abuse by Radiation Exposure

V. P. Collins* and
M. E. Gaulden+

*Houston, Texas;
+Department of Radiology, Southwestern Medical School, Dallas, Texas.

On 2 May 1974, a father was convicted of castrating his 13-year-old son by exposing him to radiation and was sentenced to 10 years in prison and a fine of $5000. The judgment was affirmed by the Court of Criminal Appeals of Texas on 10 May 1978. Since that date, the whereabouts of tne father, Kerry Andrus Crocker, have been unknown. He is presently being sought for unlawful flight to avoid incarceration.

The trial was widely reported in the press. A narrative account was presented before the 4th International Congress of the International Radiation Protection Association in Paris, France, in 1977, by Edgar D. Bailey and Martin C. Wukasch of the Texas Department of Health Resources.[1] In the lengthy affirmation of the conviction, the Court of Criminal Appeals of Texas detailed the entire series of events, the parties involved, the injuries, the evidence, the testimony, and the legal considerations.[2] The information in these assembled sources is briefly summarized here.

Kerry Andrus Crocker, a petroleum engineer, was divorced from his wife in February 1971. The divorce agreement gave the father custody of their two sons, Kirk and Patrick, on 2 weekends a month and 1 month a year. In November 1971, Crocker obtained a license authorizing possession of a 1-curie source of ^{137}Cs for oil and gas well logging. It is not recorded that this or subsequent sources were ever used for this purpose, and Crocker's business associates were unaware of his license or access to such sources. The license was amended in March 1972 to authorize possession of 2 sources of 2 curies each.

Kirk was subjected to perhaps eight exposures or attempted exposures over a 6-month period from April to October 1972, on weekends when Crocker exercised his visitation rights. These exposures occurred in the father's apartment, and on one occasion in a motel. Kirk encountered "shiny silver pellets" on at least six occasions; in the earpieces of headphones he was told to wear, in a pillow he was told to use, and in a sock he found in his bed. Repeatedly he was given a glass of orange juice in which he recognized a pill. On two occasions Kirk experienced nausea and vomiting on awakening, after probable exposure while asleep. It must be assumed that, under sedation, Kirk was exposed at such times unawares, and that the major lesions were caused by sources in contact with the skin for an unknown length of time.

The first suggestion of injury consisted of what appeared to be bruises developing to reddish brown blisters. He was seen by the family physician on 18 April 1972, about 10 days after the first suspected opportunity for exposure. The lesions were thought to be infections. They healed in about 10 days. Over succeeding weeks and months, new lesions appeared on the medial aspects of the thighs, the right ankle and right hand, and the left side of the forehead. In September 1972 he was seen by the family physician because hair was falling out from the left side of his head.

By the time the last visitation with the father and the last possible occasion of exposure in October 1972, there were persistent ulcerated lesions of the thighs and the right ankle, and Kirk was under continuing medical care. He dropped out of school on 31 October 1972, and for the next 2 years he kept up with his studies by being tutored at home. The lesions became increasingly more incapacitating, and in March 1973 he was admitted to the hospital where he remained for 3 weeks. The suspected infectious basis could not be established. Cortisone treatment gave some relief. At this time Kirk was in "incredible pain day and night." A psychiatrist consultant considered neurodermatitis related to conflict between Kirk and his father. Kirk's mother provided a list of 16 physicians who saw Kirk up until December 1973, when he was referred to a plastic surgeon, Dr. Thomas Cronin, for repair of the extensive incapacitating ulcerations. Dr. Cronin recognized the lesions as radiation necrosis.

From January 1974 to November 1978, Kirk underwent some 16 operations, 23 procedures by his mother's count. These included multiple plastic repairs and skin grafts by Dr. Cronin and several procedures conducted by Dr. Thomas Guthrie, a urologist, who reported one testicle "sloughed out" and the other effectively destroyed. Kirk was functionally castrated. The scrotum was repaired, and the testes were replaced with prostheses.

Throughout his years in high school, from 1974 to 1979, Kirk was under periodic medical-surgical care. During this time he developed a talent in speech and drama which led him into successful oratorical competition at the state and national levels. He graduated from high school cum laude and is now in his freshman year of college, and he has expressed a desire to enter law school.

He is a handsome, masculine, vigorous young man with a full range of social and scholastic activities. The injury-related findings are chiefly the extensive skin grafts of the medial aspects of the upper thighs, the perineum and scrotum, and the right ankle region. The grafts are healthy and free of any scarring that could limit motion. The heavily irradiated tissues have been completely excised.

The only residual radiation effects are a small area of telangiectasis of skin and scrotum and another of probable radiation dermatitis of the web between the thumb and forefinger of the right hand. Despite the proximity of the radiation exposure to these organs, there has been no impairment in the function of the penis, urethra, or anus. No abnormality of pelvic bones is seen on X-ray examination. All epiphyses are closed. Peripheral blood counts are normal.

The sole continuing evidence of radiation effect is the demonstration of persistent chromosomal aberrations. This aspect is under continuing study by Dr. Mary Esther Gaulden.

No numerical expression of dose can be meaningful under the circumstances of this case. For none of the lesions described is there any information on the number of sources, the amount of cesium 137, the geometry of contact, the duration of exposure, or the number of times any one area was exposed. The lesions were produced by an exposure in excess of the clinical tolerance dose for skin and subcutaneous tissue, without producing early symptoms or late detectable effect on adjacent vulnerable tissues and organs such as the anus, rectum, bladder, urethra, or penis. This, of course, is due to the rapid falloff in radiation (in accordance with the inverse square law) which makes it possible to use radiation sources clinically in surface molds or intracavitary applicators to eradicate a localized cancer without damage to adjacent normal tissues and organs.

A common loading for an intracavitary applicator for the treatment of carcinoma of the cervix might be 85 mCi of ^{137}Cs. Left in place for 48 hours, this dose could be expressed as 4080 mCi-hours. Treatment normally consists of two such applications, 2 weeks apart, for a total dose of some 8000 mCi-hours. This is of the order of exposure that would be achieved with 4 curies of ^{137}Cs in two applications of 1 hour each. Geometry and spacing could make a great difference in the surface effect. A carefully controlled placement produces a desired cancerocidal effect clinically, whereas the crude placement of high-intensity sources for the same number of millicurie-hours or curie-hours produced severe radionecrosis in Kirk. Clinical practice and experience indicates that this magnitude of dose can be directed to the uterus and cervix while not exceeding the tolerance dose to the adjacent rectum and bladder. In Kirk's case, local debridement has removed the grossly damaged tissue resulting from close contact with the radiation source and repair has been effected by grafting. In his case, as in the clinical use of radiation sources at close distance (brachytherapy), bowel, bladder, and adjacent normal tissues have received a dose well within the tolerance limits and no permanent damage or late effect need be expected.

The Factor of Child Abuse

It is remarkable how slowly the awareness of child abuse has developed since the founding of the Society for the Prevention of Cruelty to Children in 1895,[3] through the halting recognition of the significance of multiple and repetitive injuries by Caffey,[4] Silverman,[5] and Kempe.[6] The number of annual child abuse case reports has jumped from 7000 in 1967 to over 200,000 in 1974 and over a million in 1978. It is likely that this is belated recognition of an age-old problem rather than an increase in the actual incidence.[7] Injuries in childhood are commonplace, but the circumstances that might distinguish accident from physical abuse are likely to be concealed from the unsuspecting physician.

Two elements commonly found in child abuse records are present in this case. The first is that injuries or accidents are apt to be repetitive. In July 1971, Crocker took Kirk boating in Galveston Bay. He allowed or required Kirk to mount water skis behind the boat but would not allow him to wear a life jacket, despite Kirk's concern. He threw an anchor over the towrope, dragging Kirk under water until the boy could free himself. One month later, while the boy was sleeping in a mobile home on a weekend expedition with his father, a fire and explosion occurred that blew Kirk through the wall and resulted in severe burns. A second feature is that unsuspected abuse is associated with "notable behavioral and emotional problems."

Crocker was charged on one occasion with breaking and entering the office of his wife's attorney and removing her file. On another occasion he broke into his ex-wife's apartment and was found hiding in a closet. He was nobilled on this occasion because the complaint was by an "ex-wife."

Failure to seek or consider the evidence of child abuse is not limited to the medical community. The first charges brought by Kirk's mother, that her son had been abused by radiation, were considered by legal counsel to be imaginative. On a later occasion, after Crocker had been indicted, Mrs. Crocker was reluctant to have the visitation privileges continued. At a court hearing, despite unequivocal expert testimony as to the radiation injury, the presiding judge threatened the mother with jail for contempt of court if she did not release Kirk to his father in accordance with the original divorce agreement.

The Castrate Status

The usual concern for the irradiated male is whether he will experience impaired spermatogenesis or whether genetic damage will be induced. Studies can be carried out to determine whether the reduced sperm count and motility, and the chromosome aberrations encountered, are radiation-induced or have some prior etiology. In this case such radiation-caused changes have not occurred because of the total destruction of the testes. However, the castration was the result of radiation and was the charge on which the father was convicted.

There is little or no current experience with the effects of castration in children. What clinical experience does exist is based on older males with metastatic prostate cancer.[8] The associated physiological changes are clouded by competing disease and do not bear on the significance of castration in childhood.

There is a great deal of information available in the literature of veterinary medicine on castration in young males of several species.[9,10] Except for the inability to procreate, it appears that Kirk's anatomical and physiological development, with replacement hormone therapy, is likely to permit full normal activities. As of this time, Kirk is under no handicap, physically, academically, or socially, and it is likely that he will live a normal life-span.

The essential question is what may be the future effects of the total injury. The primary injury has been repaired surgically. Tissues exposed to high radiation dose have been largely removed. Neoplasm as a late effect now seems a remote possibility because severely damaged tissues have been removed. Moreover, whereas radiation-related carcinogenesis has, in the main, been related to long-continued low-level radiation exposure, the exposure in this case occurred in a limited number of brief, intensive episodes.

Concern for the possible development of leukemia is a matter for continuing study. Reports on military personnel exposed to low-level radiation at the Nevada test site in 1956 indicate an increased incidence of leukemia. The film badge exposures for eight individuals who have developed leukemia was 0 to 2977 mrem. This is rather at odds with the current impression of risks associated with clinical and occupational exposures in the same range.

Chromosomal aberrations may be an indication that leukemia will develop. At present, we have no basis for assessing a probability. It would be unfair to this young man to stigmatize his future with any firmer statement.

Comments

The distinctive feature of this instance of child abuse is not so much that it was caused by radiation, but that it was unrecognized and unsuspected for so many physicians over a period of 20 months. It is paradoxical that, where there is any hint of radiation exposure, all manner of phenomena are ascribed to it and accepted as effects, but, when any suspicion of exposure is lacking, quite standard radiation reactions are unrecognized.

The lesions demonstrated in this case are within the experience of those familiar with the medical and industrial uses of radiation, and, as demonstrated by Dr. Cronin, could be recognized instantly on gross appearance. No incident of chemical or thermal exposure capable of producing such lesions could go unnoticed, and no agent but radiation would account for a time lag in their appearance and development.

An information gap characterizes the two groups of people whose expertise would bear upon the detection and prevention of such an incident. From the first appearance of a change in skin that was taken to be a locker-room rash to the ultimate recognition of the etiology, some 16 physicians saw Kirk's lesions. It is quite possible that none of them had ever seen a radiation reaction or radiation necrosis. Similarly, the custodians of radiation sources and authorities for licensing and control are not apt to be aware of the various manifestations of child abuse or the spectrum of injuries that might be encountered in the physician's office or the hospital emergency room. Even Agatha Christie and Ellery Queen have not introduced the public to radiation as a potential lethal weapon.

In view of the nonspecific nature and the varied manifestations of radiation effects along with the availability of dangerous sources, it is probable that there have been, and will be, additional instances in which a radiation source may be put to criminal use with little chance of detection.

References

1. Bailey ED, and Wukasch MC: *Proc. 4th Int. Congr. Int. Radiat. Protection Assoc.* (Paris, France) 3:987, 1977.
2. Crocker *v.* State of Texas, 573 S.W. 2d 190 (1978).
3. Mindlin RL: Background to the current interest in child abuse and neglect. *Pediatric Annals* 5:11–14, Mar. 1976.
4. Caffey J: Multiple fractures in the long bones of children suffering from chronic subdural hematoma. *Am. J. Roentgenol. Radium Ther. Nucl. Med.* 56:163, 1946.
5. Silverman FN: The roentgen manifestations of unrecognized skeletal trauma in infants. *Am. J. Roentgenol. Radium Ther. Nucl. Med.* 69:413, 1953.

6. Kempe CH: The battered child syndrome. *JAMA* 181:17, 1962.

7. Freeman SB, and Morse CW: Child abuse: A five-year follow-up of early care findings in the emergency department. *Pediatrics,* 54:404, 1974.

8. Money J, Higham E: *Endocrinology* 3:1358, 1979.

9. Kiley M: A review of the advantages and disadvantages of castrating farm livestock with particular reference to behavioral effects. *Br. Vet. J.* 132:323, 1976.

10. Fletcher TJ, and Short RV: Restoration of libido in castrated red deer stag (*Cervus elaphus*) with oestradiol-17. *Nature* 247:616, 1974.

The 1979 Los Angeles Accident:
Exposure to Iridium 192 Industrial Radiographic Source

Joseph F. Ross,
Francis E. Holly,
Harvey A. Zarem,
Cappy M. Rothman,
and Alan L. Shabo

UCLA School of Medicine, Los Angeles, California.

The number of overexposures of industrial radiographers to ionizing radiation equals the number of overexposures of all other Nuclear Regulatory Commission (NRC) licensees, although industrial radiographers comprise only a small percentage of all NRC licensees.[1] In Southern California, it is estimated that 12 to 15 incidents with a potential for overexposure occur each year because difficulty is experienced in handling industrial radiographic sources. Many of these incidents are managed without serious overexposure, and many are believed not to be reported to the California Division of Occupational Safety and Health Administration (CALOSHA), which probably learns only of incidents in which there have been major overexposures of personnel. However, during the past two years, a single medical practitioner (JFR) has seen in medical consultation 19 individuals who were involved in five incidents of industrial radiographic overexposure. Serious overexposure accidents of this type have occurred for many years and in many parts of the world.[2-8] *These accidents are preventable,* and their continued occurrence reflects adversely on the industrial radiographic industry and on the regulatory agencies. Eradication or great reduction in the number of these tragic events could be accomplished by simple modifications of equipment, and by mandating use of improved personnel radiological safety monitoring devices that would emit not-to-be-ignored audible and visible alarm signals when more than tolerable levels of ionizing radiation are present.

We report an incident in which 11 individuals were exposed to ionizing radiation with resultant serious emotional reactions, and in one individual, grave physical damage—an incident that easily could have been prevented, with avoidance of serious suffering and great expense.

The Incident

At the conclusion of an industrial radiographic procedure, a 28-curie ^{192}Ir source became detached from the source tube of Iriditron Model #520 industrial gamma radiography exposure unit and was left by the radiographer on the floor of the engineering workshop. A workman (Case 11) placed the source in his right hip pocket and carried it there for 45 min, following which it was handled by five other workers before being returned to the radiographer. Additionally, five other plant personnel were at varying distances from the source for different periods of time. The nature of the lost source, and the fact that radiation exposure had occurred, was not realized until 21 days later. Shortly thereafter, Mr. S. Wong and Mr. D. Bunn of CALOSHA reenacted the incident, and Table 1 summarizes their estimates of the location of personnel relative to the source, and the duration of their exposure. These estimates were difficult to obtain and may be in error because of faulty memory of the personnel involved. In particular, the estimates of the duration of exposure of the fingers are gross approximations, and may be in error by a factor of two or three.

Recognition by plant personnel that overexposure to radiation had occurred resulted in severe anxiety, and certain individuals became almost hysterical. Real and imagined illnesses and symptoms were attributed to radiation exposure. For example, three weeks after the incident, Case 9 became impotent and attributed his impotence to "radiation exposure," which he believed he acquired while "taking a siesta" in the doorway of the room in which the radiographic measurements were made. The doorway was 25 feet from the source, and his exposure could not have been more than 0.2 rad. Subsequent studies demonstrated that his impotence was due to the presence of local inflammatory disease of the genital tract.

Another workman on day 32 developed severe subjective symptoms of nausea, diarrhea, lassitude, and fatigability, which he attributed to radiation exposure, an attribution that became untenable when it was discovered that he was not at work on the day of the incident. The four female employees who were exposed became very disturbed about the situation. Candid discussion of all the facts relating to exposure, clinical and laboratory findings, and expectancy in terms of acute and long-range effects of radiation was of assistance in partially allaying anxiety.

Table 1. Clinical and Exposure Data

| | | | | | Calculated radiation dose | |
Case	Sex	Age	Exposure to ^{192} Ir 28 curie	Signs and symptoms	Skin surface (R)	Whole-Body exposure body midline 10 cm (rad)
1	F	31	Fingertips: 30-60 sec Upper body: 24 in; 75 min	Fatigue & somnolence for 1 wk Erythema fingertips began 10th day Lenticular opacities observed 57th day	11,500-23,000	18-28
2	F	30	Body: 216 in; 75 min	None		0.4
3	F	18	Body: 120 in; 75 min	Fainting spells day 34		1.4
4	F	50	Body: 108 in; 75 min	None		1.7
5	M	54	Fingertips: 90-180 sec	Erythema & vesiculation 3 fingers began day 10	40,000-60,000	1-11
6	M	37	Fingertips: 60 sec Body: 168 in; 75 min	Numbness 2 fingers began day 10	23,000	0.7
7	M	27	Fingertips: 30 sec Body: 96 in; 75 min	Numbness 2 fingers began day 14	11,5000	1.8-2.1
8	M	27	Body: 30 in; 20-30 min	None		3-10
9	M	43	Body: 25 ft; 30 min	Impotence began on day 32		0.2
10	M	56	Hand: 5 in; 5 min Mid body: 12 in; 5 min	Fatigue, asthenia preceded incident no changes following	70	0.7-5.5
11	M	50	Source in right hip pocket: 45 min	Nausea: 30 min. Began 60-90 min after exposure Burning pain, erythema began after 6 hours exposure, progressing to severe burn	80,000-400,000	75-100

Radiation Dosimetry

One of us (FEH) established by direct measurement of the source that it consisted of 28 curies of ^{192}Ir. Collaboration with Mr. W. L. Beck of REAC/TS ORAU established the estimates of surface and "whole-body" radiation exposure summarized in Table 1. These studies are detailed in the article by these authors appearing elsewhere in this volume.

The physics of the dosimetry associated with small sources of a single isotope is well understood. Such calculations are routine and are done on a daily basis in every radiation oncology department. Great precision may be obtained since the exact placement of the sources is known and the exposure time is well controlled. Thus, the precision of accident dosimetry depends solely upon the reconstruction or reenactment of the incident. In this instance, where several weeks had elapsed, exposure times are only estimates, and may be in error by a factor of two or more. This is particularly the case in finger exposure estimates. Also a few centimeters uncertainty in source location (as in the case of the hip pocket) may render dose estimates at depths of a few centimeters uncertain by factors of 2 to 10. Only at depths (distances) larger than 10 and 100 cm are respective uncertainties of 100% and 10% not extant. The "whole-body" dose reported here has no meaning except in the broadest average or integral dose sense.

Clinical Observations

Although symptoms and signs of radiation exposure developed in predictable fashion in the five individuals (Cases 1, 5, 6, 7, and 11) who had direct contact with the source, the nature of these symptoms was not recognized until day 21 following the exposure.

Case 11, who had carried the source in his right hip pocket for 45 min, 60 to 90 min later became nauseated for a period of 30 min. He did not vomit. For the next two or three days, he felt "unwell" and perspired more than usual. Six hours after exposure, a burning sensation and erythema were noted on the right buttock. These symptoms increased in severity, and two days later, he sought medical care in an ambulatory care facility, where a diagnosis of "insect bite" was made. For the next 17 days, he continued to work, and treatment consisted of antihistamines, antibiotics, and local compresses. The lesion progressed to ulceration, and on day 17, he was hospitalized at the Kaiser Permanente Hospital, Fontana, as a patient of Dr. Daniel DeVore. Persistent questioning by Dr. DeVore and Dr. William Gordon during the next three days finally elicited the history of carrying an object in the hip pocket, and the diagnosis of severe radiation burn was established. By request of CA-LOSHA on day 21, this patient was transferred to the UCLA Hospital Burn Center.

On admission to UCLA, examination revealed an ulcer on the right buttock 11 × 9 cm in extent, 2 cm deep, and surrounded by a 2–4 cm wide area of intense erythema. The lesion caused continuous severe pain, necessitating administration of narcotic medication. Figures 1 and 2 illustrate the appearance of the lesion. Anterior to the larger lesion, there was an erythematous area 2.5 × 2 cm in size. Physical examination revealed the presence of bilateral supra-patellar, adductor, and extensor plantar reflexes, and unsustained knee and ankle clonus. Other neurological findings were normal. In spite of extensive neurological and radiographic studies, the nature and etiology of these findings remain unexplained. They persisted without change for 155 days. It is suspected that they are due to a preexisting condition, and are not related to radiation.

On day 94, numbness and decreased sensation of light touch developed on the skin of the distal 2 phalanges of the thumb, index, second, and third fingers of the right hand. There were no associated cutaneous or reflex changes. These symptoms gradually decreased during the next 60 days, and had disappeared by day 155. Their etiology is not known.

A marked lymphopenia was present on admission (day 24) and persisted until day 61 (Table 2). A moderate to severe normocytic, normochromic anemia was present on day 24, becoming more severe until day

Figure 1. Case 11, 31 days after exposure to ^{192}Ir radiographic source. Ulcerated radiation burn on right buttock is 11 × 9 × 2 cm. Surrounding erythema is 2 cm in width.

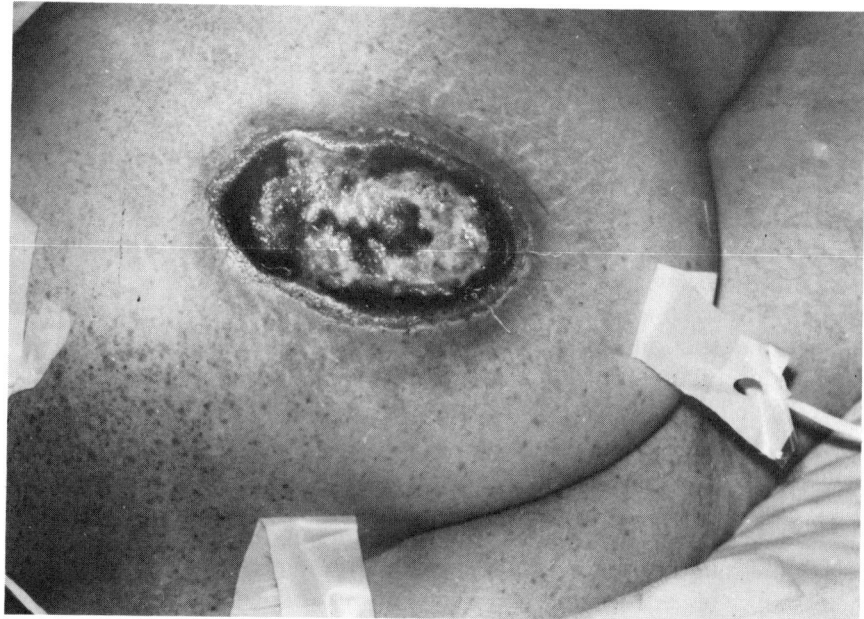

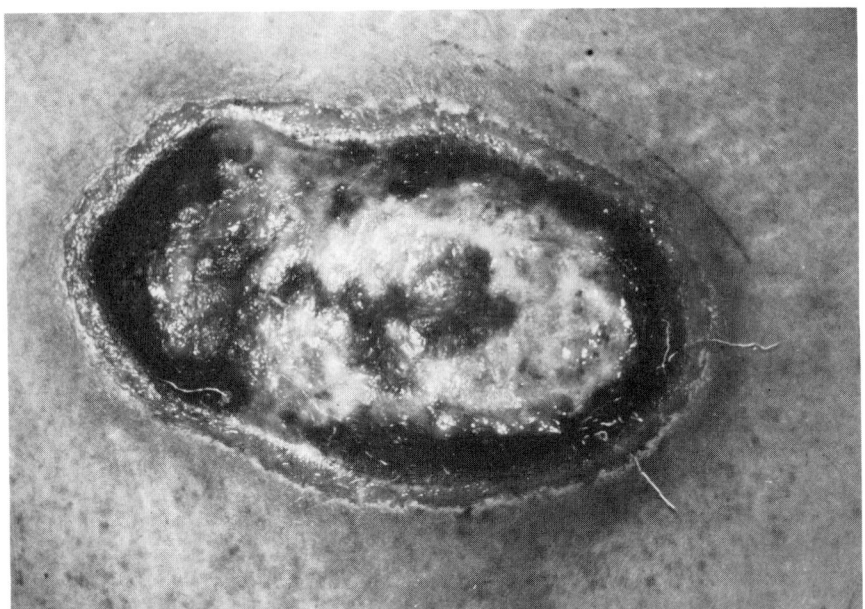

Figure 2. Case 11. Detail of Figure 1 showing fat necrosis and the surrounding intense erythema from radiation burn.

104. The blood hemoglobin concentration had returned to normal by day 155. This anemia most probably was caused by the marked inflammatory reaction of the radiation burn, although radiation effects upon hematopoiesis may have contributed to its severity. The initial reticulocyte count was slightly increased, and it never became decreased. Platelet counts were normal.

On day 28, a technetium 99 M diphosphonate tomographic scan of the entire skeleton was normal, as were radiographs of the skeleton. On day 85, an indium 111 chloride bone marrow scan showed a questionable slight decrease in marrow activity in the right hemipelvis. The marrow distribution otherwise was normal.

A computerized tomographic scan of the pelvis was performed on day 91, and the sections at 12 cm and 14 cm below the iliac crest are illustrated in Figure 3, which also indicates isodose curves. These studies showed swelling and apparent edema of the right pyriformis and gluteus maximus muscles, blurring of the neurovascular bundle on the right, swelling of the right seminal vesicle and partial obliteration of the normal tissue planes in the perirectal region. These changes are interpreted as attributable to deep exposure to the radiation source.

With the intent of increasing blood flow to the burned, ulcerated area, diminishing the adverse local effects of radiation exposure, relieving pain, and decreasing the duration of disability on day 36, the large

Table 2. Hematologic Observations[a]

Case	Day after exposure	Whole-body dose (rad)	Hgb gm%	Retic %	Leukocytes (x 10^3)			Platelets (x10^3)
					Total	Pmnis	Lymphs	
1	23	18-28	13.2	1.2	4.2	2.1	1.3	310
	36		13.0	1.1	4.1	1.4	1.9	326
	155		12.9		4.6	2.5	1.6	
5	23	1-11	15.0	1.2	6.9	4.0	2.0	215
	36		14.8	1.2	6.8	3.8	2.4	208
	155		15.3		7.6	5.4	1.5	202
8	84	3-10	16.6	1.1	10.2	6.6	2.9	300
	155		16.8	0.9	5.9	2.8	2.1	
10	35	0.7-5.5	7.0	5.0	6.5	4.4	1.2	230
	50		7.5	3.2	4.4	3.6	0.8	350
	64		9.1	2.4	4.5	2.4	1.5	
	84		11.8	1.7	5.0	3.5	1.3	
	119		12.8	1.1	5.5	3.2	1.9	
	155		14.3	1.7	6.9	4.8	2.0	178
11	20	75-100	14.1		8.7	5.1	3.5	
	24		13.2	3.0	8.1	7.1	0.8	290
	31		14.1	1.0	8.5	7.0	0.7	350
	39		11.1		8.6	6.6	1.2	
	51		12.0		9.7	7.3	1.3	450
	61		12.2		7.6	4.9	1.9	
	71		11.3		7.0	4.2	2.5	
	77		11.4		5.4	2.6	1.4	
	104		11.4		6.8	4.1	2.0	
	155		15.3		8.5	6.3	2.0	325
	Normal Range M		14-18	0.8-2.5	4.3-10	1.8-7.3	1.5-4.0	150-300
	F		12-16	0.8-4.1				

[a] Case 2, 3, 4, 6, 7, 9: All values within normal limits.

ulcerated area was excised by HAZ, and a full thickness tensor fascia lata myocutaneous flap was mobilized from the right thigh, and with its vascular pedicle intact, was sutured into the bed of the excised ulcer. Vasodilan 10 mg, three times a day, was administered by mouth from day 33 until day 104, with the intent of promoting blood flow to the skin flap and the surrounding radiated area. Initially, hypotension was produced by this medication, and it was suspected of causing neutropenia from day 75 to day 84. This cleared, even though the drug was continued.

The skin flap survived in excellent fashion, and the skin erythema cleared on its lateral aspects. Tissue necrosis and sloughing of radiated tissue adjacent to the posterior (distal) aspect of the flap occurred, but eventually this area stabilized, granulated, and on day 91 skin grafts were applied, most of which survived and epithelialized the area. The appear-

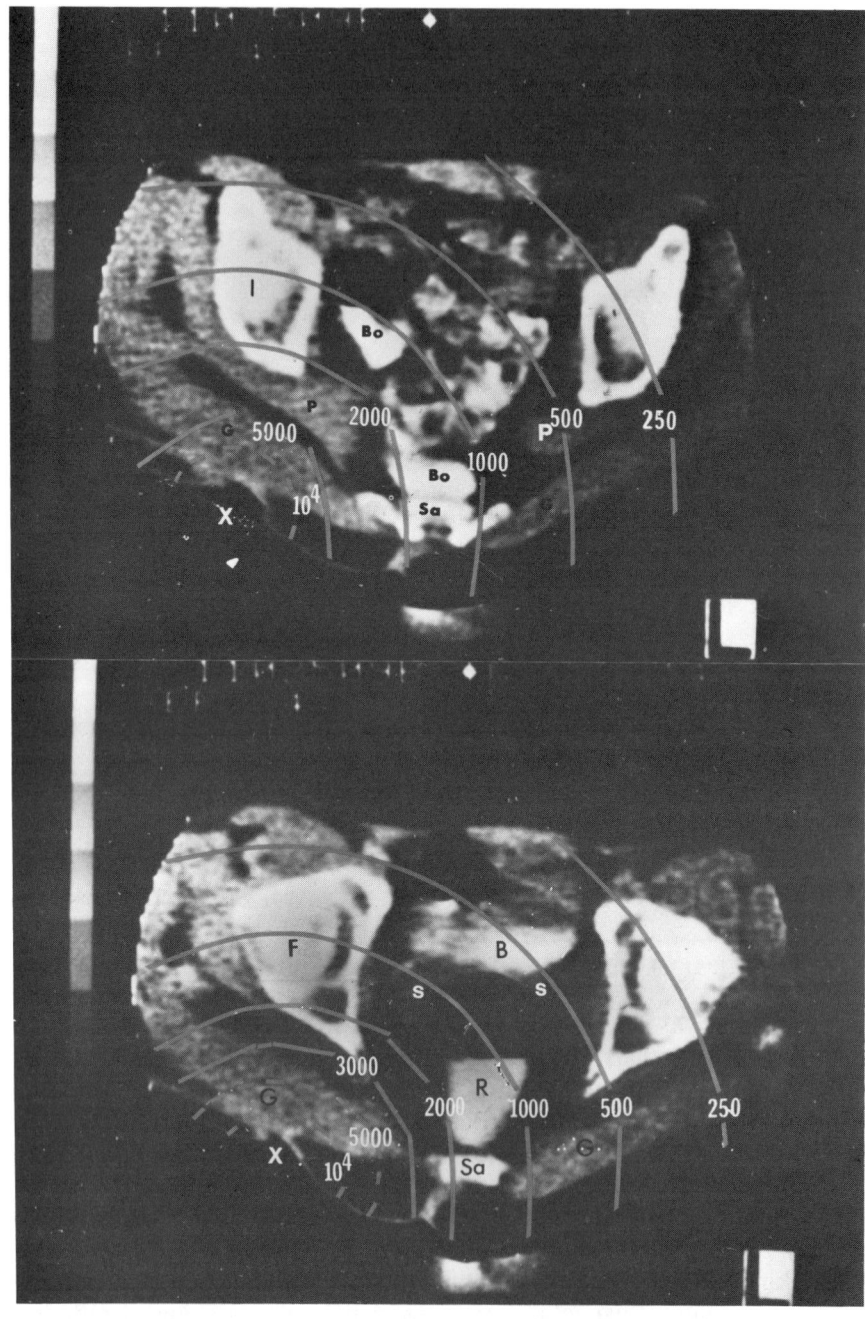

ance of the skin flap and adjacent areas on day 104 is shown in Figure 4. The erythema completely cleared, and the flap was in healthy condition. The improved circulation to the area covered by the skin flap accelerated healing of the adjacent nonulcerated radiated tissue. The smaller lesion anterior to the large ulcer was not resected, and, as shown in Figure 4, it increased in extent and developed central necrosis. Eventually it will have to be excised and treated with a skin flap. The comparison between these two lesions support the belief that radiation burns in some instances may be treated advantageously by early excision and implantation of a skin flap with intact blood supply. In Case 11, this management decreased pain and shortened the duration of disability. We emphasize that management of radiation burns must be individualized for each patient and for each lesion and, in some instances, early resection and skin flap implacement may not be indicated.

Cytogenetic studies are summarized in Table 3, and reveal chromosome abnormalities attributed to ionizing radiation at a dose estimated from the number of abnormalities at 75–100 rad whole-body radiation—an estimate identical with that based on physical measurements.

Libido and sexual potency remained normal in Case 11, although semen analyses (Table 4) showed a progressive decrease in the number and the motility of morphologically normal spermatozoa. On day 155, there were fewer than 500,000 sperm per ml of semen.

Case 11 was hospitalized for a total of 88 days, for a hospital cost of $26,000. He was discharged on day 105, 69 days after the operation. Except for increasing pain in the nonresected lesion, he feels well, but has not returned to work. Resection of the smaller lesion is contemplated within the next 30–60 days.

Case 1, a secretary who handled the source, and on whose shelf and desk it sat for 75 min, received a finger tip dose estimated at 11,500–23,000 R, and a whole-body dose of 18–28 rad (Table 1). She was asthenic, lethargic, and somnolent for a week following the incident. Erythema of the skin of the volar and lateral aspects of the terminal phalanges of the right thumb and index finger appeared on day 14. These

---

Figure 3. Case 11 CAT scan, 91 days after exposure and 55 days after surgical placement of skin flap. The upper and lower figures are 12 and 14 cm below the level of the iliac crest, respectively. There is marked asymmetry of the soft tissue of the buttocks, the right being larger than the left. The gluteus maximus and piriform muscle (P) groups are larger on the right with less sharply defined borders, and there is a partial obliteration of the normal tissue planes in the perirectal (R) region. Asymmetry of the seminal vesicles (S) could represent either edema or a normal variant. The overlying isodose regions are based on the source location (X), being stationary and in the plane of the scan. The tissue defect of the residual ulcer is evident at "X." B, Bladder; Bo, Bowel; I, Ischium; F, Femur; Sa, Sacrum.

lesions disappeared without residual abnormality in 3–4 weeks. Vesiculation did not develop. Ophthalmological examination and slit lamp biomicroscopy by ALS on day 57 revealed mild bilateral postcapsular-lens opacities. Continued follow-up of these opacities will be necessary to determine their etiology.

Complete ophthalmological examination and slit lamp biomicroscopy were performed on each case. All examinations were normal except Case 1. Follow-up examinations at 6–12-month intervals are planned.

Case 3, who received a whole-body dose of 1.4 rad, experienced fainting spells beginning on day 15. These were attributed by her to exposure to radiation, but medical evaluation indicated that similar episodes had occurred 9 and 10 years previously. A diagnosis of epilepsy was established, and she was successfully treated with dilantin.

Case 5, who handled the source for 90–180 sec, on day 10 noted erythema of the volar and lateral surfaces of the right thumb, index finger, and second finger. Deep-seated vesicles developed in these areas, but healed during the next two months; and on day 155, there were no residual skin abnormalities. He experienced no subjective symptoms.

Figure 4. Case 11, 104 days after exposure and 68 days after implantation of skin flap. Erythema above and below the graft has disappeared and healing has occurred. Necrosis posterior to the distal tip of the flap has stabilized. Skin grafts have been implanted on the granulation tissue. The small radiation burn above the skin flap that was not resected has extended in area, and central necrosis has occurred. The red area to right is the bed from which skin graft was mobilized.

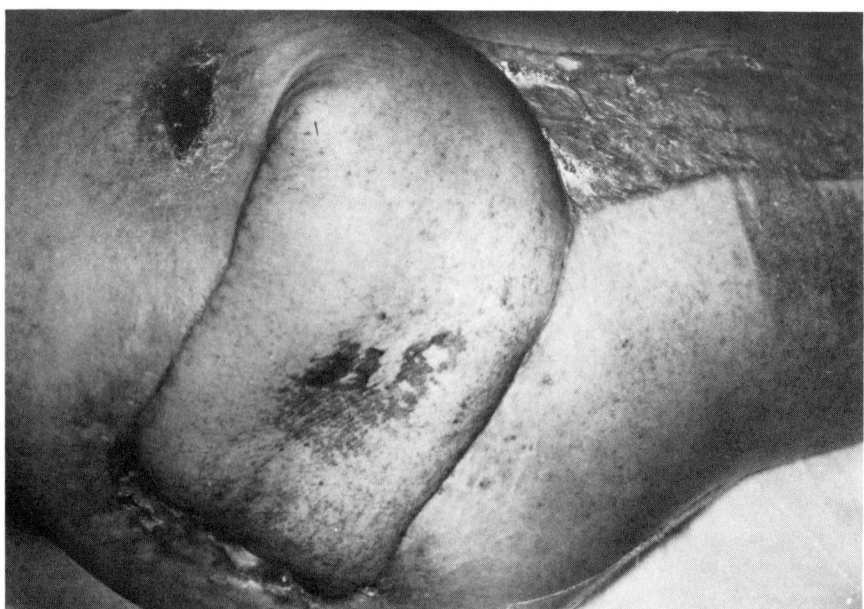

Table 3. Cytogenetic Studies

Case	Day after exposure	Whole-body exposure (rad)	Lab No. 1 100 Metaphases examined		Lab No. 2 300 Metaphases examined			Lab No. 3 600 Metaphases examined		
			Gaps	Breaks + dicentrics[a]	Acentric fragments	Dicentrics	Rings	Micronuclei per 3000 lymphocytes	Dicentrics	Dicentric frequency
1	23	18-28	0	1						
2	35	0.4	1	1						
3	35	1.4	0	0						
4	35	1.7	Premature separation of chromatids in 11 cells							
5	23	1-11	2	1						
6	30	0.7	4	1						
7	30	1.8-2.1	9	0						
8	85	3-10	2	7						
9	not done	0.2								
10	35	0.7-5.5	1	0						
11	28	75-100			20	13	2			
	30							25		
	41		5	3					50	0.0833

[a] Normal less than 3%.

Table 4. Semen Analyses

Case	Day after Exposure	Whole-body exposure (rad)	Semen vol (ml)	Number million per ml	Spermatozoa Motility 3+-4+ %	Normal morphology %
5	155	1-11	3.0	82	30	57
6	57	0.7	4.4	27	55	81
	85		4.8	57	50	65
	126		4.6	81	70	82
7	36	1.8-2.1	1.6	33	60	45
	64		4.0	28	70	73
8	155	3-10	1.7	112	40	66
9	63	0.2	2.2	102	35	63
10	56	0.7-5.5	1.5	27	35	67
	86		1.4	86	50	75
	128		1.5	123	30	69
11	21	75-100	3.5	12	20	75(?)
	31	(testes 60-150 rad)	3.0	78	15	40
	155		2.2	0.5	20	<5
		Lower limit of normal:	2.5	40	60	60

Semen analysis on day 155 was relatively normal, except for decreased motility of spermatozoa (Table 4).

Numbness, but no erythema or vesiculation occurred in *Case 6* on day 10, and in *Case 7* on day 14. Decreased concentration of spermatozoa was demonstrated in Case 6 on day 57, and in Case 7 on days 35 and 64, with a decrease in the percentage of normal sperm (Table 4).

Case 8, estimated to have a whole-body dose of 3–10 rad, experienced no adverse symptoms or abnormalities in semen, although cytogenetic studies revealed an increased number of chromosome breaks and dicentrics (Table 3). Additional cytogenetic studies are in process.

The impotence of *Case 9* already has been described. Semen analysis was abnormal, and his symptoms and abnormalities were believed to be attributable to local inflammatory disease in the genital tract.

Case 10, the radiographer, experienced severe symptoms of easy fatigability, asthenia, and hematochezia, both before and following the incident. These symptoms were due to severe iron deficiency that developed as a consequence of bleeding hemorrhoids. The anemia responded satisfactorily to oral therapy with ferrous sulphate (Table 2). No symptoms attributable to radiation exposure were described. His film badge registered 470 mrem; the dose to his fingers was 70 R, and the whole-body dose was 0.7–5.5 rad. However, when first examined on day 35, he had a lymphocyte count of 1235 cells, which on day 50 had decreased to 792. Lymphocytes did not return to normal until day 119. Semen analysis on day 56 revealed a marked decrease in the number and motility of spermatozoa. These had returned to relative normality on day 86, and complete normality on day 128. Cytogenetic studies on day 35 were reported as normal. These observations suggest that calculations of radiation dose based on the individual's statements concerning his distance from the source and the duration of exposure may be of questionable validity. Also, it is possible that his personnel radiation dosimeter might not have been worn at all times during and following the incident.

Cases 2 and 4 experienced severe anxiety and emotional distress, but there were neither physical nor laboratory abnormalities.

Laboratory Observations

During the three weeks immediately following the radiation exposure, laboratory tests were not performed. Beginning on day 20, when cases were referred for consultation, extensive evaluation of blood and chromosomes, and, in males, semen analyses were performed as promptly as possible. Nevertheless, considerable delay occurred, particularly in accomplishing semen analyses.

All cases had extensive hematologic evaluation; Table 2 details studies of cases in which the total body dose was more than 2 rad (Cases 1, 5, 8, 10, and 11). All values were within normal limits in Cases 2, 3, 4, 6, 7, and 9, and these values are not detailed in Table 2.

The anemia of Case 10 was caused by blood loss and iron deficiency. In Case 11, the hemoglobin fell to 11 gm on day 39, possibly as a consequence of local inflammatory processes associated with radiation burn.

Total leukocytes and polymorphonuclear neutrophilic leukocytes (pmnls) were normal in number in all cases. Lymphopenia of mild degree was observed in Case 1 on day 23, and was present in Case 10 from day 35 to day 119. Case 11 was lymphopenic from day 24 to day 61. Reticulocytes were not decreased in any case, and all platelet counts were normal.

In these 11 cases, the number of lymphocytes was the most sensitive hematologic indicator of exposure to ionizing radiation.

Cytogenetic Studies

The UCLA cytogenetic laboratory evaluated 48-hour cultures of peripheral blood lymphocytes on all cases except Case 9. These studies are detailed in Table 3 under Laboratory #1. The results were abnormal for Case 4, who had received an estimated whole-body dose of 1.7 rad, and on day 35 showed separation of chromatids in 11 cells. The significance of this observation is not known.

Case 8, whose estimated whole-body dose was 3–10 rad, on day 155 was found to have seven "breaks and dicentrics," a definitely abnormal finding.

The blood of Case 11, who received an estimated whole-body dose of 75–100 rad, was studied on days 28 and 30 in two research laboratories, each of which reported significant abnormalities attributed to an equivalent whole-body dose of 70–100 rad.

Additional cytogenetic studies are in process in Cases 1, 5, 8, 10, and 11. Details and interpretation of the cytogenetic studies performed on Case 11 are presented by Dr. G. Littlefield and her colleagues in a separate report in this volume.

Semen Analyses

Table 4 summarizes the results of semen analyses performed by one of us (CMR) on all seven male subjects. Significant abnormalities were observed in all individuals, except Cases 5 and 8, on whom the procedure could not be performed until day 155. The specimen on Case 9 contained many erythrocytes and leukocytes, changes believed to be attributable to genital inflammatory disease.

Case 6, whose whole-body dose was estimated at 0.7 rad, produced an abnormal semen specimen on day 57. It is improbable that this abnormality is attributable to radiation exposure. The reduction in number of spermatozoa in Case 7 probably was related to the existence of a left varicocoele.

Radiation exposure is believed responsible for the hypospermia observed in Cases 10 and 11. As noted above, the exposure of Case 10 is believed to have been greater than the estimated 0.7–5.5 rad. The estimated whole-body dose in Case 11 is 75–100 rad; the dose to his testes was estimated at 60–150 rad.

We speculate that the anxiety and emotional upset experienced by these individuals may have contributed to or been responsible for the hypospermia and some of the abnormalities of the spermatozoa.

In spite of the abnormalities in spermatozoa, except in Case 9, libido and potency were unimpaired in all male patients—even in Case 11, who developed severe hypospermia. This is attributable to the relative resistance of the Leydig cells to radiation damage.

Discussion

Prevention

This accident was preventable, and occurred in our opinion because of the acute and chronic illness and severe blood-loss anemia of the radiographer, who in contrast to many radiographers involved in such episodes had 32 years of radiographic experience and was highly regarded as a dependable, reliable professional. Regular periodic health evaluations of this man probably would have detected his illness and might have prevented the occurrence.

Industrial radiographers should have intellectual, educational, and training qualifications sufficient to ensure their ability to detect and properly manage unforeseen events and accidents. Personal observations indicate that many industrial radiographers do not have these qualifications.

Had the ^{192}Ir source been labelled as hazardous, this also would have prevented the radiation overexposure. It is anachronistic that the shielding devices in which the sources are stored should be labelled as hazardous, while the source itself has no identifying mark to indicate its dangerous nature. Personnel radiological safety monitors designed to emit a not-to-be-ignored loud noise or a brightly flashing light when dangerous levels of radioactivity are present should be required equipment for all radiographers, and their use should be mandatory.

The design of industrial radiographic equipment should be modified to make impossible the accidental disconnection of sources from the cables and source tubes used to position them. And finally, nonradiographic personnel working in areas in which industrial radiographic procedures are conducted should be informed of the potential hazards involved if radioactive materials are misplaced or improperly managed.

Medical Management

Three weeks elapsed before the true nature of the radiation burns of Cases 1, 5, and 11 was recognized. Members of the medical profession should be alert to the possiblity of such radiation accidents, and aware of the symptoms and signs of radiation exposure and radiation burns, and of the management of patients incurring radiation exposure. It is particularly important that primary care, industrial, and emergency physicians be fully informed on these subjects.

Particularly important is the recognition and consideration and sympathetic support of individuals who are terrified by the possibility or reality of radiation exposure. Full disclosure of radiation dose, clinical and laboratory findings, and the immediate and long-term effects of radiation exposure is the most effective method of management. In our experience, this approach allays anxiety, encourages cooperation, and leads to the patient's rational approach to the problem confronting him or her.

Burn Management

Conservative management which avoids irresponsible steps such as precipitate amputation are very important. When the burn is in an area in which excision of involved tissue can be accomplished, and a skin flap with a well-preserved vascular supply can be implanted as in Case 11, we believe these procedures should be accomplished as soon as practicable. Such treatment will alleviate pain, reduce duration of disability, and, because it provides improved blood supply, decrease progression of necrosis with resulting decrease in the ultimate size of the lesion. Whether or not agents to facilitate local blood supply such as Vasodilan appreciably improve prognosis is not established.

Complete ophthalmologic evaluation should be carried out in all cases as soon as possible after the exposure to establish a baseline of ocular and lens status for future reference. Whether or not an individual has lenticular opacities when exposure occurred is a matter of considerable importance.

Laboratory Studies

Our observation that transient lymphopenia, semen abnormalities, and chromosome changes occurred in individuals who had a very low radiation dose, or whose history did not indicate significant exposure to radiation, suggest that these biological changes may be more valid indicators of radiation exposure than estimations based on a subject's recollections or statements concerning exposure. It is anticipated that correlation between the numbers and characteristics of peripheral blood lymphocytes, chromosome changes and small doses of radiation will allow the use of these biological indicators for actual quantitation of low-dose radiation exposure.

Summary

Eleven engineering plant employees were exposed to a 28-curie ^{192}Ir industrial radiographic source that inadvertently had been left on the floor of the plant by a radiographer. One workman carried the source in his hip pocket for 45 min and suffered a severe burn on his buttock. This necessitated hospitalization for three months, and on day 36 following exposure, resection of the ulcer and implantation of a full thickness skin flap with intact vascular pedicle. Two workers developed radiation burns on their fingers. Acute anxiety and emotional disturbances were a prominent reaction of exposed individuals, which were partially alleviated by candid presentation of the facts of their exposure.

Clinical observations, slit lamp biomicroscopy, radiation dosimetry and depth-dose estimates, hematologic and cytogenetic studies were made on all exposed individuals. Semen analyses were performed on all seven male subjects. Lymphopenia was a sensitive indicator of significant radiation exposure, and chromosomal abnormalities were observed in three individuals. Semen abnormalities were present in five men.

Early resection and implantation of a full thickness skin flap with intact vascular supply was highly successful in alleviating pain, reducing radiation erythema, arresting progression of ulceration, and decreasing the duration of physical disability.

Prevention of such costly accidents could be accomplished by direct labeling of radioactive sources, mandatory use by all industrial radiographers of impossible-to-ignore audible alarm personnel monitoring equipment and education concerning radiation hazards to individuals working in areas in which radiographic procedures are conducted.

ACKNOWLEDGMENTS
Dr. Daniel DeVore and Dr. William Gordon, Kaiser Permanente Hospital, Fontana, established the diagnosis of Case 11 and referred the patient to UCLA Hospital. Mr. S. Wong and Mr. D. Bunn, California Division of Occupational Safety and Health Administration, reenacted the episode and provided valuable information and observations.

References

1. Public meeting on radiation safety for industrial radiographers: Remarks, questions, and answers at five NRC regional meetings, document NUREG-0495, Washington, DC, Office of Inspection and Enforcement, Division of Fuel Facilities and Materials Safety Inspection, U.S. Nuclear Regulatory Commission, 1978.

2. Saenger EL, Kereiakes JG, Wald N, Thoma GE: Clinical course and dosimetry of acute hand injuries to industrial radiographers from multicurie sealed gamma sources, in *Proceedings of the Third International Congress of the International Radiation Protection Association,* document US-AEC CPNF-730907-P1, pp. 773–782.

3. Annamalai M, Iyer PS, Panicker TMR: Radiation injury from acute exposure to an Iridium 192 source: Case history. *Health Physics* 35:387–389, 1978.

4. Yeh KY: The Peoples Republic of China accident, 1963, in *The Medical Basis for Radiation Accident Preparedness.* New York, Elsevier North-Holland, Inc., 1980.

5. Le Go R: The Algerian accident 1978: Four cases of protracted whole-body radiation, in *The Medical Basis for Radiation Accident Preparedness.* New York, Elsevier North-Holland, Inc., 1980.

6. Hirashima K: The Chiba (Japan) accident 1971: Exposure to ^{192}Iridium, in *The Medical Basis for Radiation Accident Preparedness.* New York, Elsevier North-Holland, Inc., 1980.

7. Scott EB: The Louisiana accidents 1978 and 1979, in *The Medical Basis for Radiation Accident Preparedness.* New York, Elsevier North-Holland, Inc., 1980.

8. Jockey P: The Algerian accident 1978: Acute local radiation of two children, in *The Medical Basis for Radiation Accident Preparedness.* New York, Elsevier North-Holland, Inc., 1980.

The 1978 and 1979 Louisiana Accidents: Exposure to Iridium 192

E. Benson Scott, II

West Monroe, Louisiana.

Several million photographic exposures are taken each year in Louisiana and along its coast. Very few radiation overexposures have been recorded. Over the past year and a half there have been two accidents in which four radiographers working off the Louisiana coast have been overexposed to ^{192}Ir. The first individual received significant burns to his fingers, which eventually necessitated the amputation of one finger. In the second accident, three individuals were exposed to a slightly larger total body dose of ^{192}Ir, but there were no signs of local injury.

The most significant exposure in 1978 was brought to my attention in mid-July. A 22-year-old white male presented to me with complaints of burning, swelling, erythema, and dryness of the thumbs, index fingers, and middle fingers which had been present for approximately 1 week (Figure 1). He had been working as a radiographer's technician on a barge "offshore" for 21 days and had arrived home 1 week before coming to my office. Shortly after he arrived home, the tingling and burning sensations developed in his hands and progressed slowly but unrelentingly. He had been photographing pipe welds with a gamma century exposure device and collimator housing approximately 100 curies of ^{192}Ir. He had no known incidents of overexposure but he remarked that there had been two incidents of what was believed to be dosimeter malfunction on or about 22 or 23 of June. In retrospect, it appears that the instrument had been working correctly although the sensitivity had been incorrectly set. There had been no major difficulties with the crank-out of the radioactive source other than an occasional stickiness, and the radioactive source had been returned to the shielded position without

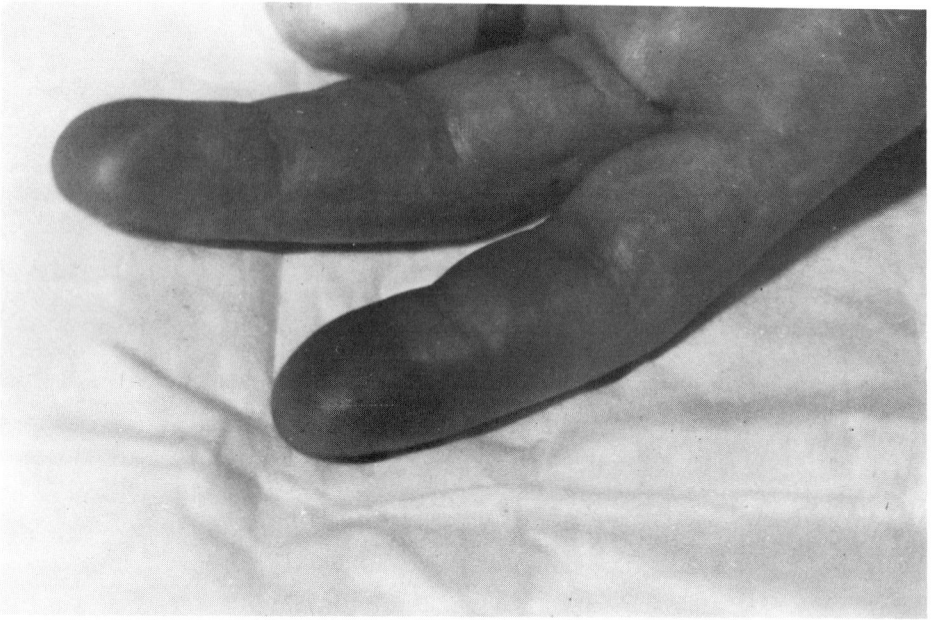

Figure 1. Left index finger, 14 July 1978.

difficulty whenever required. The patient's film badge reading for the month was 5450 mR, with daily dosimeter readings totaling 40 mR for each week.

The initial appearance of the lesions was compatible with a contact or thermal burn, but the history was incompatible because of the slow progression of the lesions. Bullae developed (Figure 2) as the patient was followed over the next several days; these became tense and spontaneously ruptured 4 to 5 weeks after the estimated time of exposure (Figure 3). During the next 3-week period, the lesions showed slow healing with granulation type tissue or wet desquamation at the base of the areas affected. Approximately 4 months after the injury, the epithelium had returned and covered all palmar surfaces but it appeared thin and friable. The patient complained of pain with motion and pain with temperature or pressure changes. Flexion of the left index finger was limited to 45° at the proximal interphalangeal joint and 15° to 20° at the distal interphalangeal joint. At 4 to 5 months after the injury, the epithelium remained intact but began to break down. The deep burning pain increased, flexion became more limited, and ulceration at the distal interphalangeal joint on the flexor surface began. The ulceration enlarged, and approximately 6 months after the injury the distal two-thirds of the left index finger was amputated because of intractable pain and progres-

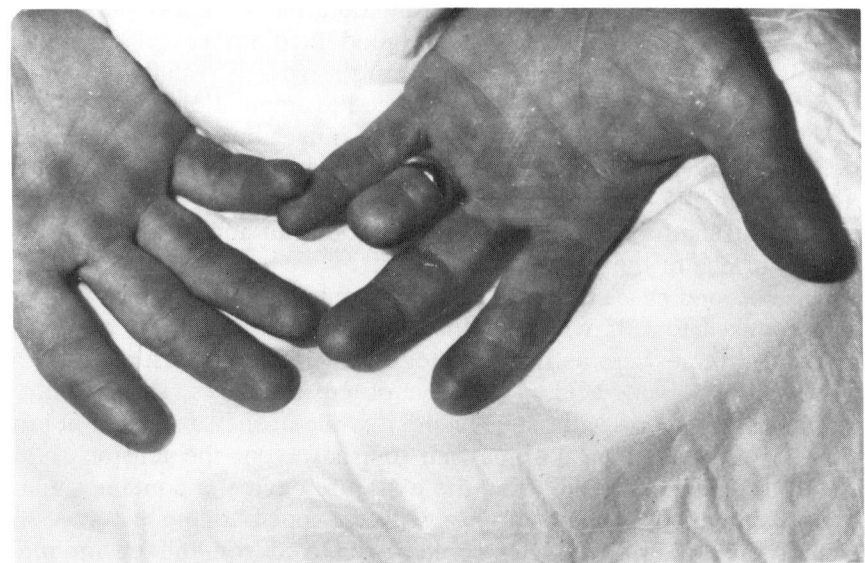

Figure 2. Both hands, early bullae formation.

Figure 3. Ruptured bullae.

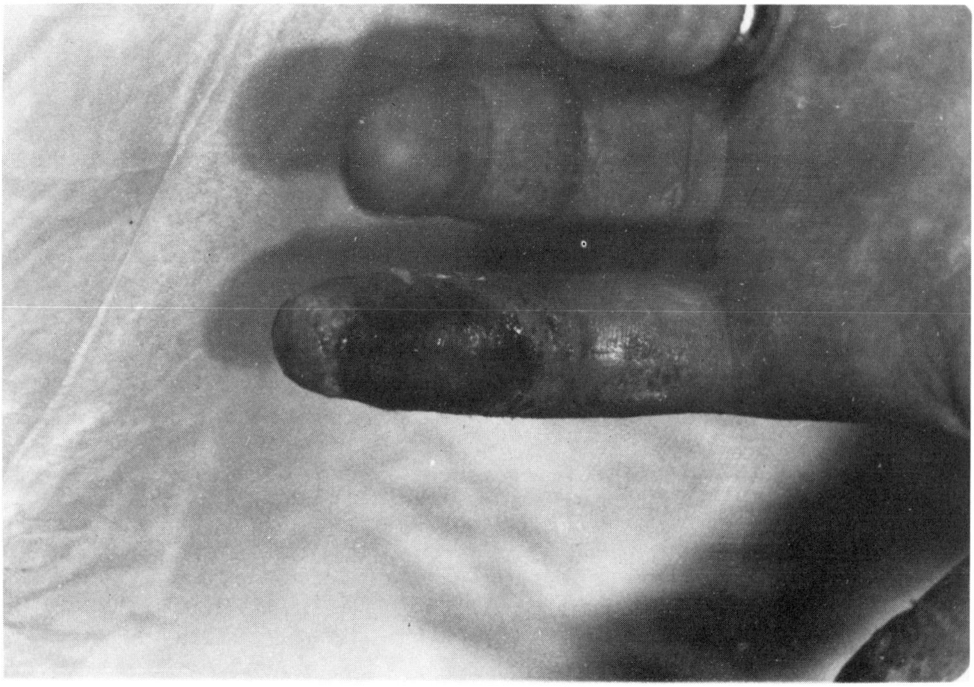

sive ulceration. The deep medial and lateral arterial vessels were intact. A preoperative arteriogram showed good medium vessel filling and perhaps a suggestion of increased size in the vessels usually associated with the distal tuft. In the 15 months since the amputation (Figure 4), the patient has had little pain in the left index finger but continues to have occasional pain in the middle finger of the left hand and both thumbs. He has been unable to use his hands for gripping or for manipulations requiring strength because of his limited ability to apply pressure to the palmar surface of the affected fingers.

In the second case, which occurred in May 1979, three radiographers were exposed to ^{192}Ir while working aboard a ship off the Gulf coast. Two of the three were actively photographing welds on a large piece of pipe which was being held by a system of tension rollers. Tension rollers are used to grip pipe without crushing it while at the same time holding it out of the water. In a somewhat unusual event the tension rollers moved, gripping and puncturing the exposure device, a container which shields and exposes the isotopes while strapped to the pipe. A few minutes passed until the device could be removed from the tension roller equipment. During this period, the container was damaged and the device

Figure 4. Amputated stump 8 months after injury.

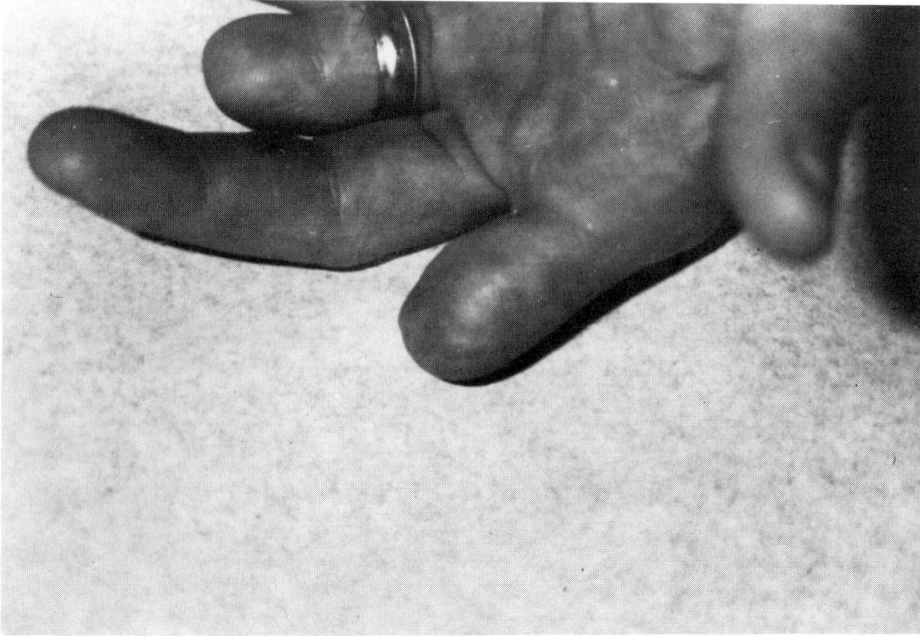

could not be turned "off" so as to completely shield the source. The container was unstrapped and handled by the two men, who called for assistance from a third member of the work crew. It was placed on a table and left there for several minutes while a rope was tied to it. The damaged device was then thrown over the side to better shield the men from the iridium source until a decision could be made as to its disposition. Later in the day the device was returned to the surface for 3 or 4 min for reevaluation and inspection. At that time those responsible believed that there was nothing more that could be done under the circumstances, and the device was again thrown overboard and kept in the water until it was returned to shore.

All three men were examined briefly and exhibited no evidence of local injury. One of the three did have mild nausea, which he felt was related to nervousness. The other two men had no systemic symptoms. Cytogenetic studies showed that their total body exposure had been quite low, less than 8 R. One man was not wearing his film badge at the time of the accident because he had been off duty when he was called to give assistance. The film badge of one of the men who had been photographing welds was lost, and the film badge of the other workman showed a reading of approximately 8 R. All three of these individuals have continued to do well since the incident with no systemic or local signs of injury. Reenacting the events gives a compatible dose curve of approximately 8 R to the body and larger doses to the hands, but less than 200 to 300 rad as a result of the manipulative ability of the workmen and their ingenuity in handling the device.

The 1978 Algerian Accident:
Acute Local Exposure of Two Children

H. Jammet, R. Gongora,
P. Jockey, and J. M. Zucker

Institut de Curie, Paris, France.

The clinical cases reported here required treatment as a result of an Algerian accident in 1978 in which a whole family was heavily irradiated. This paper concerns two children injured locally. Such a situation is exceptional enough to justify the choice of their clinical history as an example from among numerous cases we have followed at the Institut Curie. We show here how physical dosimetry and paraclinical tests enabled us to decide in favor of conservative surgery based on trophic help.

The Algerian accident began with the loss of a 25-curie ^{192}Ir source while it was being transported. Official information was promptly given to regional medical authorities so that they could recognize potential radiological burns as early as possible. As a result of an examination of two brothers suffering from skin lesions, we were able to determine that the accident occurred in the Sétif region near Algiers, and to detect by systemic blood counts those people whose whole bodies had been exposed. We shall only mention the fact that these two children had received a total body exposure as documented by significantly low blood counts but without clinical consequences.

The approximate time of the boys' exposure is known with sufficient accuracy, but the duration and extent are impossible to determine. Figure 1 shows the two boys in September 1978. They are in good general condition.

AEK, the younger, was 3 years old at the times of the accident. When he arrived at the Institut Curie, on 14 June 1978, he showed lesions of the mouth and both hands. Figure 2 shows lower lip and tongue

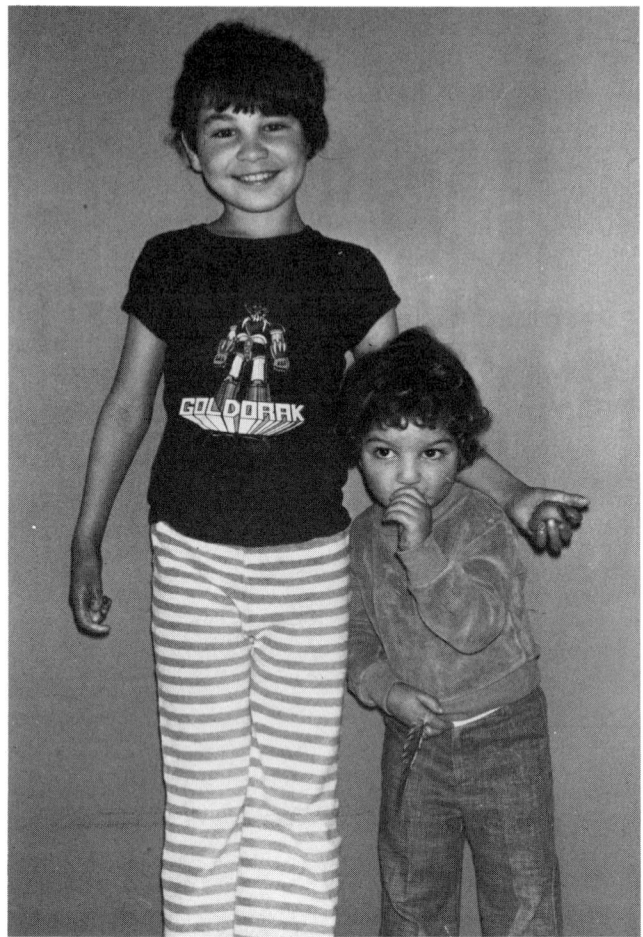

Figure 1. Picture of the two injured boys in September 1979.

ulcerations, which demonstrate that the boy had sucked the source. This fact is in accord with the electroencephalogram, which suggested a cephalic dose of 2500 rad.

Figure 3 shows a necrotic and deep ulceration of nearly 2 cm in diameter at the hypothenar on the right hand. It seems that the boy had been playing with the source-holder (Figure 4), using it as a drumstick. On the left hand (Figure 5) appears, at the same location, a much less severe lesion. Figures 6 and 7 show how the right-hand lesion developed from June to September 1978.

The failure of the lesion to heal led us to consider surgery. The choice was between radical and conservative surgery. Our choice in favor of conservative surgery was based on the results of highly specialized

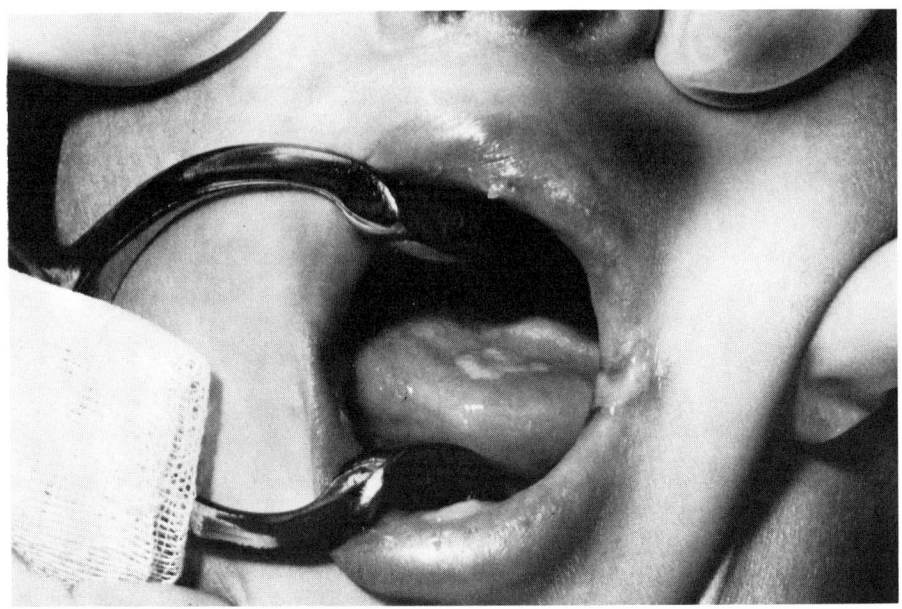

Figure 2. Initial mouth lesions of AEK, June 1978.

Figure 3. Initial lesions of the right hand of AEK, June 1978.

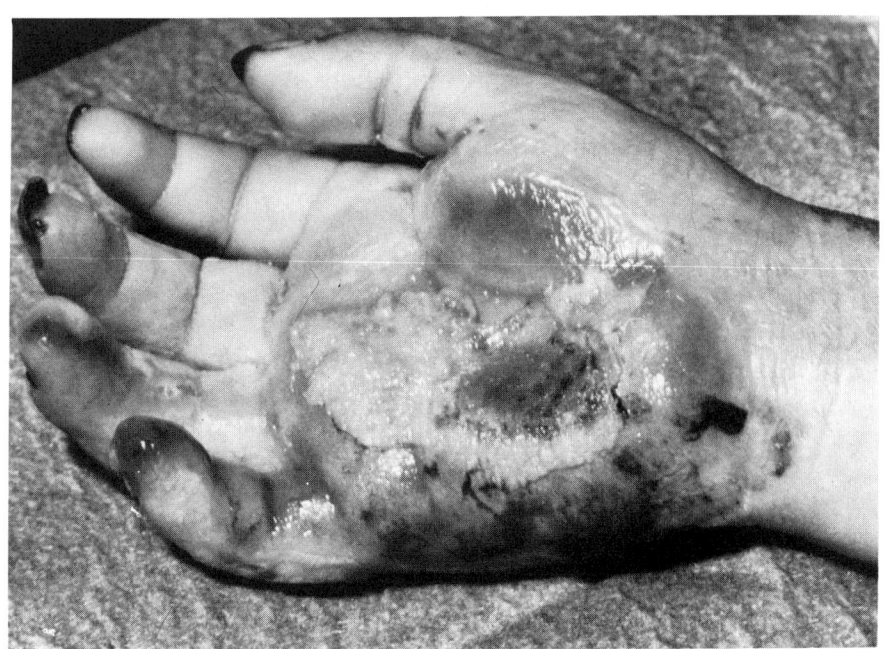

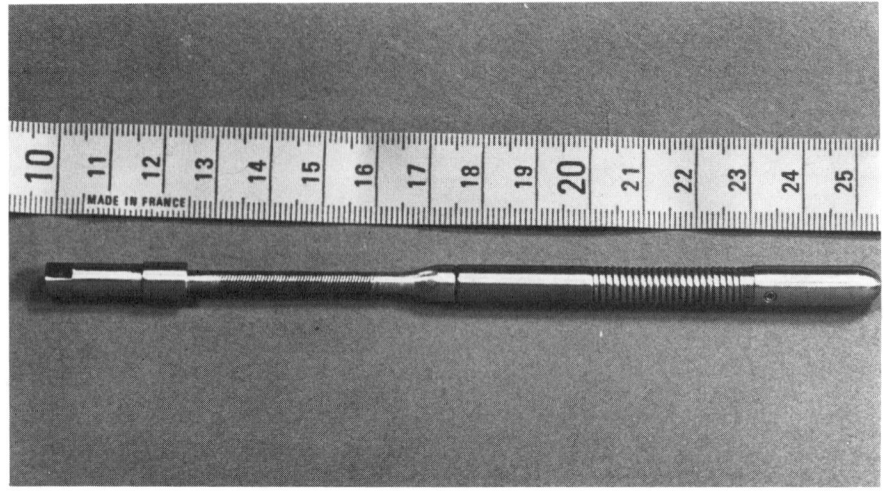

Figure 4. The ^{192}Ir source-holder responsible for the accident.

Figure 5. Initial left hand lesion of AEK, June 1978.

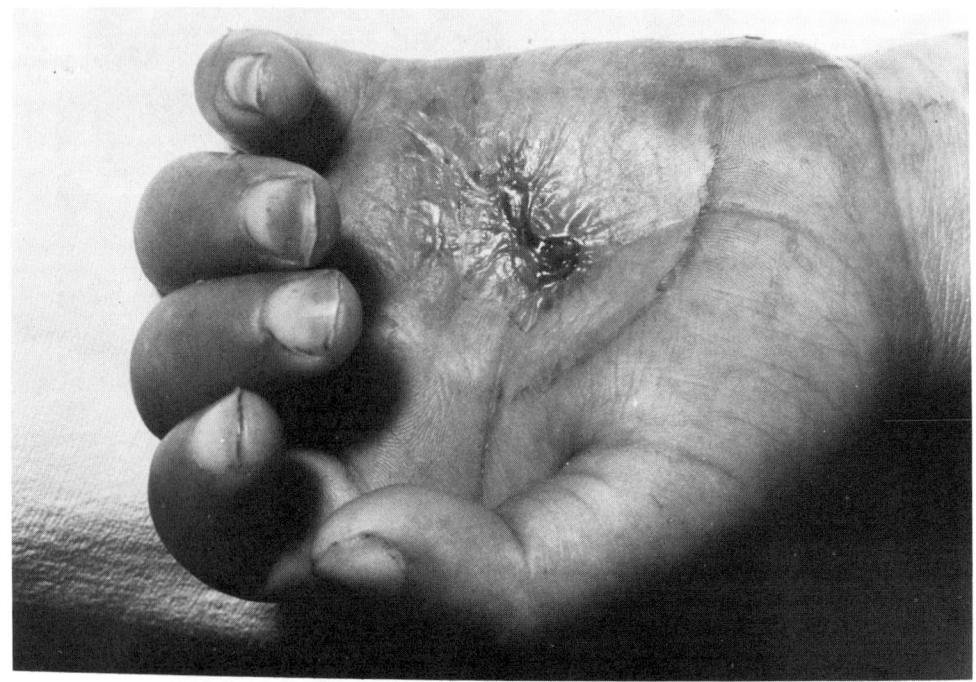

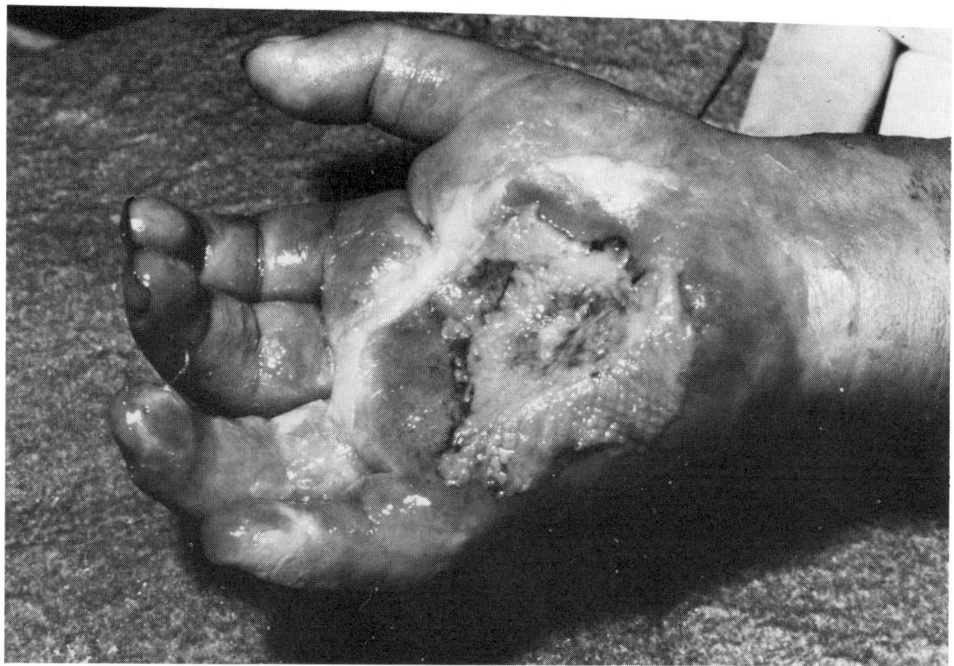

Figure 6. Right hand lesion of AEK, June 1978.

methods and dosimetry described below. Very important, too, was the asepsis of the lesions during the preoperative period.

When nothing is known about the geometry and duration of exposure, dosimetric estimation is based on clinical observation and relative physical dosimetry. The shapes of the lesions give information on the source position. In AEK's case we had evidence for a hypothenar localization. Figure 8 shows the surface dose evaluation of the right hand. The relative physical dosimetry is determined by means of a mold. Measurements were made on a mold obtained from a glove of adequate size. The depth of the dose was estimated also. For example, at 5 mm the dose is 30%.

Finally, on the basis of clinical experience and the evolution of the lesions, a dose estimation may be derived from an isodose curve. In this case, the limits of the necrosis were estimated to correspond to 1500 rad, which gives 10,000 rad for the 100% dose and 3000 rad at the metacarpus.

Figure 9 shows the liquid-crystal thermographic picture of the right hand: fingers 1 and 2 have a normal temperature; fingers 4 and 5 are cold; and finger 3 is cold also, which is an indication of a bad prognosis. The information is in agreement with the data obtained by telethermography (Figure 10).

234

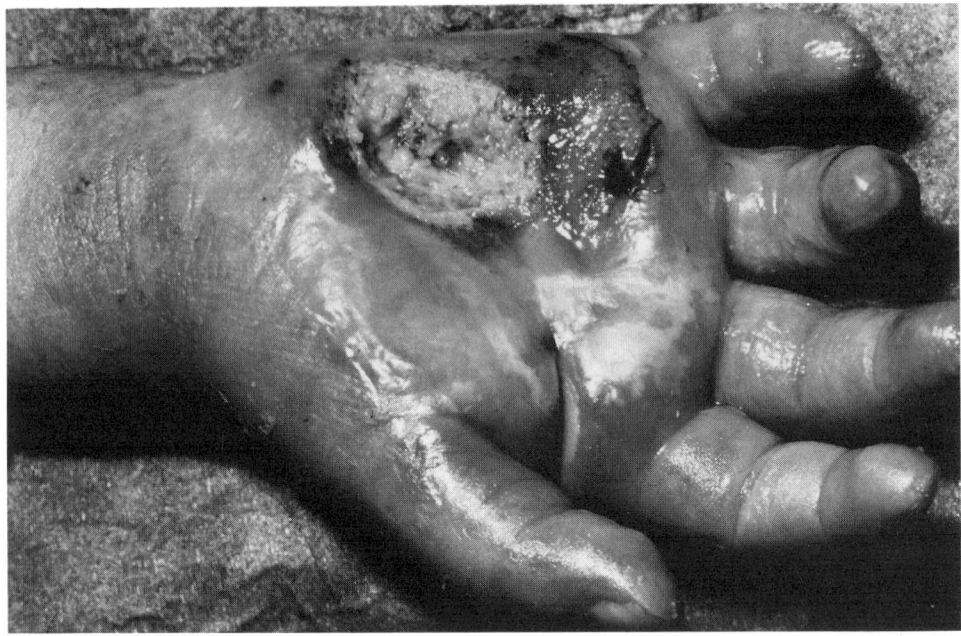

Figure 7. Right hand lesion of AEK, August 1978.

Effusivity is a parameter characterizing the ability of a medium to exchange heat with another medium. It is the square root of the product of the thermal conductivity multiplied by the volume specific heat. The "touchau" method of measuring effusivity by contact permits the in-depth localization of internal thermal anomalies, especially those due to circulatory changes. Figure 11 shows that, if one considers as normal the curve corresponding to the forefinger of the right hand, fingers 3, 4, and 5 appear to be pathological. Here again finger 3 is indicative of a negative prognosis.

The roentgenogram in Figure 12 shows a discrete osteoporosis on fingers 2, 3, 4, and 5. Bond fixation study with technetium diphosphonate indicated a high fixation by the right hand, predominantly in the metacarpal region with right-to-left ratio of 1.7, the ratio is only 1.3 at the finger level.

Figure 13 shows an arteriogram of the right hand. The diameter of the cubital artery is progressively reduced at the carpal level, and irrigation corresponding to finger 3, 4, and 5 is very poor.

At the completion of these tests in September 1975, the child complained that the lesions were very painful, and a surgical decision became necessary. In view of the deep and large necrosis, it might appear that amputation of the right hand could not be avoided. Nevertheless, dosimetry suggested that the thumb and forefinger had received only 2 to 3% of the maximum dose, and paraclinical tests indicated that fingers 3, 4, and 5 did not receive any real blood supply. Under these conditions, amputation was limited to the last three fingers with a pincer to be made from the thumb and forefinger seemed to be possible.

The solution we chose was more conservative. Taking advantage of the limits given by dosimetry and the paraclinical tests of the necrotic tissues to be removed, we decided in favor of trophic help for this hand. A thick abdominal flap was our choice for reasons of comfort and to reduce the donor area. Amputation was limited to the fifth finger.

Results are shown in Figures 14 and 15. The present status of the hand is very good, and the boy is able to use his hand. Esthetic surgery on the flap is now anticipated.

For the first year after the accident, the left hand of AEK exhibited only a small hyperkeratotic scar. It has recently developed an inflammatory process. The brain presented a cortical hyperexcitability with a right predominance. This situation must be carefully followed in view of the high dose of ^{192}Ir to which the boy was exposed.

Figure 8. Isodose distribution in relative form of the right hand of AEK.

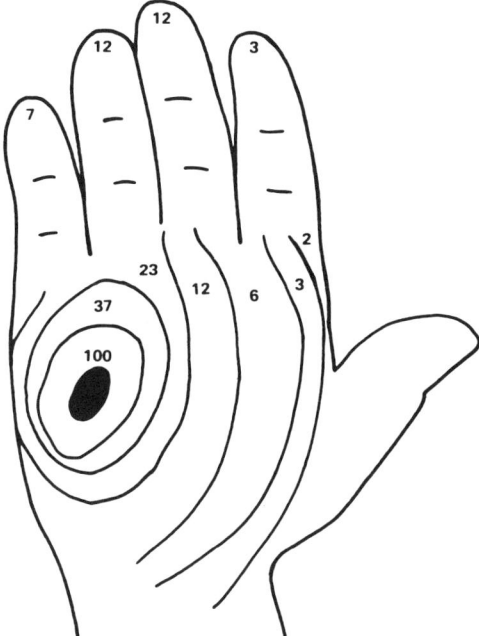

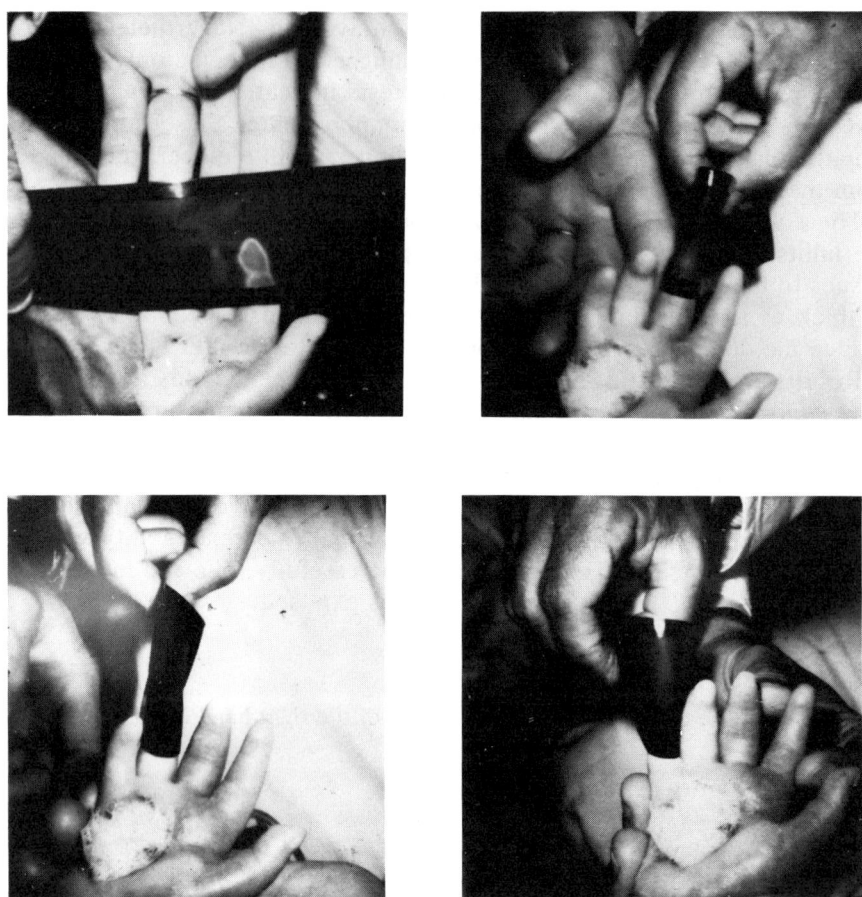

Figure 9. Liquid crystal thermography of AEK, September 1978.

The other brother, R, who was 7 years old at the time of the accident, was playing with the source under the same circumstances as AEK. At his arrival at the Institut Curie, he presented lesions of both hands and also of both buttocks and thighs.

His hand lesions appeared to be more symmetrical than those of AEK, more uniform and affected the metacarpus and fingers. Figures 16 and 17 show the hand lesions in June 1978. The buttock lesions were difficult to explain. We thought that R put the source in his school satchel, on which he sat from time to time. The relative savings of the perineal region from exposure is compatible with this hypothesis, which supposes symmetric

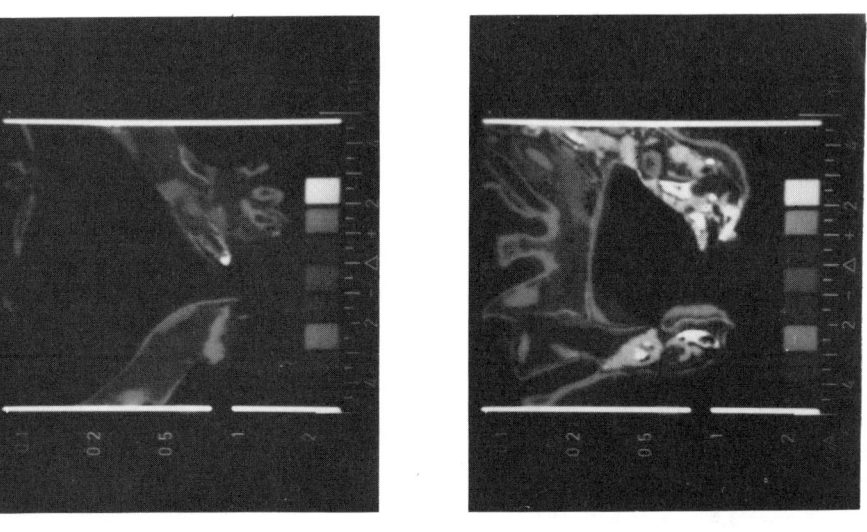

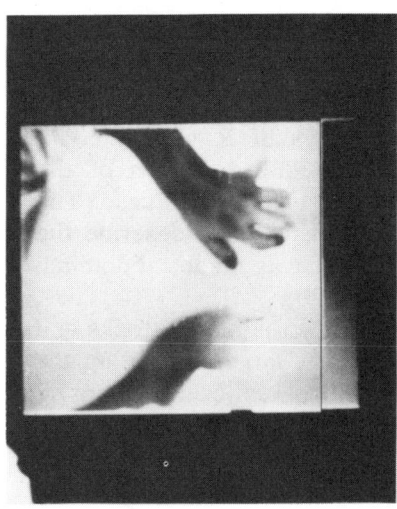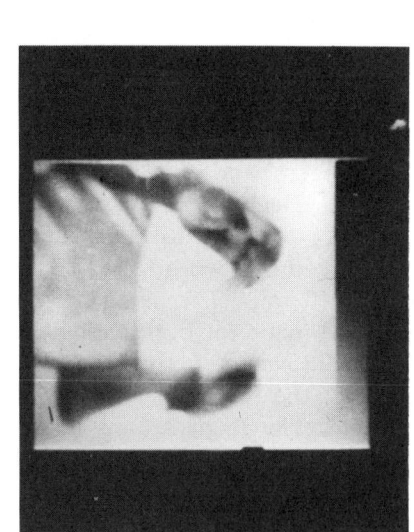

Figure 10. Telethermography of AEK, September 1978.

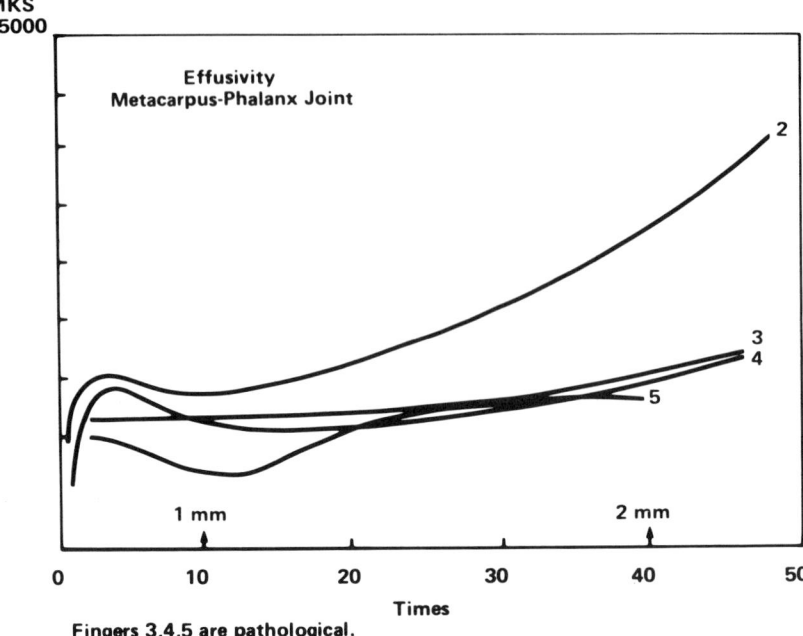

MKS
5000

Effusivity
Metacarpus-Phalanx Joint

Fingers 3,4,5 are pathological.

Figure 11. Effusivity measurements of the right hand of AEK, September 1978.

and medium distance irradiation (Figure 18). In the case of R, there was no cephalic overexposure.

The fingers and the metacarpi of both hands of R were heavily irradiated. Because the irradiation results in reduced flexion of the fingers, it is difficult to interpret the paraclinical tests in this case. The same procedures were followed as for AEK (we will not describe the results in detail). The same therapeutic decision was made; abdominal flaps were made for both hands (Figures 19 and 20).

Figure 18 shows the initial aspect of lesions affecting the buttocks and the top of the thighs of R. They were particularly large, mainly on the right side. The thigh lesions healed rapidly, but necrotic ulcerations, 7 cm in diameter, remained unhealed on the buttocks.

Our surgical strategy was quasi-experimental. On the right buttock a local flap was inserted by rotation. This procedure has the advantage that normal tissue can be placed under the sciatic pressure point. Unfortunately, because of sepsis, disruption occurred immediately and a second operation was necessary, which was successful. The naked surface was covered with a conventional skin graft.

On the left buttock adipose tissue of good quality was covered by a conventional skin graft. Cicatrization was very slow, and 60% was healing only secondarily. The result is good, but the left buttock is more fragile and less comfortable to the boy than the right (Figure 21).

A perfect knowledge of the trophic status of irradiated tissues makes it possible, when supported by precise dosimetry, to choose conservative surgery. This procedure is based on the trophic help afforded by a thick pedicle flap. A supply of blood is thus obtained that replaced the irradiated vascular tissue. This surgical approach seems to have been more effective in these two cases than the normal medical approach to radiological necrosis.

When a pedicle flap is not possible, microsurgery may be substituted;

Figure 12. Right hand roentgenogram of AEK, September 1978.

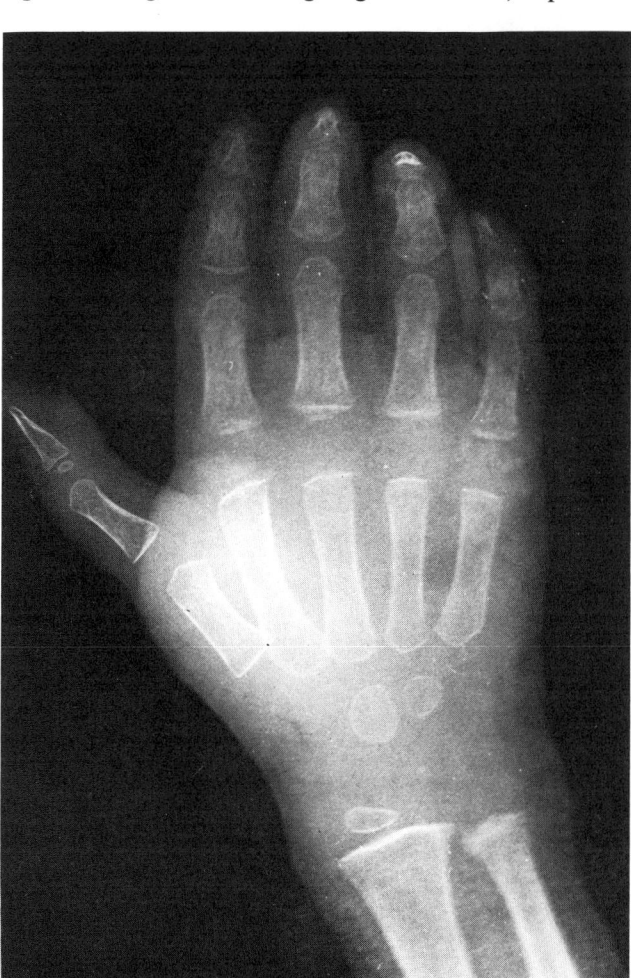

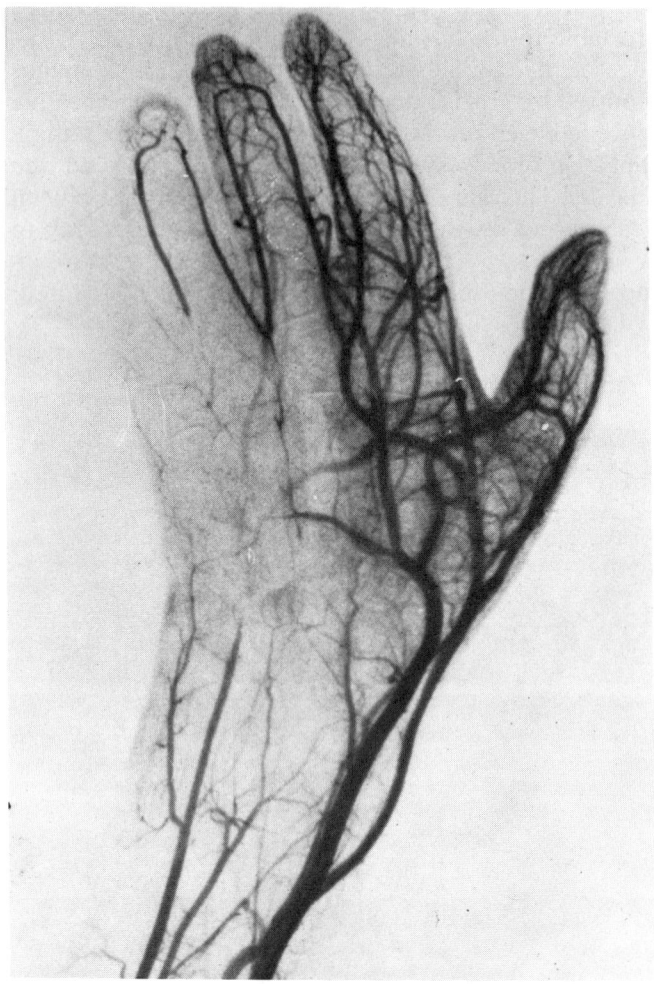

Figure 13. Right forearm arteriogram of AEK, September 1978.

a flap with a good vascular network is connected to the local protected vascularization.

These therapeutical results seem to be even more promising if one considers that, until recently, such surgery was postponed until relatively late because the surgeon was waiting prudently for a relative stabilization of the inflammatory process and for the exhaustion of the repair capacity. We should order paraclinical tests and dosimetry much more often in such cases and plan surgery earlier, at an optimal time, before the tissues are too damaged. The decision should be made on the basis of the physiopathological prognosis in view of this.

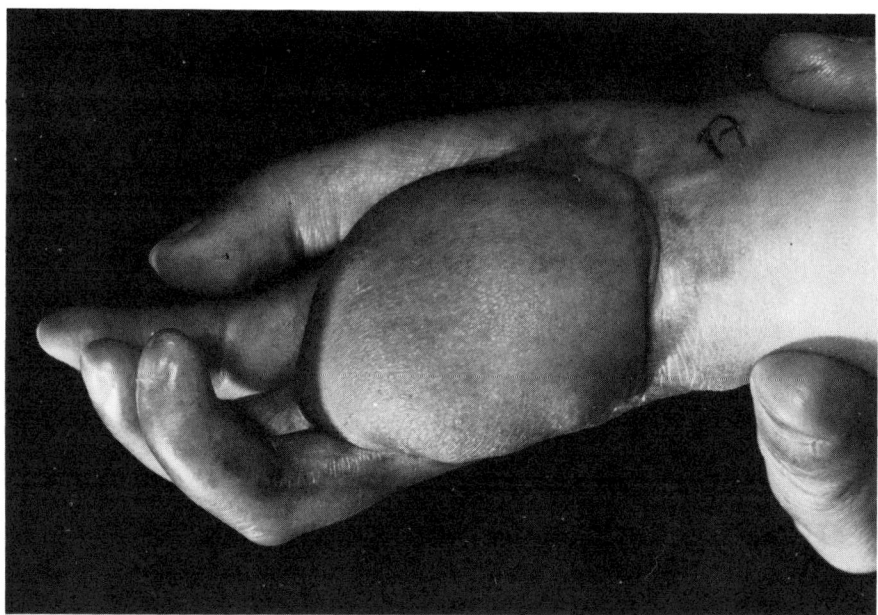

Figure 14. Actual aspect of the right hand of AEK with an abdominal flap.

Figure 15. Another view of the right hand of AEK, showing the abdominal flap.

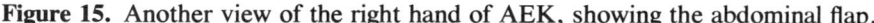

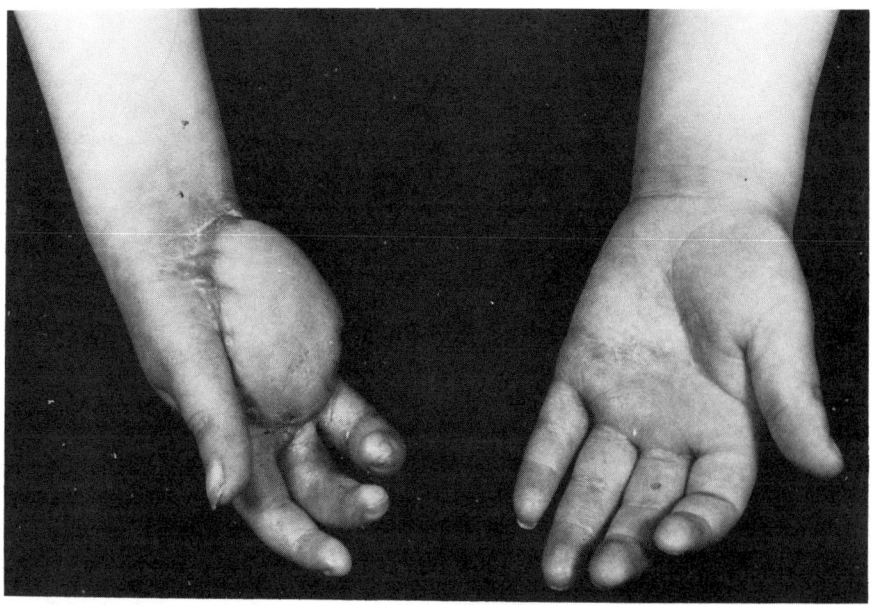

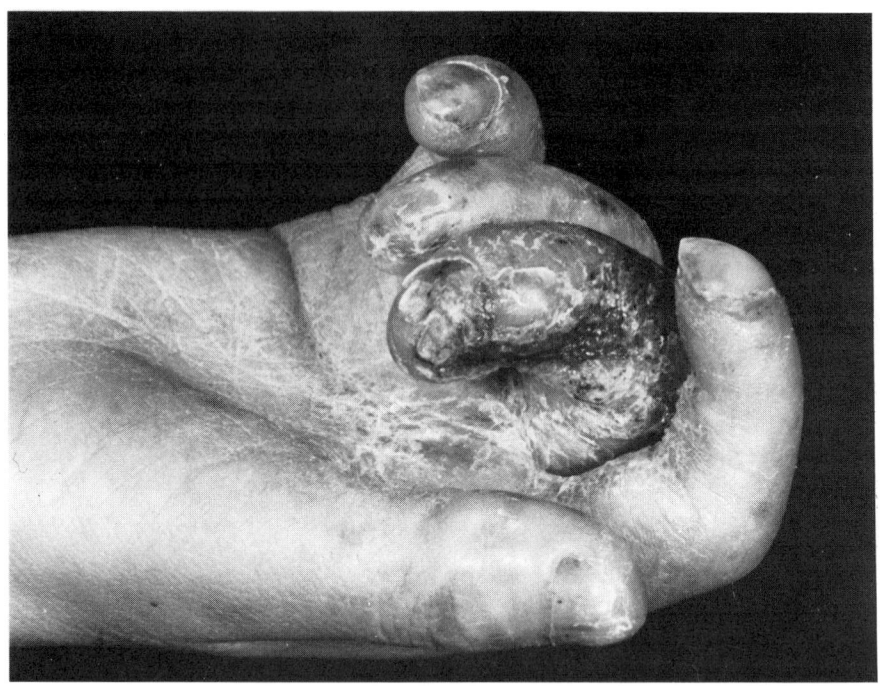

Figure 16. Right hand lesions of R, June 1978.

Figure 17. Left hand lesions of R, June 1978.

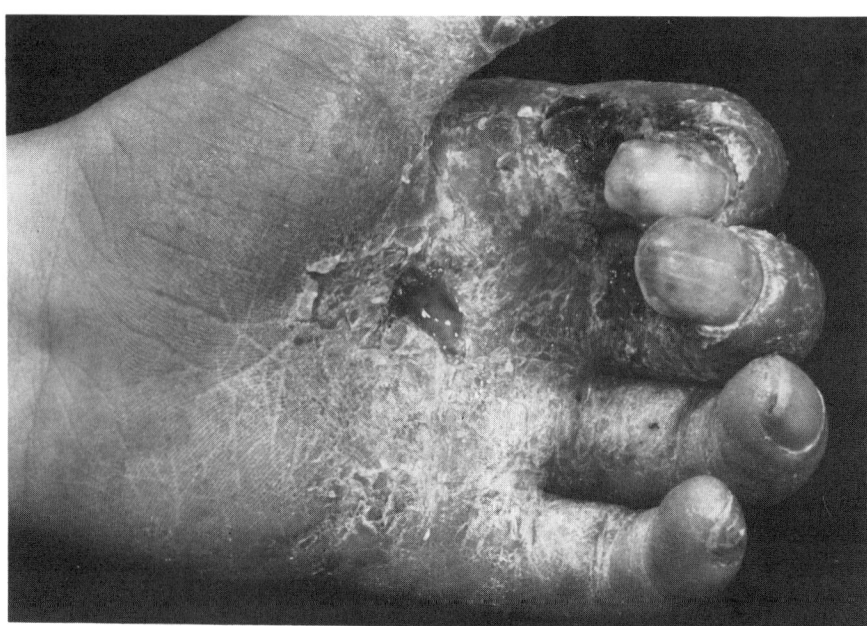

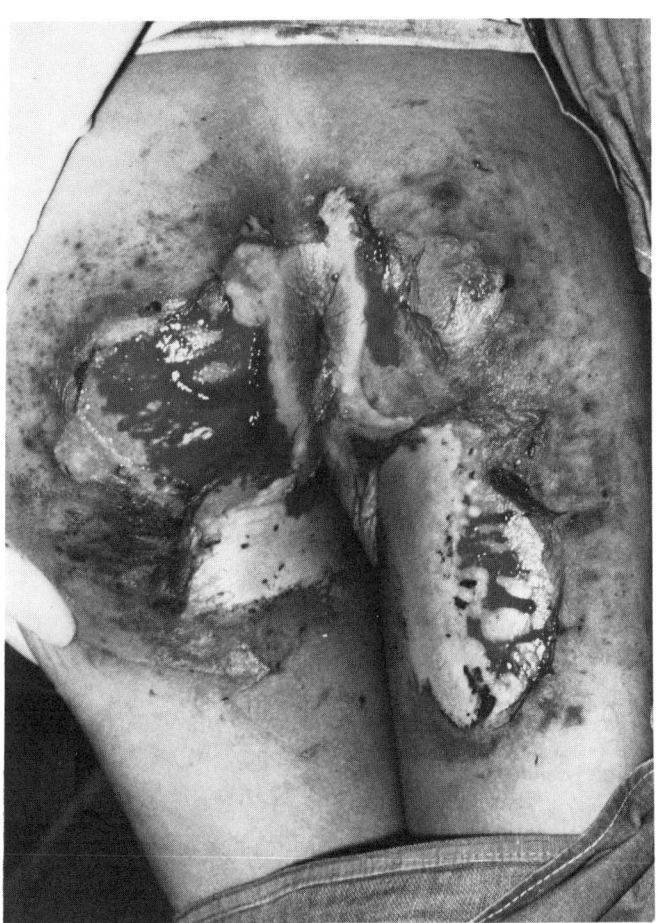

Figure 18. Buttock and thigh lesions of R, June 1978.

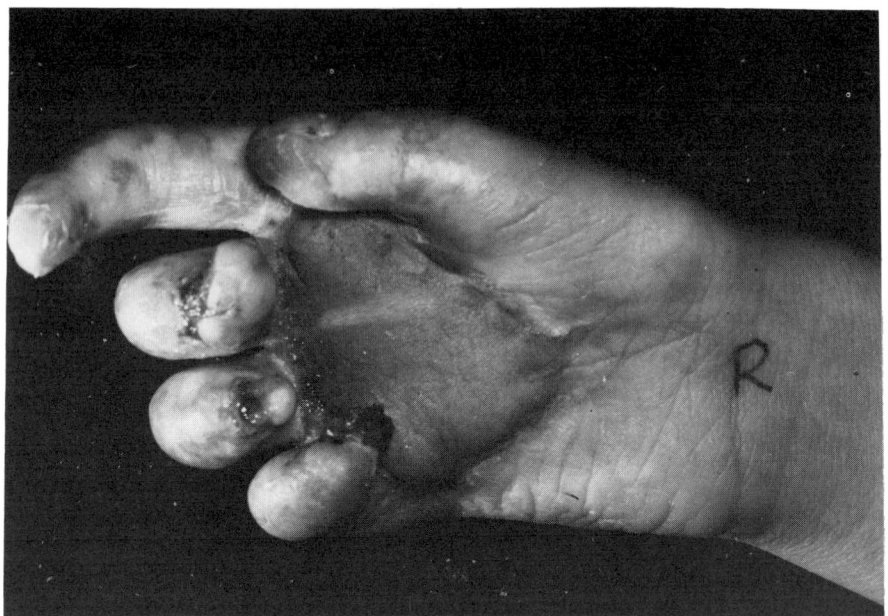

Figure 19. Actual aspect of the right hand of R with an abdominal flap.

Figure 20. Actual aspect of the left hand of R with an abdominal flap.

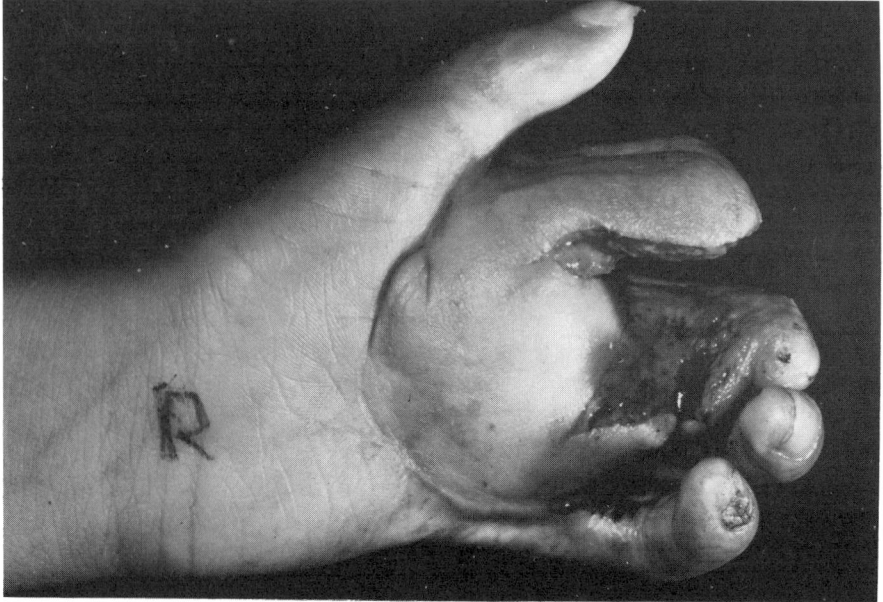

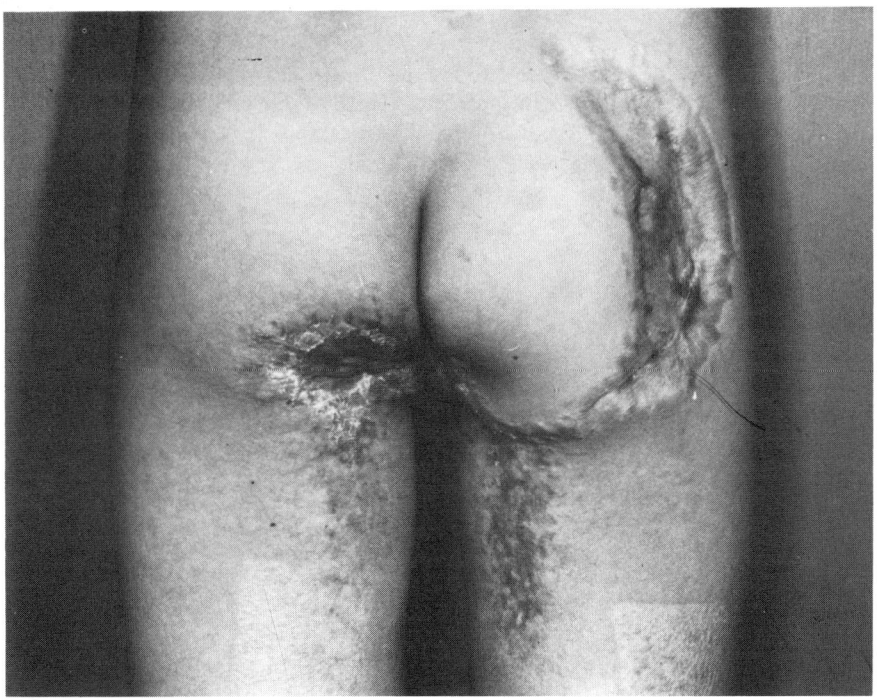

Figure 21. Actual aspect of the buttocks of R, with a flap on the right and a conventional graft on the left.

Acute X-ray Exposure of the Distal Phalanx of the Fingers

J. Connell Shearin, Jr.

Bowman Gray School of Medicine, Winston-Salem, North Carolina.

With the increasing use of X-ray in industry, an awareness of the hazards of inadvertent X-ray exposure and its biological effects has been well documented.[1] Despite the best precautionary measures, periodic acute exposures to radiation occur and these isolated instances allow us to increase our understanding of a rare injury. The total biological effect of radiation in tissues is not thoroughly understood, but it manifests itself mainly through its effects on DNA metabolism and the related destruction of associated enzymes. Since not all cells are damaged to the same extent, surviving cells will allow the tissues to repair, which is the basis of radiation therapy in oncology.

Classically, radiation injury has been grouped into three major categories: (1) acute radiation exposure over a short time period; (2) subacute radiation exposure (repeated dosage over a longer period of time); and (3) chronic radiation exposures depending on the dosages and the time relationships.

The patient described herein suffered an acute radiation injury, that is, a large dose of radiation over a short period of time. Warren has described the changes seen in skin in the classic monograph of 1943.[2] The effects of radiation on the hands have been reviewed by Knowlton et al.[3] and its current management has been clearly elucidated by Krizek and Ariyan.[4,5]

On 4 January 1978, at 11 A.M. in the morning a 28-year-old quality control inspector for an electronics component and switching firm and his assistant were adjusting a swing arm of the primary beam shutter

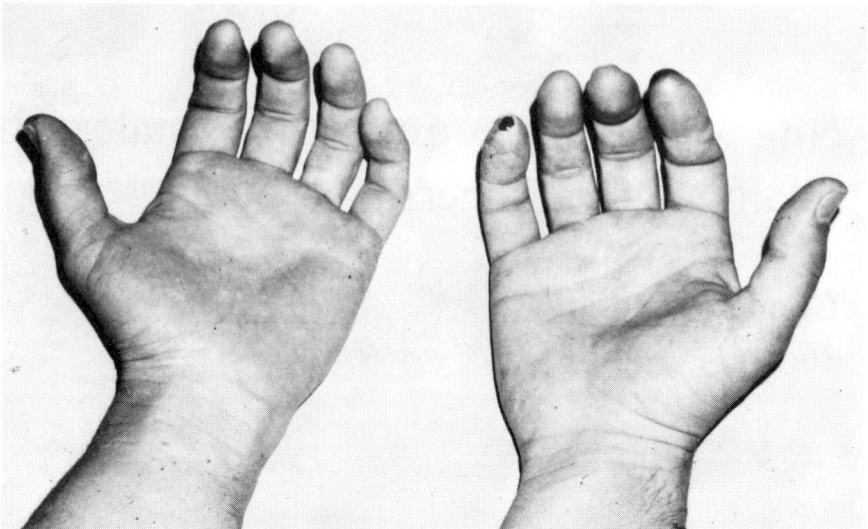

Figure 1A,B. Both sides of the patient's hands on 12 January 1979.

associated with an X-ray diffraction unit (Diano model D4014CB EA-75) used to evaluate the quality of nickel plating. The patient was holding the shutter plate in the open position by placing the right index finger inside the port aperture. After 40 to 50 sec, he felt a burning sensation in the index finger, but, since the machine was supposedly not operating with the shutter open, he removed his index finger and inserted his fifth finger to continue to hold the shutter open. He again experienced a mild burning sensation about 30 sec after inserting his little finger. He then noticed by checking precautionary devices that the machine was indeed on and producing X-rays. The X-ray diffraction unit was then turned off.

Approximately 7 hr after the exposure that patient observed numbness and a throbbing sensation in the right little finger. At 20 to 24 hr, a feeling of tightness was reported and swelling was noticed. The plant nurse confirmed the swelling but could not detect any noticeable discoloration. At approximately 48 hr after exposure the patient noticed erythema of both fingers, and at 72 hr he reported a marked increase in swelling and additional erythema with a blackening of the nailbed of both fingers.

On 8 January 1979, because the patient's fingers exhibited increased swelling, the plant nurse asked the plant consulting physician to see the patient. The physician incised both fingers, expecting to find pus; however, the discharge was a clear fluid, which continued to drain for

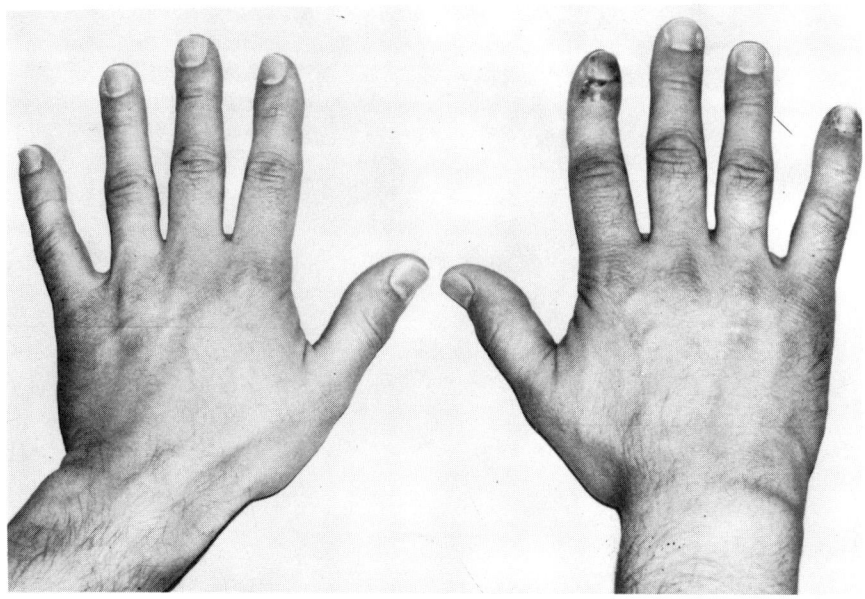

the next 2 to 3 days. The patient first sought consultation with a plastic surgeon on 12 January 1979 and at that time the fingers exhibited a moderate amount of swelling with erythema and drainage. He complained of a moderate amount of pain, with some severe pain on manipulation of the fingers. Culture at that time was negative. Because of the weeping and the slight amount of pain with total involvement of the distal phalanx including the nailbed, I instituted a conservative approach consisting of hydrotherapy, topical Betadine gauze, and splinting. Consultation was carried out with radiologists, an ophthalmologist, a urologist, a hematologist, and the cytogenetic laboratory at Oak Ridge, Tennessee. The sperm count was normal. The results of an ophthalmological examination and a hematological examination, which included a bone marrow platelet count, were within normal limits. A 2-day lymphocyte cytogenetic analysis showed no evidence of significant exposure to the whole body. On 10 January 1979 the North Carolina State X-ray Control Board surveyed the equipment and concluded that the dose to the distal phalanx was 20 k rad per second. In a second survey on 17 January, more sophisticated equipment was used that measured more sensitive low-energy X-rays. From these measurements it was estimated that the exposure rate inside the part was 9 k rad per second with an effective energy of 12 to 16 keV. At this low energy rate, it was felt that the dose

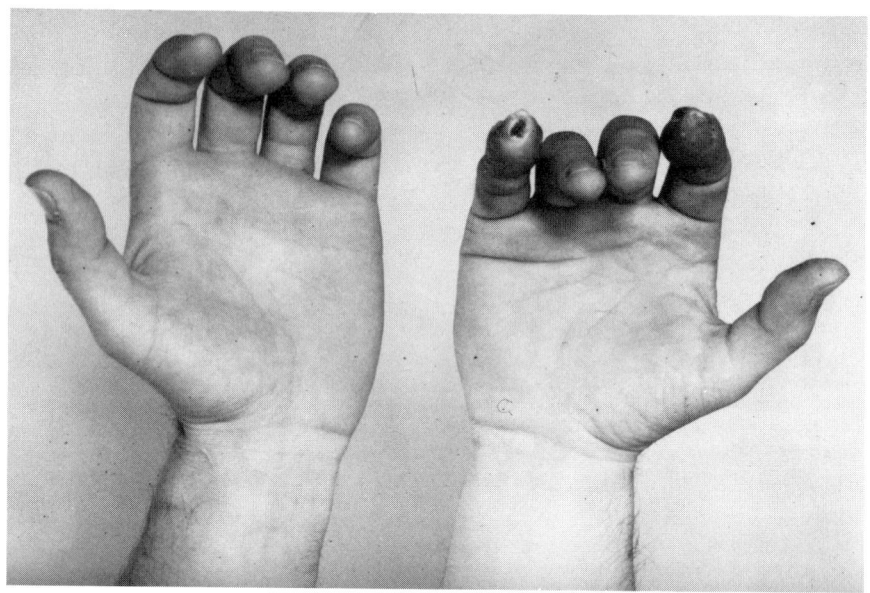

Figure 2A,B. Both sides of the hands on 24 January 1979.

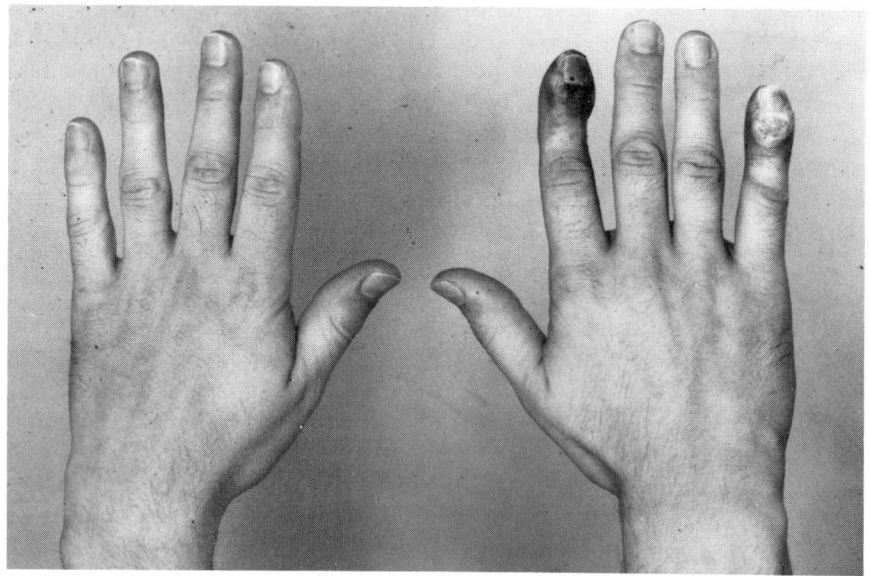

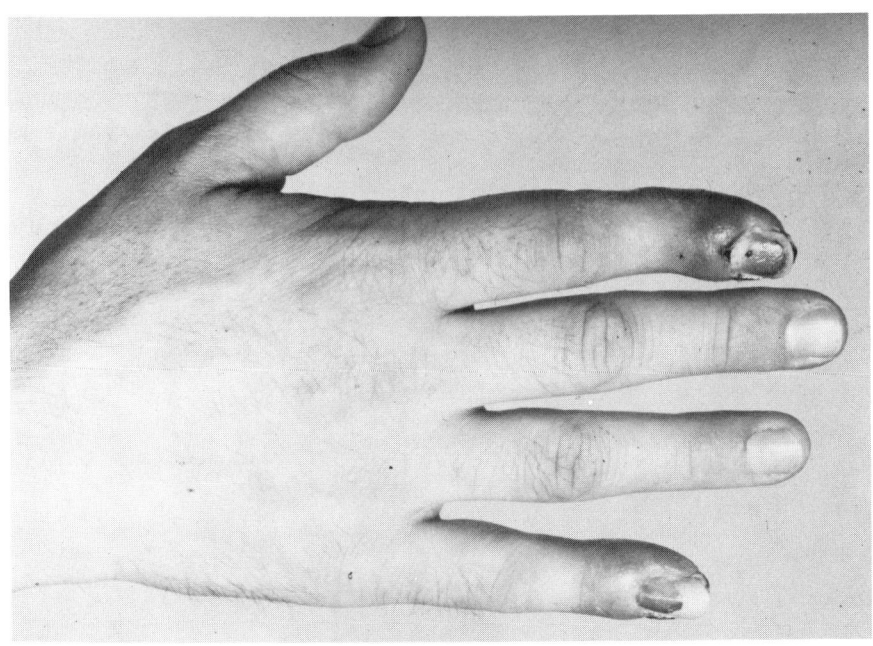

Figure 3. Right hand on 8 February 1979.

Figure 4. Right hand on 15 February 1979.

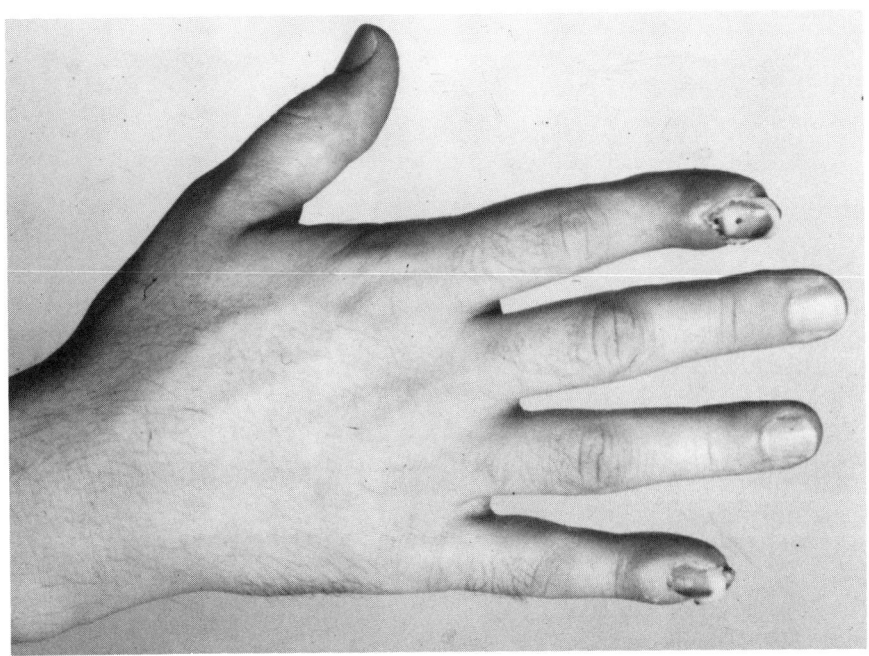

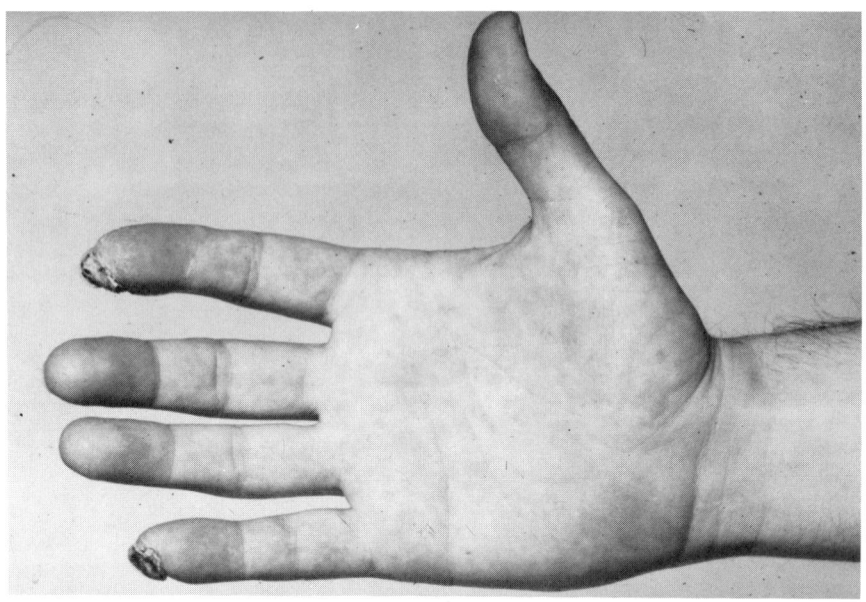

Figure 5A,B. Two views of the right hand on 5 March 1979.

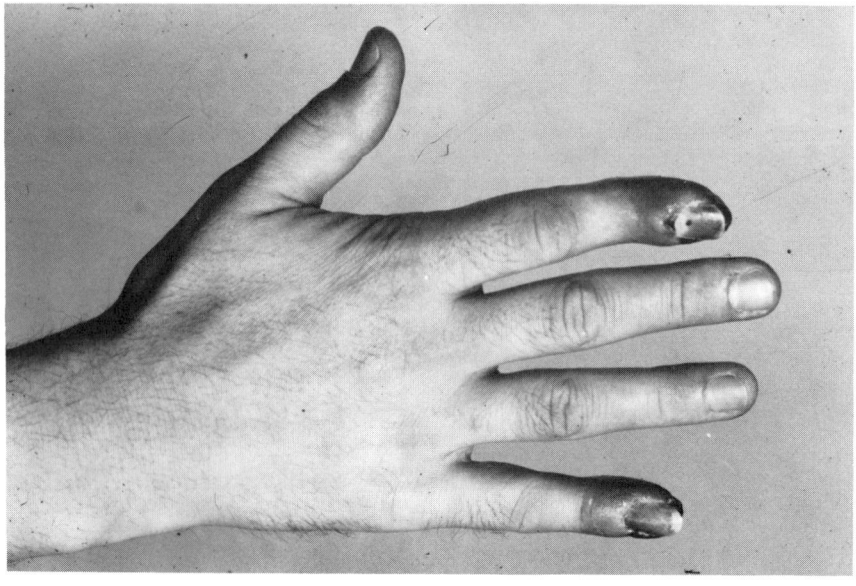

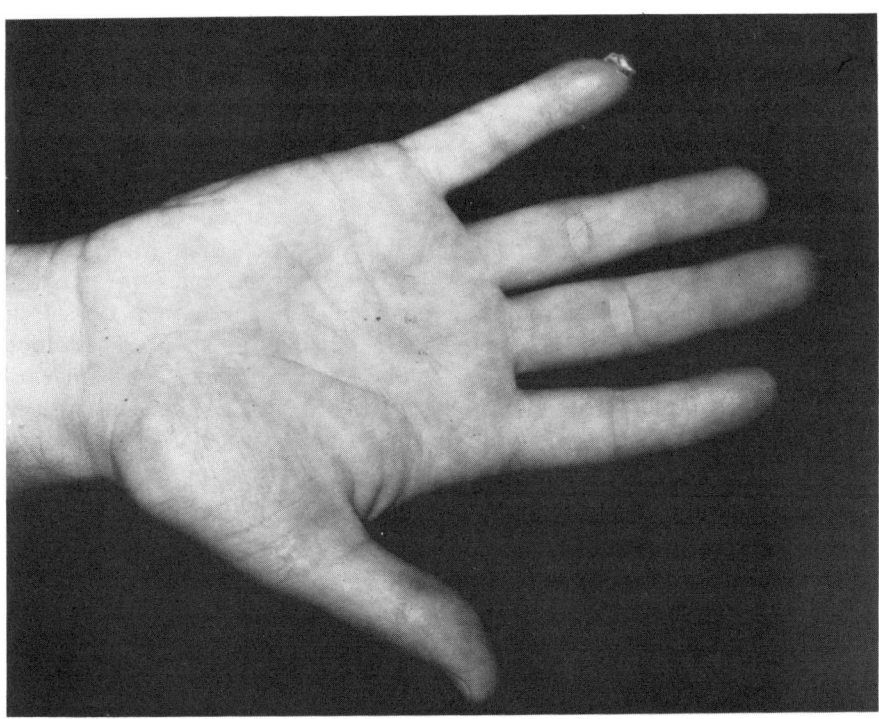

Figure 6A,B. Two views of the right hand on 6 July 1979.

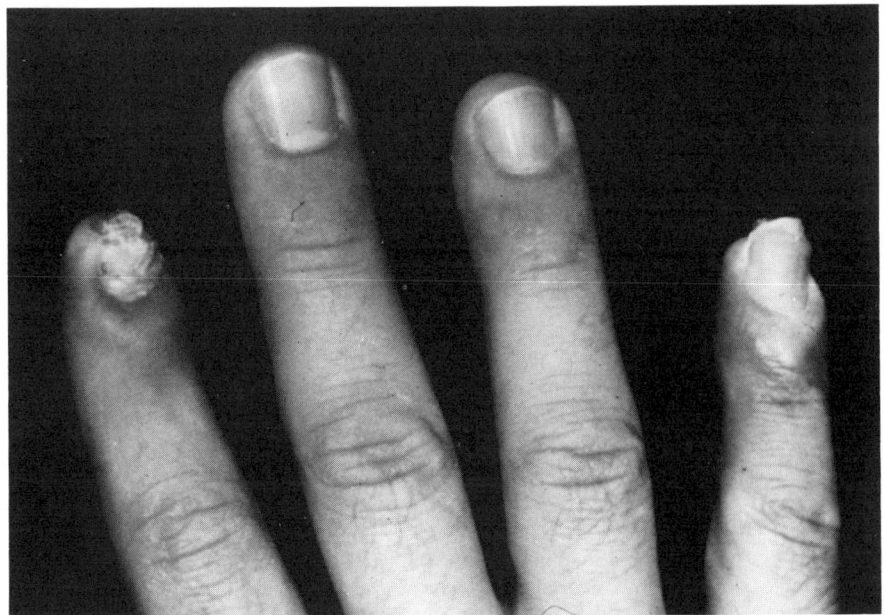

rate inside the midline of the finger was significantly less than the skin entrance exposure. If the patient's fingers were in the primary beam for 1 or possibly 2 minutes, an exposure in excess of 500 k rad of multiple low-energy X-rays could be expected.

The decision to treat the radiation injury of the distal phalanx conservatively is debatable, but a desire to maintain maximum length with possible salvation of the nailbed were considerations. The patient's decreasing amount of pain over a relatively brief time interval also encouraged conservative treatment. The fact that the exposure was felt to be from the distal tip radiating proximally and not in a dorsal or palmar direction primarily, coupled with the inability to predict which tissues would regenerate, mitigated against acute surgical excision with grafting. The patient and his surgeon wished to salvage the nailbed if at all possible. The patient will probably need some surgery in the future.

The graphic progression of this patient's lesion is depicted in Figures 1 through 6. I believe that a conservative approach in this particular incident maintained a viable digit with a viable nailbed and conserved maximum length.

Several reports indicate that conservative therapy may be the only treatment necessary for some radiation injuries.[5-10] Since this accident combined low-energy X-ray with an unusual distal tip of phalanx portal, a conservative management was used. In this particular patient, this management has proved a most satisfactory course.

The long-term effects of low dosages of this radiation to the distal phalanx are as yet unknown. The plastic surgeon and the radiation therapist who are following this particular patient are acutely aware of the potential of carcinoma development in such areas, and the patient himself was made aware of this risk. Future plans call for some selective debridement of bone with coverage of the distal phalanx of the index finger.

References

1. Upton AC: Effects of radiation on man. *Annu Rev Nucl Sci* 18:495, 1968.
2. Warren S: Effects of radiation on normal tissues. XIII. Effects on the skin. *Arch Pathol* 35:340, 1943.
3. Knowlton NP, Leifer E, Hogness JR, Hempelmann LH, Blaney LF, Gill DC, Oakes WR, Shafer CL: Beta-ray burns of human skin. *JAMA* 141:239, 1949.
4. Krizek TJ, Ariyan S: Severe acute radiation injuries of the hands. *Plast Reconstr Surg* 51:14, 1973.
5. Ariyan S, Krizek TJ: Radiation effects, biological and surgical considerations, in Converse JM (ed.): *Reconstructive Plastic Surgery*. Philadelphia, W. B. Saunders Company, 1977.

6. Brown JB, Fryer MP: Report of surgical repair in the first group of atomic radiation injuries. *Surg Gynecol Obstet* 103:1, 1956.

7. Brown JB, Fryer MP: Reconstruction of electrical injuries, including cranial losses. With preliminary report of cathode-ray burns. *Ann Surg* 146:342, 1957.

8. Brown JB, Fryer MP: High energy electron injury from accelerator machine. Radiation burns of chest wall and neck. 17-year follow up of atomic burns. *Ann Surg* 162:426, 1965.

9. Brown JB, McDowell F, Fryer MP: Radiation burns, including vocational and atomic exposures. Treatment and surgical prevention of chronic lesions. *Ann Surg* 130:593, 1949.

10. Brown JB, McDowell F, Fryer MP: Surgical treatment of radiation burns. *Surg Gynecol Obstet* 88:609, 1949.

Surgical Approaches to Radiation Injuries of the Hand

Peter J. Stern

Assistant Professor of Orthopaedic Surgery; Director, Division of Hand Surgery, Department of Orthopaedic Surgery, University of Cincinnati College of Medicine, Cincinnati, Ohio.

The first case of radiation dermatitis was reported by Daniel in 1896, a year after X-rays had been discovered.[1] The medical literature during the first half of the twentieth century is replete with reports of radiation injuries and their management,[2-6] and this rapidly led to an awareness of the dangers of ionizing radiation. Today great efforts have been made to protect individuals from accidental exposure, but injuries still occur. They result primarily from laboratory and industrial accidents as well as overexposure during therapeutic radiation.

When an accident occurs, the circumstances of the accident should be carefully reconstructed. Next, exposure time should be recorded and dosimetry studies performed by a radiation physicist. Theoretically, this data should aid the physician in estimating the extent of the damage so that his treatment can be planned accordingly. Unfortunately, precise calculations often cannot be made, and we are forced to rely on clinical judgment while managing these patients.

Regardless of the circumstances of the exposure, all radiation injuries produce some degree of obliterative endarteritis that leads to chronic ischemia and fibrosis (Figure 1). These changes may lead in turn to chronic ulceration, infection, necrosis, and poor wound healing. In the hand, in addition to skin and vascular injury, there may be damage to the bones and joints, tendons, and even peripheral nerves, making reconstruction all the more difficult.

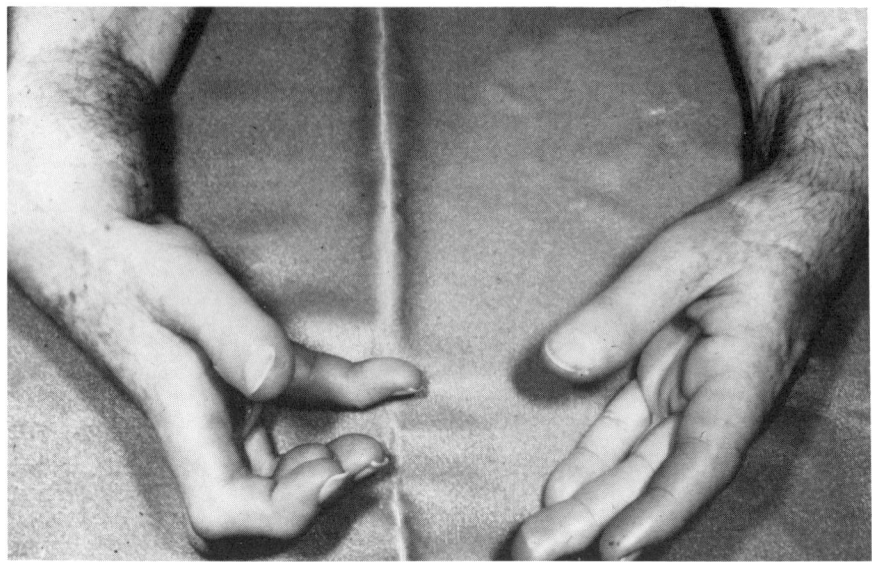

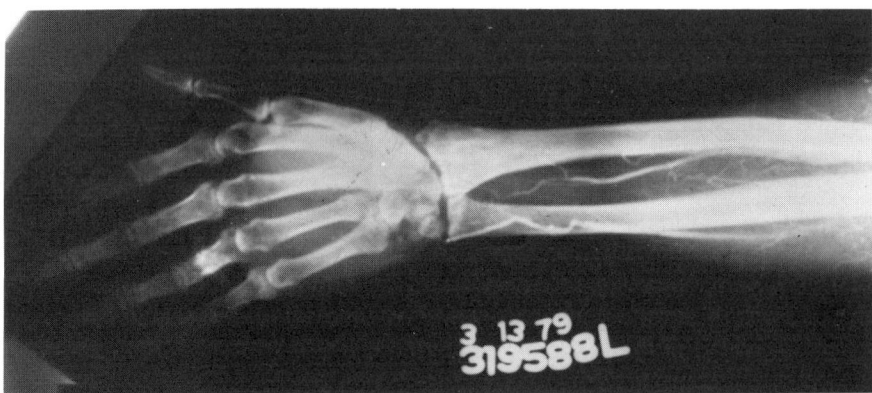

Figure 1. Radiation fibrosis. This patient was treated with a large dose of radiation for dermatitis in 1950. This photograph depicts maximum flexion. Courtesy of Dr. H. E. Kleinert.

Management of Acute Injuries

An acute radiation injury is produced when one is exposed to a high dose of radiation for a short period of time. The amount of permanent damage is highly variable and depends largely upon dose and exposure time. With massive doses, there may be initial erythema, edema, and blistering with ultimate loss of the extremity. With lower doses, there are no initial physical findings and the patient may be unaware of an injury. A week later erythema develops or it may progress to ulceration, fibrosis, and loss of tissue mass. The erythema may resolve in 4 to 8 weeks with only residual hyperpigmentation.

Initial management of acute injuries is nonoperative. These injuries tend to be progressive, and it is frequently impossible to accurately predict the amount of loss. Unlike the case for painless third-degree thermal burn, with acute radiation injuries pain is almost always present and is often severe enough to require large doses of narcotics.[7]

During the initial phase, every effort should be made to minimize contractures and to preserve joint motion. This can be accomplished through a combination of splints and physical therapy. If the hand is left unattended, the wrist will fall into a position of fixed palmar flexion, the fingers will assume an extended position at the metacarpophalangeal joint and the thumb will adduct into the palm. Resting splints in the "safe position" are designed to hold the wrist in a slightly dorsiflexed position with the metacarpophalangeal joints flexed 70° to 80° and the interphalangeal joints extended. In addition, the splint holds the thumb in palmar abduction.

Patients who have sustained massive acute radiation burns may develop gangrene which requires amputation.[8,9] Quite rightly, they have great difficulty accepting this course of action, particularly early on, when the extremity appears normal. It is better to allow the extremity to become gangrenous rather than to amputate prematurely. In delaying in this way, the patient becomes fully aware of the futility of his situation and can more easily accept the ablative procedure.

Some patients go into a subacute phase in which they develop skin necrosis with exposure of the underlying structures. It is at this stage that plans for reconstructive surgery should be formulated.[10–13] The prerequisites for surgical success include removal of all necrotic and infected tissue to the level of a good blood supply and, when this has been accomplished, to provide good soft tissue coverage for the underlying structures. Debridement must be carried down to healthy, viable tissue. If this is not done, one can expect further necrosis and infection with guaranteed failure of any subsequent procedure to provide soft tissue coverage. Furthermore, with inadequate resection, there is an increased risk of exposing vital structures such as tendons, nerves, bones, and cartilage.

In most cases, skin grafts are the easiest way to achieve coverage. Brown et al. have advocated skin grafts, particularly for patients who have been exposed to atomic radiation.[14] They reported that none of the 40 fingers exposed during the 1949 atomic testing at Los Alamos were lost with the use of the technique of resection and skin grafting. Ariyan and Krizek have noted that bleeding from the recipient wounds after debridement may be difficult to control and recommend delayed grafting 24 to 48 hr later.[12] With this technique, hematoma between the graft and the recipient site is minimized and the graft has a greater likelihood of survival. Others recommend immediate grafting. After graft application, the hand is splinted in the "safe" position. After 5 to 7 days, range of motion is begun.

Sometimes skin grafts are inadequate, and flap coverage may be required. Skin flaps are indicated to cover: (1) severely scarred areas such that, even if a skin graft took, it would later break down; (2) exposed bone, cartilage, tendon, or nerves; or (3) areas where one plans additional reconstructive surgery on tendons or nerves.

Flaps may help to improve regional blood flow after radiation injury. Krizek and Ariyan report a patient who sustained radiation injuries that were severe enough to justify the consideration of amputation.[15] An arteriogram showed a marked decreased digital blood flow with precapillary arteriovenous shunting. After a period of splinting and physical therapy, a flap was performed. An arteriogram taken 1 year later showed impressive improvement in regional blood flow.

In the past decade an exciting development has taken place in the area of reconstructive surgery. Using the operating microscope, microsutures, and microinstruments, a surgeon can sew together vessels and nerves which can barely be seen by the naked eye.[16] This allows the surgeon to move a composite of tissues with its vascular pedicle from one anatomical location to a distant one and maintain viability by anastomosing donor to recipient vessels. The distant transfer of composite tissues from one anatomical site to another has allowed the reconstructive surgeon to accomplish in a few hours what traditionally has taken weeks or months. It is now possible to transfer skin,[17] muscle,[18] bone,[19] and even toes[20] from one location to another by such techniques.

Figure 2A depicts the thumb pad of a patient who was handling radioactive iridium (^{192}Ir) when it fell out of its protective container, exposing the thumb and index finger to 1500 rad over a 1-minute period. Over the next 10 days, the patient developed painful ulcerations in the pulps of these two fingers. The ulcers failed to heal and remained painful and in addition sensation was so diminished that he was unable to perform those activities which required precision pinch. Because of persistent pain, ulceration, and poor sensation, resurfacing was indicated. Until recently, most reconstructive surgeons would have used local flaps. However, local flaps do not provide normal sensation to this critical area and it was instead elected to do a free neurovascular transfer. For this, the pad from the lateral side of the great toe and the pad from the medial side of the second toe were taken on their neurovascular pedicles and anastomosed to the digital arteries and nerves of the thumb and index finger. Although technically a demanding procedure, it can be done in a single sitting, gives excellent padding and contour to the finger, and provides good sensation (Figure 2B).

Free tissue transfer is in its embryonic stages. As our expertise in microsurgery expands, it can be expected to be a valuable part of the armamentarium of the reconstructive surgeon.

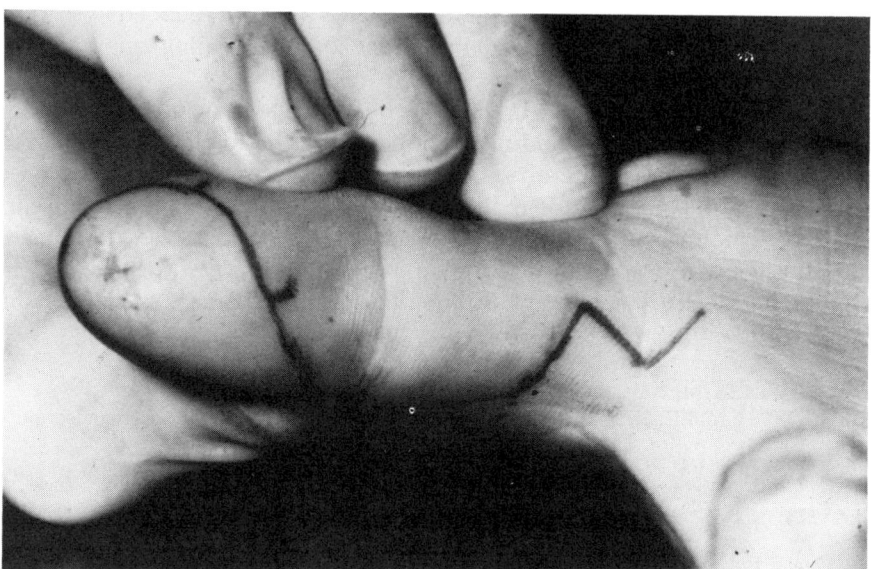

Figure 2. (A) Thumb pad fibrosis secondary to ^{192}Ir exposure. (B) Finger tips after free neurovascular transfer from toes.

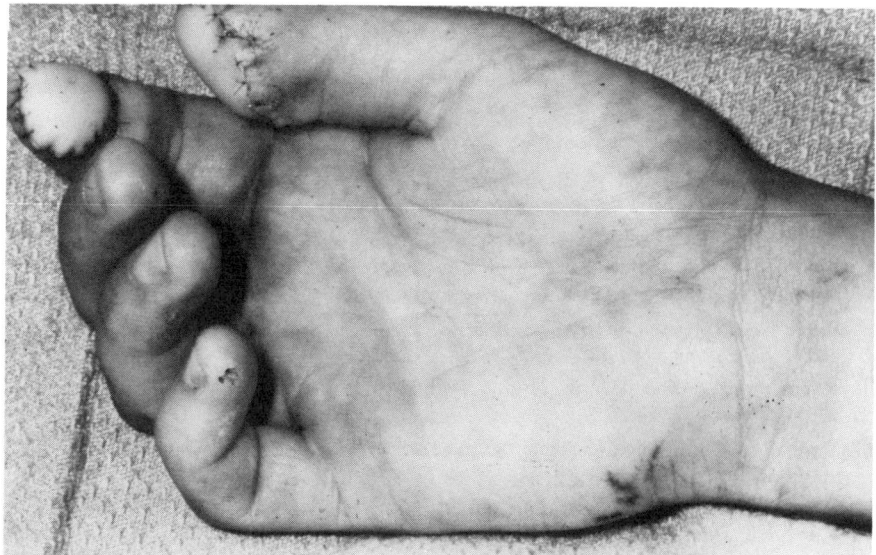

Chronic Radiation Exposure

Chronic low-dose radiation exposure produces premature aging of the skin. Skin becomes dry and wrinkles with loss of the sebaceous glands, sweat glands, and hair follicles; later there is atrophy of underlying fat and ulceration. The skin has been described as "half dead, half alive with its regenerative and recuperative powers sadly reduced."[13] It is weakly resistant to trauma and infection, and its healing qualities are quite poor.

Chronically irradiated skin should be managed as a premalignant condition. The keratoses and ulcerations should be excised and covered with split-thickness skin grafts. Chronic or proliferative ulcers should be pathologically examined for malignant degeneration. Squamous cell carcinoma, which occurs most frequently, tends to be low grade. Management varies with the location. One must do at least wide, local excision, and sometimes it is necessary to amputate a finger, a ray, or part of the hand.

ACKNOWLEDGMENT
I thank Dr. Harold E. Kleinert for providing the case examples used in this manuscript.

References

1. Daniel J: The X-rays. *New Science* 3:562, 1896.

2. Wolbach SB: The pathologic histology of chronic X-ray dermatitis and early X-ray carcinoma. *J Med Res* 21:415, 1909.

3. Porter CA: The surgical treatment of X-ray carcinoma and other severe X-ray lesions (based on an analysis of 47 cases). *J Med Res* 21:357, 1909.

4. Davis JS: Clinical illustrations of deep roentgen-ray and radium burns. *Am J Roentgenol Rad Therapy* 29:43–78, 1933.

5. Gillies HD, McIndoe AH: The role of plastic surgery in burns due to roentgen rays and radium. *Ann Surg* 101:979–996, 1935.

6. Brown JB, McDowell F, Fryer MP: Surgical treatment of radiation burns. *Surg Gynecol Obstet* 88:609–622, 1949.

7. Smith SM: Subjective experiences during A 32-year period after resurfacing hands for severe and acute radiation burns. *Plastic Reconst Surg* 51:23–26, 1973.

8. Schenck RR, Gilberti MV: Four-extremity radiation necrosis. *Arch Surg* 100:729–734.

9. Lanzl LH, Rosenfeld ML, Tarlov AR: injury due to accidental high-dose exposure to 10 MeV electrons. *Health Physics* 13:241–251, 1967.

10. Robinson DW: The hazards of surgery in irradiated tissue. *Arch Surg* 71:410–418, 1955.

11. Robinson DW: Surgical problems in the excision and repair of radiated tissue. *Plastic Reconst Surg* 55:41–49, 1975.

12. Ariyan S, Krizek TJ: Radiation effects, biological and surgical considerations, in Converse JM (ed.): *Reconstructive Plastic Surgery*. Philadelphia, W.B. Saunders Company, 1977, pp. 531–548.

13. Hansen FC, Edgerton MT: Radiation burns, in Flynn JE (ed.): *Hand Surgery.* Baltimore, Williams and Wilkins Co., 1976, pp. 383–391.

14. Brown JB, McDowell F, Fryer MP: High energy electron injury from accelerator machines. *Ann Surg* 162:426–437, 1965.

15. Krizek TJ, Ariyan S: Severe acute radiation injuries of the hands. *Plastic Reconst Surg* 51:14–22, 1973.

16. Daniel RK: Microsurgery: through the looking glass. *New England J Med* 300:1251–1257, 1979.

17. May JW, Jr., Chait LA, Cohen BE, O'Brien BM: Free neurovascular flap from the first web of the foot in hand reconstruction. *J Hand Surg* 2:387–393, 1977.

18. Manktelow RT, McKee NH: Free muscle transplantation to provide active finger flexion. *J Hand Surg* 3:416–426, 1978.

19. Weiland AJ, Daniel RK: Microvascular anastomoses for bone grafts in the treatment of massive defects in bone. *J Bone Joint Surg* 61A:98–104, 1978.

20. May JW Jr, Daniel RK: Great toe to hand free tissue transfer. *Clin Ortho* 133:140–153, 1978.

Dosimetry Studies for an Industrial Radiography Accident

F. Eugene Holly*
and William L. Beck+

*Department of Radiation Oncology, University of California at Los Angeles;
+Medical and Health Sciences Division, Oak Ridge Associated Universities, Oak Ridge, Tennessee.

Introduction

Industrial radiography is a frequently used method of nondestructive testing for many industrial products. Industrial radiography is a routine operation requiring high radiation levels and relying primarily on human diligence in observing safety procedures to prevent accidents. Consequently, there are a number of serious overexposures each year as have been reported previously.[1−6]

Iridium 192 is the most commonly used radionuclide for industrial radiography. The source activity typically ranges from 20 to 100 curies. This paper reports the dosimetry studies that were done to determine the dose to a worker who unknowingly carried such a source in his hip pocket.

On 5 June 1979, an industrial worker who was not involved with radiography and, therefore, not familiar with the appearance of a radiography source (Figure 1) found an ^{192}Ir source that had accidentally become detached and "lost" from its shielded camera. Since the source was not identified, the worker was unaware of any danger. He placed the source in the hip pocket of his coveralls and continued his work. Some time later, he took it to the plant manager. Approximately three weeks elapsed prior to the discovery that his injury was due to radiation.

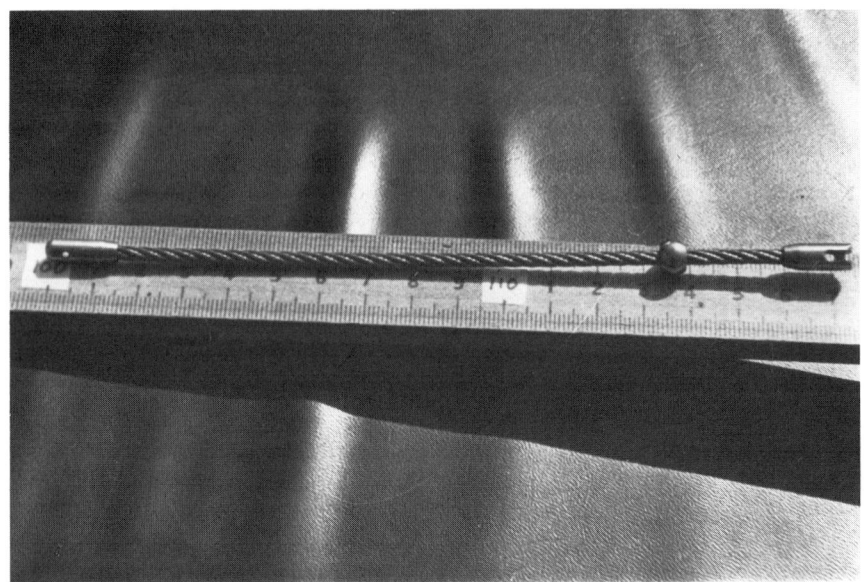

Figure 1. ^{192}Ir source capsule assembly, Model No. 200-520-008, Automation Industries, Inc.

His clinical course is described in the paper by Ross and Holly in this book.[7]

The worker initially estimated that the source was in his pocket for approximately two hours. However, after an extensive investigation, representatives of the California Occupational Safety and Health Department estimated the source time to be about 45 min. Reconstruction using the actual clothing demonstrated that the source was probably in contact with or no further than 1 or 2 cm from the skin of the worker's hip during the exposure.

Dosimetry Studies

Activity/Exposure Determination

The manufacturer quoted the source activity as 103.0 curie (3.81 TBq) on 8 January 1979. Using a half-life of 74.2 days,[8] the expected activity on the date of the accident would have been 25.6 curie (1.04 TBq) to 33 curie (1.22 TBq).

More precise measurements were required for the clinical management of this injury and to provide archival information for similar accidents. A Baldwin-Farmer 0.6-cc ionization chamber with a ± 3% calibration accuracy (traceable to the National Bureau of Standards) was exposed, in air, at distances of 10 and 20 cm from the source. The positioning error was estimated to be less than ± 0.5 cm. These measurements indicated an average exposure rate on 5 June 1977, of 2250 Roentgens per min or 13.5 R/hr at distances of 1 cm and 1 m, respectively. The standard deviation of eight such measurements was less than 3%. This corresponds to a source activity of 28 ± 2 curie (1.04 ± 0.007 TBq), with the uncertainty reflecting possible positioning errors. This activity determination was based on an Exposure-Rate-Constant of 4.8 R-cm²/millicurie-hr as reported in NCRP Pamphlet 40.[8] Although estimates of the Exposure-Rate-Constant for ¹⁹²Ir range from 4.3 to 5.0 R-cm²/millicurie-hr,[9,10] the value of 4.8 was selected to be consistent with the exposure estimation methods of NCRP 40. The exposure and dose calculations of this paper are based on the actual exposure rate measurements and are independent of the exact source activity.

Spectral Distribution

The presence of impurities, especially those with long half-lives and high radiation energies, can significantly alter the absorbed doses. Impurities contained in some commercial ¹⁹²Ir sources are ¹⁹⁴Ir (62% natural abundance), ⁵¹Cr, ⁵⁶Mn, ⁵⁹Fe, and ⁶⁰Co—the latter two being the most troublesome as the source decays due to their longer half-lives and higher photon energies.

Figure 2 shows the energy spectrum obtained at a distance of six feet with a 3 × 3 inch NaI spectrometer and slit collimation. This spectrum indicates that the source has no contaminants that would significantly influence absorbed dose distributions.

Depth-Dose Calculations

The absorbed dose (D_d) at depths from 1 cm to 25 cm in tissue with the source in surface contact was calculated by

$$D_d = \frac{0.96 \, A\Gamma}{(d + 0.24)^2} f(d)$$

where A = source activity in curies (A is the exposure rate at 1 cm), Γ = exposure rate constant, 0.96 = rads/Roentgen, d = depth in tissue in cm, 0.24 = estimated encapsulation thickness, f(d) = scatter and attenuation polynomial of Shalek and Stovall[10] for d ≤ 15 cm or exp(−.035d) for d ≥ 15 cm.

Since there is a likelihood that the source may have been at a distance of up to 2 cm from the surface, depth doses were also calculated for these circumstances using standard depth-dose improvement factors with the greater distances from the surface. These values are tabulated in Table 1 and compared in Figure 3 with actual measurements.

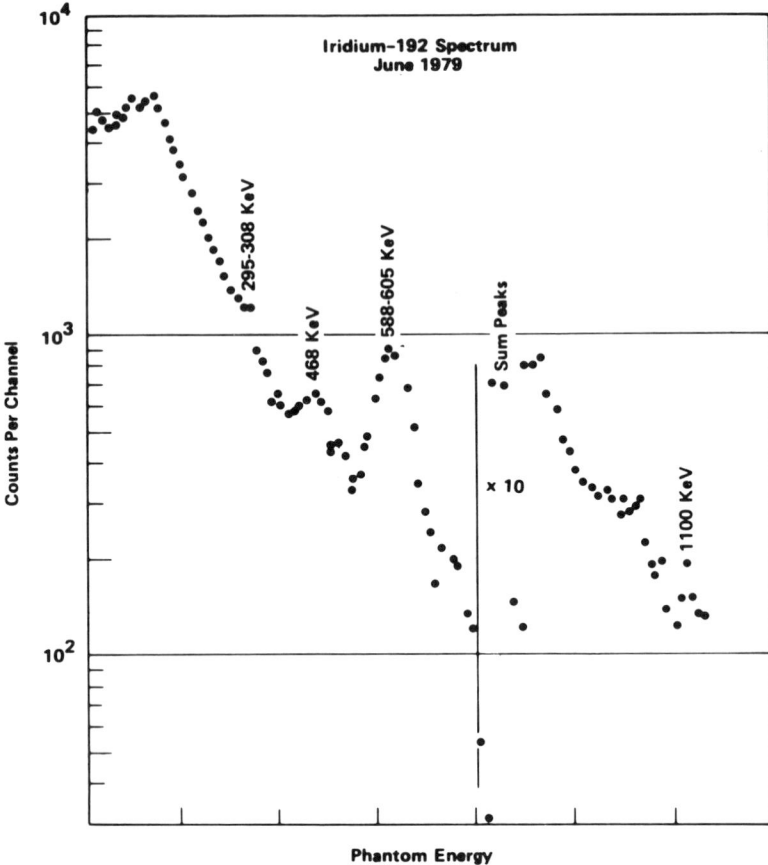

Figure 2. Field measurement of energy spectrum of ^{192}Ir source 6.5 months after production. The measurement was at 6 feet with a 3 × 3-inch NaI spectrometer with slit collimation. Scatter, self-absorption in the source, and differential collimator absorption obliterate low-energy photon peaks; however, the spectrum is identifiable as ^{192}Ir with a possible trace contamination of ^{59}Fe or ^{60}Co.

Phantom Depth-Dose Measurements

Precalibrated calcium fluoride (bulb) thermoluminescent dosimeters (TLD's) were placed in a 31 × 31 × 31 cm *water phantom* at the owner's site to measure the actual dose rate at varying depths. Three separate experimental trials were made with one, including a central ionization chamber measurement for an additional calibration check. These results are compared in Figure 3 with the calculations.

An Alderson Rando phantom was used as a *patient analog* (Figure 4). This standard-man-sized phantom is constructed of isocyanate rubber, equivalent to tissue in interactions with ionizing radiation. A human skeleton and density-adjusted lungs are contained within the otherwise solid phantom. The phantom is sliced into transverse sections 2.5-cm thick with holes of 5-mm diameter arranged in a 3 × 3-cm grid to provide positions for TLD's (Figure 5). When not in use as a dosimeter site, the holes are filled with removable plugs of tissue-equivalent material.

Dosimeters were placed in the phantom at locations corresponding to the femoral artery, piriformis muscles, and eye lens. Dosimeters were also at positions near the surface and along the body midline. The latter covers a range of depths from 1 to 24 cm. These results are also compared with calculations in Figure 3.

Results

Dosimeters placed on the surface of the Alderson Rando phantom at distances of 1, 5, and 10 cm from the point of source contact measured exposures [28 curie (1.04 TBq), 45 min] of 80,000 R, 4100 R, and 760 R, respectively.

Dosimeters placed on the eye lens and at the location of the testes yielded doses of 9 and 95 rad (90 and 950 mGy).

An "average midline dose" was estimated to be 68 rad (cGy) by averaging the response of 48 dosimeters placed at 5-cm intervals uniformly along the body midline. Although not directly comparable to this average midline dose, two independent groups have made estimates of the "equivalent whole-body dose" by cytogenetic dosimetry. The results of Dr. Norman (private communication) were reported as follows: "The equivalent whole-body dose estimated from the acentric fragments is about 100 ± 22 rad. From the dicentrics plus rings, I estimate a dose of 70 ± 18 rads. The two estimates are not significantly different. I place

Table 1. Calculated Doses Based on a 45-Min Exposure to 28 curie (1.04 TBq)

Depth in tissue (cm)	Rad/45 min, Source "d" cm from surface[a]		
	d = 0.24	d = 1.24	d = 2.24
1	52,000	16,000	7,600
2	19,000	9,000	5,800
3	9,000	5,200	3,400
4	5,200	3,400	2,400
5	3,400	2,400	1,800
6	2,400	1,800	1,400
8	1,300	1,050	860
10	820	680	600
15	320	280	250
25	80	70	60

[a] Encapsulation is assumed to be 0.24cm.

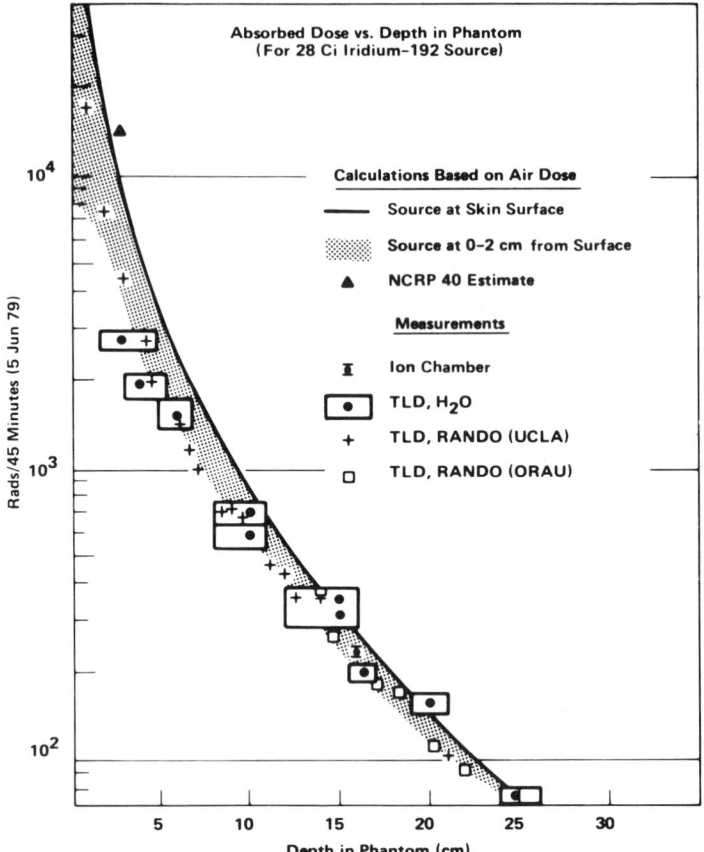

Figure 3. Absorbed dose vs. depth. The heavy black line indicates maximum theoretical 45-min exposure with source-surface contact. The shaded area indicates theoretical exposure with the source at 0–2 cm from the surface. The results of three independent TLD experiments are shown. The on-site water phantom measurements are depicted with large uncertainties due to possible positioning errors. Measurements in the Alderson Rando phantom (+ UCLA, □ ORAU) have a ±10% uncertainty. In all instances, calculations of depth dose based on surface contact would have resulted in safe-side or maximum estimates.

the equivalent whole-body dose in the range of 70 to 100 rad. The estimate based on our count of micronuclei—25 in 3000 lymphocytes—falls within this range." Littlefield's[12] results, which are reported in detail in this book, estimated the whole-body equivalent dose as 91 rad (cGy).

Of particular concern was the dose to the deep femoral artery (profunda femoris), which is the major supplier of blood to the leg. In an Argentinian accident involving a lost source carried in the pants pockets,

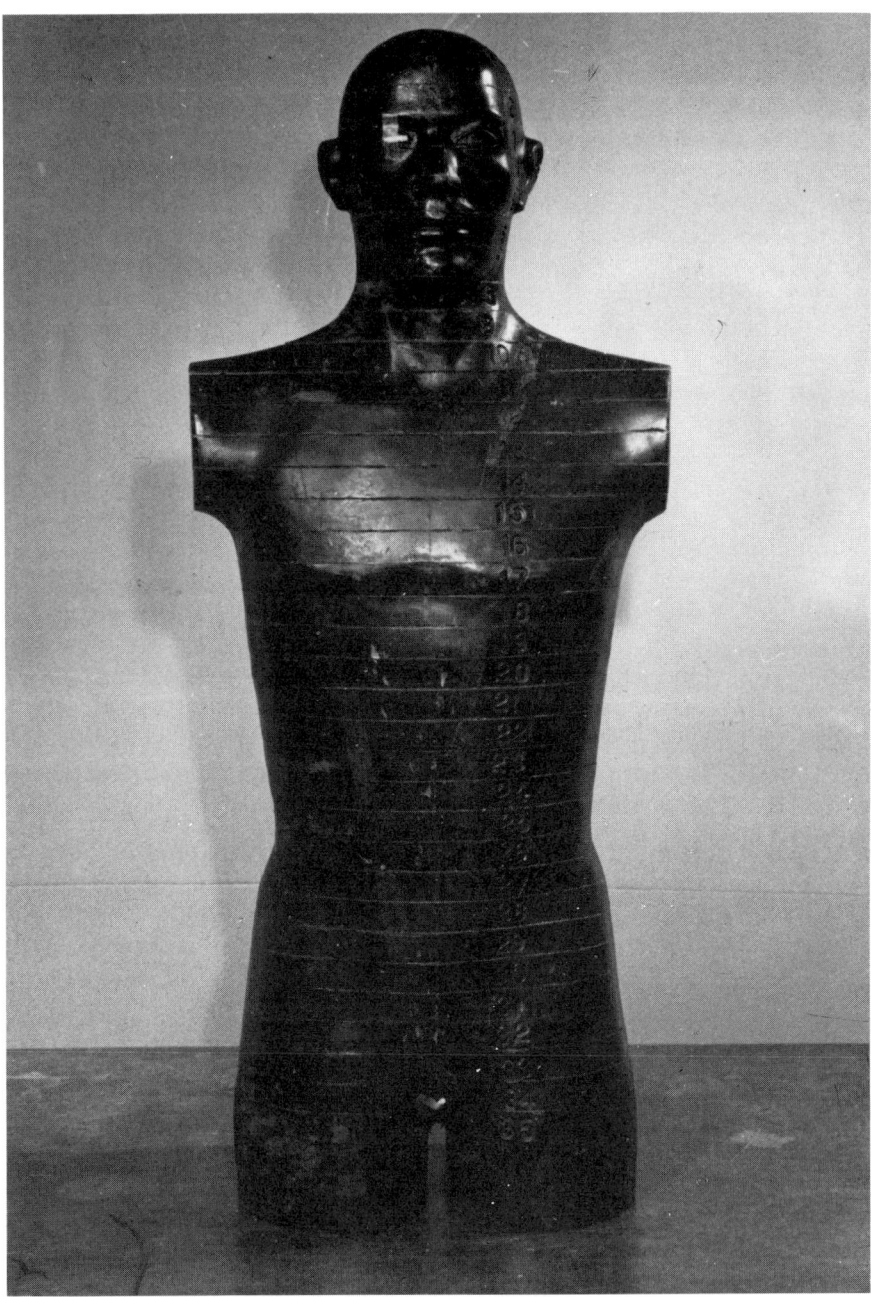

Figure 4. The Alderson Rando dosimetry phantom.

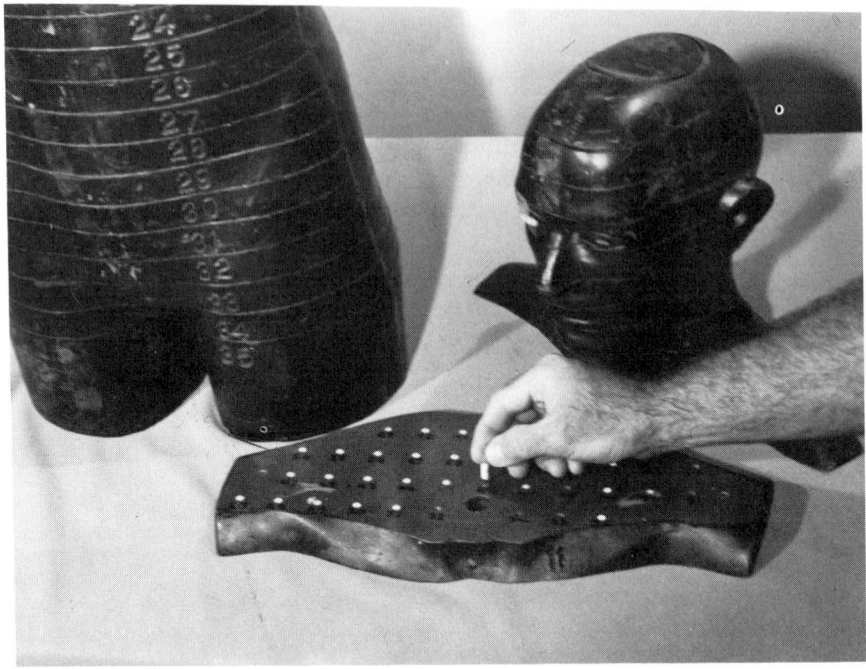

Figure 5. A LiF dosimeter being inserted into a thoracic section of the Alderson Rando phantom.

the victim lost both legs.[13] The workman's deep femoral arteries received a much larger dose than in this accident for two reasons. First, he carried the source for several days, and, second, the source was carried in each of the front pant pockets, which placed the source nearer to these important arteries. Our estimate of the dose to the deep femoral artery in this accident is 180 rads (1.8 Gy).

Interpretations of computerized transaxial tomography (CTT) performed approximately three months after the accident revealed, in addition to extensive local damage, possible damage to the piriformis muscle and the neurovascular bundle immediately anterior. Dosimeters in corresponding phantom locations received 700–2000 rad (7–20 Gy) at positions ranging from the posterior muscle to the anterior neurovascular bundle as judged from the CTT studies.

Accident Scenarios

It was not the purpose of this paper to investigate or explain how this particular accident happened. However, as there have been several serious accidents that have occurred because radiography sources have been "lost" from their shields, we would like to describe two scenarios that may explain how sources have become detached.

A typical radiography camera is shown in Figure 6. The shielding container is in the center of the photograph. The cable with the crank device is the source drive cable which allows remote operation. It attaches to the camera on the locked end, and it also attaches to the source. Coiled closest to the camera is a flexible metal tube called the source tube. This attaches to the other end of the camera; and during operation, the source moves from the shield to the opposite end of the source tube and remains there until the exposure is completed. Figures 7–9 show the proper procedure for attaching the drive cable to the source cable (Figure 1). In Figure 7, the "hook" of the drive cable and the "eye" of the source cable can be seen. Figure 8 shows how the drive cable must be turned 90° to the source cable in order to make the hook-and-eye connection. After this connection is made, the drive cable must be aligned with the source cable in order to connect the drive cable to the camera via the threaded connector (Figure 9). When these steps are completed properly, the drive cable can push the source out of its shield to make exposures and pull the source back into the shield at the end of

Figure 6. A typical radiography camera.

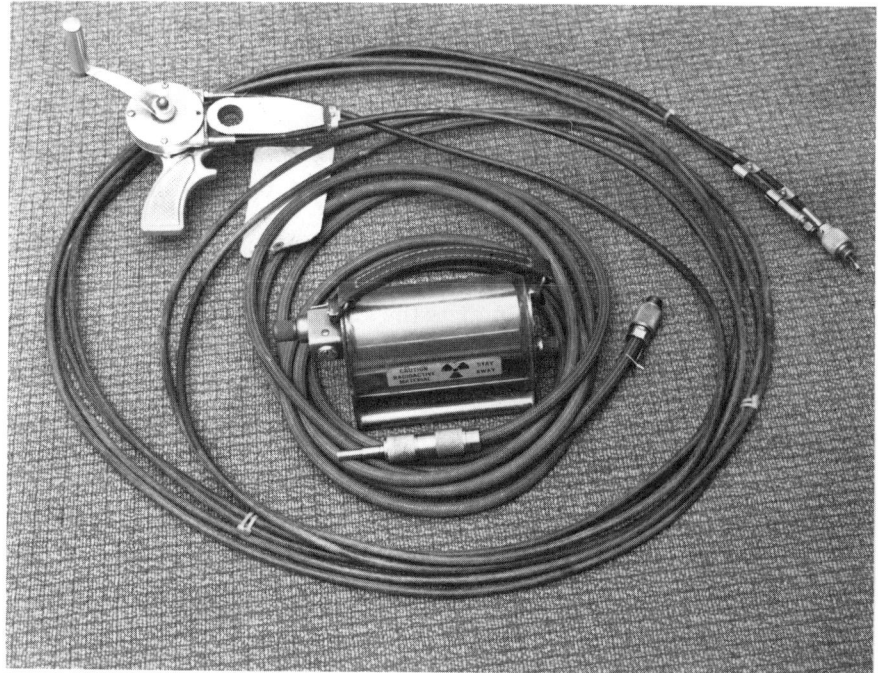

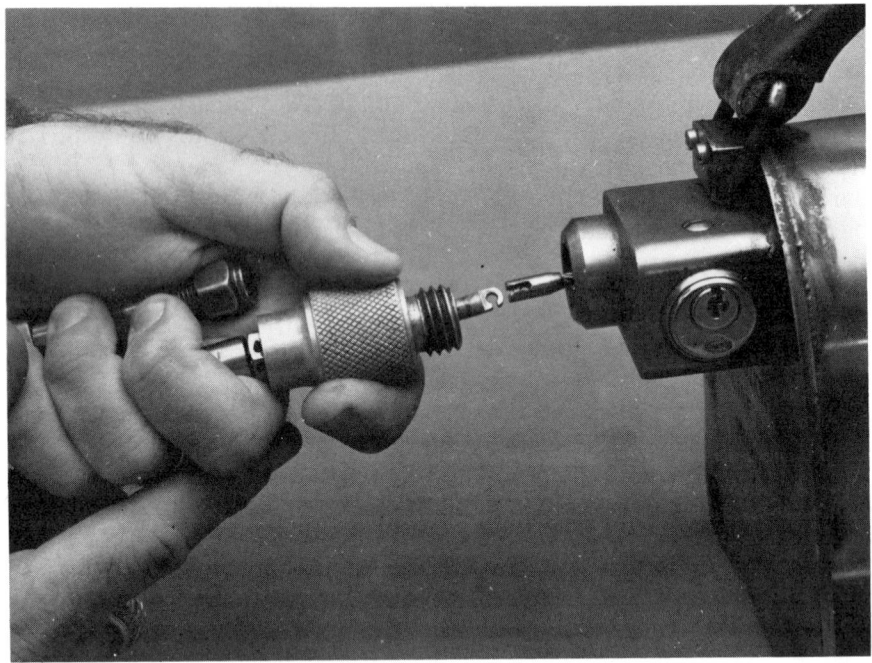

Figure 7. The hook-and-eye cable connection. The hook is on the drive cable, and the eye is on the source cable.

the required exposure time. However, if the hook-and-eye connection is not made, the drive cable assembly can still be attached to the camera. The drive cable can still push the source out of the shield, but it cannot pull it back into the shield; the source will remain in the source tube cable. Even if the hook-and-eye connection is made but the source tube is not used, the source may rotate 90° and become disengaged from the drive cable when the connection exits the camera. In either instance, the source will be left in the exposure position, even though the radiographer thinks that it is in the shielded camera because he has returned the drive cable. If he fails to make a proper radiation survey of the camera or to disconnect the drive cable to confirm the location of the source, he will not be aware of this malfunction. The source may then be "lost" and result in accidental exposure to the radiographer and other individuals.[1-7, 12, 13]

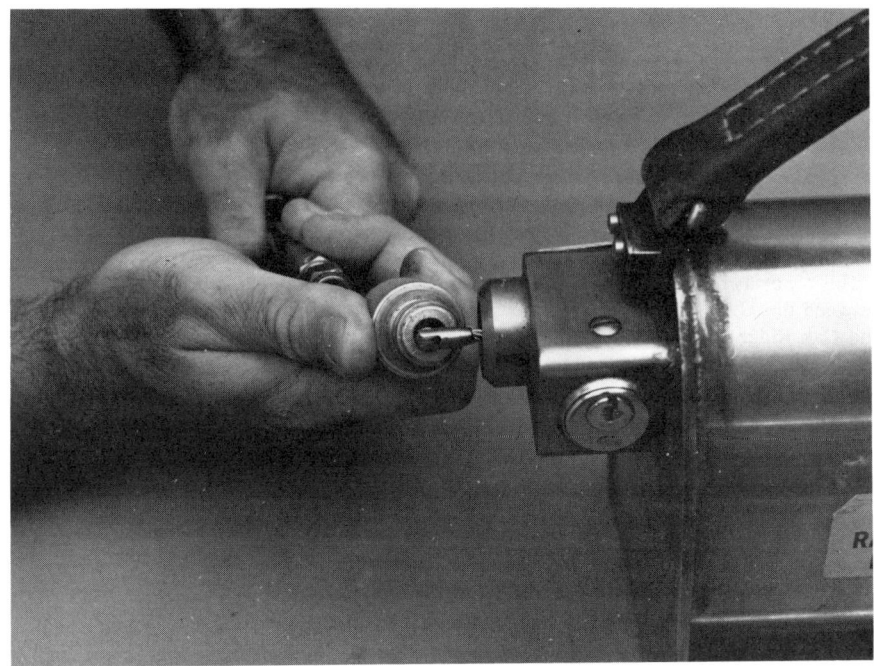

Figure 8. The drive cable must be turned 90° to the source cable in order for the connection to be made.

Figure 9. The drive cable and the source cable must be aligned before the threaded drive cable connection to the camera can be made.

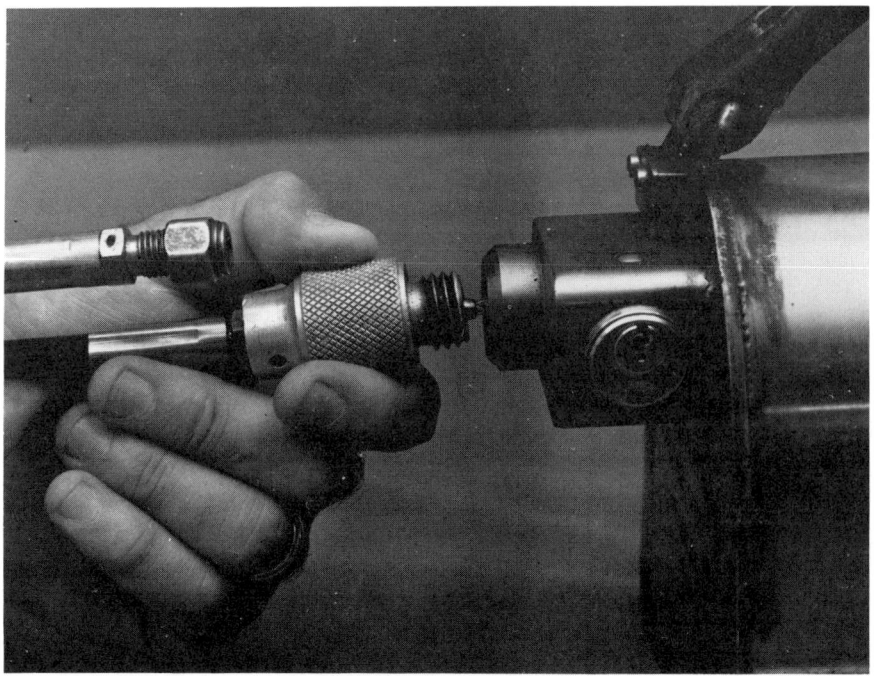

ACKNOWLEDGMENTS

The authors wish to express their appreciation to Dr. Amos Norman, Department of Radiological Science, the University of California at Los Angeles, and to Dr. Gayle Littlefield, Medical and Health Sciences Division, Oak Ridge Associated Universities, for allowing us to use the results of their cytogenetic dosimetry; and to Mr. Ed Gupton, Director of Personnel Dosimetry, Oak Ridge National Laboratory, for providing a cross calibration for thermoluminescence measurements used in this report.

This report is based on work performed in part under Contract No. DE-AC05-760R00033 between the U.S. Department of Energy, Office of Health and Environmental Research, and Oak Ridge Associated Universities, and in part by the UCLA Center for the Health Sciences.

References

1. Annamalai M, Iyer PS, Panicker TMR: Radiation injury from acute exposure to an iridium 192 source: Case history. *Health Physics* 35:887–389, 1978.

2. Kumatori T, Hirashima K, Ishihara T, Kurisu A, Sugiyama H, Hashizume T: Radiation accident caused by a ^{192}Ir radiographic source, in *Proceedings of the Symposium on the Handling of Radiation Accidents*. Vienna, pp. 35–42, 1977.

3. Brown JK, McNeil JR: Biological dosimetry in an industrial radiography accident. *Health Physics* 21:519–522, 1971.

4. Maxfield WS, Porter GH: Accidental radiation exposure from Iridium-192 Camera, in *Proceedings of the Symposium on the Handling of Radiation Accidents*. Vienna, p. 459, 1969.

5. Catlin RJ: Radiation accident experience—causes and lessons learned, in, *Proceedings of the Symposium on the Handling of Radiation Accidents*. Vienna, p. 437, 1969.

6. Biles MB: Characteristics of radiation exposure accidents, in *Proceedings of the Symposium on the Handling of Radiation Accidents*. Vienna, p. 3, 1969.

7. Ross J, Holly E: The 1979 Los Angeles accident: Exposure to an iridium 192 industrial radiographic source, in *The Medical Basis for Radiation Accident Preparedness*. New York, Elsevier North Holland, Inc., 1980.

8. Protection against radiation from brachytherapy sources. *NCRP Pamphlet No. 40*, National Council on Radiation Protection and Measurements, March 1, 1972.

9. Glasgow GP, Dillman LT: Specific gamma constant and exposure rate constant of [192]Ir. *Medical Physics* 6:49–52, 1979.

10. Shalek RJ, Stovall M: Dosimetry in implant therapy, in Attix, Roesch, and Tochlin (eds.): *Radiation Dosimetry*. New York, Academic Press, 1969.

11. Alderson SW, Lanzl LH, Rowllins M, Spira J: An instrumental phantom system for analog computation of treatment plans. *Am J Roentgenol Radium Therapy and Nucl Med* 87:185–195, 1962.

12. Littlefield LG, Joiner EE, DuFrain RJ, Hübner KF, Beck WL: Cytogenetic dose estimates from *in vivo* samples from persons involved in real or suspected radiation exposures, in *The Medical Basis for Radiation Accident Preparedness*. New York, Elsevier North Holland, Inc., 1980.

13. Beninson D, Placer A, Vander E. Estudio de un caso de irradiacion humana accidental, in *Proceedings of the Symposium on the Handling of Radiation Accidents*. Vienna, pp. 415–429, 1969.

Discussion for Section II

W. K. SINCLAIR: A number of incidents, mostly in industrial radiography, have been presented, and I haven't heard any reference to either personnel monitors or area monitors where exposures might have been prevented or reduced by warning many of the exposures. They are recommended, I believe; are they not used?

E. B. SCOTT: In the accident that I've been associated with, most of the time there has been some question about the function of the monitoring devices. In the gentleman whose fingers I showed, there was a question whether the dosimeter and the scanning devices were working at all. They did go off scale, but, as it turned out, the instrument was set on the wrong sensitivity. In the other accidents mentioned earlier, a short cut is often taken, or the devices aren't always used. As I mentioned, people working in the marshlands and on barges don't really have very good ways of doing things. They traipse through the mud all day long, and sometimes they lose or misplace their film badges, or they change clothes, and it stays in other clothes. I don't think it's a lack of what should be there; it's a physical problem of keeping everything in the right place and in the right perspective to the sources.

W. J. BECK: I want to respond to Dr. Sinclair's comment on whether or not there are monitors around the radiography situation. Normally, the only monitoring device used in industrial radiography are survey instruments. However, commercially available warning devices called "personal radiation alarms" or "chirpers" are very effective.

They warn the worker of high radiation levels by beeping at a rate proportional to the radiation intensity. They cost only about $100 and should be required for working with any device that produces high radiation fields.

D. L. MCNEILL: Dr. Ross recommends early surgery to stop ulcerative growth, and Dr. Scott recommends later surgery; what are the criteria for graft surgery in early and late operations?

J. F. ROSS: Dealing with the finger or the thumb, it's different from the buttock. The man's buttock was obviously going to keep on ulcerating for months, as the small lesion has done. It was decided that if left alone it would not increase in size, and he would have a disability of 6 to 12 months longer than if it was incised and grafted with a flap. The control lesion that was not resected is getting bigger and breaking down and will have to be resected, so at least in this instance, I think it was appropriate to resect it. If it's a finger, I think it's a different matter, but even then we've seen fingers that have had skin flaps put on. It didn't necessitate the removal of a digit. I think it would be justifiable to try before you amputate a digit, and I think it's up to an experienced plastic surgeon to determine just what he's going to do.

E. B. SCOTT: I did not intend to suggest early surgery or late surgery. The two injuries in question both involved index fingers but were produced in different types of accidents. The surgery was also performed for different reasons. It is easy to say one must take each case individually, but I feel that the decision involves looking at all angles and picking the best for that situation. I think Dr. Ross may be better able to give the criteria for grafts and grafting procedures.

C. SHEARIN: With the treatment of radiation burns, the primary problem is a progressive endarteritis; in frostbite or thermal burns you do not have that problem. I don't think the patient I presented with the index finger burn is out of the woods yet. He had almost a quarter of a million rad of low energy, and the physicist told me that within 4 mm of the skin 60% of this was gone and by the time it reached the bone, all the energy would have been absorbed. We elected with this particular individual to watch him to see what would happen. But I think I should have skin grafted this fellow's finger with a palmal, dorsal, or whatever graft or a flap earlier. I think Dr. Stern mentioned that in these individuals you must establish a new blood supply. Although these lesions appear to heal initially, they usually reoccur and break down unless some new tissue is brought in.

W. CARPAY: Dr. Shearin, could you give more detailed information about the conservative therapy you give your patients for the treatment of pain, in local application of ointments, and methods of systemic treatment.

C. SHEARIN: Regarding pain, the patients usually all complain of fairly severe pain that frequently requires hospitalization and often necessitates parental analgesics such as morphine or demerol. The pain is described as unrelenting and very severe and probably is best relieved by surgical debridement with application of split thickness skin grafts. This should be done at a time when there is no evidence of infection present, and in the tissue so affected, bacterial counts should be less than 10^5 per gram of tissue.

The local application of any topical ointment is adequate as long as the patient does not show an allergic reaction to it, since an allergy would compound the problem. I think that ointments with some antibacterial action probably are best. During the first week or ten days radiation injuries can be treated with Silvadene, Sulfamylon, Betadine, Neosporin, etc., as long as the area is cleaned twice daily with sterile water and saline before the application. For a prolonged period of time, however, the answer is probably skin grafting to establish adequate cover and healthy tissue.

In answer to systemic treatment of local radiation injuries, I am not aware of anyone who was given specific systemic treatment for prevention of necrosis of the fingers or hands or of the skin of this area. The basic injury is one to the adventitial cells of the endothelium supplying the dermis, and no amount of systemic therapy is going to prevent this. Radiation injury is different from a burn injury or ischemic injury in the fact that the lesion is progressive over many years. The disease involves the cytoplasm and nucleic acids in the cell, with progression of fibrosis and thickening of the adventitial cells that results in poor blood supply to the area of involvement. Some physicians would advocate systemic antibiotic coverage over the acute period of radiation injury in addition to the previously mentioned topical ointments. As far as I know, no one has yet used any arterial infusions or systemic drugs such as Vasodilan, aspirin, heparin, Dextran, Persantin, etc., to treat these specific lesions. This would probably be futile; however, I have no evidence or studies to document this.

G. A. PODA It seems everyone talks about arteritis in local injuries, yet no one has discussed medical treatment to either prevent or diminish this. Antihistamines, aspirin, or prednisone help prevent the original erythema; reserpine, aspirin, or other antiprostaglandins could help reduce arteritis. Nerve blocks might increase circulation. Has any of these or other procedures been attempted? If not, why not?

J. F. ROSS: The patient with the buttock burn was given a material called Vasodilan. The plastic surgeons used it on the man, and they thought that it definitely improved the circulation in the surrounding area. They gave it to him prior to the surgery and continued it after the surgery. However, there were some side effects. His blood pressure went way down; he got tachycardia and high fever, which I believe could have been attributable to this medication, but this was the first time that they had used it. They were convinced it was effective, and they could use it in future cases in which there is blocked impairment of the vascularization.

P. J. STERN: I think the problem is that the entry has already been created and that these measures would only be temporizing. It would certainly be reasonable to try them, and I think the suggestion is a good one.

E. L. SAENGER: Thank you Dr. Stern. Are there any other questions or comments? It may at times be difficult to obtain an estimate of the biological effect of radiation to a portion of the body when the exposure occurs in several fractions separated by several days in time. In radiation therapy, this end is achieved by use of an equation initially derived by F. Ellis in which a term, nominal standard dose, is calculated. The equation is:

$$D = (NSD)\ T^{0.11}\ N^{0.24}.$$

where D is the tolerance dose of normal tissue, T is the overall treatment time in days, and N is the number of fractions. Note that no corrections are made for the field size. A more extensive treatment of this methodology can be found in E. J. Hall's *Radiobiology for the Radiologist* (2nd edition, Harper and Row, Hagerstown, North Dakota, 1978). This approach to complex dosimetry and biological effects therefrom may not be strictly applicable to the acute and subacute radiation injury from accidents, but its use may provide useful approximations to determine extent of injury and prognosis.

I might also comment on remarks made by Dr. Ross that the Nuclear Regulatory Commission files, at least as far as licensees in nonagreement states are concerned, show a very striking decrease in the number of severe radiation exposures of the type we've discussed. Of course, that doesn't reflect what goes on in the state of California, but since so many things don't reflect what goes on in the state of California, this is not hard to understand. I visited the NRC several weeks ago, and I reviewed these things. The NRC and others are taking more time to have training programs for the radiographic technicians, who are really, I think, essentially high-school graduates with rather short training periods. In the state of California, they have a short training program, and then they are licensed. I'm not entirely clear about it, by maybe this licensing procedure should be evaluated more completely. I don't know, Dr. Ross, whether you care to comment on what I just said.

J. F. ROSS: I should like to ask if the privilege of the floor might be given to Mr. Christenson, who is a specialist in these things and knows all about licensing. Mr. Christenson is the president of a company that employed the 32-year-duration employee, who got sick and made the mistake. Could you comment about the licensing about California radiographers?

W. A. CHRISTENSON: The licensing in California is conducted by the state as authorized by NRC. The state carries it to the point where a company such as mine has to appoint a radiation safety officer who is approved by the state in conjunction with his documentation that is presented. This documentation outlines the company's and the radiation safety officer's total program for the handling of radioisotopes. All of the reporting to the state is done by the radiation safety officer. All of the communications from the state to our company are addressed to our radiation safety officer. We are surveyed annually by the state health department, radiation division. They come in and survey all the records, occasionally go out in the field to check the various companies, and submit again to the radiation safety officer. I see one of these men once a year for 2 minutes, telling me that everything is fine.

E. L. SAENGER: Thank you Mr. Christenson. We appreciate your candor for discussing this very difficult question.

M. E. GAULDEN: I would just like to discuss the business of the industrial radiographers. The ones I've had the most experience with are the men who work in the oil fields, and I think we have to take more into consideration than just the courses. Let me give you an example. The last patient I discussed with you, the oil field worker with the very high frequency of dicentrics, gave the safety board lots of trouble, because they apparently could not impress him with the dangers of radiation. He was not impressed with it until he was informed that he was sterile. One of the things that has to be taken into account by the NRC is not only training programs but the psychology of the men that are dealing with these things. These men have great machismo; anything they can't see, feel, taste, or hear they just cannot conceive of doing them any harm. So I think that aspect really has to be taken into account, because with these men it goes in one ear and out the other.

E. L. SAENGER: Thank you Dr. Gaulden. I think that is a very pertinent remark, having dealt with some of these folks.

R. PARKER: I'd like to make a comment on this. I can see it from two vantage points. One is as a previous director of a state registrar program of the state of Louisiana in the period of its conception, in 1964, until 1971, and more recently as a consultant health physicist on both the medical and industrial side. I am surprised at how people are viewing the recent radiography exposures. I can personally attest that there have been numerous exposures; in fact, I can add to the number of cases that have been reported, but apparently were not that well known in the 50s and 60s. There were numerous case studies. At the same time I would like to point out that we proposed to NRC, in 1969-1970, the necessity to place some additional responsibility on the individual industrial radiographer. The present registrar system places all the responsibility on a radiography company, and, if something goes wrong, the company takes the blame. The only thing the company can do is to fire that individual or take disciplinary action. The employment market is so strong for the individual radiographer that he can leave that company and walk down the street to another job. The radiography agencies cannot take any disciplinary actions against a single individual, and until this registrar policy is changed I think there will continue to be trouble.

SECTION III:

Radiation Accidents:
The Medical Response
to Acute Radiation Exposure

Introductory Remarks:
The Importance of the Initial Response

Thomas A. Lincoln

Corporate Medical Director, Union Carbide Corporation, New York, New York.

The speakers in this session on medical response will discuss preparedness for a radiation accident and the diagnostic and therapeutic management of patients who have been overexposed. Two other related items of secondary interest need to be discussed briefly. They are the delay in initiating appropriate care and the general state of ignorance about the management of radiation injuries of most practitioners.

An example of what can happen occurred recently and has been or will be reported in greater detail by others at this meeting. A worker was exposed to a high level of gamma radiation in an irradiator. The potential seriousness of the exposure was not appreciated by the worker's supervisor who only advised him to go to the emergency room at the local hospital if he developed any symptoms. Several hours after his exposure, he developed nausea and vomiting and, as instructed, went to the emergency room. He told his story to the physician who ignored it and diagnosed an acute gastroenteritis and sent the patient home with some antinausea medication. No calls to the plant were made. No blood counts were obtained. Later that night, because his symptoms worsened, the workman returned to the same hospital emergency room where he was seen by a different physician. As before, he told the same story and was given essentially the same treatment. Adequate care was not begun for many hours after the exposure.

Thus, twice in one 24-hr period, emergency room physicians did not believe the history a patient gave, ignored the classical signs of the acute radiation syndrome, and failed to get a blood count which could have been of great value in estimating the seriousness of the exposure.

Providing an adequate medical response to a patient who has been potentially overexposed to radiation is difficult. Too few physicians have had any experience, and therefore the number that have been personally challenged is small. They have had almost no stimuli to learn about diagnostic techniques or to become skilled in treatment. As a consequence, when a potential overexposure occurs, several hours and even several days may pass before adequate care is initiated. Many of our colleagues in clinical medicine apparently believe that there is no sense of urgency.

The first physician who sees a patient who has been in a radiation accident plays a crucial role. He or she should see to it that responsible people at the scene of the accident obtain all the information possible about the details of the potential overexposure. Accidents often occur late on Friday afternoons or on days before a holiday. Plant personnel who could contribute valuable information about the details of an accident may leave town at the start of a holiday weekend or go off on shopping trips as soon as the plant shuts down. Precious time may thus be lost before proper care is begun, because the individual who potentially has been exposed frequently does not know precisely what happened to him and is not familiar with the technical details, which often can only be obtained from supervisors. The people who have this information must be alerted quickly and their locations and phone numbers for the next several days must be recorded. They must remain available to provide additional information. The primary physician probably will not know what questions to ask until he has established contact with an expert consultant.

Reconstructing the precise chain of events in an accident is frequently difficult even when an investigation is begun immediately. Estimates of the amount of time a person was in a specific location need to be made by all observers, including the patient. Making these estimates 24–48 hr later is less than adequate. Memories are short!

The immediate collection of important biological specimens after an accident can be of considerable importance. Efforts should be made to obtain a urine specimen which reflects the existing body burden before the accident and before excretion of the new contaminant has begun. Getting a prompt blood count to establish a base line can be of great value.

When internal contamination with radionuclides has occurred, the rapid use of blocking agents, displacement therapy, isotopic dilution, and chelating agents may reduce the uptake of the radionuclide into tissues; once uptake has occurred, it may be extremely difficult to remove the contaminant.[1]

Efforts to inform the primary physician-contact of his (or her) responsibilities have been less than successful. Very few radiation accidents occur, and, as a result, many physicians fail to acquire experience. Postgraduate continuing education is valuable, but few emergency room physicians have much interest. They believe that their skills are needed to handle more common problems. Committee 37 of the National Council of Radiation Protection and Measurements is preparing a report on the "Management of Persons Contaminated with Radionuclides,"[2] which should be an essential reference in every hospital emergency room. The International Atomic Energy Agency has published a *Manual on Early Medical Treatment of Possible Radiation Injury* in its safety series.[3] This report also should be in every emergency room.

The physicians who are attending this meeting are the consultants who will provide the expert advice or definitive care. They are here to sharpen their skills. That is excellent, but let us not forget the need to alert and train more physicians who will provide the initial care. We have a missionary responsibility which I feel we have neglected. When you go home, share what you learn today with your colleagues. The general and emergency room physicians need to be better informed. Remember that, in order for you to be of maximum effectiveness when you are called in consultation, your colleague who refers his case to you must have done his initial care correctly.

References

1. Lincoln TA: Importance of initial management of persons internally contaminated with radionuclides. *Journal of the American Industrial Hygiene Association,* 37:16–21, 1976.
2. "Management of Persons Contaminated with Radionuclides." Committee 37. Bethesda, Md., National Council of Radiation Protection and Measurements, in press.
3. Nenot JC, Lushbaugh CC, Lincoln TA: *Manual on Early Medical Treatment of Possible Radiation Injury.* Safety Series No. 47. Vienna, International Atomic Energy Agency, 1978 (available in the United States at UNIPUB, 345 Park Avenue South, New York, N.Y. 10010).

Published 1980 by Elsevier North Holland, Inc.
K. F. Hübner and S. A. Fry, eds. The Medical Basis for Radiation Accident Preparedness

REAC/TS:
Its Role as a Specialty Referral Center and Training Site

Robert C. Ricks

Oak Ridge Associated Universities, Medical and Health Sciences Division, Oak Ridge, Tennessee.

Shortly after its completion in 1976, REAC/TS, the Radiation Emergency Assistance Center and Training Site, and its operational philosophies were described in a paper by Lushbaugh et al.[1] In the 40 months of operation since then, REAC/TS and its programs for radiation-accident response, radiation-accident management training courses, accident registries, cytogenetic dosimetry, and diethylenetriaminepentaacetic acid (DTPA) distribution and therapy has established itself as an internationally recognized center for all phases of radiation-accident management. In this paper I examine the current role REAC/TS plays in emergency medical response to radiation accidents and summarize training activities conducted within the facility. Other aspects of the REAC/TS program, emphasizing the registries and cytogenetic dosimetry, will be presented elsewhere in this symposium (see papers by Fry and Littlefield).

The Specialty Referral Center Concept

Modern, state-of-the-art emergency medical response at times requires personnel and services unavailable at many community hospitals and major medical centers. Such services are well-defined, mandating the need for highly specialized equipment and a staff trained in all aspects of their respective emergency or intensive care service. This specialization has led to the establishment of referral centers which provide these unique services. The specialty referral center concept is illustrated in Figure 1. In the majority of situations, a specialty referral center is physically attached to a local hospital, thereby facilitating easy transfer

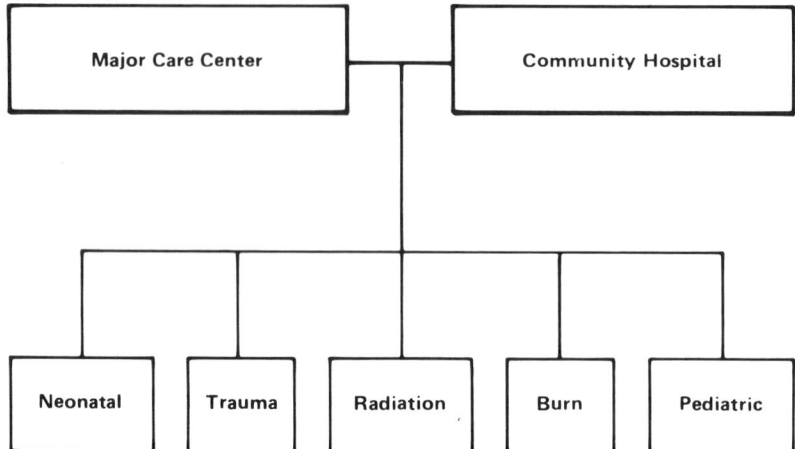

Figure 1. Block diagram illustrating the specialty referral center concept and the interrelationship between these centers and conventional hospitals.

of patients. REAC/TS, located within the Oak Ridge Hospital of the Methodist Church in Oak Ridge, Tennessee, is a leading specialty referral center in the United States for the treatment of radiation-accident victims. However, REAC/TS is only one of several such centers strategically located within the continental United States. Others include the Hanford Environmental Health Foundation, Richland, Washington, and the E. I. du Pont Savannah River Plant at Aiken, South Carolina. In addition, there are several major medical centers that have been identified for their expertise in radiation-accident management. Although these specialty referral centers for radiation-accident victims exist, the great majority of radiation accidents involving personnel injury or contamination do not require the use of such facilities. Generally speaking, most radiation-accident victims can be adequately cared for at the local hospital if the staff has received sufficient training in radiation-accident management. Opportunities for such training will be reviewed later in this paper.

Since specialty referral centers for radiation are limited in number, those existing have gradually assumed regional response roles. Although REAC/TS will accept patients from areas remote from Oak Ridge, the facility serves primarily the local and southeastern United States. In this respect, REAC/TS provides medical backup for radiation-accident management to the three local Union Carbide Nuclear sites and their combined 15,000 atomic workers in Oak Ridge, as well as a variety of nuclear facilities in the Southeast. This backup support is arranged through letters of agreement between the Department of Energy (DOE),

Oak Ridge Operations (ORO), and the requester. Figure 2 summarizes the agreements for medical support currently in existence. The non-DOE contractors constitute the largest group and are primarily nuclear power-generating stations in the Southeast. Inquiries pertaining to these agreements should be directed to the Energy Programs and Support Division, Department of Energy, Oak Ridge Operations, Federal Office Building, Oak Ridge, Tennessee 37830.

REAC/TS Emergency Response Concept

The operation of REAC/TS is comparable to that of any other emergency response facility. A radiation-accident response team with adequate backup support is on 24-hr callout duty. The facility is staffed Monday through Friday, 8:00 A.M. to 4:30 P.M., and there are two remote beepers (operating through the Oak Ridge Hospital switchboard) for afterhours, weekends, or holiday contact.

As with any emergency response group, REAC/TS maintains the necessary staffing required to receive, survey, and treat radiation-accident victims. The staff consists of physicians, nurses, health physicists, research scientists, an emergency coordinator, and ancillary support groups. A written plan for response action organizes these personnel into well-defined subgroups, each with specific assignments. The radiation emergency response team concept for REAC/TS is illustrated in Figure 3. During emergency response status, approximately 24 persons provide in-house support to the medical director. The response team can be expanded to about 50 persons when support personnel from the Oak Ridge Hospital, Union Carbide Medical Health Division teams, and DOE-ORO are requested. The Oak Ridge Associated Universities (ORAU) support groups from central supply, technical maintenance, and administration provide added assistance as needed.

Figure 2. Summary of assistance agreements establishing REAC/TS as a medical backup facility for radiation-accident management; DOD, Department of Defense; TVA, Tennessee Valley Authority.

Categorical Listing	Number
Oak Ridge Associated Universities	8
DOE Contractors	7
Non–DOE Contractors	26
U.S. Navy Submarine Program	3
U.S. Reactor Power Program (TVA)	2
U.S. DOE/DOD Groups	3
Total	49

REAC/TS RADIATION EMERGENCY RESPONSE TEAM CONCEPT

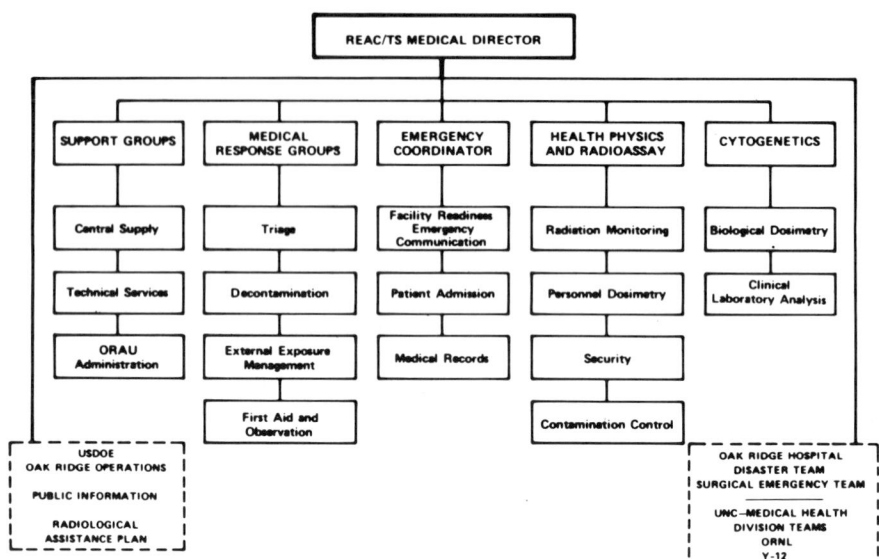

Figure 3. Block diagram illustrating the organization of the REAC/TS emergency response team for radiation-accident management; ORNL, Oak Ridge National Laboratory; UNC, University of North Carolina.

Each aspect of emergency response to radiation accidents is practiced through regularly scheduled drills. These drills, designed to convey as much realism as possible, assist each individual of the staff to identify his role and to determine how it interrelates with the roles of others during actual radiation-accident response configurations. Drills are designed to involve ancillary support groups, particularly the Oak Ridge Hospital surgery department that provides all emergency surgical support to REAC/TS.

REAC/TS Training for Radiation-Accident Management

Another vitally important mission of the REAC/TS program is to disseminate information and current methodology for the medical management of radiation accidents to medical response groups remote to the Oak Ridge area. This training is vitally important to meet the needs of potential radiation-accident victims, even though such accidents are quite limited in number. The primary mechanism for disseminating this information is through training courses for medical, paramedical support, and health physics personnel. Indeed, the REAC/TS training program constitutes one of the most unique features of the overall program.

Three different training activities are scheduled each fiscal year. The first course, *Medical Planning and Care in Radiation Accidents,* is designed for physicians who provide medical services to the nuclear industry, as well as city, county, and state health officers, who may be called upon to provide first aid or medical care in the event of a radiation accident. The curriculum includes fundamentals of radiation and radiobiology, radiation detection and measurement, care of radioactively contaminated injuries, evaluation and treatment of internal radioactive contamination, and the acute radiation syndromes. Included are demonstrations of equipment and facilities used to evaluate and treat radiation injuries. The course is of 5 days duration and is acceptable for credit in category 1 of the Physician's Recognition Award by the American Medical Association. A second course, *Health Physics in Radiation Accidents,* is also of 5 days duration and is designed for health physicists who may be called upon to respond to accidents involving radioactive materials and personnel injury. The major topics covered are a review of radiation physics, principles of radiation detection and internal dosimetry, protective clothing and equipment, radiological emergency procedures, and the role of the health physicist in a medical environment. Lectures are complemented by demonstrations, laboratory exercises, and a simulated radiation accident drill. This course is approved by the American Board of Health Physics for continuing education units and recertification of health physics personnel. A third course, *Handling of Radiation Accidents by Emergency Personnel,* is of 2.5 days duration and is approved by the American College of Emergency Physicians and the Tennessee Nurses Association for continuing education credit. The course is designed primarily for emergency room physicians and nurses who may be called upon to administer initial hospital aid to a radiation-accident victim. The course emphasizes the practical aspects of handling a contaminated victim and deals with the fundamentals of radiation, how to detect and measure it, how to prevent the spread of contamination, how to reduce the radiation dose to the victim and attending personnel, and how the medical physicist treats contaminated accident victims. Lectures are complemented by demonstrations, laboratory exercises, and a simulated accient drill.

In each of these three training endeavors, participation is limited, thereby providing for optimum student–faculty ratios and the opportunity for everyone to participate in laboratory and drill activities. The teaching faculty serving these training courses includes both REAC/TS personnel and nationally recognized experts in radiation-accident management, many of whom are participating in this symposium. By background

REAC/TS Training Activities
November, 1976–September, 1979

Course Title	No. of Courses	No. of Persons Trained							
		MD	PhD	Nurse	Adm.	EMT	HP	Other	Total
Medical Planning and Care in Radiation Accidents	6	110	4	8	1	––	––	3	126
Health Physics in Radiation Accidents	4	––	8	––	––	––	70	––	78
Handling of Radiation Accidents by Emergency Personnel	8	36	––	66	15	13	2	24	156
Sum Totals	18	146	12	74	16	13	72	27	360*

*Includes 14 Foreign Nationals From Taiwan, Sweden, Mexico, Canada, and Brazil.

Figure 4. Summary of REAC/TS training course activities covering the period of facility operation from its beginning in 1976 to the end of fiscal year 1979; EMT, emergency medical technologists [treatment (military)]; HP, health physicists.

training, the faculty includes M.D.'s, Ph.D.'s, certified health physicists, registered nurses, licensed practical nurses, as well as other professional biologists, chemists, and physics personnel.

Laboratory exercises and accident drills are designed to provide meaningful, realistic information and the opportunity to practice techniques for emergency response to radiation accidents. Course participants complete written examinations and critique forms at the close of each respective course. Critique summaries and test scores are mailed to respective course participants and are used to evaluate and update training activities. Also, a semiannual newsletter published by REAC/TS is mailed to all former course participants. The REAC/TS training course activities are summarized in Figure 4.

References

1. Lushbaugh CC, Andrews, GA, Hübner KF, Cloutier RJ, Beck WL, Berger JD: REAC/TS: A pragmatic approach for providing medical care and physician education for radiation emergencies, in *Diagnosis and Treatment of Incorporated Radionuclides* (Proceedings of the International Atomic Energy Agency–World Health Organization Seminar, Vienna, 1975). Vienna, International Atomic Energy Agency, 1976, p. 565.

Medical Management of Accidental Total-body Irradiation

Gould A. Andrews

Division of Nuclear Medicine, University of Maryland Hospital, Baltimore, Maryland.

Proper care can undoubtedly make the difference between death and survival for a significant group of patients who have received high dose total-body exposures in radiation accidents. This statement is based upon a small experience; accidents have not been many, and most of them have involved doses of radiation too low to be life-threatening,[1,2] but the effectiveness of therapy has been well demonstrated in marrow depression of other causes. This discussion will be based mainly on exposures that occur rapidly—in less than an hour—and it will deal with the management during the first six weeks or so; this is the period that is crucial in determining the outcome. (The effects that may be manifested years later—an increased incidence of leukemia and cancer—are presented elsewhere in this symposium.) Persons subjected to protracted exposure over a period of days or weeks constitute a special group and will be discussed briefly. Similarly, brief consideration will be given to another special group—those who have a very high-dose injury to a local area of the body along with significant whole-body exposure.

The assumption is that accidents involve small numbers of persons, under conditions of adequate availability of medical care. If exposures of large numbers occur, and medical resources are limited, it will be necessary, obviously, to provide a hasty diagnostic assessment and to channel therapeutic resources to the group for which treatment is likely to determine survival, with lower priorities for the minimally or moderately exposed and for the presumably hopeless.

Patterns of Injury

The degree of injury is generally proportional to radiation dose. Contrary to statements sometimes made, we do not find any remarkable variability in the response of different persons to a given dose and only a moderate degree of biological variation, except for rare instances of hypersensitivity associated with preexisting disease.

A set of total-body radiation syndromes has been described for man, relating symptoms, laboratory changes, and outcome to the severity of injury. There has been very little human experience with the effects of high-radiation doses, except in Japan where the data are incomplete and complicated by combined injury effects. Thus some of these human syndrome descriptions are based on inadequate data, or are partially extrapolated from results in experimental animals. We can, however, make plans on the basis of this incomplete information, while hoping that we will never have better.

Subclinical injury requires little description. A known history of exposure can be based on radiation monitors and demonstrated levels of exposure in the environment. Sensitive laboratory changes consist of small numbers of chromosome changes, which are expensive to demonstrate because of the large number of cells that must be analyzed. A delayed fall in sperm count may also show quite low doses. Less sensitive and less specific is the slight decrease in absolute lymphocyte count. In all of these tests sequential values from serial tests are likely to improve sensitivity, and in all, the possible effects of factors other than radiation cause difficulties in interpretation.

The *hematopoietic syndrome* is represented by fairly plentiful data in man. It consists of alterations in hematopoiesis due to damage of stem cells in marrow and lymphatic tissue. The changes may vary from mild to lethal. A decrease in lymphocytes occurs promptly, most of it taking place within 24 hr after exposure (Figure 1). The level of this early lymphopenia is one of the best indicators of severity of radiation injury. The level of neutrophil granulocytes shows a very early rise, usually limited to the first 48 hr or less; the degree of its elevation has not been correlated with the extent of injury (Figure 2). (In the neurovascular syndrome, granulocytosis is very pronounced and persists until death.) In the dose range that produces the hematopoietic syndrome, after the early rise, granulocyte numbers fall to fairly low levels at about day 10, and there is then a transient, abortive rise at around day 15, perhaps due to mitoses of a genetically damaged population that cannot continue to reproduce. (The absence of an abortive rise is an unfavorable sign.) Then a steady fall in granulocyte count begins, with the nadir at about day 30 after exposure. If the patient survives, this is followed by spontaneous

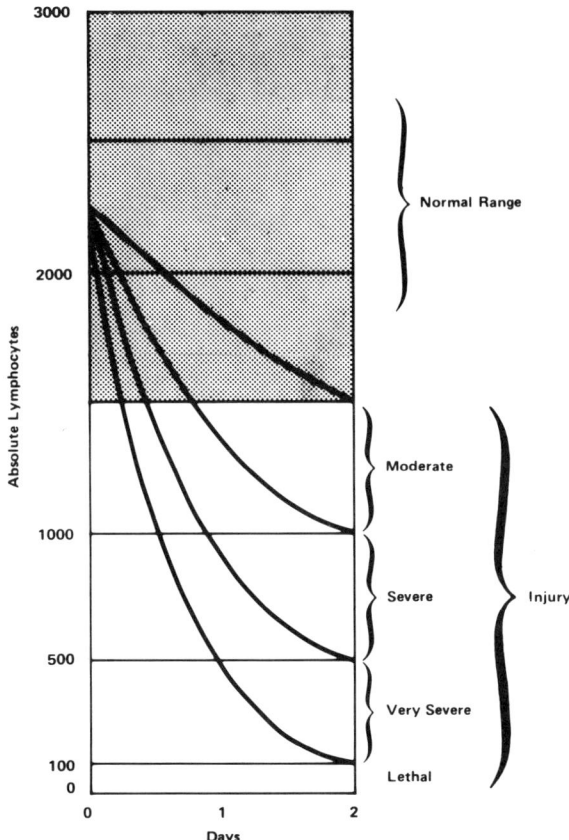

Figure 1. Patterns of early lymphocyte response in relation to dose.

recovery, beginning in the fifth week. The platelets may show a rise in the first 2 or 3 days after exposure, then a gradually accelerating decrease with the nadir also reached at about day 30. During recovery the platelets are likely to bounce up well above normal levels.

There are several remarkable aspects to this series of blood changes (Figure 2). One is the pronounced delay in reaching the nadir in granulocytes and platelets. This cannot be accounted for entirely on the basis of the time periods involved in normal blood cell kinetics; much more rapid patterns are seen with some marrow-damaging cancer-chemotherapeutic agents. The radiation changes do appear to be at least indirectly related to normal intervals of cell dynamics, however, and occur much more rapidly in small experimental animals than in man. The time

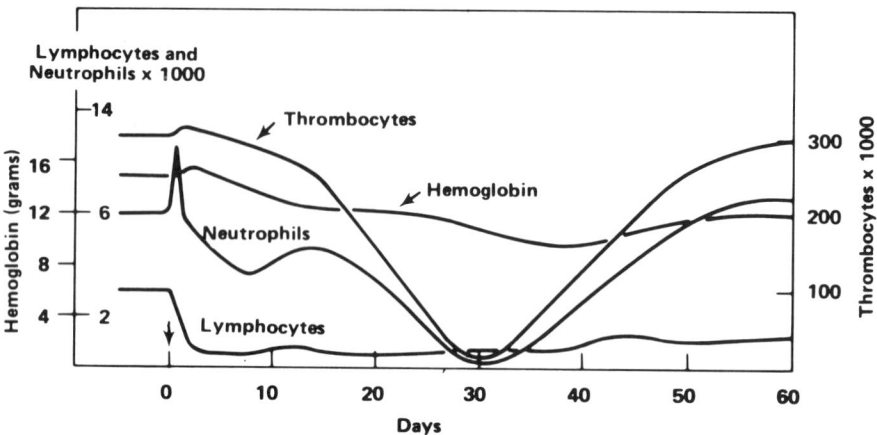

Figure 2. Typical chart of blood values in fairly severe hematopoietic syndrome.

sequence is not altered in relation to radiation dose as much as might be expected. With exposure levels causing a severe hematopoietic syndrome, the onset of pronounced granulocyte and platelet depression is earlier, but the time of recovery is only slightly delayed.

The so-called *gastrointestinal syndrome* is not well documented in man. It has been believed to result mainly from radiation inhibition of mitosis of the cells in the crypts of the intestine, with electrolyte loss from the mucosa, and extensive bacterial invasion there. Clinically it is characterized by severe, persistent nausea, vomiting, and diarrhea, in addition to manifestations of a very profound hematopoietic syndrome. Death is estimated to occur during the second week after exposure. However, studies of total-body radiation given clinically to facilitate marrow grafts (at dose rates below those likely to occur in accidents) suggest that in man quite high doses can be given without producing this syndrome.[3]

The *neurovascular syndrome* occurs when extremely large doses of total-body irradiation are received, and it has been seen in two persons accidentally irradiated. It is characterized by pronounced neurological disturbances, after an early interval of mental alertness. Intractable hypotension is a prominent feature and may be the major basis for the neurological changes rather than direct radiation damage to the brain as was earlier proposed.[4] There is early onset of severe nausea, vomiting, and bloody diarrhea. Lymphocytes fall promptly to near-zero levels, and pronounced leukocytosis develops early and persists until death at perhaps 2 to 5 days after exposure.

Classification of Cases

The severity of total body injury and the radiation dose may be estimated from the following[5,6] information:

1. Clinical responses.
2. Laboratory values, mainly hematologic and cytogenetic.
3. Data from film badges and monitors.
4. Estimation of source size, location of patient during exposure, and duration of exposure. A mock-up of the accident with a dosimeter-bearing human phantom may prove useful.
5. For those accidents in which the radiation source includes a neutron component it is useful to establish a neutron-gamma ratio, if possible, and to measure induced radioactivity by performing radioassays on:
   a. Blood samples (along with chemical determination of blood sodium concentration), so that an activation value may be obtained for sodium 24. It is important to recognize that during the very early hours after exposure one may also detect significant amounts of chlorine 38, half-life 37 min.
   b. Whole body. Again, mainly for sodium 24, and possibly chlorine 38. There may also be radioactivity induced in metals, especially gold, present as a result of dental work.
   c. Hair and nails, in which stable sulfur is activated to ^{32}P.
   d. Jewelry, coins, metal rims of glasses, wrist watches, buttons, and other metal in clothing, in which activation of metals may be measured. It is necessary to record the exact location of these articles on the body of the patient so that dose distribution may be obtained. (It is of course necessary to distinguish between induced activity and contamination. The obvious differences are that external contamination is always uneven and much of it can be removed with the clothing. Internal contamination may not be so easily distinguished, but it can be identified on the basis of body distribution, blood radioactivity measurements, excretion, and, if necessary, determination of energies and half-lives.)

For the estimation of the severity of injury and the planning of therapy, clinical and biological indicators are more important than dosage measurements. The physical dosimetry for most accidents is less than optimal, even with the best of efforts, particularly because it is impossible to estimate the duration of exposure with reasonable accuracy.

The presence or lack of nausea and vomiting tends to separate the exposed into high-dose (possibly fatal) and low-dose (probably nonfatal) categories. Psychogenic vomiting has not proved to be a common occurrence in unexposed persons frightened by their proximity to an accident. The vomiting due to radiation exposure is likely to begin between 20 min and 3 hr after exposure, and early onset suggests a high radiation dose. Individual episodes of vomiting may come on suddenly without preceding nausea. Diarrhea is a less useful symptom in indicating degree of injury and is probably more likely than vomiting to be caused by emotional responses; however, very prompt and explosive diarrhea, especially if bloody, is likely to indicate a fatal dose.

Redness of the conjunctivae may appear fairly promptly after a dose of 150 rad or more, and redness of the skin is likely to appear within a few hours after doses of 500 rad or more, but both of these manifestations have highly variable thresholds. If caused by radiation of relatively low energy they may seem more ominous than they really are, since they may be present with a realtively low dose to the bone marrow and other internal organs.

Laboratory values are of great usefulness. Early lymphocyte changes at various levels of damage are shown in Figure 1, and a typical example of a quite severe hematopoietic syndrome in Figure 2. The lymphocyte decrease is the best early indicator of degree of injury, and the levels of granulocytes and platelets, which are most clearly correlated with clinical infection and hemorrhage, are the most important guides for later therapeutic needs.

Epilation is a relatively late clinical effect, usually beginning on day 17 to 20; any considerable loss of hair usually means a dose of 200 rad or more. Because it occurs so late this manifestation is of little value as a clinical indicator.

Considerations in Treatment

An obvious general medical banality is the statement that the treatment should be suited to the needs of the individual patient, but in the field of radiation accidents this platitude is worth emphasizing, because in some accidents the exposed patients, with varying levels of exposure, have been considered as a group and treated somewhat similarly.

Several factors contribute to pronounced apprehension in accident victims, including the general public's alarm about radiation injury, and the multiple consultants and questioners that always converge. There is also the isolation, some of it resulting from appropriate or inappropriate concern about the hazards to others from radiation in or on the patient's body, and some of it due to later protective measures against infection. For the patient with a life-threatening exposure, the best management of these problems is the assignment of one sympathetic physician to be in charge. This physician's role should be clearly established with the patient and with all other persons involved; he or she should be present when the patient is questioned by anyone concerned with the accident and should be empowered to exclude or eject questioners who might be harmful.

Whatever the level of exposure, there are no known early measures that can be taken to reduce the late effects on the incidence of leukemia and cancer. This hazard should be discussed frankly with the patient and put in perspective. For example, if we use the data summarized by McLean,[7] indicating that 1 rad of radiation to a million people would produce 125 of these diseases, and if we use a linear extrapolation to a much higher dose in a single person, we arrive at figures like these: 100 rad will produce a 1.25% increased likelihood, and 500 rad, 6.25%. This can be compared with the normal incidence in the non-irradiated of something in the neighborbood of 15 to 20%. Furthermore the physician can discuss measures for reducing the risk of cancer by avoidance of smoking and other carcinogens, and for reducing mortality by early diagnosis. For accident victims who wish to have children later, the possibility of hereditary effects should be discussed. The data from the atom bomb victims in Japan give considerable reassurance on this score, and it appears that no radiation accident victim should fear later parenthood, although it is prudent, on the basis of animal data, to suggest that a period of at least several months should elapse after the accident before this project is undertaken.

Persons exposed at low, nonthreatening levels mainly need reassurance. Some laboratory follow-up such as weekly blood counts for 5 weeks may be justified to document the absence of significant injury. Continued work activity as close as possible to the normal routine is probably desirable in most instances; such activity may tend to minimize psychic stress.

Patients with clearly fatal exposures need, of course, comfort-giving measures, close attention (not avoidance) by the physician, and the amount of information that they want and are able to handle.

Since very few accident victims have received unquestionably fatal radiation doses, the major management concern is with the intermediate group, and especially with those whose injury would be fatal if not effectively treated.

A helpful guide is to plot the daily level of lymphocytes, granulocytes, and platelets, and to make similar plots, on the same scale, from published reports of other accident patients exposed in the same general dose range. Thus the individual patient can be compared with his peers and any deviation from the early estimate of level of injury becomes apparent. This is not meant to imply that hematologic values are the only thing to consider, but they are important.

The problem, simply defined, is to keep the patient alive for about five weeks, when marrow recovery will have begun. Total destruction of hematopoietic stem cells from acute radiation injury would probably require an extremely large radiation dose, such that damage to other tissues would also be in the lethal range. Death with severe pancytopenia, occurring three to five weeks after exposure, does not mean that all stem cells are lost; it means that the patient could not be kept alive long enough for recovery to take place.

Unlike the contaminated patient, the one with total-body radiation injury does not present an urgent requirement for emergency therapy; time is available to decide where the best management can be provided. Since the main treatable manifestation is bone marrow injury, the ideal spot for treatment is an institution set up to deal with this problem. Such facilities are usually located at active hematology centers and institutions specializing in cancer. Here, patients with similar problems of pancytopenia are commonly treated: patients with marrow failure, patients with leukemia or lymphoma who have almost complete destruction of marrow function due to their disease, and patients who because of extensive chemotherapy and radiation treatment may present a similar picture. A valuable source of data are patients given intentional total-body irradiation and marrow transplantation as treatment for leukemia or aplastic anemia. It is fortunate that much active work is going on with these problems, work that can be applied to the rare radiation accident patients who need such care. The accidentally irradiated patient can probably be handled best by a collaboration involving physicians active in this type of work and physicians experienced in radiation accidents.

The two prominent mechanisms of death after acute radiation exposure are infection and hemorrhage, with the former a more formidable problem than the latter. The two tend to develop simultaneously and to be synergistically and rapidly progressive. For example, areas of hemorrhage in the lungs provide foci favorable to bacterial growth, while infectious lesions of the intestinal wall may precipitate bleeding there.

The experience in dealing with patients suffering from accidental total-body irradiation is limited and needs to be supplemented with information from the related types of clinical experience listed above, and, to some extent, with information from experiments in animals. When treating patients with severe pancytopenia the clinician must be prepared for a sudden unfavorable turn of events, with very rapid clinical deterioration, particularly as may happen in septicemia due to Gram-negative organisms. It is also important to keep in mind that special conditions may apply—for example, the ineffectuality of some antibiotics in the absence of adequate numbers of granulocytes.

While it is useful to derive information from patients with cancer and hematologic disorders, we should also emphasize the ways in which radiation accident patients differ from them. The accident patient starts out with a healthy marrow and needs only to be kept alive for five weeks. Much is at stake since he will be virtually normal if he survives. Second, the accidentally irradiated patient usually has normal bacterial flora at the outset, not influenced by previous stays in a hospital environment; thus he is less likely to harbor drug-resistant strains of bacteria. Third, the accident victim usually begins with good general health and nutrition, little likelihood of previous sensitization to antibiotics, and no previous therapy with adrenal cortical steroids. Fourth, the person exposed in a radiation accident is unlikely to have radiation-induced fever beginning days or weeks after exposure, and any fever that occurs is probably indicative of infection (although possible drug reaction may be a consideration). This is unlike the situation in the leukemia or cancer patient who may have fever due to the underlying disease.

Bone Marrow Transplantation

With the present state of knowledge, there is no adequate basis for stating the proper use of homologous marrow grafts in radiation accidents. The potential for benefit was well demonstrated in the Pittsburgh accident patient who happened to have an identical twin donor.[8] This rare event, with almost zero probability of recurrence, was useful in showing that the injection of healthy stem cells works in man as expected from animal studies, and that the lesion is not elsewhere—in the marrow stroma, for example. The only other clinical experience known was in the Yugoslav accident, in which the marrow was probably given too late to be of benefit but was, at least, apparently not harmful.[9] The possible availability of stored autologous marrow previously obtained from the accident victim has been extensively considered but has important limitations as a practical method of dealing with the problem of radiation accidents.[10]

Transplantation from a homologous donor carries the risk of serious graft-versus-host reaction. Furthermore, grafts require 10 to 14 days for the injected cells to give rise to enough progeny to help the patient. Thus the attempted transplantation would need to be done early, not more than a week after exposure, to be useful. The delayed benefit from marrow is in contrast to the immediate results that can be obtained from donor granulocytes and platelets given when they are required. As has been previously implied, it appears unlikely that a graft would rescue a patient with zero living stem cells, and the benefit of the procedure would probably be as a more effective means of tiding the patient over the temporary period of pancytopenia.

In our present state of knowledge it appears that a trial of early marrow graft might be wise for a person who has a well-matched donor and who is believed to have received an otherwise almost certainly lethal exposure. It would not appear appropriate to add early immunosuppressive measures to the irradiation already received. If a graft-versus-host reaction later develops, it should probably be treated like those seen in hematologic disorders treated with grafts.

Infections and Hemorrhage

Multiple factors may contribute to the susceptibility to infection that occurs in the irradiated mammal, but the level of circulating granulocytes appears by far the most important, and the main hazard of infection occurs during the phase of most profound granulocytopenia. Bodey et al. have shown that in leukemic patients the rate of infection correlates extremely well with the severity of granulocytopenia.[11] Other factors, less well-defined in relation to infection, include lymphopenia and the radiation-induced suppression of immune responses.

There are special features of the infections that occur in patients with severe granulocytopenia and immunosuppression. Organisms normally nonpathogenic can cause fatalities. Infections tend to develop rapidly and may cause prompt death. Prominent organisms are *Pseudomonas aeruginosa* (often acquired in hospital environment), *Escherichia coli, Klebsiella-enterobacter* species, and *Staphylococcus aureus.* At the same time, there is a deficiency in the usual exudative responses to infection. Erythema may be lacking in involved skin and mucous membranes. Pneumonitis may occur with a normal chest X-ray, and meningitis without nuchal rigidity. Infections in these patients are difficult to treat and may be unresponsive, because of the lack of granulocytes or for other reasons, to the standard forms of therapy.

After exposure to total body irradiation there is a period during which granulocyte levels may be near normal. During this period it is desirable to culture mouth, nares, throat, sputum if obtainable, skin sites, vagina, urine, and feces; a search for infections around the teeth should be made. Techniques of culture should be very complete, to detect the unusual organisms that may be important. Any obvious pathogens should be treated with specific antibiotics at this early stage, during the first week after exposure.

The use of laminar flow sterile environment facilities has been the subject of extensive work, and their value has been clearly demonstrated.[12,13] They are especially appropriate for radiation accident victims, who usually need only a short but critical period of protection from infection. An ordinary hospital environment, because of the presence of antibiotic-resistant organisms, should be avoided. If the patient can be kept under reasonably clean conditions at home, it may be feasible to postpone the use of the laminar flow facility until marrow depression is fairly definite.

White cell and platelet transfusions may be of great supportive value during the period of marrow depressions.[14,15] Immediately after the incident the patient should have HLA typing of blood cells, and the family members who might be potential donors of granulocytes and platelets should also be typed, and arrangements should be made for their availability to serve as donors. It may be ideal to use a single, well-matched donor for repeated donations of white cells and platelets; this can involve significant stress to the donor. When to start platelet injections is a matter of clinical judgment; obvious clinical bleeding or a platelet count below 40,000/mm³ might be considered reasonable indications. The presence of infection is likely to increase the need for platelets.

A typical plan for treating a potentially lethal hematologic syndrome is suggested in Table 1. Adaptations would, of course, be made for particular circumstances. Improved methods of management will continue to become available as a result of studies on the other types of patients who need treatment for impaired bone marrow function. Better combinations of antibiotics and other therapeutic agents can be expected.

Supplemental support with immune globulin preparations is not well established but may be an area of significant future development.

Table 1. Suggested Plan for Control of Infection

Immediately after diagnosis of exposure to 100 rad or more:

Avoid hospitalizing patient except in sterile environment facility. Look for preexisting infections and obtain cultures of suspicious areas — consider especially carious teeth, gingivae, skin, and vagina. Culture a clean-caught urine specimen. Culture stool specimen for identification of all organisms; run appropriate sensitivity tests for *Staph. aureus* and Gram-negative rods. Treat any infection that is discovered. Start oral nystatin to reduce *Candida* organisms. Do HLA typing of patient's family, especially siblings, to select HLA-matched leukocyte and platelet donors for later need.

If granulocyte count falls to less than 1500/mm³:

Start oral antibiotics — vancomycin 500 mg liquid P.O. q. 4 hr, gentamycin 200 mg liquid P.O. q 4 hr, nystatin 1 x 10⁶ units liquid P.O. q. 4 hr, 4 x 10⁶ units as tablets P.O. q. 4 hr. Isolate patient in laminar flow room or life island. Daily antiseptic bath and shampoo with chlorhexidine gluconate. Trim finger and toenails carefully and scrub area daily. For female patients, daily Betadine douche and insert one nystatin vaginal tablet b.i.d. Culture nares, oropharynx, urine, stool, and skin of groins and axillae twice weekly. Culture blood if fever over 101 degrees F.

If granulocyte count falls to less than 750/mm³:

In the presence of fever (101° F) or other signs of infection give antibiotics while awaiting results of new cultures (especially blood cultures). The regimen suggested is ticarcillin 5 gm q. 6 hr I.V., gentamycin 1.25 mgm/kg q. 6 hr I.V. For severe infection not responding within 24 hrs, give supplemental white cells, and if platelet count is low give platelets from preselected matched donors. When cultures are reported, modify antibiotic regime appropriately. Watch for toxicity from antibiotics, and reduce medications as soon as practicable.

When granulocyte count rises to over 1000/mm³ and is clearly improving:

Discontinue isolation and antiseptic baths, antibiotics; continue nystatin for 3 additional days.

Protracted Exposure

In a few radiation accidents, especially with unidentified, unshielded industrial radiographic isotope sources, the exposure has extended over days or weeks. In these, the time for development of the manifestations of injury is somewhat prolonged and recovery is greatly delayed; while a significantly greater radiation dose can be tolerated, once there is obvious evidence of damage, the prognosis for good recovery is much poorer than with the acute doses. The same general types of therapy already discussed may be adapted to the needs of these patients, but the results are likely to be less successful and the complications of therapy more serious. Marrow transplantation is not likely to be helpful.

In the patient who also has total-body irradiation injury, local areas of unusually high-dose exposure obviously present special sites for possible hemorrhage, necrosis, and entry of bacteria. When the local area is on an extremity, amputation may eventually be required, and there is a need for better methods of determining the ultimate extent of amputation, so that protracted series of operations can be avoided.[16] When the area of local injury is on the torso, extensive skin grafts may be needed. Obviously, severe pancytopenia would be very undesirable at the time of any major surgical procedure. After acute radiation injury the surgery can usually be delayed until hematopoietic recovery is under way. However, when the exposure, and therefore the marrow depression, are protracted, as has happened with the accidents involving industrial sources, an extremely difficult situation is presented and surgery may need to be done under adverse circumstances, with the support of antibiotics, donor leukocytes, and platelets.

Recovery Phase

In patients with acute total-body exposure the recovery of granulocyte and platelet levels is quite rapid after the fifth week. Persistent fatigue may be out of proportion to any organic findings and not clearly related to anxiety and psychological stress. Common sense suggests that the patient should be encouraged to return to normal life activities and work habits as rapidly as he can comfortably do so, with frequent supportive interviews by the physician.

Future work with radiation, if desired by the patient, should not be automatically precluded. The occurrence of another serious accident is obviously exceedingly unlikely, and if a repeated exposure does take place the threshold for early morbidity or mortality is not likely to be greatly altered, although the chances of delayed effects would, of course, be further increased approximately in proportion to dose. Assuming no further accidents, the small, generally acceptable occupational exposure does not significantly change the outlook. These comments might not be applicable to the patient with prominent local radiation injury, for example, to the hands. In all cases, individual factors would be important, of course.

Therapy can be highly effective in the hematologic syndrome of total body radiation injury, even when the injury is very severe. Specialized resources are needed and are available at medical centers that treat patients with marrow depression of other etiologies.

ACKNOWLEDGMENTS
The author is indebted to Dr. C. Lowell Edwards of the Rockford School of Medicine, Rockford, Illinois, and to Dr. Stephen C. Schimpff of the Baltimore Cancer Research Center, for extensive assistance in the preparation of this paper.

References

1. Thoma, GE Jr., Wald N: The diagnosis and management of accidental radiation injury. *J Occup Med* 1:421–447, 1959.

2. Andrews GA, Balish E, Edwards CL, Kniseley RM, Lushbaugh CC: Possibilities for improved treatment of persons exposed in radiation accidents, in *Handling of Radiation Accidents*. Vienna, International Atomic Energy Agency, 1969, pp. 119–135.

3. Thomas ED, Storb R, Clift RA, Fefer A, Johnson FL, Neiman PE, Lerner KG, Glucksberg H, Buckner CD: Bone marrow transplantation. *N Eng J Med* 292:832–843, 895–902, 1975.

4. Fanger H, Lushbaugh CC: Radiation death from cardiovascular shock following a criticality accident. *Arch Path* 83:446–460, 1967.

5. *Personnel Dosimetry for Radiation Accidents*. Vienna, International Atomic Energy Agency, 1965.

6. *Assessment of Radioactive Contamination in Man*. Vienna, International Atomic Energy Agency, 1972.

7. McLean AS: Radiation accidents: Reflections and reminiscences, in *Handling of Radiation Accidents*. Vienna, International Atomic Energy Agency, 1977, pp. 3–17.

8. Thomas E, Donnall R, Robert H: Isogeneic marrow grafting in man. *Exp Hematol* 21:16–17, 1971.

9. Andrews GA: Criticality accidents in Vinca, Yugoslavia, and Oak Ridge, Tennessee. *JAMA* 179:191–197, 1962.

10. Nelson BM, Andrews GA: Autologous stem-cell banks for restoring hemopoiesis, in Lett JT, Adler H, (eds.): *Advances in Radiation Biology*. New York, Academic Press, 1976, pp. 325–338.

11. Bodey GP, Buckley M, Sathe YS, Freireich EJ: Quantitative relationship between circulating leukocytes and infections in patients with acute leukemia. *Ann Int Med* 64:328–340, 1966.

12. Buckner CD, Clift RA, Sanders JE, Meyers JD, Counts GW, Farewell VT, Thomas ED: Protective environment for marrow transplant recipients. *Ann Int Med* 89:893–901, 1978.

13. Schimpff SC: Infection prevention during granulocytopenia. *Curr Clin Topics Infec Dis:* in press.

14. Schimpff SC: Therapy of infection in patients with granulocytopenia. *Med Clin N Am* 61:1101–1118, 1977.

15. Schiffer CA: Principles of granulocyte transfusion therapy. *Med Clin N Am* 61:1119–1131, 1977.

16. Schenck RR, Gilberti MV: Four-extremity radiation necrosis. *Arch Surg* 100:729–734, 1970.

Published 1980 by Elsevier North Holland, Inc.
K. F. Hübner and S. A. Fry, eds. The Medical Basis for Radiation Accident Preparedness

Current Approaches to the Management of Internally Contaminated Persons

George L. Voelz

Los Alamos Scientific Laboratory, Los Alamos, New Mexico.

The use of radionuclides in industry, research, nuclear power, and medicine is increasing. As a result, there may also be increased possibility of human exposure to internal depositions of radionuclides. Preventative measures should continue to reduce the number of these exposures, but it is important that the physician-in-charge uses the available techniques and drugs to reduce these internal depositions. This paper summarizes important considerations in the management of these cases and outlines some available major therapeutic regimens.

Basis for Treatment

The need for treatment in an individual exposure case should be based on an understanding of the consequences or risk of late effects on the health of the individual. If discomfort, side effects, or risk accompany the therapy, it is especially important to understand the need and basis for treatment. Our understanding of the dose-effect relationship due to radiation is limited, especially at lower doses and at the dose rates often associated with internal despositions. I know of few data which demonstrate that current treatment regimens for internal radionuclides are effective in reducing health effects. The benefits of treatment are assumed to be present, based on a reduction in the amount of radionuclide present in an organ. The benefit of therapy is, therefore, understood no better than our imperfect understanding of radiation risk at low dose and dose rates. The basis for treatment is thus based on "as low as readily achievable" dose. On this basis, at some point therapy will yield a diminished return.

With proper application of currently available treatments, it is possible to reduce the internal dose by a factor of about 2 to 10 for some of the radionuclides. To be sure, the goal of reducing dose is a worthy objective. That health effects do result from radiations caused by internal radionuclides has been amply demonstrated in radium dial painters, uranium miners, thoratrast-injected persons, and the Marshallese Islanders exposed to radioactive iodine in fallout. In all these cases the exposures were orders of magnitude above those permitted by the regulatory guidelines applied to the radiation worker.

The value of treatment of cases with smaller exposures, for example, below the so-called permissible guidelines, is not known. Currently, the decision for treatment in such cases is based on the perception of risk by the physician responsible for the case and his patient. The physician must make a judgment concerning the ultimate benefit versus the potential harm or side effects of the therapy, a judgment common to all medical practice.

All treatments for internal radionuclides are most effective if applied within minutes to a few hours after exposure, a period when limited information upon which to base a treatment decision is available. The earliest information after the accident will consist perhaps of some scanty information on the accident, probable identification of the major radionuclides by history or early spectrometric data, a few radiological measurements (contamination surveys, air concentrations, and nasal smears), and no clinical symptoms or signs except possible trauma from an accident. The absence of clinical features places the physician at a great disadvantage in trying to determine the need for immediate treatment. Fortunately, the treatment procedures to be considered early have essentially no risk, and so errors of therapy omission are likely to be more serious than those of commission.

The cessation of treatment is another decision that is dependent on the experience and judgment of the physician-in-charge. This decision is based on the relative risks and effectiveness of the particular treatment. This question arises primarily in connection with possible continuing use of mobilizing or chelating agents. This decision is not as crucial as the decision to initiate treatment and can be made after due deliberation on the results and after consultation.

Therapeutic Treatments

For the past several years, Committee 37 of the National Council on Radiation Protection and Measurements (NCRP) has been studying the subject of the management of persons accidentally contaminated with radionuclides. The committee members include George L. Voelz, chairman; Thomas A. Lincoln; Herta Spencer; Niel Wald; H. David Bruner;

and Victor Smith. A comprehensive report[1] of their study will be published in NCRP Report 65 in early 1980. The therapeutic measures described below are discussed in more detail in that report.

Reduction of internally deposited radionuclides can be accomplished by the use of two general processes: (i) reduction of absorption and internal deposition and (ii) enhanced elimination or excretion of absorbed nuclides. Both are achieved more effectively when therapy is begun at the earliest time after exposure.

Treatment is most effective if the absorption of contaminants into the systemic circulation is prevented although the administration of diluting and blocking agents is nearly equally effective in some instances because it enhances the elimination rates of the radionuclide or reduces the quantity of radionuclide incorporated in tissue. Therapeutic measures that use mobilizing agents or chelating drugs are less effective when the radionuclide has already moved into the tissue cells.

Wound Irrigation and Excision

After emergency first aid to control hemorrhage and treat shock, any potential radioactive contamination in wounds must be located. Weak beta- and alpha-emitters present special problems unless special instrumentation is available. An example of such equipment is the thin, unshielded NaI(Tl) detector[2] used to measure plutonium in wounds at the Los Alamos Scientific Laboratory. It will detect as little as 0.07 nanocurie of ^{239}Pu with a single 500-sec count. This screening instrument, unfortunately, cannot be used easily to evaluate wounds with complicated geometry or mixtures of radionuclides. All such wounds and those with more than 2 nanocuries of plutonium activity are measured with a Si(Li) detector. Longer analysis times are necessary, but the X-ray and gamma-ray lines of interest are easily resolved, identified, and quantified.

Irrigation of the wound with sterile water or saline, free bleeding, and occluding venous return with a tourniquet have been advocated for immediate action.[3] A pulsating water jet lavage has been used with some additional success.[4]

After thorough wound irrigation, long-lived radionuclides, such as plutonium and americium, may be removed by excision of the wound area. A block excision of a small wound area is often more effective than lesser wound debridements. Primary closure of the wound is performed after the results of a check for residual activity are satisfactory. Use of a skin biopsy punch is a convenient way to excise small puncture wounds. All removed tissue, gauze sponges, and irrigation water, if possible, should be retained for radiochemical analysis.

Reduction of Gastrointestinal Absorption

Gastrointestinal absorption can be reduced either by washing out or by the use of medications selected for specific elements. These medications combine with the radionuclides so that they are less available for absorption and are then eliminated in the stool. Such treatments are summarized below.

Use of a nasogastric or gastric tube to empty the stomach (stomach lavage) would generally be used in the highly unusual circumstance where the known intake of a large quantity of radionuclides will pose a significant threat to the present or future health and where it has occurred recently enough that the material is in the stomach.

In most cases, stomach lavage would be the procedure of choice but may not always be successful. Emetics act by stimulating the gastric mucosa, by stimulating the vomiting center in the brain (medulla), or by a combination of the two. Their use is contraindicated if the state of consciousness is impaired or after the ingestion of corrosive agents. Apomorphine hydrochloride and ipecac are the most likely drugs to consider for this use.

Selection of a purgative to speed the elimination of the contents of the intestinal tract should include the consideration of the speed of action. Of particular concern is the effect of relatively insoluble radionuclides that may remain for many hours in the colon and rectum. These portions of the gastrointestinal tract will receive the largest radiation doses but the damage can be reduced by prompt removal of the radionuclides from the intestinal tract. Some purgatives may have special advantages because they produce a less soluble compound of the radionuclide. Magnesium sulfate, for example, is a saline cathartic that can produce relatively insoluble sulfates with some radionuclides, for example, radium, and thus reduce absorption. Use of enemas will empty the colon in a few minutes and may also be a consideration in some cases. Purgative drugs taken orally, such as biscodyl, castor oil, or phenolphthalein, require several hours before taking effect, but these have faster action than others.

The basis for oral administration of strong cation- or anion-exchange resins to aid in the removal and reduced absorption of radionuclides from the gastrointestinal tract has weakened because of increasing evidence of toxic side effects. Activated charcoal would seem to be a potentially useful substitute.

Ferric ferrocyanide (Prussian blue) has been found effective in accelerating the removal of cesium, thallium, and rubidium by the fecal route in animals.[5-9] Prussian blue is essentially nonabsorbed from the gastrointestinal tract and has low toxicity. One gm of Prussian blue given three times per day from several days up to 3 weeks is well tolerated in man.[10] The compound has been used in man to remove cesium.[6,11,12] It reduces the biological half-time of ^{137}Cs to a third of the usual value.

Aluminum-containing antacids are effective in reducing intestinal uptake of radioactive strontium. A single oral dose of 100 ml of aluminum phosphate gel given immediately after exposure will decrease the intestinal absorption of radioactive strontium by about 85%.[13-15] A single dose of aluminum hydroxide gel, 60 to 100 ml, given immediately after exposure will reduce the uptake by about 50%. Both drugs are nontoxic and well tolerated. A mixture of aluminum and magnesium hydroxide can also be considered as a possible agent to reduce gastrointestinal absorption.

Alginates, salts of alginic acid, are jelly-like substances obtained from the brown algae known as kelps. These substances inhibit the intestinal absorption of radioactive strontium by 80 to 90%.[16] The principal disadvantage to their use is the viscosity of the material which makes it difficult to swallow.

Barium sulfate is a highly insoluble salt used as a contrast medium for roentgenographic examination of the gastrointestinal tract. Except for constipation, no adverse effects have been observed. The principal indication for barium sulfate in this application is as an immediate antidote for ingested strontium and radium. Formation of insoluble sulfates of these elements will markedly decrease their intestinal absorption.

Significant amounts of phytates are found in grains and grain cereals, particularly in oats and soya bean products. Phytates contain phosphorus, as phytic acid phosphorus, which combines with calcium, magnesium, zinc, and iron to form insoluble salts. Absorption of these elements from the intestinal tract may be reduced by the administration of phytates.

Blocking and Diluting Agents

A blocking agent saturates a specific tissue with the stable element, thereby reducing the uptake of the radionuclide. Isotopic dilution is achieved by the administration of large quantities of the stable element or compound so that, on a statistical basis alone, the opportunity for incorporation and exposure of the radionuclide is lessened. Displacement therapy is a special form of dilution therapy in which a nonradioactive element of a different atomic number successfully competes with the radionuclide for uptake sites.

The use of a stable iodide to prevent the uptake of radioactivity in the thyroid is an example of an effective blocking agent. A dose of 300 mg of potassium or sodium iodide achieves maximal blocking and will stop further uptake of radioiodine by the thyroid. Six drops of a saturated solution of potassium iodide in a glass of water is a convenient form of administration also. The iodide should be administered as soon after exposure as possible because, once iodine is in the gland, its turnover is slow. The biological half-time in the gland is about 120 days.[17] Only about 50% of the uptake is blocked if the iodide administration is delayed 6 hours, and little effect can be achieved if administration is delayed more than 12 hours.[18] If stable iodide has been given promptly, it should be continued at about 30 mg/day for a week or two to prevent the small amount of radioiodine that leaves the gland from being recycled.[19]

Stable strontium is useful as a diluting agent for radiostrontium. It is available as tablets (strontium lactate, 300 mg, to be given two to five times a day) or intravenous solutions (strontium gluconate, 600 mg of strontium per day infused with 500 ml of 5% glucose in water over 4 hr). The tablets are well tolerated if given with meals and are nontoxic at this dose. This agent can be given daily for several weeks.

Phosphate can be used to decrease the intestinal absorption of radioactive strontium. It may also be useful as a diluting agent in case of medical misadministration of ^{32}P. Oral phosphates can be given in inorganic (sodium or potassium phosphate) and organic forms (sodium glycerophosphate). Vomiting, diarrhea, or both, may occur from phosphate administration in doses exceeding 2 gm per day. Phosphate is used as a saline cathartic. Intravenous phosphate infusion is an unlikely drug candidate for use in treating radionuclide uptakes. Rapid intravenous administration can cause severe hypotension, renal failure, and myocardial infarction. Serum calcium and electrocardiograms must be monitored during such infusion.

In cases of exposure to tritium, a high level of fluid uptake by mouth will increase tritium excretion. Fluid forcing should be continued for at least 1 week or until further reduction in dose is limited. The half-time of tritium in the body can be reduced from the normal 10 to 12 days to 5 days or less by forcing at least 3 to 4 liters of fluid per day. The radiation dose may thus be reduced by a factor of 2 or more by careful management.

Orally and intravenously administered calcium increases the urinary excretion of radioactive strontium and calcium in man. Zinc administered orally can be used for isotopic dilution in cases of exposure to ^{65}Zn.

Mobilizing Agents

Mobilizing agents are compounds that increase a natural turnover process, thereby inducing a release of some forms of radioisotopes from body tissues. This results in an enhanced rate of elimination of these radioisotopes. These agents are more effective if they are given soon after exposure, but some still produce an effect if given within about 2 weeks.

When radioactive iodine has already been taken up by the thyroid, treatment with stable iodine is not effective. Antithyroid drugs may be considered in these cases if the radioactive dose is high enough to justify the use of these drugs with their potentially dangerous side effects. Propylthiouracil and methimazole directly interfere with the oxidation of the iodide ion and block the formation of thyroid hormone. These drugs are absorbed from the gastrointestinal tract within 20 to 30 minutes; their blocking action on thyroid hormone formation, however, lasts only about 6 to 8 hours. Administration of the drug every 8 hours would probably be required for maximum effectiveness. In three human volunteers, 40 mg of methimazole given daily starting several days after ^{131}I administration reduced the biological half-time about 50% and the effective half-time about 25%.[20] If the thyroid already has an ample supply of stable iodine, the response of the thyroid to these drugs is greatly reduced.[21]

Ammonium chloride, given orally (1 to 2 gm four times a day), is effective in mobilizing radiostrontium deposited in the body. Its effectiveness can be enhanced by simultaneous use of intravenous calcium gluconate, 500 mg of calcium in 500 ml of 5% glucose in water over 4 hours, on 3 to 6 consecutive days.[22] An estimated reduction in the body burden of radiostrontium between 40 and 75% may be obtained if treatment is started soon after exposure. Ammonium chloride frequently causes gastric irritation, nausea, and vomiting and should not be used in persons with severe liver disease.

Diuretics are untested for the treatment of internal radionuclide deposition. Enhanced excretion of sodium, chloride, potassium bicarbonate, magnesium, and water in the urine occurs with induced diuresis. Some corresponding radionuclides that could be associated with radiation accidents are ^{22}Na, ^{24}Na, ^{38}Cl, ^{42}K, and ^{3}H.

Studies on the effect of expectorants and inhalants on inhaled radioactive particles have been disappointing.[23] None provides effective action that would be dependable or particularly useful in treating persons after the inhalation of radioactive particles. There is need for further scientific study to confirm the initial studies with animals; for this purpose the use of some of these agents, such as oral ammonium chloride or inhaled sodium chloride solution aerosol, can be justified for a therapeutic trial.

Injections of parathyroid extract promote the urinary excretion of calcium and phosphorus. Removal of radioactive strontium from the body can be induced as a result of the increased excretion of calcium and strontium which results from bone breakdown caused by parathyroid extract. Parathyroid hormone has been used effectively to treat an accidental overdose of radiophosphorus, ^{32}P, in man.[24]

Chelating Agents

A number of chemical compounds enhance the elimination of metals from the body by chelation, a process by which organic compounds (ligands) exchange less firmly bonded ions for other inorganic ions to form a relatively stable nonionized ring complex. This soluble complex can be excreted readily by the kidney. A properly selected and administered chelating drug will enhance the excretion of some radioactive elements and thus reduce their residence times in the body. Therapy with a chelating agent is most effective when it is begun immediately after exposure while the metallic ions are still in circulation and before they have been incorporated into cells.

The calcium salt of ethylenediaminetetraacetic acid (calcium edetate, $CaNa_2EDTA$ or CaEDTA) is the most common form of chelator used in man, primarily to treat lead poisoning. It can also be used to chelate zinc, copper, cadmium, chromium, manganese, and nickel. It has some effectiveness for the transuranium metals, such as plutonium and americium, but $CaNa_2DTPA$ (described next) has been found to be more effective by an order of magnitude for those radionuclides.

The edetates are nephrotoxic and must be used with extreme caution in patients with preexisting renal disease. Transient bone marrow depression, mucocutaneous lesions, chills, fever, muscle cramps, and histamine-like reactions (sneezing, nasal congestion, and lacrimation) have also been described.

In the treatment of lead poisoning, CaDTPA is usually administered by intravenous injection in 250 to 500 ml of 5% glucose in water or isotonic saline. The maximal dose is 75 mg/kg of body weight daily given in two divided doses, up to a maximal dose of 375 mg/kg weekly. The maximal dose for a total regimen normally should not exceed 550 mg/kg. Doses of about one-half of those listed above may be effective for radioactive metals. The infusion time should be about 1 hour for each 1 gm of EDTA. Urine should be tested for albumin before and after EDTA administration. Treatment should be discontinued if albuminuria occurs.

The powerful chelating agent diethylenetriaminepentaacetic acid (pentathamil, DTPA) is generally more effective in removing heavy-metal, multivalent radionuclides than CaEDTA. It is effective for the transuranium metals (plutonium, americium, curium, californium, and neptunium), the rare earths (cerium, yttrium, lanthanum, promethium, and scandium), and some transition metals (zirconium and niobium).

CaDTPA also binds trace metals present in the body, such as zinc and manganese. It is the reduction in these two trace metals that probably accounts for the toxicity to high doses in animal experiments. Doses over 2000 μmol/kg (the clinical human dose range is 10 to 30 μmol/kg) can produce severe lesions of the kidneys, intestinal mucosa, and liver, and may be lethal.[25] Increased toxicity from fractionated dose schedules has been demonstrated in experiments with beagle dogs in which injections at the human dose levels, 5.8 μmol/kg of CaDTPA given every 5 hours, were fatal as early as 4 days after the onset of treatment.[26] The most significant injury occurs in the intestinal epithelium. No untoward effects in rats was noted with doses of 100 μmol/kg given twice weekly over a 44-week period.[23] Teratogenicity and fetal death have occurred in mice given five daily injections of 720 to 2880 μmol/kg given throughout gestation.[27,28] Daily doses of 360 μmol/kg in mice, about ten times the human daily dose, produced no harmful effects.[27]

The zinc salt of DTPA is less toxic than CaDTPA and therefore is advantageous to use for longer-term treatments and especially for fractionated treatments.[26] ZnDTPA also did not cause teratogenicity or fetal death in experiments with mice.

No serious toxicity in man has been reported as a result of CaDTPA administration in recommended doses. Long-term, low-dose administrations in man, 1 gm per week, showed no adverse effects after 4 years.[29]

CaDTPA is more effective than ZnDTPA in rats when given promptly after exposure to ^{239}Pu, ^{252}Cf, or ^{241}Am.[30,31] This finding led to the general recommendation that CaDTPA be used during the first 24 to 48 hours after exposure and then that ZnDTPA be used for continuing treatments.

The effectiveness of DTPA in enhancing the excretion of plutonium is markedly affected by the chemical form of the plutonium. For both wounds and inhaled particles, the absorption of relatively insoluble plutonium compounds, such as plutonium oxide, into the circulation occurs over many days and weeks. DTPA is not effective in these cases because of the small amount of plutonium present soon after exposure in the blood or intracellular fluids. Soluble compounds, such as plutonium nitrate, have relatively rapid uptake and translocation, and so the plutonium is more available early after exposure for chelation. Data from persons treated with CaDTPA soon after exposure (on the first day) indicate that about 60 to 70% of the soluble forms of plutonium is removed as compared to cases without CaDTPA treatment.[32]

Both CaDTPA and ZnDTPA are available as an investigational new drug in the United States and can be obtained through the Radiation Emergency Assistance Center and Training Site, Oak Ridge, Tennessee. These drugs have been administered by both intravenous injection and aerosol inhalation. The intravenous form consists typically of 1 gm of CaDTPA or ZnDTPA in 250 ml of normal saline or 5% glucose in water given over 1 hour in a single daily dose. The dose may be repeated on 5 to 6 successive days. The aerosol form usually consists of 1 gm1 of CaDTPA or ZnDTPA placed in a nebulizer. The entire volume is usually inhaled in 15 to 30 minutes. Administrations by inhalation can also be repeated daily. It is prudent not to use the inhalation route in persons with preexisting pulmonary disease. The drug is contraindicated if significant leukopenia, thrombocytopenia, or kidney dysfunction exists. Urinalysis should be normal prior to each treatment. Hall et al.[32] have developed a model for plutonium excretion after DTPA treatment that suggests an optimal dosage schedule is provided with treatments on days 1, 2, 4, 7, and 15 after exposure.

Dimercaprol (BAL) forms stable chelates with mercury, lead, arsenic, gold, bismuth, chromium, and nickel. Although seldom the agent of first choice, dimercaprol should be useful in accelerating removal of ionic metals that are attracted to sulfur.

Unfortunately, dimercaprol is toxic; approximately 50% of subjects receiving 5 mg/kg intramuscularly will experience toxicity.[33] There is frequently increased blood pressure and tachycardia. Other unpleasant but not dangerous reactions are nausea, vomiting, headache, a burning sensation in the mouth, conjunctivitis, chest pain, and a feeling of anxiety. Sterile abscesses occasionally develop at the site of injection.

The drug is given by intramuscular injection. The doses for stable arsenic and gold intoxication are 2.5 mg/kg or less administered at 4-hour intervals during the first 2 days, twice on day 3, and once daily for 5 to 10 days.[33]

Penicillamine, an amino acid derived from the degradation of penicillin, chelates with copper, iron, mercury, lead, gold, and possibly other heavy metals. It is superior to dimercaprol and CaEDTA for the removal of copper. The incidence of adverse effects with penicillamine is low. The most common and serious are hypersensitivity reactions manifested by a maculopapular or erythematous rash. One fatal case of granulocytopenia has been reported.

Penicillamine is given by mouth, 250 mg four times a day, on an empty stomach between meals and at bedtime. The dose may be increased to 4 or 5 gm daily in divided dose. If the person has a penicillin sensitivity, the drug should be given cautiously. If adverse reaction occurs, discontinue. Blood cell counts should be taken and urinalysis should be done every 3 days during the first 2 weeks of therapy and at least every 10 days thereafter.

Deferoxamine (DFOA) has been used effectively in the treatment of iron storage diseases and acute iron poisoning. If given promptly, DFOA surpasses CaDTPA in the enhancement of excretion of plutonium (IV) compounds.[30,34–38] Its effectiveness declines rapidly, which makes its clinical use for this purpose questionable.[39] The combination of DFOA and CaDTPA yields better results than either drug separately.[30]

DFOA is given by intramuscular injection, 1 gm initially, followed by 500 mg every 4 hours for two doses. Then 500 mg can be given every 4 to 12 hours to a maximal total dosage of 6 gm in 24 hours. Intravenous administration (the same dosage) should never exceed 15 mg/kg of body weight per hour. Toxic reactions, usually manifested as a generalized erythema, flushing, tachycardia, urticaria, or sudden hypotension, are serious enough to contraindicate use of DFOA in the treatment of mild iron poisoning. Its use for radionuclides should be considered only under circumstances of serious exposure.

Lung Lavage

Deposition of radioactive particles in the lung is one of the more common types of accidental exposure of humans to radionuclides. Insoluble particles, once inhaled into the lung, may be mobilized and translocated to other organs at a low rate over many months or years.

Lavage of the tracheobronchial tree has shown promise as a treatment technique for individuals who have inhaled relatively insoluble radionuclides.[40,41] The procedure requires placement of an endotracheal tube into the trachea and major bronchi while the patient is under general anesthesia so that the lungs can be lavaged with isotonic saline.

Dogs treated after inhaling insoluble radioactive particles have shown reductions in their lung burdens from about 25 to 50% (average, 44% in eight dogs) after five lavages of each lung.[41-43] Radiation pneumonitis and early deaths were prevented in 75% of the treated dogs in contrast to the untreated dogs.[43] The same regimen of ten lavages removed 35 to 49% of ^{239}Pu and ^{238}Pu, polydisperse aerosols of different chemical characteristics.[44] Sixty to 90% of the lung burdens of plutonium oxide in baboons were removed by treatment with ten pulmonary lavages.[45]

In one case in which a person had inhaled a ^{239}Pu aerosol, three lavages at 8, 12, and 17 days removed about 13% of the estimated initial lung burden.[46] The aerosol proved to be more soluble than was assumed initially and this may have reduced the efficacy of lavage therapy.

Possible use of this experimental technique in man requires a careful risk-benefit assessment. The risk lies primarily in the administration of a general anesthetic. The overall mortality risk may be 0.2 to 0.5% for each procedure. Thus, this procedure should be considered only in high exposures in which a reduction 25 to 50% of the dose could be expected to prevent acute or subacute effects, such as radiation pneumonitis or fibrosis. The risk from the procedure is immediate, whereas late effects of radiation exposure to the lung may occur many years later.

Therapy for Selected Radionuclides

The treatments listed above summarize the available therapy for internally deposited radionuclides. Examples of their use for some of the more common radionuclides that may be encountered are given in Table 1.

Table 1. Therapy for Selected Elements

Nuclides	Therapy	Comment
Transuranium elements: americium, californium, curium, neptunium, plutonium	CaDTPA or znDTPA	CaEDTA may be used if DTPA is not immediately available, but it is less effective. DFOA may be considered for high plutonium exposures if DTPA is not available. Excise contaminated wounds.
Rare earths: cerium, lanthanum, promethium, scandium, yttrium	CaDTPA or ZnDTPA	CaEDTA may be used if DTPA is not immediately available. Consider need for stomach lavage and purgatives
Cesium	Prussian blue	Consider need for lavage and purgatives.
Cobalt	Penicillamine	Therapeutic trial of penicillamine is useful. Consider need for stomach lavage and purgatives.
Iodine	KI or NaI, or SSKI	Success depends on early administration after exposure.
Phosphorus	Aluminum hydroxide	Consider stomach lavage. Severe overdosage may be treated with parathyroid extract and oral phosphorus.
Radium	Magnesium sulfate Alginates Ammonium chloride Calcium	No effective therapy after absorption Consider stomach lavage early.
Strontium	Aluminum phosphate gel Strontium or calcium Ammonium chloride	Barium sulfate and alginates are alternatives to block GI uptake. Consider stomach lavage early.
Tritium	Forced fluids	

References

1. "Management of Persons Accidentally Contaminated with Radionuclides," Committee Report No. 37. Washington, D.C., National Council on Radiation Protection and Measurements, in press.
2. Vasilik DG, Martin RW, Umbarger CJ: A sensitive, yet simple, plutonium wound monitor. *Health Physics* 35:557, 1978.
3. Norwood, WD: Therapeutic removal of plutonium in humans. *Health Physics* 8:747, 1962.

4. Grower MF, Bhaskar SN: Effect of pulsating water jet lavage on radioactive contaminated wounds. *J Dent Res* 51(No.2):536, 1972.

5. Nigrovic V: Enhancement of the excretion of radiocesium in rats by ferric cyanoferate (II). *Int J Radiat Biol* 7:307, 1963.

6. Richmond, CR: Accelerating the turnover of internally deposited radiocesium, in Kornberg HA, Norwood WD (eds.): *Diagnosis and Treatment of Deposited Radionuclides*. New York, Excerpta Medica Foundation, 1968, p. 315.

7. Stather JW: Influence of Prussian blue on metabolism of ^{137}Cs and ^{86}Rb in rats. *Health Physics* 22:1, 1972.

8. Richmond CR, Drake GA, London JE: Enhanced removal of radiorubidium from rodents and beagles with ferric ferrocyanide (abstract). *Radiat Res* 55:546, 1975.

9. Ducousso R, Causse A, Pasquier C: Comparative affects of acetazolamide and Prussian blue on ^{137}Cs retention in the rat. *Health Physics* 28:75, 1975.

10. Stromme A: Increased excretion of ^{137}Cs in humans, in Kornberg HA, Norwood WD (eds.): *Diagnosis and Treatment of Deposited Radionuclides*. New York, Excerpta Medica Foundation, 1968, p. 329.

11. Madshus K, Stromme A, Bohne F, Nigrovic V: Diminution of radiocesium bodyburden in dogs and human beings by Prussian blue. *Int J Radiat Biol* 10:519, 1966.

12. Madshus K, Stromme A: Increased excretion of ^{137}Cs in humans by Prussian blue. *Z Naturforsch*. 23b:391, 1968.

13. Spencer H, Lewin I, Samachson J: Radiostrontium absorption in man. *Lancet* 1:156, 1967.

14. Spencer H, Lewin I, Belcher MJ, Samachson J: Inhibition of radiostrontium absorption by aluminum phosphate gel in man and its comparative effect on radiocalcium absorption. *Int J Appl Radiat Isotopes* 20:507, 1969.

15. Spencer H, Lewin I, Samachson J, Belcher MJ: Effect of aluminum phosphate gel on radiostrontium absorption in man. *Radiat Res* 38:307, 1969.

16. Hesp R, Ramsbottom, B: Effects of sodium alginate in inhibiting uptake of radiostrontium by the human body. *Nature* 208:1341, 1965.

17. Bernard SR, Fish BR, Royster GW, Farabee LB, Brown PE, Patterson GR: Human thyroid uptake and bodily elimination of ^{131}I for the case of single and continual ingestion of bound iodine in resin-treated milk. *Health Physics* 9:307, 1963.

18. Ramsden D, Passant FH, Peabody CO, Speight RG: Radioiodine uptakes in the thyroid. Studies of the blocking and subsequent recovery of the gland following the administration of stable iodine. *Health Physics* 13:633, 1967.

19. Von Henreich HG, Gabbe EE, Meineke B, Whang OH, Kuhnau J: Quantitative *in vivo*-unter suchungen zur vollstandingen hemmung der gesamtkorper—inkorporierung und retention der [131]I—beim menschen. *Atomkernenergie* 11, 1/2:83, 1966.

20. Janaka S, Mochizuki Y, Yabumoto E, Iinuma TA, Kumatori T, Yamane T, Akiyama T, Matsusaka N: Protection of thyroid gland and total body from radiation delivered by radioactive iodine, in Kornberg HA, Norwood WD (eds.): *Diagnosis and Treatment of Deposited Radionuclides*. New York, Excerpta Medica Foundation, 1968, p. 298.

21. Gilman AG, Murad F: Thyroid and antithyroid drugs, the *The Pharmacological Basis of Therapeutics* 5th ed., Goodman LS, Gilman AG (eds.), New York, Macmillan Co., Inc., 1975, p. 1410.

22. Spencer H, Samachson J, Hardy, Jr. EP, Rivera J: Effects of intravenous calcium and of orally administered ammonium chloride on strontium-90 excretion in man. *Radiat Res* 26:695, 1965.

23. Bair WJ, Smith VH: Radionuclide contamination and removal, in *Progress in Nuclear Energy, Series XII Health Physics.* New York, Pergamon Press, 1969, vol. 2, p. 157.

24. Cobau CD, Simons CS, Meyers MC: Accidental overdosage with radiophosphorus: therapy by induced phosphate diuresis. *Am J Med Sci* 254:451, 1967.

25. Planas-Bohne F, Lohbrier J: Toxicological studies on DTPA, in Kornberg HA, Norwood WD (eds.): *Diagnosis and Treatment of Incorporated Radionuclides.* IAEA Publication No. STI/PUB/411. Vienna, International Atomic Energy Agency, 1976, p. 505.

26. Taylor GN, Williams JL, Roberts L, Atherton DR, Shabestari L: Increased toxicity of Na_3Ca DTPA when given by protracted administration. *Health Physics* 27:825, 1974.

27. Fisher DR, Mays CW, Taylor GN: Ca DTPA toxicity in the mouse fetus. *Health Physics* 29:780, 1975.

28. Fisher DR, Scott EC, Mays CW, Taylor GN: Ca DTPA-induced fetal death and malformation in mice. *Teratology* 14:123, 1976.

29. Slobodien MJ, Brodsky A, Ke CH, Horm I: Removal of zinc from humans by DTPA chelation therapy. *Health Physics* 24:327, 1973.

30. Volf V: Plutonium decorporation in rats, in *Diagnosis and Treatment of Incorporated Radionuclides.* IAEA Publication No. STI/PUB/411. Vienna, International Atomic Energy Agency, 1976, p. 307.

31. Seidel A: Removal of [252]Cf and [241]Am from the rat by means of Ca DTPA and Zn DTPA, in *Diagnosis and Treatment of Incorporated Radionuclides.* IAEA Publication No. STI/PUB/411. Vienna, International Atomic Energy Agency, 1976, P. 323.

32. Hall RM, Poda GA, Fleming RR, Smith JA: A mathematical model for estimation of plutonium in the human body from urine data influenced by DTPA therapy. *Health Physics* 34:419, 1978.

33. Levine WG: Heavy metals and heavy-metal antagonists, in Goodman LS, Gilman AG (eds.), *The Pharmacological Basis of Therapeutics,* 5th ed., New York, Macmillan Publishing Co., 1975, p. 920.

34. Rosenthal MW, Lindenbaum A: Effect of desferrioxamine–methane sulfonate (DFOM) on removal of plutonium *in vitro* and *in vivo. Proc Soc Exp Biol Med* 117:749, 1964.

35. Smith VH: Prevention of plutonium deposition by desferrioxamine-β. *Nature* 209:899, 1964.

36. Taylor DM: The effects of desferrioxamine on the retention of actinide elements in the rat. *Health Physics* 13:135, 1967.

37. Volf V: The effect of combinations of chelating agents on the translocation of intramuscularly deposited [239]Pu nitrate in the rat. *Health Physics* 29:61, 1975.

38. Volf V, Seidel A, Takada K: Comparative effectiveness of Ca DTPA, desferrioxamine-β, and their combination in removing transuranium elements from rats. *Health Physics* 32:155, 1977.

39. Catsch A, Harmuth-Hoene AE: New developments in metal antidotal properties of chelating agents. *Biochem. Pharmacol* 24:1557, 1975.

40. Pfleger RC, Wilson AJ, Cuddihy PG, McClellan RO: Bronchopulmonary lavage for removal of inhaled insoluble materials from the lung. *Dis. Chest* 56:524, 1969.

41. Pfleger RC, Wilson AJ, McClellan RO: Pulmonary lavage as a therapeutic measure of the lung. *Health Physics* 16:758, 1969.

42. Boecker BB, Muggenburg BA, McClellan RO, Clarkson SP, Mares FJ, Benjamin SA: Removal of [144]Ce in fused clay particles from the beagle dog by bronchopulmonary lavage. *Health Physics* 26:505, 1974.

43. Muggenburg BA, Mauderly JL, Boecker BB, Hahn FF, McClellan RO: Prevention of radiation pneumonitis from inhaled cesium 144 by lung lavage in beagle dogs. *Am Rev Resp Dis* 111:795, 1975.

44. Muggenburg BA, Mewhinny JA, Miglio JJ, Slauson DO, McClellan RO: The removal of inhaled ^{239}Pu and ^{238}Pu from beagle dogs by lung lavage and chelation treatment, in *Diagnosis and Treatment of Incorporated Radionuclides*. IAEA Publication No. STI/PUB/411. Vienna, International Atomic Energy Agency, 1976, p. 341.

45. Nolibe D, Nenot JC, Metivier H, Masse R, Lafuma J: Traitement des inhalations accidentelles d'oxyde de plutonium par lavage pulmonaire *in vivo*, in *Diagnosis and Treatment of Incorporated Radionuclides*. IAEA Publication No. STI/PUB/411. Vienna, International Atomic Energy Agency, 1976, p. 373.

46. McClellan RO, Boyd HA, Benjamin SA, Cuddihy RG, Hahn FF, Jones RK, Mauderly JL, Mewhinny JA, Muggenburg BA, Pfleger RC: Bronchopulmonary lavage and DTPA treatment of an accidental inhalation ^{239}Pu exposure case, in *Fission Product Inhalation Program Annual Report, 1971–1972*, Report LF-45. Albuquerque, N.M., Lovelace Foundation for Medical Education and Research, 1972, p. 287.

Published 1980 by Elsevier North Holland, Inc.
K. F. Hübner and S. A. Fry, eds. The Medical Basis for Radiation Accident Preparedness

Decontamination and Decorporation: The Clinical Experience

George A. Poda

E. I. du Pont de Nemours and Company, Savannah River Plant, Aiken, South Carolina.

For the sake of brevity, I shall not give a historical account of decontamination techniques used over the past 25 years or so; rather, I will briefly touch on recent clinical usages in a major transuranium-processing facility. The contaminants of clinical concern at the Savannah River Plant are isotopes of uranium, plutonium, americium, curium, and californium. The processes of decontamination and decorporation of the actinides are often very difficult to separate in clinically dealing with a contaminated individual. During this procedure, health physics and medical personnel work as a team.

We have a plan for heavily contaminated persons. To minimize the time of exposure, a decontamination unit is placed in the manufacturing area of the plant. This unit (Figure 1) consists of a hot-water tank with hose plus a box which contains protective clothing and survey instruments to be used by the helpers; also present are a venous tourniquet, detergents, scrub brushes, sanitary pads, hair clippers, a blanket, and a change of clothes for the one exposed. The gross contaminant can be quickly removed by using the materials in the decontamination unit and the contaminated person is then taken into the second-stage unit, the health physics decontamination unit, where he can shower and do a more finite job of cleansing. If hair won't clean up here, it can be removed and more sophisticated means can be used to cleanse the nose and skin. Should this fail, the contaminated person is taken by ambulance to the third-stage step, the medical decontamination unit (Figure 2).

Thus far, we have not needed to use drastic approaches. Rather, some common-sense techniques have been used, quite successfully.

Hair is scrubbed and scrubbed with detergent and water; if heavily

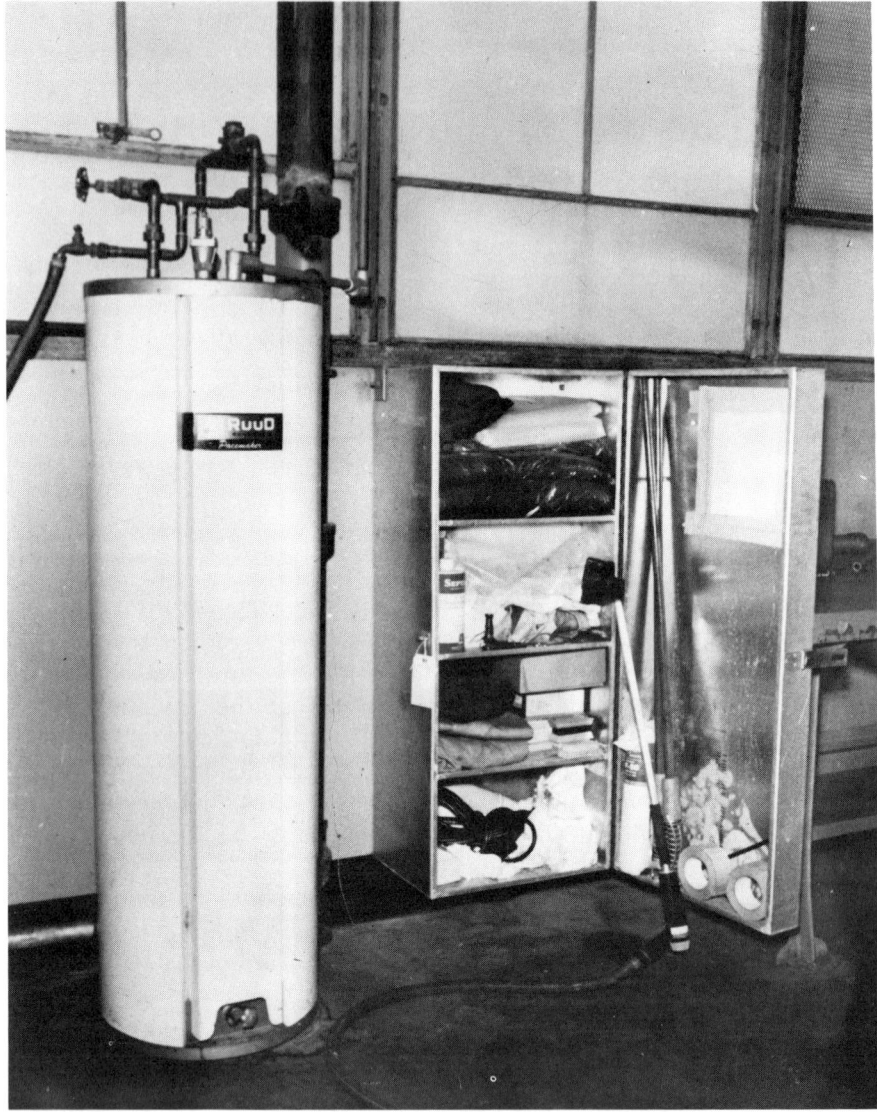

Figure 1. First-stage decontamination unit in the work area of the plant.

contaminated, the person bends over a sink and has help so that he does not spread contaminant all over the entire body. If the contamination is not heavy, a total shower is quite successful. We have removed hair only once and this on the chest to ensure a true lung count. Close clipping of the hair sufficed.

For nasal contamination, the individual is told to blow his nose. Then, if needed, a 500-ml saline intravenous is used, minus the needle, and, with the person leaning over a sink, a nose douche is used. After use, the whole unit is discarded.

Skin is generally washed first with a surgical soap gently maneuvered with sanitary pads and next with a stronger laundry detergent in like manner; if this also is unsuccessful, sodium hypochlorite (simple laundry bleach) in a 1:4 dilution is applied several times. For very stubborn cases, I have used a full-strength bleach but this must be quickly rinsed off. Should the skin become red or sting, we find it advisable to stop and wait a while.

Fingernails and the pads of fingers may not respond unless fine emery cloth is used. I have had no trouble decontaminating finger nails. Finger pads may need to be sanded smooth of all skin whirls before the contaminant is entirely removed. If this fails, the hand is placed in a rubber glove and the glove is left on for 8 to 16 hr to allow perspiration

Figure 2. Medical decontamination unit (third stage) consisting of a shielded tank which protects persons working on the exposed individual while they are either further decontaminating him or, if necessary, surgically removing any embedded matter.

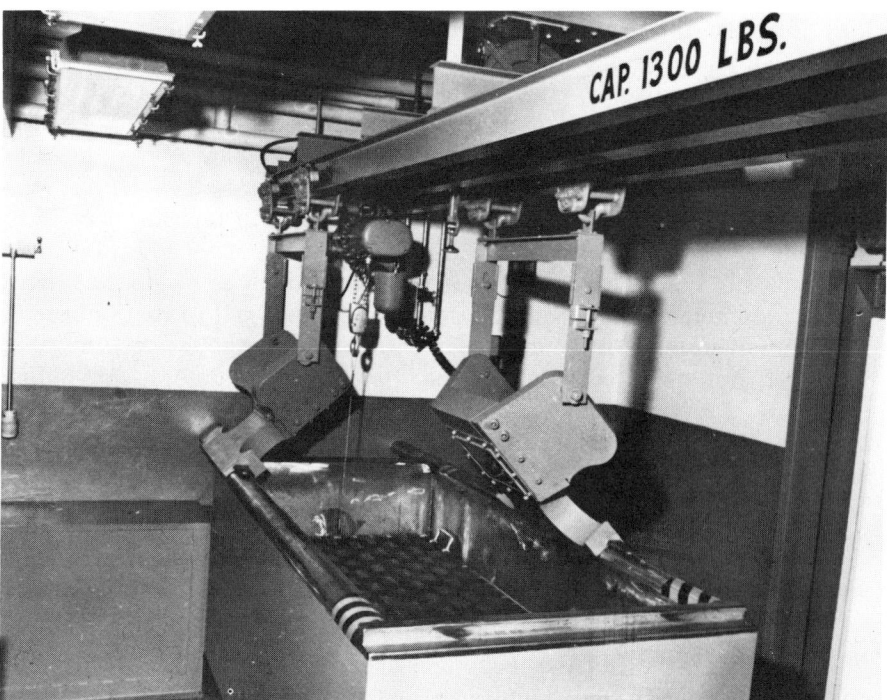

to decontaminate by normal means. The hand emerges water-logged but usually clean.

If the contaminated person has simple wounds such as punctures or lacerations, a venous tourniquet is applied first to promote bleeding; the lacerations are then cleansed with a pad, surgical soap and water. Should this fail, we use the bleach technique.

Some wounds may still require debridement. Puncture wounds of finger pads or fleshy areas are best treated by removing a core of tissue with a dermatology biopsy punch,[1] snipping the end, touching the surfaces with a silver nitrate stick, and applying a firm dressing.

Small contaminated burns are cleansed in like manner, and then a solution of 2% silver nitrate is applied. Any remaining surface contaminant seems to fall off in the eschar. If, however, contaminant is dissolved in acid, it becomes fixed in the skin and won't come off until the skin regenerates. We apply an enzyme cream to expedite the process—dead skin comes off in days rather than weeks. Avulsed tissue can be cleansed in saline, but, if after this treatment it is still contaminated, it can be cleansed in sodium hypochlorite and applied as a primary graft as it will be clean and yet viable.

Inhaled contaminations usually present the greatest challenges. In order to deal with this contaminant, we must determine such things as: the contaminant, how much was inhaled, is it soluble or insoluble, for how long did the person inhale it, does he suffer from hay fever or chronic pulmonary disease? All these factors need be considered. A simple nasal swab only tells us that contaminant went at least up the nostrils. Sputum coughed up may or may not tell much more. If, after obtaining a careful history, one concludes that some of the material reached the lungs, the procedure outlined below is used. Since some of the actinides seem to be more soluble in acid than in neutral or basic solution, a single dose of 100 grains of soda bicarbonate followed by 15 gm of calcium lactate is given orally to neutralize gastric juices, then 1 gm of the chelate DTPA (the dicalcium trisodium salt of diethylenetriaminepentaacetic acid) is given. If the contaminant is known to be insoluble, no chelation is entertained; but, if it is soluble, a single dose of chelate is given within the hour. I prefer to administer the chelate by the aerosol route as it seems more effective in smaller absorbed quantity and seems to be eliminated more slowly than when given intravenously. This is then followed by one ounce of Fleet's phosphosoda, which causes evacuation of the gastrointestinal tract within a very few hours. Experience has indicated that fecal samples collected during the first few days after inhalation contain 60% of the contaminant entering the nasopharynx which is translocated into the gastrointestinal tract. Although not quantitative, examination of the feces is a useful indicator of the amount of contaminant still in the body. The health physics unit then carefully monitors bioassay samples, and these values, the lung count, and other factors determine whether further chelation is called for. Naturally, a complete blood count and urinalysis are done before and after treatment.

Since about 1952 or 1953, we have had six incidents at the Savannah River Plant which were treated with EDTA (ethylenediaminetetraacetic acid). Out of 184 contaminated individuals, 145 received single chelations of DTPA (Table 1), either aerosol or intravenous (the rest got multiple chelation or no chelation). One person[2] received a total of 123 doses of DTPA over a 2.25-year period. He developed anosmia and hypogeusia, which cleared spontaneously 100 days after his last chelation. Several of the others received two or three doses of DTPA. Some persons experienced multiple incidents of contamination.

One person has received seven doses of the zinc salt of DTPA. The first three were given by aerosol, but because he objected to the metallic taste and dryness of the throat, the remaining doses were given intravenously. This man also had general achiness for a few hours after the second aerosol administration, but no aftereffects from the intravenous injection.

Once the bioassay tells us an individual has over 10% of body burden, we offer to chelate. The Hall formula,[3] developed at the Savannah River Plant, is used to determine the frequency of chelation. We have also on occasion chelated persons who have inhaled insoluble particles. Urinary excretion data indicate that all actinides are somewhat soluble in the lungs.

These are some of our clinical experiences that I wish to share, in the hope that they may be of some use to others and also in the hope that others may discover and share with us even better methods of dealing with radioactive contamination.

Table 1. Generalized Effects of Chelation by DTPA Aerosol (1 gm): Single Versus Weekly Treatment

	Percentage of inhaled transuranium elements (transportable) excreted in urine		
Week	No treatment	Single treatment	Weekly treatment
1	0.64	39.	39
2	.24	11.	15.
3	.17	5.6	9.4
4	.13	2.8	6.0
5	.11	1.4	4.2
6	.094	0.70	3.1
7	.084	0.35	2.4
Total (7 weeks)	1.5	61.	79.

References

1. Vernon PB, Hall RM, Poda GA: Monitoring decontamination and bioassay of a plutonium-contaminated injury. *Health Physics* 12:1539–1543, 1966.
2. Jolly J Jr, McClearen HA, Poda GA, Walke WP: Treatment and evaluation of a plutonium-238 nitrate contaminated puncture wound—a two-year case history: *Health Physics* 23:333–341, 1972.
3. Hall RM, Poda GA, Fleming RR, Smith JA: A mathematical model for estimation of plutonium in the human body from urine data influenced by DTPA therapy. *Health Physics* 34:419–432, 1978.

Discussion for Section III

E.L. SAENGER: A legend states that if one shaves the eyebrows, there is a relatively high probability that they will not grow back. Is this statement true? If so, what shall we do?

G.A. PODA: Women have been doing it for years. It is not very often necessary. At one of the REAC/TS courses the question was answered. About 50% of them will not grow back entirely, but they will have enough that they can use an eyebrow pencil and be fine.

R. V. DORN: In partial answer to the general question regarding shaving of eyebrows, this seemingly trivial problem has become serious on occasion. There have been successful lawsuits for malpractice when the eyebrow has been shaved, even when this was felt to be necessary for proper medical care (e.g., cleaning and suturing of a brow laceration). Plastic surgeons, for example, will frequently not shave the eyebrow to aid in skin repair because of these successful lawsuits. Just some food for thought!

E. L. SAENGER: Dr. Voelz, would the effect of blocking doses of stable iodide be affected by a continued release of radioiodine; that is, should blocking doses be given over a period of days, and, if so, what would its efficiency be?

G. L. VOELZ: After the initial blockage, which is 300 mg for sodium iodide, there will be a recycle problem, with the radioactive iodine being reabsorbed. Therefore it should be followed with a daily dose of iodide, which can be as low as 30 mg per day; so 30 to 100 mg, or something in that range, a day for one to two weeks will prevent the recycle and should be at least partially effective for a week or more in reducing exposure to continuous levels of radioiodine.

W. S. DINGLEDINE: Some have proposed the prophylactic use of iodide for nuclear reactor workers (in special circumstances), as well as the use of ^{127}I immediately post-exposure. Has the prophylactic use of T_4 been considered?

G. L. VOELZ: I think these are all possibilities. Actually, as far as I know, we have no data on the effectiveness of those, but I think there are a variety of possibilities here, and probably we should have a good thyroid expert take a look at what might be the most effective. I am not in favor of the general prophylactic use of iodide for nuclear reactor workers, because in most cases use of respirators and protective clothing are better means of preventing uptake. From a philosophical viewpoint, I see less reason to use T_4 than stable iodide. KI has a long shelf life, is economical, safer, and effective if used immediately after exposure.

J. TAYLOR: Do you recommend use of chelation therapy during the period of physiological stabilization of an insoluble, inhaled particulate to minimize circulatory translocation from the lung.

G. VOELZ: There is no single or simple recommendation that answers the question of the value of chelation therapy following inhalation of particulates. The quantity of the inhaled radionuclides in the blood, extracellular fluids, and soft tissues is the portion that is available for chelation. Thus the rate of solubilization and transfer of radionuclides from the lung determines whether chelation will be worthwhile. If the particles are relatively insoluble, resulting in a slow transfer rate to the blood, the chelation will not be effective. The only way to find out, early after exposure, is to give the chelation drug and measure the excretion rate of the radionuclides in the urine. The activity is a measure of the enhanced elimination rate. The physician must decide whether this is or isn't sufficient to warrant continuing the therapy.

M. SCHECTER: How does the surgeon protect himself and the operating team when treating a contaminated wound? How does one clean potentially contaminated anaesthetic machines and equipment?

G. A. PODA: A surgeon is primarily kept from getting contaminated by the usual techniques of decontamination; removal of clothing and rinsing. Usually, most of these things will not go through rubber gloves. If you're anticipating doing this kind of surgery, finger monitors can be worn on your fingers so that you can be monitored by a good physicist who can set a program for you and and tell you how much radiation you're getting. You notice on one of the slides I've presented that we have a facility where a surgeon anticipating high dosage can be protected. Most of the radium shields, or something like that in a hospital, can be modified for such use in an emergency room. Gene Saenger has written a lot about how you protect your hospital from gross contamination of many patients, and he might be the one to answer that one for you.

E. L. SAENGER: I think there are two approaches. One, which we published some years ago, was to use the autopsy room of a hospital and this sometimes creates an emotional problem; it is an area that is not crucial to the daily operation of the hospital. The principal problem is not to bring a patient in through the emergency room— the usual emergency room—if he is previously identified as being contaminated. Simply, have another route into the hospital.

We have solved this in our hospital on a number of occasions by using a garage; we now have a relatively inexpensive suite that would in no way compare with the DOE's suite, which has both high- and low-level decontamination areas. Other hospitals have done this simply by having a room in the basement in which they could put a patient and carry out simple decontamination. It seems to me to be inappropriate to stand them up at a wall outside of the hospital and rinse them down with a firehose. This has been advocated by some hospitals that I have visited.

I would comment that decontamination of an anesthetic device can be very difficult, particularly if your exposure is to actinides. I think the need for using it is extremely rare, and you may decide that it is expendable; you may have to discard it after you're through.

F. M. BARLOTTA: Under what circumstances would you recommend bone marrow transplantation for a total-body radiation accident victim?

G. A. ANDREWS: I don't believe that the decision can be based entirely on criteria that are set up in advance. We are working without any adequate data base and extrapolating from other situations. I think that in Dr. Wald's patient, who received the bone marrow from his identical twin, the graft may have been life saving, but if the patient could have been kept alive by other means, I feel sure that his own marrow would have regenerated.

When a homologous donor is used, we do not have a good estimate of the risk of death from a graft-versus-host reaction. If this were known to be a low probability, I would be more eager to attempt grafts. In general, a graft attempt appears indicated when a good donor is available, the exposure has not been protracted, and the dose truly life threatening.

H. C. ALLEN: A comment in response to a previous question to Dr. Voelz. TSH should not be used too early, for it would increase the thyroid uptake of radioactive iodine. It should serve as a very useful purpose 24 to 48 hours after exposure, for it would increase the rate of release of radioactive thyroxine and triiodothyroxine by decreasing the effective half-life by approximately 50%, from six days to two or three days, thereby reducing the radiation dose to the thyroid gland significantly.

S. MILLER: Would you advise distribution of potassium iodide or sodium iodide to the general public, as has been done in Toronto, Canada?

G. L. VOELZ: There was a report by the National Council on Radiation Protection and Measurements about this specific problem, and we have the chairman and expert on this subject in the crowd, so I'll call on Dr. Saenger again. Gene, do you want to say what your committee did about this problem?

E. L. SAENGER: It's not clear from this question whether he means it should be distributed prior to the accident or whether there should be some type of emergency technique to distribute it after the accident. We were very careful in our report since we didn't give any specific instructions as to how this was to be distributed or under what circumstances. We left this up to the discretion of public health authorities. Subsequently, there has been a great deal of interest in this matter, and various techniques have been worked out for prior distribution of iodide blocking agents. The initial idea the FDA had was that it would be sold as an over-the-counter drug very much as you could buy nose drops or antiacids or whatever, and that each household, company, or school could stock this. This seems to me to be a very practical solution to the problem. Other alternatives had been that the plant would distribute this sort of drug slightly ahead of this wave of radioiodine; it would be stocked in police stations, schools, factories, etc. I don't think that anyone has really had a practical solution to the problem. Our very distinguished visitors from other countries are facing this problem. They have a public to deal with, and they have a very firm nuclear energy program, and I would be very much interested in hearing from people from the United Kingdom, Germany, and France as to how they are approaching this problem.

M. C. WILLS: A comment was made that KI pills have been distributed to the general population in the Toronto region, near a nuclear power generating station to be used in the unlikely event of an iodine release. This is not the case. There is no prior distribution of pills to the general population, and at present there are no plans to do so.

z. DEANOVIC: A question to Dr. Andrews. What do you think about the possibility to preserve the bone marrow *auto*transplant (in a "bone marrow bank") in persons with a greater exposure risk?

G. A. ANDREWS: The techniques are available for storing frozen stem cells, and it appears highly likely that they could be maintained alive for fairly long periods. Obtaining the cells involves considerable discomfort and possibly slight risk to the donor. Multiple marrow aspirations are needed, and this requires general or spinal anesthesia, or heavy pain-relieving medication. Stem cells can also be obtained from circulating blood, but the yield is low and a large volume must be processed. The long-term storage would involve significant expense.

Radiation accidents are rare and most occur in quite unexpected situations; therefore it is not generally feasible to establish a high-risk group. If an unusual situation should arise, in which a small number of people were known to have a high, unavoidable risk, preparations for the autograft would appear practical, but it is difficult to conceive of such a situation. Under present conditions, if a radiation worker had some of his stem cells stored, they would be very much more likely to be useful in treating later incidental cancer or leukemia, unrelated to his occupation, than in treating a radiation accident.

J. MCCONKEY: Is hyperalimentation used as a treatment modality for those total-body-exposure patients with gastrointestinal symptoms?

G. A. ANDREWS: I am not aware of any special attention that has been directed toward nutrition. In most patients with the hematopoietic syndrome, even when it is severe, the vomiting stops within two or three days, and subsequently the appetite is not greatly impaired; however, some do lose weight and may well benefit from extra nutritional support. Malnutrition does not play any obvious role in the prolonged fatigue seen after hematologic recovery; at least there is no lack of appetite or tendancy to lose weight. For the few patients who have received extremely high radiation doses and who have died within days, I doubt that much attention has been paid to nutrition. Probably greater consideration will be given to this aspect of supportive care in the future.

K. ROOS: Can the water used in decontamination be put in the general outflow without any step? What is the general policy?

G. A. PODA: I gather he is referring to the concern about the water that you use for decontamination getting into the general sewage. We have an underground, 5,000 gallon holding tank. All the contaminated water goes down there and is handled as contaminated material. In local hospitals, when I've been asked what to do, I suggest that they use a bi-valve system in their autopsy room or wherever, one line going into a plasticized tank. The other line will flow into the standard sewer system, so when they're using contaminated water they can store it; when they're not, they can use the sewer system. That's the way we've been handling it.

SECTION IV:

The Role of Cytogenetics in Biological Dosimetry

Published 1980 by Elsevier North Holland, Inc.
K. F. Hübner and S. A. Fry, eds. The Medical Basis for Radiation Accident Preparedness

Cytogenetic Methods in Diagnosis of Acute Radiation Injuries

E. Komarov

World Health Organization, CH-1211 Geneva 27, Switzerland.

Most of the speakers in this conference mention the cytogenetic methods as more or less routine methods in use in various countries and laboratories. I suppose it is a very good sign, and I think we can draw a conclusion from this meeting. Namely, cytogenetic methods are established methods in the diagnosis of radiation injury in man.

I would like to elaborate on the historical development of this methodology. In 1961, WHO held a meeting on "Diagnosis and Treatment of X-irradiation Injury in Man." At this meeting practically no mention was made of the use of the cytogenetic method for diagnosis. In 1971, jointly with the Atomic Energy Agency, the WHO held a meeting on biochemical indicators of radiation injury in man and described in detail the biochemical indicators. The meeting came to the conclusion that cytogenetic methods would be the most sensitive methods for the diagnosis of radiation injury. Also, the UNSCEAR report on genetic effects of radiation was issued in 1969 with recommendations to develop the cytogenetic method for the assessment of radiation effects in man; namely, individuals exposed to radiation in accidents in their occupational environment and in medical diagnosis and treatment. I could also add a fourth group, the general public. All agree in the UNSCEAR recommendation and report of 1969.

The WHO decided to appoint some kind of coordinator of the research programs on use of chromosome aberration as a biological indicator of radiation damage in man; the WHO usually assigns the highest priority to treatment of infectious diseases, rather than irradiation injury. We invite various institutions from various countries to participate in such a coordinated program and an international study. Throughout this program of activity I visited many laboratories and one of the first I visited was the National Radiation Protection Board in Great Britain headed by Dr. Dolphin, who felt that such activity should be promoted. This research was finally developed to the extent that man can now use this diagnostic method not only for radiation accidents but also the occupational exposure of the personnel.

I also visited Oak Ridge in 1972, and we discussed future development of this program of activities. One development, which was very important for this program was the modification of the technique to use peripheral blood lymphocytes to study somatic chromosome aberrations. This was a breakthrough for biological monitoring. We can say today that this method is fully approved in the diagnosis of radiation accidents and evaluation of occupational personnel; we still need a lot of work in the occupational field. Should we use data from medical exposures to help the people who work in the field of radiation accidents? This information might be important to some extent in studying the effect of internal exposure.

The last and most difficult problem is the use of this methodology for population studies. I don't think we should recommend the use of cytogenetics to evaluate, for example, the population exposure in the case of the Three Mile Island Accident. We can make some kind of study on populations of surrounding areas, but the value of such data will be doubtful because we know that—for the time being—the detection level for chromosome aberrations is not less than 10 rad. Of course, we should discuss the possibility of the use of cytogenetic methods for evaluation of possible chronic effects on the environment and chronic effects on the population.

I would like to mention to you that the program in WHO has always had good support from various international institutions: the International Atomic Energy Agency and from National Laboratories. To maintain these activities, we established a system of collaborating laboratories in cytogenetics for the evaluation of radiation and other environmental effects. At the present time we have three such collaborating centers. One center is NPB Population Cytogenetic Laboratory in Edinborough. The second center is in Moscow, the Institute for Medical Genetics, and the third one is a Cytogenetic Laboratory in Ottawa. These centers are reference centers that provide advice on methodology and applications, and training in cytogenetic methods. A manual on the study of chromosome aberrations in man was developed and published in 1973 and is still a very valuable publication.

We are not only involved in the evaluation of the radiation environmental effects, but also in the evaluation of all of the effects of environmental pollutants. There is a possibility for the use of cytogenetic methods for the evaluation of the environmental pollution. We are also considering some kind of integral monitoring system that could be used for evaluation of health and biological effects on the population. We still need more data and more precise evaluations of use of cytogenetic methods in partial-body irradiation in cases of internal emitters. We should look into the possibility of studying combined effects of chemicals and radiation, and consider other sources of information. Our judgments are presently based on evaluation of the chromosome aberration in lymphocytes and in bone marrow. Rarely do we have data on chromosome aberration in skin fibroblasts, but sometimes it is very useful. We heard here of one such case. Also, an attempt was made to use the hair roots as a source of information, but we don't have any good results with this method, and it is not confirmed in some laboratories.

Today we can use cytogenetics as a diagnostic tool. We cannot give any kind of evaluation of the significance of cytogenetic changes for the induction of cancer, leukemia, or for genetic effects of the population. Therefore, for the moment we should limit ourselves to diagnostic applications of cytogenetic methods.

Published 1980 by Elsevier North Holland, Inc.
K. F. Hübner and S. A. Fry, eds. The Medical Basis for Radiation Accident Preparedness

The 1976 Hanford
Americium Accident

K. R. Heid,* B. D. Breitenstein,+
H. E. Palmer,* B. J. McMurray,*
and N. Wald‡

*Pacific Northwest Laboratory, Richland, Washington;
+Hanford Environmental Health Foundation, Richland, Washington;
‡University of Pittsburgh, Pittsburgh, Pennsylvania.

,

Introduction

On 30 August 1976, at 2:55 A.M., a 64-year-old nuclear chemical operator was injured by the chemical explosion of an ion exchange column used for americium recovery. The explosion occurred in a waste treatment facility operated under the auspices of the United States Energy Research and Development Administration (now the Department of Energy) in the state of Washington. The primary materials in the resin column were concentrated nitric acid, cation exchange resin, and americium. As a result of the impact of flying acid and debris, the operator sustained chemical burns of the face, eyes, neck, and right shoulder, as well as lacerations and embedded foreign bodies in these areas. He was heavily externally contaminated with americium and inhaled a significant quantity of the element.

Patient Care and Data Analysis

Initial Medical Care and Findings

The injured operator was assisted from the scene of the accident by coworkers, who were also contaminated with americium but to a much lesser extent. A health physics technician and a fellow operator, in protective clothing and respirators, removed the operator's contaminated clothing and began decontamination by flushing his face and eyes with water. Two registered nurses assigned to the area, wearing protective equipment, continued decontamination. An ambulance designed to handle contamination cases than transported him 40 km (25 miles) to the Emergency Decontamination Facility (EDF)[1] in Richland, Washington, where he arrived about 2 hours after the accident. Upon his arrival at the EDF, 1 gm of calcium diethylenetriaminepentate (Ca DTPA) was administered intravenously, and the operator was decontaminated further with soap and water in a shower. Removal of superficial foreign matter from the face and neck and irrigation of the eyes with normal saline were carried out by attending physicians and nurses. Surgical and opthalmological consultations were obtained.

Physical examination revealed chemical burns of the face, scalp, neck, and shoulder, with more severe involvement of the right than the left side. The surfaces of the eyes were hyperemic. The eyelids were swollen, and marked eyelid spasm was present. Crude testing indicated that vision was intact in both eyes. The blood pressure was 115/60 and the pulse 60/min with an occasional dropped beat (this condition had been present before the accident). The remainder of the examination was essentially normal.

Administration of DTPA was continued, with several doses given daily for the first month (Figure 1). DTPA chelates americium and other heavy metals, minimizing their deposition in the body and promoting their excretion in urine.[1] Since long-term therapy with this agent was anticipated, it was deemed advisable to switch at an early date from Ca DTPA to Zn DTPA. The rationale for the change to Zn DTPA was that prolonged frequent administration of Ca DTPA has been shown to cause major bodily depletion of Zn. At high levels of administration, the adverse effects observed have been more severe in experimental animals treated with Ca DTPA than in those treated with Zn DTPA.[2-6] Zn DTPA had been used clinically abroad but had not previously been approved for human use in the United States. The United States Food and Drug Administration provided permission to use Zn DTPA in this case.

Fluid intake was encouraged to promote urinary excretion. Liquid and

---

[1]The EDF is a detached facility adjacent to the Richland community hospital. It was built in 1963 by the United States Atomic Energy Commission as an emergency support facility for the Hanford production site. The EDF consists primarily of a large windowless room with supporting facilities for radiation and contamination control. The room has thick shielding walls and two heavily shielded enclosures to protect attending personnel against penetrating radiation; such protection was not necessary in this case. The ventilation system provides heating and cooling, and it exhausts through two banks of high-efficiency particulate air filters. All radioactive liquid wastes are collected in a holding tank. Storage space and change and wash rooms for support personnel are also present in the facility.

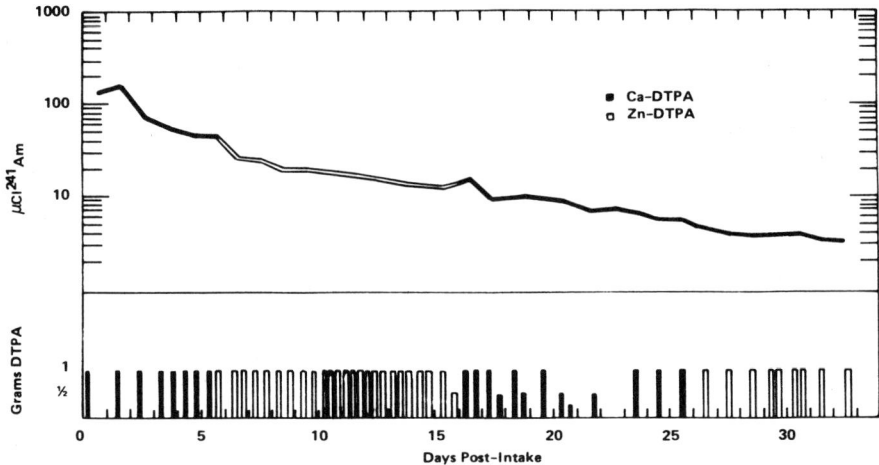

Figure 1. Early urinary excretion and DTPA administration.

solid intake and output were recorded, and all urinary and fecal specimens were collected separately for radiobioassay. The chemically burned areas on the face, neck, and right shoulder were left exposed; no dressings or external medications were used. Ophthalmic steroid-antibiotic ointment was instilled into each eye several times daily.

Facial contamination was monitored during the first few days by means of alpha radiation survey meters. However, since much of the contamination was embedded in the tissues of the face, primarily about the right eye and in the wound on the forehead, it soon became necessary to use more sophisticated equipment to measure the total burden present in the face. Based on measurements made using a sodium iodide detector, about 3000 microcuries of americium were estimated to have been deposited on the face, with an additional 300 microcuries embedded in the facial tissues. Another detector was used to measure the 3-, 17-, and 60-keV photons. The ratio of these emissions was used to estimate an average depth of 0.7 mm for the facial deposition.

One surgical effort using local anesthesia had been attempted during the first week to remove some of the larger and more deeply embedded foreign bodies from the face; a gamma-detecting probe was used to locate the deposited material. This effort proved unsuccessful because the larger foreign bodies identified by X-ray examination were apparently no more radioactive than the surrounding skin and subcutaneous tissue.

Decontamination Procedures

Decontamination procedures were undertaken twice daily for the first week after the accident; after this time, the same procedures were used once daily. During the decontamination procedure the patient, clothed in a disposable plastic suit, sat in a shower room that was filled with steam to promote sweating. The steaming was followed by a bath during which he was scrubbed and rinsed by properly protected attendants. During the bath, the patient's body was flushed with a DTPA solution[2] while he protected his eyes with soft washcloths. (Antibiotic ophthalmic ointment was applied to the eyes prior to the bath.) The DTPA solution was flushed off with water. Detergent soap (pHisohex®) was then scrubbed on the body and rinsed off with water. Because the patient's facial skin was tender from the chemical burns, he washed his face, including the area around his eyes, using diluted baby shampoo on soft toweling. The face was then flushed, and the procedure repeated several times. A Water-Pik® was used to clean the ears and the surrounding skin.

Baths as described were discontinued after two months, but daily showers for decontamination and general hygiene were continued. All decontamination solutions and wash liquids were collected in a holding tank, analyzed, and found to contain a total of about 4500 microcuries of americium. The hair of the patient's head and eyebrows was shaved during the first week because it could not be decontaminated. The hair and eyebrows subsequently grew back normally.

Long-term Medical Care and Findings

For the first four months, daily superficial debridement of the patient's face and neck was performed without anesthesia to remove scales, crusts, scabs, and extruded foreign bodies. The frequency of debridement was then decreased. Over a period of several months, metallic, plastic, cloth, and glass foreign bodies measuring up to 0.5 cm were extruded spontaneously or teased out with tweezers as they reached the skin surface.

An indolent superficial ulcer that occurred in the area of highest americium concentration (below the medial aspect of the right eyebrow) healed after 1 year, leaving a scar. Foreign matter was spontaneously extruded from the area prior to complete healing.

During the first month after the accident, multiple daily doses of Ca or Zn DTPA were administered intravenously; the patient was then given single 1-gm doses of Zn DTPA daily until July 1977, when the frequency of administration was reduced to three times per week.

Laboratory studies were conducted daily during the first three months and less frequently afterwards. They included complete blood counts, urinalyses, and blood chemistry (SMA 12/60) and fecal occult blood studies. The results of the studies were normal except that the peripheral

---

[2]Ca DTPA was used in the external decontamination solution, mixed initially in proportions of one-third DTPA (25%) solution and two-thirds normal saline. Later, Shubert's solution[7] (a DTPA solution with other chelates) was prepared and used for external decontamination.

blood lymphocyte count declined from 1860/mm³ on the day of the accident to 530/mm³ 1 week later. The average lymphocyte count was 943 (range: 590–1640) for the next eight months and 1522 (range: 728–3170) for the following 15 months. Previous lymphocyte counts had been 1520 in January 1976, 2332 in 1973, 2805 in 1970, and 3151 in 1967. Serial chest X-rays, pulmonary function tests, and electrocardiograms have shown no significant findings.

Special studies included several analyses of peripheral blood lymphocyte chromosomes, a facial skin biopsy, and a bone marrow examination. Radiation-induced cytogenetic lesions in lymphocytes were observed. (Variation in the frequency of radiation-damaged lymphocytes as a function of time after the accident will be the subject of a separate report.) The skin biopsy revealed scattered alpha "stars"; all other changes were compatible with the patient's age. The bone marrow examination was performed two weeks after the accident and was normal. None of these studies indicated the need for a change of therapy.

The staff psychologist was involved early in the care of the patient and has continued to provide advice to the staff and care to the patient and his family.

After 2.5 months of treatment in the windowless room of the EDF, the patient was transferred to a 9-m-long (30-foot-long) travel trailer adjacent to the EDF, which provided a transitional, controlled environment before his return home. While the patient, his wife, and their dog lived in the trailer, wastes were collected and measured for radioactivity, and routine surveys of the environment were made. From mid-November 1976 until his discharge in late January 1977, no americium contamination was found in the trailer.

The principal medical problem since the accident has involved the patient's eyes, which suffered corneal nitric acid burns and contained a few superficial corneal and conjunctival foreign bodies; the latter were excised or spontaneously extruded over a period of several months. In addition, a traumatically induced cataract began to develop in the left eye several months after the accident and was surgically removed in February 1978. The cataract had none of the characteristics usually associated with radiation induction. The patient was fitted with glasses and has been able to obtain a renewal of his state motor vehicle driver's license. His visual acuity has been improved by the use of special eyeglass covers with multiple perforations that reduce distortion caused by the chemically induced corneal irregularities.

Radioisotope Dosimetry Evaluation

Early measurements *in vivo* were difficult to make accurately because of the gross external contamination. Interpretation of the measurements was further complicated by the fact that the intake resulted from both inhalation and solubilization of the americium embedded in the facial tissue. Special equipment and techniques that will be described in a later report were improvised, and measurements of the americium deposited in the patient's chest, liver, and bone were initially obtained three days after the accident.

A cone-shaped, collimated sodium iodide (NaI) detector 1 mm thick and 5.1 cm in diameter was used to measure the isotope of americium 241 in each lung and in the liver. A lead shield was placed between the patient's head and chest to eliminate scattered radiation from the face, which otherwise greatly increased the count rate in the detector.

Forty microcuries of americium were measured in the lungs on day 3 after the accident, indicating a dose rate of 11 rad/day to the lungs. Subsequently, routine measurements of lung activity were made to determine the rate of clearance from the lungs (Figure 2). After 300 days, the activity remaining was largely attributed to americium in the ribs. The cumulative average dose to the lungs through 1978 was estimated to be 200 rad.

Figure 2. *In vivo* chest counts.

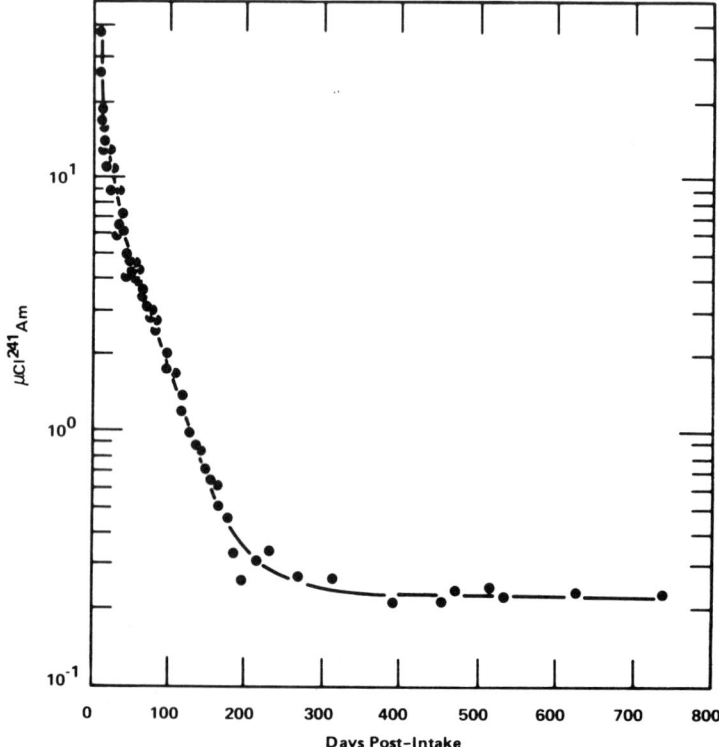

The liver burden on day 3 post-intake was 40 microcuries. Clearance from the liver was rapid (Figure 3) and the activity remaining after 300 days was also considered to reside in the ribs. The DTPA chelation therapy was largely responsible for the rapid clearance, which reduced this dose rate from 7 rad/day on day 3 to less than 0.03 rad/day at the end of 1978. The cumulative dose to the liver through 1978 was estimated to be 160 rad.

Initially, the activity in a small section of bone directly below the knee cap was measured using an NaI detector, and was related to the total bone burden using a model based on data from baboon studies.[8] Through this technique, the bone burden on day 3 post-intake was estimated to be 40 microcuries. Subsequently, the counting procedure was calibrated by distributing americium sources uniformly on the inner bone surfaces of a cadaver leg. Using this technique, the estimated bone burden for day 3 was revised to 70 microcuries, which indicates a dose rate of about 3 rad/day. By day 30 post-intake, the bone burden had decreased to approximately 25 microcuries (1 rad/day) and has remained at that level. The estimated cumulative bone dose was about 860 rad through 1978, and we expect the dose to continue at a rate of 1 rad/day. Without DTPA therapy, the bone burden would be expected to increase substantially over time because of the translocation of americium from the soft tissue of the face.

The dose to the lens of the eye was calculated to evaluate the possibility that the cataract that developed was due to radiation. The maximum initial dose rate of about 4 rad/day decreased sharply with time. The estimated cumulative dose to the lens of the eye was 140 rad through 1978. This is significantly less than the 500 rad or more associated with cataract formation.

Bioassay Data and Effectiveness of DTPA Therapy

All urinary and fecal specimens were collected and analyzed for americium content prior to the patient's discharge home and, subsequently, on an intermittent basis. Treatment with DTPA, which was started within three hours of the accident and has continued ever since, drastically alters the usual patterns of americium excretion. Therefore, the bioassay data could not be used to estimate the systemic burden. However, these data were useful in determining the effectiveness of the DTPA therapy and the need for continuing treatment.

The amount of americium initially available for deposition in the body may be estimated by adding to the amount excreted in the urine and feces the quantity estimated to remain in the bone, liver, and facial skin. The calculated total is about 1100 microcuries of americium. (See Table 1 for a summary of the deposition and excretion data.) Using models derived from animal experimentation, we estimate that a total of 760

352

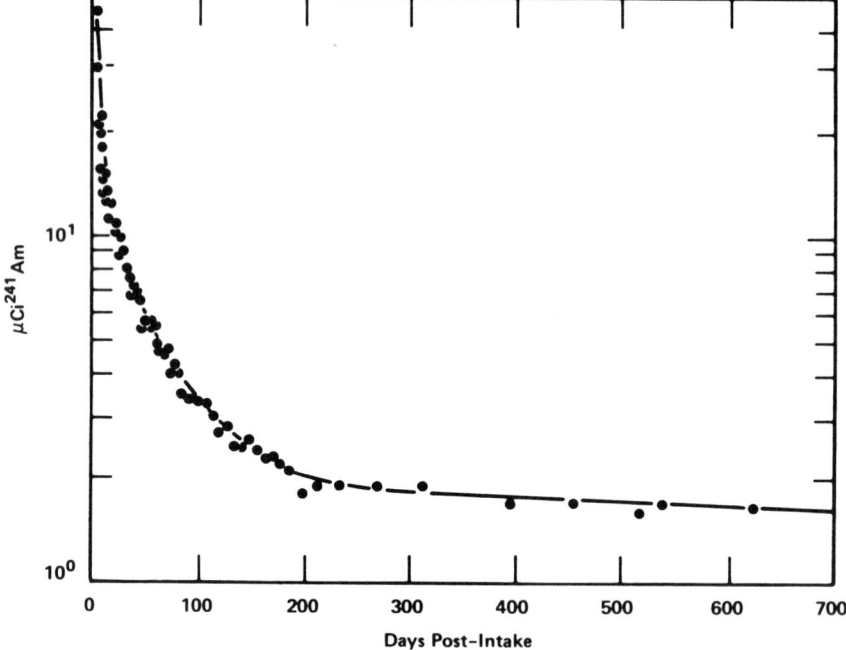

Figure 3. *In vivo* liver counts.

microcuries would have been deposited in bone and liver if DTPA therapy had not been available. Since only about 25 microcuries were retained (see Figure 4), we believe that the DTPA was better than 95% effective in reducing the anticipated body burdens. The early data on urinary excretion, shown in Figure 1, indicate that Zn DTPA was as effective as Ca DTPA in the decorporation of americium. Neither clinical

Table 1. Fate of Americium in Microcurie Quantities

	Time Post-Intake					
	Day 1	Day 3	Day 10	Day 60	1 Year	2 Years
Burdens						
Facial skin	300		300	150	35	20
Chest		40	15	5	2	1.5
Bone		70	30	25	25	25
Liver		40	16	4	0.2	0.2
Cumulative Excretion						
Urine	150	400	600	840	880	890
Feces	0	130	180	185	190	200

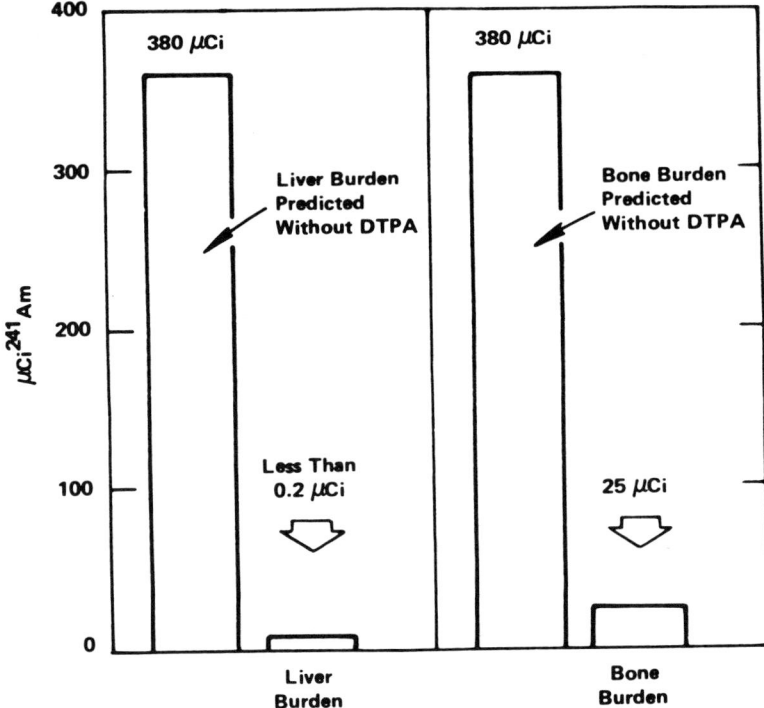

Figure 4. Effectiveness of DTPA in reducing liver and bone burdens.

nor laboratory findings showed evidence of toxicity from the use of DTPA.

Current Clinical Status

More than two years after the accident, the patient is experiencing no symptoms definitely attributable to the radiation exposure. There is no evidence of functional impairment in the bone, lung, or liver; the cumulative doses to these organs are, respectively, 860, 200, and 160 rad. The patient continues to have visual difficulty as previously outlined, but the condition is stable.

Case Management

Team Approach to Decision-making

A team approach was used to arrive at decisions regarding treatment and arrangements for the patient's care after his discharge. The team, which consisted of the patient, staff and consulting physicians and radiobiologists, the staff psychologist, health physicists, nurses, and radiation monitors, met frequently and many of the procedures and methods used were based on the consensus of the assembled group. Including the patient in the decision-making process was invaluable, not only in obtaining his concurrence in the choice and application of procedures but also in giving us the benefit of his knowledge, based on his long experience in the industry. His understanding, willing cooperation, and concern that his experience benefit others were exemplary.

Public Relations

The case aroused national and international interest, both in the scientific community and in the communications media. In the days immediately after the accident, time demands by the media were great and required careful control to prevent interference with the proper care of the patient. The situation was further complicated by the need to secure the patient's privacy and prevent the dissemination of privileged information. From the beginning, public relations professionals worked closely and effectively with the medical and scientific staff. The importance of carefully organizing the public relations aspects of such an emergency cannot be overemphasized.

Conclusions

1. Unusually high levels of americium deposition have not caused any demonstrably harmful effects in the patient during a two-year period of observation.
2. Prompt and intensive chelation therapy proved extremely effective in this case. Zinc DTPA appeared to be as effective as Ca DTPA in removing americium from the body and preventing its translocation. No toxicity from the DTPA therapy was observed over a two-year period.
3. The "total" person must be treated. Not only must medical and health physics concerns be considered, but also the psychological effects, the impacts on family and friends, and the response of the patient to extended inactivity.
4. The use of a team approach to decision-making was highly successful and helped surmount the many difficulties encountered in this case.
5. The use of a transitional discharge regime (EDF, trailer, home) was beneficial psychologically and assured adequate control of contamination from bodily sources (i.e., contaminated skin flakes or scales, and excretion products).
6. Careful organization of the handling of public relations under the stress of an emergency is well worth the effort.

ACKNOWLEDGMENTS
Many scientists and health professionals at Hanford and across the United States contributed valuable recommendations on the management of the case. Individual contributions will be acknowledged in several papers being prepared for publication in the near future. We also wish to acknowledge the cooperation of the patient, who throughout his long and trying experience has done everything possible to ensure that his experience will be used to benefit others in the future.

This was prepared for the U.S. Department of Energy under Contract EY-76-C-06-1830.

References

1. Lloyd RD, McFarland SS, Taylor, GN, Williams, JL, Mays CW: Decorporation of ^{241}Am in beagles by DTPA. *Radiat Res* 62:97–106, 1975.

2. Taylor GN, Williams JT, Roberts L, Atherton DR, Shabestari L: Increased toxicity of Na$_3$Ca DTP when given by protracted administration. *Health Phys* 27:285–288, 1974.

3. Seidel A: Removal from the rat of internally deposited ^{241}Am by long-term treatment with Ca-Zn DTPA. *Radia Res* 61:478–487, 1975.

4. Planas-Bohne F, Olinger H: On the influence of Ca DTPA on the Zn- and Mn-concentrations in various organs of the rat. *Health Phys* 31(2):165–166, 1976.

5. Lloyd RD, Mays CW, McFarland SS, Taylor GN, Atherton DR: A comparison of Ca DTPA and Zn-DTPA for chelating ^{241}Am in beagles. *Health Phys* 31:281–284, 1976.

6. Ohlenschlager L: Efficiency of Zn-DTPA in removing plutonium from the human body. *Health Phys* 30:249–250, 1976.

7. Wald N, Wechsler R, Brodsky A, Yaniv S: Problems in independent medical management of plutonium-americium contaminated patients, in *Diagnosis and Treatment of Deposited Radionuclides*, Kornberg HA, Norwood D (eds.): Excerpta Medica Foundation, 1968, p. 579.

8. Rosen JC, Cohen N, Wrenn ME: Short-term metabolism of ^{241}Am in the adult baboon. *Health Phys* 22:621–626, 1972.

Published 1980 by Elsevier North Holland, Inc.
K. F. Hübner and S. A. Fry, eds. The Medical Basis for Radiation Accident Preparedness

In Vitro Human Cytogenetic Dose-Response Systems

Russell J. DuFrain, L. Gayle Littlefield, Eugene E. Joiner, and Edward L. Frome

Radiation Emergency Assistance Center/Training Site (REAC/TS), Medical and Health Sciences Division, Oak Ridge Associated Universities, Oak Ridge, Tennessee.

Introduction

To provide dosimetry for radiation accident management, *in vitro* dose-response models are used for deriving biological estimates of the doses received by the individuals involved in accidents. The actual dose estimates are made by comparing the frequency of specific cytogenetic aberrations in the cultured blood lymphocytes of the individual involved in the accident with the frequency observed in human lymphocytes irradiated *in vitro*. The central assumption in this line of reasoning is that if the important *in vivo* exposure conditions can be duplicated *in vitro*, the quantitative response of the lymphocytes, at least in chromosome aberration induction, will be identical. If this basic assumption is true, and there are many reports of studies with experimental animals[1-5] and in man[6-9] that indicate that it is, we have a relatively simple method for accurately estimating the radiation dose absorbed by the lymphocytes of an exposed individual. For most accidental exposures this dose to lymphocytes can be assumed to be an "equivalent whole-body" dose.[10-12]

Three kinds of factors influence the accuracy of the *in vitro* dose-response relation determinations and thus the accuracy of the estimated dose for individuals involved in radiation accidents. These are the biological aspects of the human lymphocyte and the *in vitro* culture system; statistical and mathematical aspects of the data collection and analysis for dose estimation; and the physical conditions of the *in vitro* radiation exposure. Each of these topics will be briefly discussed in one of the three following sections. Finally, examples of *in vitro* dose-response curves generated by the cytogenetics group at Oak Ridge Associated Universities (ORAU) in response to the needs for dose estimates in specific radiation accidents involving americium 241[13] and iridium 192[14] exposures will be presented.

Biological Aspects

The induction of chromosome aberrations in peripheral blood lymphocytes is used as a quantitative measure of radiation dose in both the *in vitro* dose-response systems and the estimation of dose in exposed individuals.[10−12,15−26] Fortunately, these lymphocytes are uniform in radiosensitivity,[18,27] relatively long-lived[28−31] and circulate rapidly throughout the body.[10] The cells are synchronized in a post-mitotic pre-DNA synthetic (G_0) state, which leads to the uniform radiosensitivity and the induction of chromosome type abnormalities.[32,33] Although a variety of lesions are induced by radiation,[32,34] a two-break asymmetrical chromosome type exchange, the dicentric chromosome with accompanying fragment, is now accepted as the standard for human radiation dosimetry.[35] Because human T lymphocytes are long-lived,[29−31] blood can be drawn for dosimetry up to several weeks after exposure without significant loss of the lesion bearing lymphocytes.[8,36] The rapid circulation of the lymphocytes through the body tends to integrate the dose and makes possible estimates of whole-body equivalent dose following exposure to penetrating low-LET radiation.[8,12] These factors are important aspects of the lymphocyte system, and along with the ease of obtaining blood samples and the standardized lymphocyte culture methods[37−40] are primary reasons that the peripheral lymphocyte has become the human biological dosimeter.

The techniques for culturing peripheral blood lymphocytes and obtaining appropriate material for cytogenetic evaluation have been described and discussed in detail elsewhere by several authors[26,37−41] and will only be briefly touched on here. In the system used by the cytogenetics group at ORAU,[41] leukocyte rich plasma obtained from settled venous blood collected in vacuum tubes is added to tissue culture medium (Medium 199) that is supplemented with cell-free autologous plasma. The culture is supplemented with phytohemagglutinin, a mitogenic agent that induces a blastic transformation of the lymphocytes and a resumption of mitotic activity, and grown at 37°C for two days. In cytogenetic dosimetry, culture time is an important factor[20,37,42−44] since lymphocytes cultured for longer than two days traverse several cell cycles,[27,45] which reduces the frequency of dicentric chromosomes,[46−48] the lesions upon which we base our dose estimate. Recently, Scott[27] has shown that lymphocytes in their first mitosis after *in vitro* radiation exposure have the same dicentric/cell frequency regardless of the time of harvest. However, for such analyses 5-bromodeoxyuridine (BrdU) must be added to the cultures to distinguish between metaphases in their first or subsequent *in vitro* division.[49] The cultures are treated with a spindle blocking agent, terminated, and prepared for microscopic observation as previously described.[41] Staining is routinely accomplished with a 5% Giemsa solution or in the case of cells which incorporated BrdU, a fluorescence plus Giemsa (FPG) technique[49] is used to identify cells that replicated their DNA more than one time during the *in vitro* culture period.

The resulting preparations are scanned at low power (100×) for mitotic figures. Adequately spread metaphases are analyzed in detail at 1250×. Only metaphases with 45 or 46 centromeres are accepted for lesion evaluation, and all chromosome aberrations are recorded, with the exception of the gap (a staining discontinuity of less than the width of the chromatid). Metaphases from the cells grown in BrdU supplemented medium are scored if the chromatids are uniformly dark, indicating one *in vitro* DNA synthesis.[49]

When *in vitro* dose-response curves for chromosome aberration induction in irradiated lymphocytes are generated, it is absolutely essential that the *in vivo* conditions are mimicked as closely as possible. For example, for *in vitro* exposure to penetrating forms of radiation, whole blood maintained at 37°C[37,39] is irradiated under conditions of venous oxygen tension;[50,51] whereas, for particle emitting nuclides the blood is mixed with tissue culture medium containing the isotope[52,53] and subsequently washed before culture. The culture and harvest procedures are identical to those described above.

Mathematical Aspects

Several mathematical considerations are important in developing the *in vitro* dose response systems and in applying these results to actual cases of accidental exposure. Initially, the appropriate underlying distributions for the aberration data need to be determined and confirmed. Radiation biology studies have historically shown that energy deposition events, which result in chromosome aberrations, are random in cells exposed to radiations and that in most instances the data collected were counts. Because of the random, quantal nature of the events, the dispersion of chromosome lesions in cells is adequately described by a Poisson distribution in which the mean is equal to the variance.[54] The main ramification of this is that statistics based on the normal distribution where the mean and variance are assumed to be independent are not appropriate for analysis. In a recent report by Edwards,[55] the analysis of over 50,000 metaphases from irradiated human lymphocytes showed that the Poisson distribution adequately described the dispersion of dicentrics for low-LET and some forms of high-LET radiation. We recently found that in samples of 100 metaphases from alpha-particle-irradiated lymphocytes the variations in total dicentrics (i.e., dicentrics/100 cells) can be adequately described by the Poisson distribution, although the distribution in individual metaphases is overdispersed.[53] Partial-body exposures to low-LET radiation and non-uniform irradiation from internal deposition of radionuclides also lead to overdispersion of dicentrics[17,56–61] as does neutron irradiation.[12,56,62] For a detailed discussion of the statistical methods used in this type of dispersion analysis, see the appendix of the detailed review by Savage[63] or other, more technical treatment.[64,65]

A second mathematical problem involves determination of the number of metaphases that need to be evaluated. A practical and financial aspect of this problem is that a trained observer can average scoring about 50 metaphases per working day. In a previous analysis,[66] we have shown that evaluation of 200 to 500 metaphases is usually sufficient for dose estimation in medically significant accidental exposures. This is in agreement with the number of evaluations recommended by the British NRPB.[67] For the *in vitro* dose-response relation, determination of the number of different doses to be evaluated and the number of cells per dose, both vary depending on the dose levels of interest and the quality of the radiation. Values used range from a few hundred cells at four or five doses to 10 to 20 thousand cells for some low dose low-LET determinations.[39] We are currently evaluating methods for optimizing the effort in cell scoring for *in vitro* dose response parameter determinations. Some of the problems encountered in this analysis are different shapes of dose response curves for different qualities of radiation (Figure 1), dependence of some of the dose-response parameters on rate of dose for some qualities of radiation, but not for others (Table 1), and optimization of parameters and their variances for nonlinear, non-normally distributed, quadratic curves with nonzero intercepts. Another mathematical problem involves the determination of appropriate methods for model verification for data with the attributes described above. This is essential if the shapes of *in vitro* dose-response curves are to be verified and used for extrapolations. Some questions about the quadratic dose response for low-LET penetrating radiation continue to arise[68,69] and are refuted[70] but cannot be completely put to rest until better statistical model testing methods are developed.

A final statistical problem under current investigation involves the estimation of variation in the amount of exposure to radiation when cytogenetic dosimetry is performed. Or more simply, "How do we derive a confidence interval for our dose estimates?" The mathematics involved becomes tedious, but basically two methods have been proposed.[66,67] A maximum likelihood method is described by Edwards.[67,70] Its salient

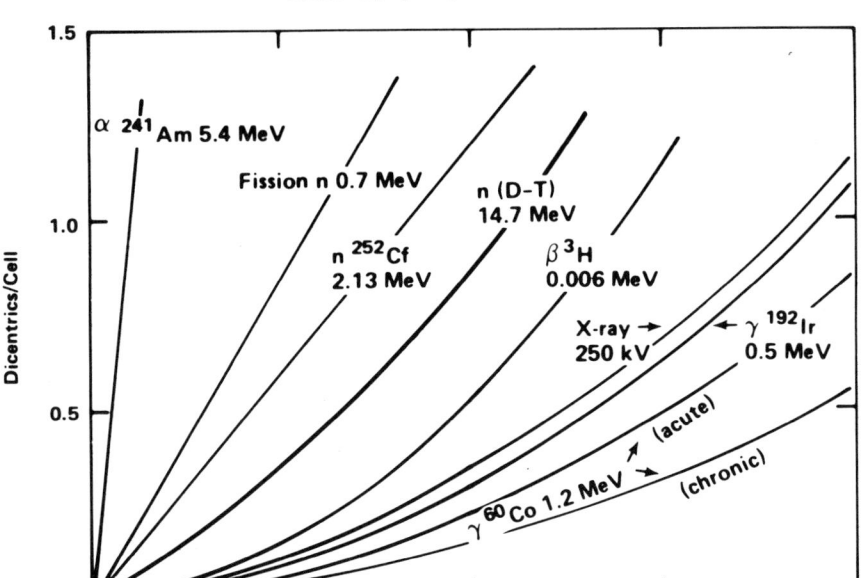

Figure 1. A series of generalized dose-response curves for dicentric chromosome induction when human lymphocytes are irradiated *in vitro*. Coefficients for the Y = αD and Y = αD + βD² equations used to generate the curves are given in Table 1 (denoted by *a*).

feature is the fact that the large amounts of data collected in the generation of *in vitro* dose-response curves render their parameters so little variance that estimated confidence intervals for exposure are based on the Poisson variances of the dicentric/cell frequencies observed in the lymphocyte samples from the exposed individuals. We recently described an alternative method requiring dose-response curves with somewhat less data.[66] It is valid for linear or quadratic polynomials that pass through the origin and assumes the dicentric/cell yield for both the dose-response curve and the unknown exposure follow the Poisson distribution.

Several other statistical and mathematical considerations are in need of investigation, but for the sake of brevity will only be mentioned. What is the role of individual variation in cytogenetic dose estimation?[25,43] Can the dose-response models be extrapolated to environmental or background-dose levels?[71] What are adequate sample sizes for internal contamination and localized exposures?[60,67] These few examples ade-

Table 1. Coefficients Reported for Dose-Response Relationships for Human Lymphocytes Irradiated in Vitro

Type of radiation	$a \times 10^{-4}$	$\beta \times 10^{-6}$	Reference
^{60}Co γ 1.2 & 1.3 MeV[a]	1.6	5.0	Lloyd 1975 (39)[b]
^{60}Co γ 1.2 & 1.3 MeV[a] (chronic)	1.8	2.9	Lloyd 1975 (39)
^{60}Co γ 1.2 & 1.3 MeV	3.9	8.2	Brewen 1972 (8)
^{60}Co γ 1.2 & 1.3 MeV	0.9	6.8	Sasaki 1971 (22)
^{60}Co γ 1.2 & 1.3 MeV	2.7	4.8	Bauchinger 1979 (75)
^{60}Co γ 1.2 & 1.3 MeV (chronic)	2.7	3.0	Bauchinger 1979 (75)
^{60}Co γ 1.2 & 1.3 MeV	5.7	3.2	Brenot 1974 (76)
^{137}Cs γ 0.67 MeV	6.8	0.7	Brewen 1971 (74)
^{192}Ir γ 0.59, 0.47 Mev[a]	3.2	6.1	this chapter
^{3}H β 0.006 MeV[a]	3.1	12.0	Bocian 1977 (52)
e^{-} 15 MeV (microseconds)	0.9	6.1	Purrott 1977 (77)
e^{-} 15 MeV	0.6	5.7	Purrott 1977 (77)
e^{-} 3 MeV	2.6	3.5	Schmid 1974 (78)
X-ray 30 kV	11.1	8.7	Virsik 1977 (79)
X-ray 150 kV	−0.2	7.4	Virsik 1977 (79)
X-ray 180 kV	4.0	2.6	Liniecki 1973 (50)
X-ray 180 kV	9.1	6.3	Bocian 1977 (52)
X-ray 200 kV	7.5	7.1	Sasaki 1971 (22)
X-ray 220 kV	7.8	4.2	Schmid 1972 (24)
X-ray 220 kV	7.9	5.4	Schmid 1976 (80)
X-ray 250 kV	5.6	5.5	Bender 1969 (20)
X-ray 250 kV	3.6	6.7	Vulpis 1974 (81)
X-ray 250 kV[a]	4.8	6.2	Lloyd 1975 (39)
X-ray 250 kV	6.3	6.5	Carrano 1975 (73)
X-ray 1.9 MeV	0.9	4.3	Norman 1966 (82)
− π ions (plateau)	13.4	2.8	Purrott 1978 (83)
− π ions (peak)	23.4	4.8	Purrott 1978 (83)
D-T neutrons 15.0 MeV	14.1	3.8	Bauchinger 1975 (84)
D-T neutrons 14.7 MeV[a]	26.2	8.8	Lloyd 1976 (62)
D-T neutrons 14.1 MeV	25.0	3.7	Sasaki 1971 (22)
D-Be neutrons 7.6 MeV	47.8	6.4	Lloyd 1976 (62)
D-Be neutrons 6.2 MeV	33.8	−	Biola 1974 (85)
^{252}Cf neutrons 2.13 MeV[a]	60.0	−	Lloyd 1978 (72)
D-Be neutrons 2.0 MeV	74.5	−	Sasaki 1971 (22)
Fission neutrons 1.5 MeV	64.8	−	Biola 1974 (85)
Fission neutrons (Nereide)	87.4	−	Biola 1974 (85)
Fission neutrons (Crac)	90.1	−	Biola 1974 (85)
Fission neutrons (IRT-200)	26.6	−	Todorova 1973 (86)
Fission neutrons 0.7 MeV	84.9	−	Scott 1969 (56)
Fission neutrons 0.90 MeV	72.8	−	Lloyd 1976 (62)
Fission neutrons 0.85 MeV	78.4	−	Carrano 1975 (73)
Fission neutrons 0.70 MeV[a]	83.5	−	Lloyd 1976 (62)
^{241}Am $\propto$ 5.5 MeV[a]	489.8	−	DuFrain 1979 (53)

[a] Values used to generate curves in Figure 1.

[b] Numbers in parentheses () refer to source.

quately illustrate the need for further studies aimed at developing and testing appropriate statistical models and methodologies.

Physical Aspects

The two primarily physical aspects of radiation exposure of human lymphocytes pertain to radiation quality and delivery. Radiation quality can be roughly divided into two components as far as cytogenetic dosimetry is concerned. These are low-LET penetrating radiations and high-LET radiations, which may be penetrating as is the case for certain types of neutrons or of limited range in the case of alpha particles. In general, the high-LET radiation results in linear dose-response curves such as those reported for americium 241 alpha particles,[53] californium 252 neutrons,[72] 0.85 MeV fission neutrons,[73] and 0.7 MeV and 0.9 MeV fission neutrons.[62] The linear dose-response model $Y = \alpha D$ (Y is dicentric/cell; alpha is the slope coefficient of the curve; and D is the dose in rads) is adequate for describing this data. As the energy of neutrons increases their LET decreases and the $Y = \alpha D$ model needs a second term, becoming quadratic with $Y = \alpha D + \beta D^2$ necessary to adequately describe the relation. This has been demonstrated for 7.6 and 14.7 MeV-neutron irradiation of human lymphocytes.[62] The cytogenetic explanation for the quadratic dose-response curve is that some dicentrics are caused by single energy deposition events, while others are caused by the interaction of two events (thus increasing with the square of the dose). As a rule, as the neutron energy increases the LET falls and the energy deposition becomes less dense along the track of the neutron leading to the $Y = \alpha D + \beta D^2$ relation. Dose-response relations for acute doses of low-LET radiation are described by the $Y = \alpha D + \beta D^2$ function for the same reason (the energy deposition events are more widely scattered). The alpha and beta coefficients have been derived by numerous authors for X-rays and ^{60}Co-gamma rays and are in general agreement when the methods used for dose-response curve generation are well controlled.[39] The coefficients of dose have also been derived for ^{3}H beta particles,[52] ^{137}Cs gamma rays,[74] and will be given for ^{192}Ir-gamma rays in this report. Table 1 is a listing of the coefficients of dose for several qualities of radiation reported when exposure is under *in vivo* simulating conditions, and induced dicentrics or dicentrics plus centric rings per cell are recorded as the response. For the 9 radiations denoted by an "a," generalized dose-response curves are shown in Figure 1. For dose estimation in exposed individuals, the dose-response curve corresponding to the quality of radiation seen in ʾhe accident should be used, or if an appropriate curve is not availabl·, one of similar radiation type and energy should be selected.

The other major physical factor involved in cytogenetic dose-response relationship determination is the dose rate,[87] which is important for low-

LET but not for most high-LET radiation.[88] In the quadratic equation the βD^2 component is dependent on dose rate because it is presumed to result from an interaction of events and is thus lower when the events are temporally further apart.[75,80,87] When the dose rate for low-LET radiation decreases to near environmental levels, the βD^2 term is apparently eliminated as was recently demonstrated so clearly for the occupational exposure of shipyard workers in England.[89]

When the dose rate is important in human cytogenetic dosimetry, a newly developed method for determining the dependency of dicentric frequency on rate can be applied.[75] This study showed that by using the mean interaction time of primary breaks of about 110 min and the G function of Lea,[80] $\{G(\chi) = (2/\chi^2) [\chi-1 + \exp (-\chi)]\}$, a theoretically predicted dose-response curve of dicentrics/cell on dose could be generated for 1.7 rad/min-exposed lymphocytes from data collected at 50 rad/min. Then they demonstrated that the predicted curve and an experimentally derived curve from 1.7 rad/min exposures did not differ statistically.[80] Thus, if the individual exposure rate in a radiation accident involving low-LET radiation is substantially different from the rate used in the generation of the calibration curve, a theoretical curve can be generated and used in dose estimation. However, the upper limit on dose estimation will always be a value estimated on the basis of the linear or αD component. Again, the study of shipyard workers provides evidence to support this line of reasoning.[89]

In vitro Dose-response Curve Generation

Following the Richland, Washington, accident[13] and our initial evaluations of the cytogenetic aberrations induced in the survivor's lymphocytes by the massive americium 241 contamination,[61] we developed a method for the in vitro irradiation of human lymphocytes with ^{241}Am alpha particles.[53] Briefly, the method involves mixing human blood with soluble ^{241}Am dissolved in dilute nitric acid and tissue culture medium, which allows a short, but precisely measured exposure period, extensively washing the blood, and subsequently culturing the lymphocytes by standard methods. The dose-response curve that resulted from this study is shown redrawn in Figure 2; the dicentric induction dose-response equation ($Y = 4.9 \pm .42 \times 10^{-2}$ D) was calculated by a weighted least squares method appropriate to the type of data collected.[90] The distribution of a type of two-break asymmetric exchange (dicentric) is presented in Table 2. This tabulation shows the overdispersion of the dicentrics when compared with the expected Poisson values. The probability values shown in Table 2 were calculated by Fisher's method,[64] which is the most exact and thus appropriate statistical method for this particular case. The overdispersion noted here is also a characteristic of

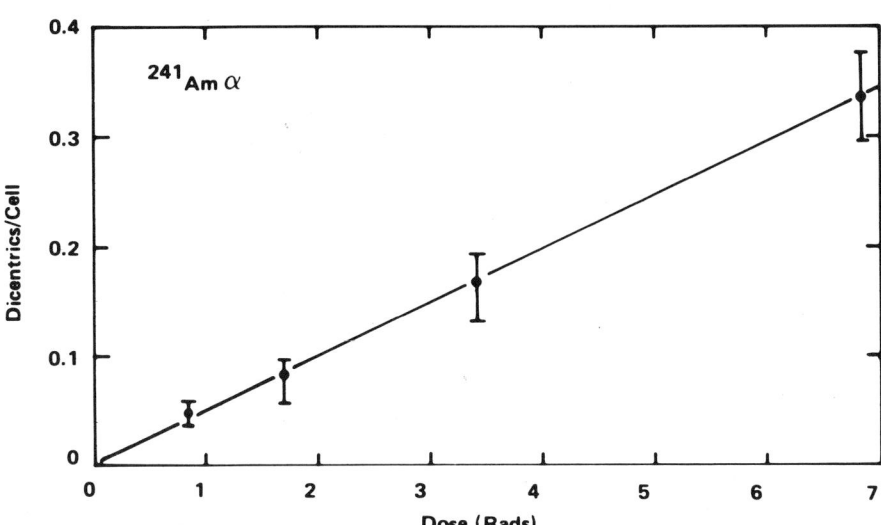

Figure 2. A dose-response curve for dicentric chromosome induction in human lymphocytes by alpha particles from ^{241}Am. The uncertainties shown on the data points are standard errors based on the assumption of a Poisson distribution. Doses were calculated from specific activities as described in detail elsewhere.[53]

other high-LET radiations, such as fast neutrons.[55] Subsequent studies in our laboratory with higher doses of radiation from ^{241}Am alpha particles have consistently shown this overdispersion of dicentrics when the Poisson distribution is used as a basis for comparison. Unfortunately, these higher doses lead to a saturation of the dose-response curve, probably because of cell death.

To use this derived relationship for point and 95% confidence interval estimates, we use the methods described previously,[66] which are illustrated in Figure 3. For the point estimate from the $Y = \alpha D$ equation we simply substitute 4.9×10^{-2} for alpha, the observed dicentrics per cell value from the survivor's lymphocyte cultures for Y, and solve for the radiation dose, D. Determination of the interval estimate for 95% confidence requires the number of dicentrics observed, the number of cells scored and values from the variance-covariance matrix derived from the dose-response curve data.[66] Then it is simply a matter of substituting the values into a pair of likelihood equations, determining the unknowns in a pair of second-order-polynomial equations, and extracting the roots of the quadratic form of a polynomial [Equation 13 in Frome and DuFrain[66]]. These roots represent the upper and lower boundaries of the confidence interval.

Table 2. A Distributional Analysis of Alpha-Particle-Induced Dicentric Chromosomes

Dose	Dicentrics	Cells	$\overline{X}$	Frequency of cells with number of dicentrics							Probability[a]
				0	1	2	3	4	5	6	
0.85 rad	19	400	.0475	Exp. 381	19	0	0	0	0	0	
				Obs. 386	10	3	1	0	0	0	<.001
1.71 rad	15	200	.0750	Exp. 185	15	0	0	0	0	0	
				Obs. 187	11	2	0	0	0	0	<.002
3.42 rad	33	200	.1650	Exp. 169	29	2	0	0	0	0	
				Obs. 178	14	5	3	0	0	0	<.001
6.84 rad	67	200	.3350	Exp. 143	48	8	1	0	0	0	
				Obs. 160	23	12	2	2	0	1	<.001

[a] Calculated from Fisher's exact test for a Poisson Distribution.[64]

Figure 3. The americium 241 dose-response curve with 95% confidence interval belts for 400 metaphases evaluated. The method of point and interval estimation for an observed 155 dicentric equivalents in 400 evaluated metaphases is shown.

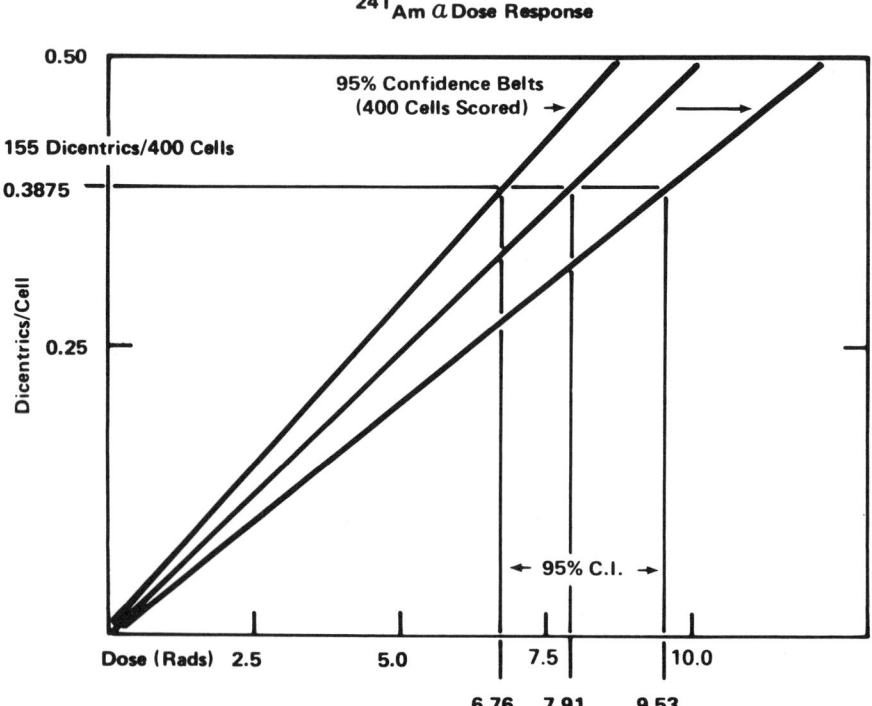

As an example, we will use the data from the 3-month blood samples from the ^{241}Am contamination accident.[61] A total of 155 dicentric equivalents were observed in the 400 metaphases evaluated, giving a rate of 0.3875 dicentrics per metaphase scored, which when divided by the 4.9×10^{-2} dicentric/cell/rad coefficient gives a point estimate of 7.91 rad. For a 95% confidence interval the appropriate values are substituted into the equations given by Frome and DuFrain[66] and result in the quadratic form: $0 = 23.303 - 379.642\chi + 1501.563\chi^2$, which when solved for χ gives roots of 6.76 and 9.53 that in rads are the lower and upper bounds of the 95% confidence interval for the dose estimate. All of these curves and values are shown on Figure 3. These derived values pertain to the estimated average radiation dose absorbed by the circulating blood lymphocytes. For a discussion of the interpretation and significance of these estimated values see Littlefield et al.[61]

In conjunction with the accidental exposure to a high localized dose of ^{192}Ir gamma radiation,[14] the cytogenetics laboratory of ORAU obtained a blood sample for cytogenetic dosimetry 44 days after the accident.[61] A rapid survey of the appropriate scientific literature revealed that no ^{192}Ir-gamma-radiation dose-response curve for human lymphocytes existed. Because of this finding and the fact that accidental exposures to ^{192}Ir appears to be widespread,[23,35,61,91] we set out to generate a dose-response curve for ^{192}Ir gamma radiation, although we expected that the dose-response relationship would be similar to other low-LET penetrating types. Our expectations were confirmed as the dose-response curve (Figure 1) for the gamma radiation from ^{192}Ir falls between the X-ray and ^{60}Co gamma curves of the British NRPB.[39]

To generate the dose-response curve shown in Figure 4, we used our standard lymphocyte culturing methods after exposure of heparinized whole venous blood maintained at 37°C. Tubes of blood and water filled tubes containing thermoluminescent dosimeters (TLDs) were placed in an arc 12.5 cm from the point where a 24.0 curie ^{192}Ir radiography source (Automation Industries model 520-008) would emerge from its shield. The calculated exposure rate of 12.3 R/min., as confirmed by the TLD's, was given to various tubes to total doses of 50, 100, 200, and 400 rad. After the exposure, lymphocyte cultures were initiated and supplemented with BrdU so that only first division metaphases would be scored for dicentrics.[27] The scoring of dicentrics in first division metaphases was partitioned to minimize the variance of the alpha and beta coefficients in the quadratic dose-response equation by using some exploratory statistical methodology. The technique involves scoring 50 metaphases at each dose, estimating parameters (i.e., coefficients) by a weighted least squares method, and determining how many more metaphases should be scored at each dose (minimum at each dose 100) to reduce the variation in the estimated alpha and beta coefficients of the quadratic equation. The data from the first 800 metaphases evaluated by this method was

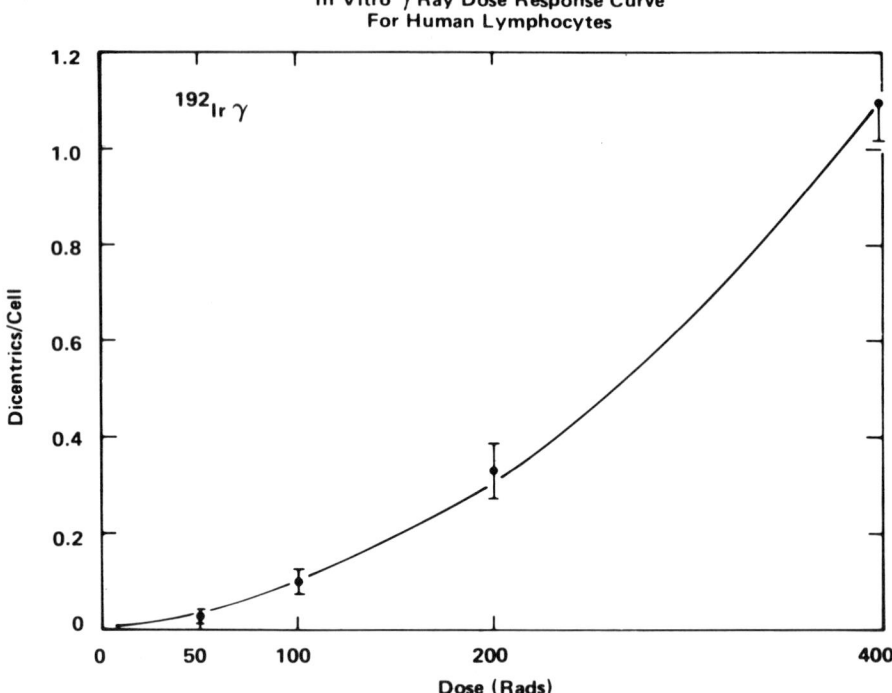

Figure 4. A dose-response curve for dicentric chromosome induction in human lymphocytes by gamma rays from Iridium 192. The uncertainties shown on the data points are standard errors based on the assumption of a Poisson distribution. Dose determination is described in the text.

used to prepare Figure 4. The $Y = \alpha D + \beta D^2$ equation parameters and their variances were calculated by an extension of the method described for the linear model.[66] The values are $\alpha = 3.18 \pm 1.80 \times 10^{-4}$, and $\beta = 6.09 \pm 0.72 \times 10^{-6}$. Table 3 contains the observed and expected distribution of dicentric chromosomes in the evaluated metaphases, showing that the Poisson distribution adequately describes the dispersion in the data, as expected. This observation tends to confirm that evenly applied doses of penetrating low-LET radiation give rise to cellular distributions of dicentrics that are random and are not significantly different than predicted by a Poisson process where the variance is dependent on and equal to the mean.

The newly generated dose-response curve for ^{192}Ir gamma radiation, based only on metaphases from first division cells,[27] was used to determine both the point and 95% confidence interval estimates[61] for the individual exposed to the high, localized dose of radiation from

Table 3. A Distributional Analysis of Gamma-Ray-Induced Dicentric Chromosomes

Dose	Dicentrics	Cells	$\overline{X}$		Frequency of cells with number of dicentrics						Probability[a]
					0	1	2	3	4	5	
50 rad	7	300	.023	Exp.	293	7	0	0	0	0	
				Obs.	293	7	0	0	0	0	>.90
100 rad	20	200	.100	Exp.	181	18	1	0	0	0	
				Obs.	180	20	0	0	0	0	>.67
200 rad	33	100	.330	Exp.	72	24	4	0	0	0	
				Obs.	74	20	5	1	0	0	>.12
400 rad	218	200	1.090	Exp.	67	73	40	15	4	1	
				Obs.	59	80	46	14	1	0	>.89

[a] Probabilities calculated from unit normal deviate values.[63]

^{192}Ir.[14] The methods used to make these determinations are given in great detail elsewhere[66] and a discussion of the significance and interpretation of the findings will be given in the subsequent presentation in this book.[61]

These two human *in vitro* dose-response curves adequately demonstrate the currently available techniques for determining the dose-response relations of the $Y = \alpha D$ and $Y = \alpha D + \beta D^2$ types and give examples of the form of the data generated. An example of dose estimation and 95% confidence interval determination for ^{241}Am alpha-particle irradiation of human lymphocytes from an individual involved in an actual ^{241}Am-contamination accident is presented. The frequency distributions generated in these dose-response studies demonstrate the basic cytogenetic response difference between high-and low-LET forms of radiation and the kinetics of dicentric induction. Information about the dispersion of lesions in irradiated lymphocytes may be of considerable importance when the particular circumstances surrounding an accidental radiation exposure cannot be adequately determined. This is in addition to the use of the lesion frequency estimation of equivalent whole-body dose.

ACKNOWLEDGMENTS

The authors would like to thank Dr. C. C. Lushbaugh for his encouragement on cytogenetic dosimetry studies and for his critical review of an early draft of this report. We also wish to recognize the assistance of S. Colyer and J. Batson for scoring, W. L. Beck for iridium 192 dosimetry, and E. Ayres for the technical illustrations.

This article is based on work supported by the Division of Biomedical and Environmental Research and NICHHD Grant HD-08828.

References

1. Brewen JG, Gengozian N: Radiation-induced human chromosome aberrations. II. Human *in vitro* irradiation compared to *in vitro* and *in vivo* irradiation of marmoset leukocytes. *Mutat Res* 13:383–391, 1971.

2. McFee AF, Banner MW, Sherrill MN: Induction of chromosome aberrations by *in vivo* and *in vitro* gamma irradiation of swine leukocytes. *Int J Radiat Biol* 21:513–520, 1972.

3. Clemenger JFP, Scott D: A comparison of chromosome aberration yields in rabbit blood lymphocytes irradiated *in vitro* and *in vivo*. *Int J Radiat Biol* 24:487–496, 1973.

4. Preston RJ, Brewen JG, Jones KP: Radiation-induced chromosome aberrations in Chinese hamster leukocytes. A comparison of *in vivo* and *in vitro* exposures. *Int J Radiat Biol* 21:397–400, 1972.

5. Bajerska A, Liniecki J: The yield of chromosomal aberrations in rabbit lymphocytes after irradiation *in vitro* and *in vivo*. *Mutat Res* 27:271–284, 1975.

6. Norman A, Ottoman RE, Sasaki M, Veomett RC: The frequency of dicentrics in human leukocytes irradiated *in vivo* and *in vitro*. *Radiology* 83:108–110, 1964.

7. Buckton KE, Langlands AO, Smith PG, Woodcock GE, Looby P, McLelland J: Further studies on chromosome aberration production after whole-body irradiation in man. *Int J Radiation Biol* 19:369–378, 1971.

8. Brewen JG, Preston RJ, Littlefield LG: Radiation-induced human chromosome aberration yields following an accidental whole-body exposure to ^{60}Co γ-rays. *Radiat Res* 49:647–656, 1972.

9. Schmid E, Bauchinger M, Bunde E, Ferbert HF, Lieven HV: Comparison of the chromosome damage and its dose-response after medical whole-body exposure to ^{60}Co γ-rays and irradiation of blood *in vitro*. *Int J Radiat Biol* 26:31–37, 1974.

10. Bender MA, Gooch PC: Types and rates of X-ray induced chromosome aberrations in human blood irradiated *in vitro*. *Proc Nat Acad Sci (USA)* 48:522–532, 1962.

11. Norman A, Sasaki MS, Ottoman RE, Veomett RC: Use of chromosome abberations to estimate X-ray and gamma-ray dose to man, in *School of Aviation Medicine Technical Report*, SAM-TR-67-112, 1967. (Also published as AD-66713).

12. Dolphin GW: Biological dosimetry with particular reference to chromosome aberration analysis, in *Handling of Radiation Accidents, Proceedings of a Symposium*, Vienna, International Atomic Energy Agency, 1969, pp. 215–224.

13. Heid KR, Breitenstein BD, Palmer HE, McMurray BJ, Wald N: The 1976 Hanford accident, in *The Medical Basis for Radiation Accident Preparedness*. New York, Elsevier North Holland, Inc., 1980.

14. Ross JF, Holly FE: The 1979 Los Angeles accident: Exposure to an iridium 192 industrial radiographic source, in *The Medical Basis for Radiation Accident Preparedness*. New York, Elsevier North Holland, Inc. 1980.

15. Tough IM, Buckton KE, Baikie AG, Court-Brown WM: X-ray-induced chromosome damage in man, *Lancet* ii:849–851, 1960.

16. Sasaki M, Ottoman RE, Norman A: Radiation induced chromosome aberrations in man. *Radiology* 81:652–656, 1963.

17. Bender MA, Gooch PC: Somatic chromosome aberrations induced by human whole-body irradiation: the "Recuplex" criticality accident. *Radiat Res* 29:568–582, 1966.

18. Evans HJ: Dose-response relations from *in vitro* studies, in Evans HJ, Court-Brown WM, McLean AS (eds.): *Human Radiation Cytogenetics: Proceedings of an Interna-*

tional Symposium, Edinburgh, 1966. Amsterdam, Elsevier North Holland, 1967, pp. 20–36.

19. Brown JK, McNeill JR: Aberrations in leukocyte chromosomes of personnel occupationally exposed to low levels of radiation. *Radiat Res* 40:534–543, 1969.

20. Bender MA, Brewen JG: Factors influencing chromosome aberration yield in the human peripheral leukocyte system. *Mutat Res* 8:383–399, 1969.

21. Bender MA: Human radiation cytogenetics, in Augenstein LG, Mason R, Zelle M (eds.): *Advance in Radiation Biology,* Vol. 3. London, Academic Press, 1969, pp. 215–275.

22. Sasaki MS: Radiation-induced chromosome aberrations in lymphocytes: possible biological dosimeter in man, in Sugaharo T, Hug O (eds): *Biological Aspects of Radiation Protection; Proceedings of the International Symposium, Kyoto, 1969.* Berlin, Springer, 1979, pp. 81–91.

23. Brown JK, McNeill JR: Biological dosimetry in an industrial radiography accident, *Health Physics* 21:519–522, 1971.

24. Schmid E, Bauchinger M, Hug O: Chromosomenaberrationen menschlicher Lymphocyten nach Röntgenbestrahlung *in vitro.* I. Qualitative und quantitative aspekte der Dosiswirkungsbeziehung. *Mutat Res* 16:307–17, 1972.

25. Silberstein EB, Ewing CJ, Bahr GK, Kereiakes JG: The human lymphocyte as a radiobiological dosimeter after total-body irradiation. *Radiat Res* 59:658–664, 1974.

26. Bauchinger M: Chromosome aberrations in human lymphocytes as a quantitative indicator of radiation exposure, in Evans HJ, Lloyd DC (eds.): *Mutagen-Induced Chromosome Damage in Man.* New Haven, Yale University Press, 1978, pp. 9–13.

27. Scott D, Lyons CY: Homogeneous sensitivity of human peripheral blood lymphocytes to radiation-induced chromosome damage. *Nature* 278:756–758, 1979.

28. Buckton KE, Jacobs PA, Court-Brown WM, Doll R: A study of the chromosome damage persisting after X-ray therapy for ankylosing spondylitis, *Lancet* ii:676–682, 1962.

29. Buckton KE, Court-Brown WM, Smith PG: Lymphocyte survival in men treated with X-rays for ankylosing spondylitis. *Nature* 214:470–473, 1967.

30. Santos Mello R, Kwan D, Norman A: Chromosome aberrations and T-cell survival in human lymphocytes. *Radiat Res* 60:482–488, 1974.

31. Prosser JS: Survival of human T and B lymphocytes after X-irradiation. *Int J Radiat Biol* 30:459–465, 1976.

32. Evans HJ: Chromosome aberrations induced by ionizing radiations, *Int Rev Cytol* 13:221–321, 1962.

33. Bender MA, Griggs HG, Bedford JS: Mechanisms of chromosomal aberration production. III. Chemicals and ionizing radiation. *Mutat Res* 23:197–212, 1974.

34. Sax K: Chromosome aberrations induced by X-rays. *Genetics* 23:494–516, 1938.

35. Dolphin GW: A review of *in vitro* dose-effect relationships, in Evans HJ, Lloyd DC (eds.): *Mutagen-Induced Chromosome Damage in Man.* New Haven, Yale University Press, 1978, pp. 1–8.

36. Preston RJ, Brewen JG, Gengozian N: Persistence of radiation-induced chromosome aberrations in marmoset and man. *Radiat Res* 60:516–524, 1974.

37. Purrott RJ, Lloyd DC: The study of chromosome aberration yield in human lympho-cytes as an indicator of radiation dose. I. Techniques. National Radiological Protection Board, Harwell, England, NRPB-R2, 1972.

38. Buckton, KE, Evans HJ (eds.): Methods for the analysis of human chromosome aberrations. Geneva, World Health Organization, 1973.

39. Lloyd DC, Purrott RJ, Dolphin GW, Bolton D, Edwards AA, Corp MJ: The relationship between chromosome aberrations and low-LET radiation dose to human lymphocytes. *Int J Radiat Biol* 28:75–90, 1975.

40. Evans HJ, O'Riordan ML: Human peripheral blood lymphocytes for the analysis of chromosome aberrations in mutagen tests. *Mutat Res* 31:135–148, 1975.

41. Littlefield LG, Joiner EE: Cytogenetic follow-up studies in six radiation accident victims — 16 and 17 years post-exposure, in *Late Biological Effects of Ionizing Radiation*, Proceedings of the Symposium, Volume 1. Vienna, International Atomic Energy Agency, 1978, pp. 297–308.

42. Buckton KE, Pike MC: Time in culture. An important variable in studying *in vivo* radiation-induced chromosome damage in man. *Int J Radiat Biol* 8:439–452, 1964.

43. Sharpe HBA, Scott D, Dolphin GW: Chromosome aberrations induced in human lymphocytes by X-irradiation *in vitro:* the effect of culture techniques and blood donors on aberration yield. *Mutat Res* 7:453–461, 1969.

44. Lloyd DC, Dolphin GW, Purrott RJ, Tipper PA: The effect of X-ray-induced mitotic delay on chromosome aberration yields in human lymphocytes. *Mutat Res* 42:401–412, 1977.

45. Sasaki MS, Norman A: Proliferation of human lymphocytes in culture. *Nature* 210:913–914, 1966.

46. Conger AD: The fate of metaphase aberrations. *Radiat Botany* 5:81–96, 1965.

47. Sasaki MS, Norman A: Selection against chromosome aberrations in human lympho-cytes. *Nature* 214:502–503, 1967.

48. Carrano AV, Heddle JA: The fate of chromosome aberrations. *J Theor Biol* 38:289–304, 1973.

49. Perry P, Wolff S: New Giemsa method for the differential staining of sister chromatids. *Nature* 251:156–158, 1974.

50. Liniecki J, Bajerska A, Karniewicz W: The influence of blood oxygenation during *in vitro* irradiation upon the yield of dicentric chromosomal aberrations in lymphocytes. *Bull Acad Pol Sci Ser Sci Biol* 21:69–76, 1973.

51. Prosser JS, White CM, Edwards AA: The effect of oxygen concentration on the X-ray induction of chromosome aberrations in human lymphocytes. *Mutat Res* 61:287–295, 1979.

52. Bocian E, Ziemba-Zak B, Rosiek O, Sablinski J: Chromosome aberrations in human lymphocytes exposed to tritiated water *in vivo*. *Curr Top Radiat Res* 12:168–181, 1977.

53. DuFrain RJ, Littlefield LG, Joiner EE, Frome EL: Human cytogenetic dosimetry: A dose-response relationship for alpha particle radiation from [241]Americium. *Health Physics* 37:279–289, 1979.

54. Haight FA: *Handbook of the Poisson Distribution.* New York, J. Wiley & Sons, 1967, p. 168.

55. Edwards AA, Lloyd DC, Purrott AJ: Radiation induced chromosome aberrations and the Poisson distribution. *Radiat Environ Biophys* 16:89–100, 1979.

56. Scott D, Sharpe H, Batchelor AL, Evans HJ, Papworth DG: Radiation-induced chromosome damage in human peripheral blood lymphocytes *in vitro*. I. RBE and dose-rate studies with fast neutrons. *Mutat Res* 8:367–381, 1969.

57. Lloyd DC, Purrott RJ, Dolphin GW: Chromosome aberration dosimetry using human lymphocytes in simulated partial body irradiation. *Phys Med Biol* 18:421–431, 1973.

58. McFee AF, Banner MW, Sherrill MN: Chromosome aberrations in the leukocytes of partial-body-and whole-body-irradiated swine. *Radiat Res* 60:165–172, 1974.

59. McFee, AF: Chromosome aberrations in the leukocytes of pigs after half-body or whole-body irradiation. *Mutat Res* 42:395–400, 1977.

60. Lloyd DC: The problem of interpreting aberration yields induced by *in vivo* irradiation of lymphocytes, in Evans HJ, Lloyd DC (eds.): *Mutagen-Induced Chromosome Damage in Man.* New Haven, Yale University Press, 1978, pp. 77–88.

61. Littlefield LG, Joiner EE, DuFrain RJ, Hübner KF, and Beck WL: Cytogenetic dose estimates from *in vivo* samples from persons involved in real or suspected radiation exposures, in *The Medical Basis for Radiation Accident Preparedness.* New York, Elsevier North Holland, 1980.

62. Lloyd DC, Purrott RJ, Dolphin GW, Edwards AA: Chromosome aberrations induced in human lymphocytes by neutron irradiation. *Int J Radiat Biol* 29:169–182, 1976.

63. Savage JRK: Sites of radiation induced chromosome exchanges. *Curr Top Radiat Res* 6:129–194, 1970.

64. Fisher RA: The significance of deviations from expectation in a Poisson series. *Biometrics* 6:17–24, 1950.

65. Rao CR, Chakravarti IM: Some small sample tests of significance for a Poisson distribution. *Biometrics* 12:264–282, 1956.

66. Frome EL, DuFrain RJ: Estimation of the amount of exposure to an environmental clastogen using human cytogenetic dosimetry, in Davis HT, Prairie RR, Truit T (eds): *1978 DOE Statistical Symposium,* Albuquerque, NM, 1979, US Department of Energy CONF-781108, 1979, pp. 169–172.

67. Lloyd DC, Purrott RJ, Prosser JS, Edwards AA, Dolphin GW, White AD, Reeder EJ, White CM, Cooper SJ, Stephenson BD, Tipper PA: *Doses in Radiation Accidents Investigated by Chromosome Aberration Analysis. VIII. A Review of Cases Investigated: 1977.* National Radiological Protection Board, Harwell, England, NRPB-R70, 1978.

68. Luchnik NV: Do one-hit chromosome exchanges exist? *Radiat Environ Biophys* 12:197–204, 1975.

69. Luchnik NV, Sevankaev AV: Radiation-induced chromosomal aberrations in human lymphocytes 1. Dependence on the dose of gamma rays and an anomaly at low doses. *Mutat Res* 36:363–378, 1976.

70. Edwards AA: The evidence for one-hit chromosome exchanges. *Radiat Environ Biophys* 14:161–165, 1977.

71. Upton AC: Radiobiological effects of low doses: implications for radiological protection. *Radiat Res* 71:51–74, 1977.

72. Lloyd DC, Purrott RJ, Reeder EJ, Edwards AA, Dolphin GW: Chromosome aberrations induced in human lymphocytes by radiation from ^{252}Cf. *Int J Radiat Biol* 34:177–186, 1978.

73. Carrano AV: Induction of chromosomal aberrations in human lymphocytes by X-rays and fission neutrons: dependence on cell cycle stage. *Radiat Res* 63:403–421, 1975.

74. Brewen JG, Luippold HE: Radiation-induced human chromosome aberrations: *in vitro* dose rate studies. *Mutat Res* 12:305–314, 1971.

75. Bauchinger M, Schmid E, Dresp J: Calculation of the dose-rate dependence of the dicentric yield after Co γ-irradiation of human lymphocytes. *Int J Radiat Biol* 35:229–233, 1979.

76. Brenot J, Chemtob M, Chmelevsky D, Fache P, Parmentier N, Soulie R, Biola MT, Haag J, Le Go R, Bourguignon M, Courant D, Dacher J, Ducatez G: Aberrations chromosomiques et microdosimetrie, in Booz J, Ebert HG, Eickel R. Walker A (eds.): *Proceedings of the 4th Symposium on Microdosimetry,* Verbania, Italy, 1973. Euratom Report EUR 5122 (Vol. 1), 1974, pp. 545–583.

77. Purrott RJ, Reeder EJ, Lovell S: Chromosome aberration yields induced in human lymphocytes by 15-MeV electrons given at a conventional dose rate and in microsecond pulses. *Int J Radiat Biol* 31:251–256, 1977.

78. Schmid E, Rimpl G, Bauchinger M: Dose-response relation of chromosome aberrations in human lymphocytes after *in vitro* irradiation with 3-MeV electrons. *Radiat Res* 57:228–238, 1974.

79. Virsik RP, Harder D, Hansmann I: The RBE of 30 kV X-rays for the induction of dicentric chromosomes in human lymphocytes. *Radiat Environ Biophys* 14:109–121, 1977.

80. Schmid E, Bauchinger M, Mergenthaler W: Analysis of the time relationship for the interaction of X-ray-induced primary breaks in the formation of dicentric chromosomes. *Int J Radiat Biol* 30:339–346, 1976.

81. Vulpis N: Impiego della "dosimetria da aberrazioni cromosmiche" nella irradiazione acuta parziale: Studio *in vitro* mediante culture miste di linfociti umani. *Radiobiol Radioter Fis Med* 25:195–211, 1974.

82. Norman A, Sasaki MS: Chromosome-exchange aberrations in human lymphocytes. *Int J Radiat Biol* 11:321–328, 1966.

83. Purrott RJ: The assessment of the therapeutic potential of high-LET beams by means of chromosome aberrations induced in human lymphocytes, in Evans HJ, Lloyd DC (eds.): *Mutagen-Induced Chromosome Damage in Man.* New Haven, Yale University Press, 1978, pp. 22–32.

84. Bauchinger M, Schmid E, Rimpl G, Kuhn H: Chromosome aberrations in human lymphocytes after irradiation with 15.0-MeV neutrons *in vitro.* I. Dose-response relation and RBE. *Mutat Res* 27:103–109, 1975.

85. Biola MT, Le Go R, Vacca G, Ducatex G, Dacher J, Bourguignon M: Efficacite relative de divers rayonnements mixtes gamma, neutrons pour l'induction *in vitro* d'anomalies chromosomiques dans les lymphocytes humains, in *Biological Effects of Neutron Irradiation; Proceedings of the Symposium, Neuherberg, 1973.* Vienna, International Atomic Energy Agency, 1974, pp. 221–223.

86. Todorov S, Bulanova M, Mileva M, Ivanov B: Aberrations induced by fission neutrons in human peripheral lymphocytes. *Mutat Res* 17:377–383, 1973.

87. Purrott RJ, Reeder E: The effect of changes in dose rate on the yield of chromosome aberrations in human lymphocytes exposed to gamma radiation. *Mutat Res* 35:437–444, 1976.

88. Purrott RJ: Chromosome aberration yields in human lymphocytes exposed to fractionated doses of negative π mesons. *Int J Radiat Biol* 28:599–602, 1975.

89. Evans HJ, Buckton KE, Hamilton GE, Carothers A: Radiation-induced chromosome aberrations in nuclear-dockyard workers. *Nature* 277:531–534, 1979.

90. Frome EL, Kutner MH, Beauchamp JJ: Regression analysis of Poisson-distributed data. *J Am Stat Assoc* 68:935–940, 1973.

91. Lloyd DC, Purrott RJ, Prosser JS, White AD, Dolphin GW, Reeder, EJ, Martin LC, Priseman SJ, Gray SA: Doses in radiation accidents investigated by chromosome aberration analysis. IX. A Review of Cases Investigated, 1978. National Radiological Protection Board, Harwell, England, NRPB-R83, 1979.

Published 1980 by Elsevier North Holland, Inc.
K. F. Hübner and S. A. Fry, eds. The Medical Basis for Radiation Accident Preparedness

Cytogenetic Dose Estimates from *In Vivo* Samples from Persons Involved in Real or Suspected Radiation Exposures

L. Gayle Littlefield, Eugene E. Joiner, Russell J. DuFrain, Karl F. Hübner, and William L. Beck

*Radiation Emergency Assistance Center/Training Site (REAC/TS),
Medical and Health Sciences Division, Oak Ridge Associated Universities,
Oak Ridge, Tennessee.*

Introduction

In 1964 Bender reported that the frequencies of radiation-induced chromosome lesions in cultured lymphocytes from men having recent exposures to gamma and mixed gamma/neutron radiations showed good correlations with the coefficients for aberration induction obtained from human blood irradiated *in vitro*.[1] This observation focused attention on the potential use of radiation-induced chromosome lesions in lymphocytes as a method for human biological dosimetry. During the ensuing 15 years, numerous studies in experimental animals and man further defined the variables that affect aberration yield in irradiated mammalian and human cells,[see 2–4] and firmly established the utility of cytogenetic techniques for dose estimation in persons having relatively homogeneous exposures to a large portion of the body.[5–9] Although the advantages of the use of the method are widely recognized, cytogenetic dosimetry has not been extensively applied except in scientific instances of known overexposures.[see 9] A notable exception is the routine application of the technique by the cytogenetics unit of the National Radiological Protection Board (NRPB), U.K., where dose estimates have been made in over 390 persons[10] since the inception of their program in 1969.[5]

In May of 1976, our laboratory first offered cytogenetic dosimetry as an adjunct to clinical consultations in persons referred to the Radiation Emergency Assistance Center/Training Site (REAC/TS)[11] because of known or suspected overexposures to radiation. Since that time we have responded to requests for dosimetry in 46 persons and initiated follow-up studies in 21 individuals to gather information about the persistence of chromosome lesions in human lymphocytes after exposure. In this communication we summarize the results of this experience in applying cytogenetic techniques for dose estimation in persons with suspected radiation exposures.

Protocols for Blood Handling and Lymphocyte Culture

Whole blood samples are collected in sterile vacutainer tubes containing 10 units/ml sodium heparin. When samples are to be shipped to the laboratory from distant sites, the tubes are surrounded by refrigerator coolant packs and packaged in an insulated container. In our experience, aberration frequencies in cultures initiated from shipped blood samples received up to 24 hr after collection are not significantly different from those observed in cultures initiated immediately after blood collection. Upon receipt of blood in the laboratory, lymphocytes are cultured as previously described.[12] During the first two and one-half years of our studies, replicate cultures containing approximately 1.0 ml leukocyte-rich plasma and 1.0 ml leukocyte-free autologous plasma were established on each REAC/TS patient. Currently, we are initiating additional cultures supplemented with 10 μg/ml 5-bromodeoxyuridine (BrdU) from each patient for fluorescence plus Giemsa (FPG) staining[13,14] and assessment of first, second, and third division metaphases.[15,16] Since the presence of BrdU in culture medium does not affect the frequency of radiation induced chromosome lesions in cultured lymphocytes,[9,17] the use of this technique allows positive identification of metaphases in their first *in vitro* division, thereby eliminating errors introduced by scoring second or third divisions.[18] All cultures are incubated at 37°C for 46 hr, exposed to colchicine for 4 hr, and harvested at 50 hr. For routine dosimetry estimates, 300 first division metaphases having chromosome counts of 45 or 46 are analyzed for asymmetrical radiation induced lesions (i.e., deletions, and ring and dicentric chromosomes with and without accompanying fragments). Both the percentage of metaphases bearing lesions and the distribution of lesions in damaged cells are recorded for each culture.

Dose Calculation

We use the frequency of dicentrics/cell for calculations of "equivalent whole-body dose," since significant variability in dicentric induction is not noted between donors when human blood is irradiated *in vitro*.[19,20]

and since this lesion is estimated to occur with a frequency of less than 1 in 4000 lymphocyte metaphases from non-irradiated persons.[3] We employ coefficients derived from *in vitro* dose-response curves generated in our laboratory for calculating dose in persons exposed to alpha radiation from americium 241 (^{241}Am)[20] and for gamma radiation from iridium 192 (^{192}Ir).[21] Published coefficients are used for X-ray,[22] cobalt 60 (^{60}Co), gamma,[22] and neutron[23,24] exposures. We have previously determined that the yields of dicentrics we observe at several doses of X and ^{60}Co gamma radiation are not significantly different from these reported yields, thereby allowing use of published coefficients for these radiation qualities. Limits of error on dose estimates are determined by maximum likelihood methods as previously described.[25]

Categories of Persons with Suspected Radiation Exposures

In their extensive applications of cytogenetic techniques for biological dose estimates, the cytogenetics group at the NRPB have described four main categories of persons for whom cytogenetic studies are frequently requested.[10] These include possible non-uniform exposures in which the relationship between dose to the film badge and to the body is uncertain; suspected overexposure to persons not wearing a dosimeter; overexposure where satisfactory estimates of whole-body dose can be made from physical measurements; and chronic internal and external exposures. To date, our experience with dosimetry at Oak Ridge is quite similar to that of the British group, with all persons studied fitting into one of the four categories described above. In addition, our laboratory is also conducting long-term follow-up studies in persons with radiation exposures.

A summary of studies conducted by the REAC/TS cytogenetics staff since May 1976 is shown in Table 1. During the last three years cytogenetic evaluations have been initiated in 67 persons, 46 of whom were suspected of having recent exposures. A total of 18,902 metaphases have been analyzed from cultures from these individuals, a task requiring approximately 378 scorer days for microscopic evaluations. We have responded to requests for dosimetry studies from DOE and other government facilities, state regulatory agencies, and private individuals. Patients have been referred to us from 14 different states. The occupations of the 46 persons for whom dosimetry estimates were requested are shown in Table 2. Seventeen of these persons had real or suspected exposures to various radionuclides used in industrial radiography "cameras," while the second largest group of persons with suspected exposures worked within the nuclear industry. Malfunction or misuse of radiography cameras or inadvertent uncovering or removal of point sources from their shielding devices were the primary causes of exposures of the industrial radiographers. The types of accidental exposures were varied in the other groups of individuals (i.e., "nuclear industry

Table 1. Summary of Cytogenetic Studies Conducted by REAC/TS Cytogenetics Staff May 1976 — July 1979

	No. persons studied	No. metaphases analyzed
Dosimetry estimates	46	13,738
Follow-up evaluations	21	5,164
Total	67	18,902

workers," persons in academic or research professions), but generally resulted from misuse or malfunction of radiation equipment or improper handling, packaging, or containment of radioisotopes. Of the 46 persons on whom dosimetry estimates were made, 34 had known or questionable exposures to external radiation, while 12 were suspected of having internal contamination with various radionuclides (Table 3). Whole-body counts or bioassay data were available for 10 of the 12 persons with "internal contamination." Film badge or other physical estimates of dose were available in only 13 of the 34 persons having possible external exposures. Results of cytogenetic analyses in these 46 individuals revealed that the majority had received equivalent whole-body doses of 0–10 rad, while two persons had estimated doses in excess of 90 rad (Table 4).

Cytogenetic and Physical Dose Estimates in Persons with Suspected External Exposures

As noted, physical estimates of dose (i.e., from film badge readings, mock-ups of accidents) were available for 13 persons (Table 5). In an additional person, referred to REAC/TS because of possible internal

Table 2. Occupation of Persons with Suspected Exposures

Occupation	Number of persons
Academic/research	7
Nuclear industry	9
Industrial radiographer	17[a]
Health physicist	4
X-ray technician	3
Other	6

[a] Includes persons with suspected exposures to ^{192}Ir, ^{60}Co, and neutrons from Americium-Beryllium surveying instruments.

Table 3. Types of Suspected Exposures of Persons Referred to REAC/TS for Cytogenetic Dosimetry

	Internal Contamination		External Exposures (Whole body/partial body)		
Isotope	Number of persons	Whole-body[a] counts	Radiation quality	Number of persons	Film[b] badge
^{241}Am	5	5	"mixed"	11	5
Radium	1	1	^{192}Ir	11	4
Uranium	2	2	^{137}Cs	2	0
Tritium	3	1	X-ray	3	1
Krypton	1	1	^{60}Co	2	2
			Neutron	5	1
Totals	12	10		34	13[c]

[a] Number of persons for whom whole body or body fluid counts were available.

[b] Number of persons for whom film badge or other physical estimates of dose were available.

[c] Includes two erroneously high film badge readings.

contamination with ^{241}Am, five dicentrics were observed in 400 lymphocyte metaphases (Case 1). Whole-body counts were negative for ^{241}Am; however, medical history for the five-year period preceding the cytogenetic evaluation revealed that this person had received extensive diagnostic radiation with an entrance exposure estimated at 100 R and an estimated accumulated dose of 10–40 rad. Cytogenetic findings in this person are included in Table 5 because of his extensive external exposure.

In persons having suspected whole-body exposures to external radiation (Group A), cytogenetic dose estimates generally showed good correlations with physical estimates of dose. In only two instances did we fail to observe aberrations in 300 lymphocyte metaphases and, in both persons, film badge readings suggested exposures of less than 11 R. Two additional persons were referred to us for evaluation because of suspected erroneous exposures of their film badges (Cases 8,9). In both instances high film-badge readings were encountered in routine readouts, and in neither case was there reason to suspect that the persons received an overexposure. Cytogenetic evaluations in these two persons verified that dose to their film badges did not represent dose to their body. In circumstances such as these, cytogenetic evaluations provide unique and valuable information, both to the employer and to the individual who may feel great concern because of the uncertainties of exposure.

Cytogenetic evaluations were also conducted in five persons having

Table 4. Equivalent Whole-Body Dose Estimates[a]

	0-10 rad	11-20	21-30	31-40	41-50	>90
Number of cases:	33	8	2	1	0	2

[a] Equivalent whole body dose estimates for X or gamma radiation (in rads) were calculated for all persons including those individuals internally contaminated with alpha-emitting radionuclides.

known exposures of a portion of the body to determine whether they also received a significant whole-body dose. Aberrations were not noted in two persons having extensive exposures of the fingers (Cases 10,11), while lesions were observed in a third person having a similar exposure. It is not surprising that cytogenetic evidence of exposure is not consistently obtained in persons receiving exceedingly high doses to localized areas of the extremities, since in these instances it might be anticipated that only a minute fraction of the circulating lymphocyte pool actually received radiation exposure.

Evidence of a significant whole-body exposure was obtained in cytogenetic studies in a person having a severe overexposure of the right hip and lower torso in the recent ^{192}Ir accident (Case 14). The clinical details of this accident are presented in this book by Ross,[26] and the physical dosimetry by Holly and Beck.[27] Blood samples drawn 30 days after the accident were received in our laboratory 13 hours after shipment from California. Lymphocyte cultures initiated both with and without BrdU were harvested at 50 hr for analyses of radiation-induced chromosome lesions. Three hundred first division metaphases were scored from slides stained with the FPG technique and an additional 300 metaphases were analyzed from cultures that had not been substituted with BrdU. Significant differences in aberration frequencies were not observed in the two sets of cultures; thus the data were pooled for tabulations of lesion frequencies (Table 6). Thirty-six of the 600 metaphases scored contained 49 dicentric or ring chromosomes, of which 44 had accompanying fragments. A total of 48 dicentrics were observed for a frequency of 0.08 dicentrics/cell. Using the coefficients of aberration induction derived in our laboratory from *in vitro* exposures of human lymphocytes to [192]Ir[21] (i.e., $Y = 3.2 \pm 1.8 \times 10^{-4}D + 6.1 \pm 0.7 \times 10^{-6}D^2$), this dicentric- yield estimates an equivalent whole-body dose of 91.4 rad with a 95% confidence interval of 70.7 to 116.2 rad (Figure 1).

Actually the dose received by this individual was highly non-uniform, with those regions of the body proximal to the ^{192}Ir source receiving exceedingly high doses and distant areas receiving minimal exposures (Table 7). Although the cytogenetic equivalent whole-body dose estimate is in reasonable agreement with the estimated average body midline dose of 75 rad, it is apparent that different body compartments received a

Table 5. Comparison of Cytogenetic and Physical Dose Estimates in Persons with Suspected External Exposures

Case No.	Occupation	Cytogenetic equivalent whole-body dose estimate (rad)[a]	Physical whole-body dose estimate[b]	Dose to extremity
		A. Suspected whole-body exposures		
1.	Health physicist[c]	20.0 29.7 (repeat culture)	10-40 rad	—
2.	Reactor worker	32.3	15.4 rad	—
3.	Reactor worker	0[d]	10.6 rad	—
4.	Reactor worker	14.0	14.7 rad	—
5.	Reactor worker	14.0	14.3 rad	—
6.	Industrial radiographer	14.7	32.0 R	—
7	X-ray technician	0	7.8 R	—
		B. Suspected film badge exposures		
8.	Industrial radiographer	0	40 R neutron 1.3 R gamma	—
9.	Industrial radiographer	0	72.5 R personal film badge 500 R film badge in truck	—
10.	X-ray technician	0	?	about 100,000 R to finger
11.	Health physicist	0	?	about 1,200 R to tips of fingers
12.	Cyclotron operator	20.7 17.2 (repeat culture)	15.5 rad	132 R to hand
13.	Industrial radiographer	4.9	?	about 6000 R to finger
14.	^{192}Ir accident victim	91.4	65 rad (midline dose)	80,000 R at 1 cm (hip)

[a] Equivalent whole-body dose estimates were based on a minimum of 300 metaphases analyzed and were calculated using coefficients for the specific radiation quality involved in each exposure incident.

[b] Physical dose estimates from film badge readings, mock-up of accident, or medical history.

[c] Patient initially suspected of having internal contamination with ^{241}Am, which was not detected in whole-body counting; it was subsequently learned that he had had extensive diagnostic X radiation estimated at 10-40 rad.

[d] When no dicentrics were observed in 300 metaphases, doses of 0 rad are reported.

Table 6. Frequency of Dicentrics and Rings in Cultured Lymphocytes from a Patient Accidentally Exposed to ^{192}Ir[a]

Metaphases scored	Metaphases with lesions	Metaphases with centric rings and dicentrics	Total number of centric rings and dicentrics
600	48(8.0%)[b]	36(6.0%)	49

	Frequency of cells with 0, 1, 2, 3, etc. Centric Rings and Dicentrics							Probability[c]
	0	1	2	3	4	5	6	
Observed	564	28	6	1	0	0	1	<.001
Expected[d]	553	45	2	0	0	0	0	

[a] Patient exposed to a 28-curie source of ^{192}Ir for approximately 45 min on 5 June 1979; blood samples obtained for cytogenetic evaluation 5 July 1979.

[b] Includes metaphases with asymmetrical exchanges, and terminal and interstitial deletions.

[c] Probabilities calculated from unit normal deviate values.

[d] Expected distribution based on Poisson statistics.

wide variation of doses. When the cytogenetic findings are considered in terms of distributions of lesions, the data from cultured lymphocytes from this patient also provide evidence of the non-uniformity of his exposure. It is well known that chromosome lesion induction is random in human lymphocytes receiving uniform exposures to low-LET radiation and that the distribution of lesions in irradiated cells is described by a Poisson distribution.[20,28–30] Overdispersion of two-break lesions (with respect to the Poisson distribution) in cultured lymphocytes from persons exposed to low-LET radiation is thus indicative of a localized or non-uniform exposure.[2,5,31] When the frequency of metaphases with 0, 1, 2, etc., rings and dicentrics from this patient were compared to the expected values from the Poisson distribution, the test statistics demonstrated a highy significant overdispersion (Table 6). These findings indicate that a portion of his lymphocytes received excessive doses of radiation and suggest that the radiation he received after exposure to ^{192}Ir was not uniformly distributed over his body.

Cytogenetic Findings in Persons Internally Contaminated with Radionuclides

Whole-body counts or bioassay data were available on 10 of 12 persons evaluated because of possible internal contamination with various radionuclides. Positive counts were obtained on five individuals, one of whom had positive urinary counts following inhalation of tritium gas, while the other four were internally contaminated with [241]Am in amounts ranging from less than one maximum permissible body burden to an estimated initial burden of 3000 microcurie (i.e., the individual accidentally contaminated in the Hanford accident of September 1977. See report of the accident by Breitenstein,[32] this volume). The cytogenetic findings in these individuals is compared with their estimated body burdens in Table 8. Extensive chromosome damage was observed in 50-hr lymphocyte cultures initiated 30 days after the accident on blood samples from the Hanford patient (Case I). In this preparation, 14% of the lymphocyte metaphases contained centric rings and dicentrics, with many cells having multiple lesions. In 50-hr cultures established 90 days after the accident 400 metaphases were analyzed, of which 21% contained asym-

Figure 1. *In vitro* dose-response curve for dicentric induction in human lymphocytes exposed to iridium 192.[22] The 95% confidence intervals are based on the analysis of 600 metaphases. Also shown are the methods for point and interval estimation of dose in the recent iridium-accident victim using the observed dicentric frequency of 48 dicentric equivalents in 600 lymphocyte metaphases from this patient.

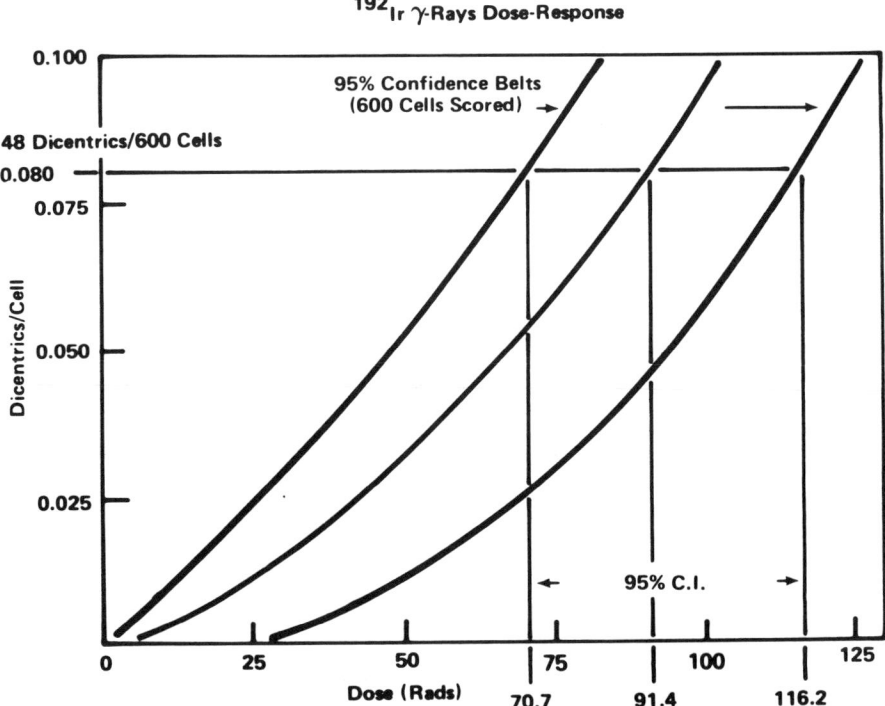

Table 7. Dose Estimates from Phantom Mock-up of ^{192}Ir Accident[a]

Organ or Tissue	Dose (rad)
Body midline	65
Femoral artery	180
Testes	90
Lens of eye	10
Skin exposure at 1 cm	80,000 R

[a] Dose estimates calculated from exposure of an Alderson Rando phantom to an Automation Industries model no. 520-008 radiography source containing a 22.0-curie iridium 192 source. Harshaw type TLD-100 LiF dosimeters were used to measure dose to phantom, and dose estimates were corrected to a source strength of 28 curie and an exposure time of 45 min.

metrical exchanges. Two or more rings and dicentrics were observed in 39 metaphases. An example of a metaphase having multiple two-break lesions from the 90-day culture is shown in Figure 2. Metaphases having multiple two-break lesions were also noted in two other persons having minor body burdens of ^{241}Am (Cases II and III). In cultures from each of these individuals two metaphases with asymmetrical exchanges were noted in 500 cells scored, and, in each instance, one of the damaged

Table 8. Cytogenetic Findings in Persons Internally Contaminated with Radionuclides

Case	Isotope	Body burden	Metaphases scored	Metaphases with centric rings/ dicentrics	Total number centric rings/dicentrics[b]
I[a]	^{241}Am	3,000 microcurie (facial skin)	178[c] 400[d]	25 83	47 164
II	^{241}Am	0.4 nanocurie	500	2	3
III	^{241}Am ^{137}Cs	1.1 nanocurie 12,000 nanocurie	500	2	3
IV	^{241}Am	40 nanocurie (lung)	300	0	0
V	^{3}H	46 microcurie/liter (urine)	300	0	0

[a] Date of accident 8/30/76, body burden day 1, 3000 microcurie ^{241}Am (facial skin).

[b] Multicentrics converted to dicentric equivalents by the factor (N-1), where N is the number of centromeres.

[c] Date of culture 9/29/76.

[d] Date of culture 11/30/76.

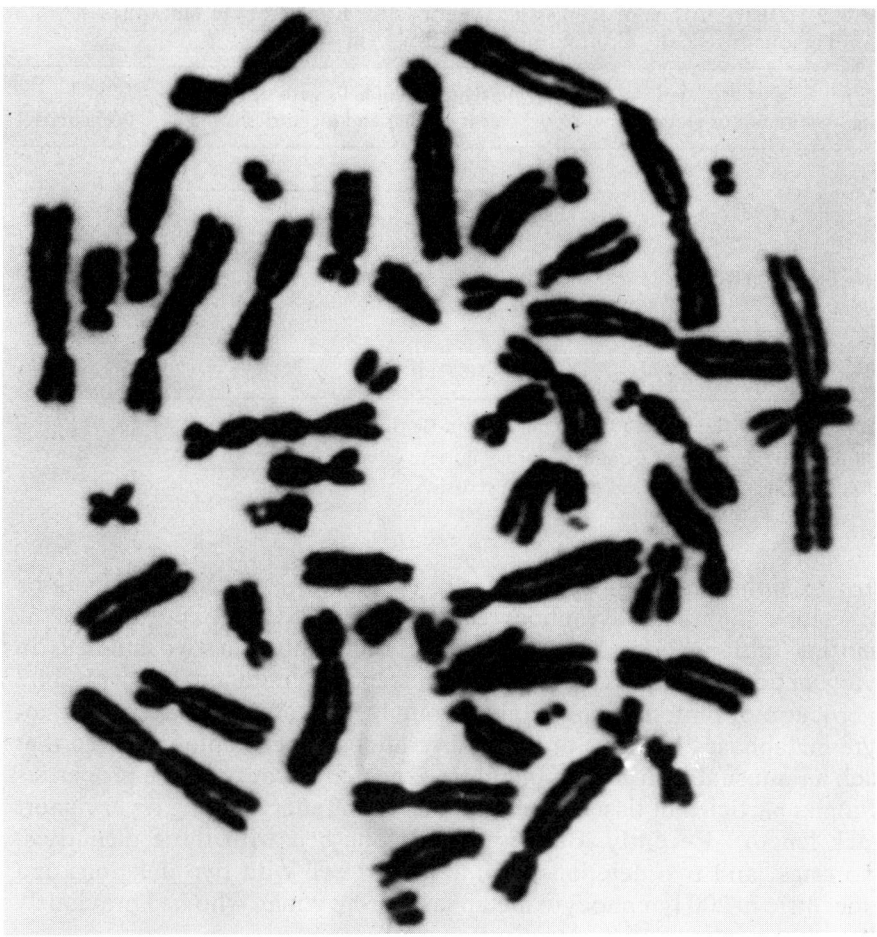

Figure 2. Metaphase with multiple radiation-induced chromosome lesions from the 90-day sample from the Hanford americium 241 accident victim.

cells contained two rings or dicentrics. Typical radiation induced lesions were not observed in metaphases from a fourth person internally contaminated with americium 241 (Case IV) nor in cultures from the individual having a minor body burden of tritium (Case V).

When the distribution of two-break exchanges in lymphocytes from the three patients internally contaminated with americium 241 was compared with expected distributions based on Poisson statistics, lesion frequencies were found to be highly overdispersed (Table 9). Similar increases in the proportion of metaphase having multiple two-break lesions were observed in metaphases of human lymphocytes exposed *in*

Table 9. Distributions of Rings and Dicentrics in Lymphocyte Metaphases from Persons Internally Contaminated with ^{241}Am

Case	Number of metaphases		Frequency of cells with 0, 1, 2, etc. centric rings and dicentrics								Probability[b]
			0	1	2	3	4	5	6	7	
I	400[a]	obs.	317	44	18	10	6	2	1	2	
		exp.[c]	266	109	22	3	0	0	0	0	< .001
II	500	obs.	498	1	1						
		exp.	497	3	0						< .001
III	500	obs.	498	1	1						
		exp.	497	3	0						< .001

[a] Distribution of lesions in 90-day sample from Hanford accident victim.

[b] Probabilities calculated from unit normal deviate values.

[c] Expected distribution based on Poisson statistics.

vitro to alpha radiation from ^{241}Am[20] (Table 10). Unusual distributions of lesions in human lymphocytes following *in vivo* exposures to α-emitting radionuclides have previously been noted in two studies. In cytogenetic evaluations of a patient internally contaminated with 14.2 microcurie of plutonium in a finger wound,[32] 11 of 21 damaged lymphocyte metaphases had two or more aberrations. These authors noted that such an unusual distribution might be expected because of the properties of alpha particles in tissues (i.e., deposition of energy along a very short track length). Recently, Bender[9] noted one cell with three dicentrics, two rings, and two deletions, and a second cell with two deletions and a dicentric in 200 lymphocyte metaphases from a man who had previously

Table 10. Comparison of Distributions of Lesions in Human Lymphocytes Exposed to Alpha Radiation from ^{241}Am

Exposure	Number cells	Frequency of cells with 0, 1, 2, etc., centric rings and dicentrics								Probability[b]
		0	1	2	3	4	5	6	7	
In vivo[a]	400	317	44	18	10	6	2	1	2	< .001
In vitro[c]	200	159	23	13	2	2	0	1	0	< .001

[a] Data from a 90-day sample Hanford ^{241}Am accident victim.

[b] Probabilities calculated from unit normal deviate values.

[c] Data from *in vitro* dose-response curve of DuFrain et al.[21]

worked in a uranium mill. Our data from *in vitro* exposures of human lymphocytes to ^{241}Am, as well as our findings in the Hanford patient and two other persons having measurable body burdens of ^{241}Am, provide additional evidence that multi-hit lesions are a characteristic finding in cultured lymphocytes exposed to α-emitting radionuclides.

Estimates of equivalent whole-body dose from chromosome lesion frequencies are not as meaningful in a clinical sense in persons internally contaminated with particle-emitting radionuclides as in individuals exposed to external radiation. Because most radionuclides tend to localize, specific regions of the body may receive extensive doses, while other areas will receive little or no radiation exposure. Thus, aberrations recovered in lymphocytes may be more indicative of "dose" to the circulating lymphocyte pool than of equivalent dose to the body. However, estimations of dose using *in vitro* dose-response coefficients are valuable in comparing relative doses of persons having differing body burdens of internal emitters. Using the coefficients of aberration induction derived from the *in vitro* exposure of human lymphocytes to soluble ^{241}Am[20] and to 250 kVp X-rays[22] we can compare equivalent whole-body doses of alpha and X-radiation in four persons having internal contamination with α emitters (Table 11). Based on the frequencies of dicentrics observed in cultured lymphocytes, our findings estimate that these four persons received equivalent doses ranging from 7.64 (Case III) to 214.69 rad (Case I) of X-radiation. Because of the increased efficiency of α particles in inducing chromosome lesions in lymphocytes,[20] these same dicentric frequencies estimate considerably lower doses of α radiation [i.e., 0.08 (Case III) to 7.91 rad (Case I)].

Table 11. Comparisons of Doses in Four Persons Internally Contaminated With a-Emitters

| | | | | Dose (rad) | |
| | | | | | Equivalent[b] |
Case	Isotope	Estimated Body Burden	Dicentrics/ cell	α^a	X-ray dose
I	^{241}Am	3000 μCi (facial skin)	.39^c	7.91	214.69
II	^{241}Am	1.1 nCi	.006	0.12	11.02
III	^{241}Am	0.1 nCi (lung)	.004	0.08	7.64
IV	^{239}Pu^c	14.9 μCi	.028	0.57	39.02

^{a} Coefficients of DuFrain et al.[21] used in calculations.

^{b} Coefficients of Lloyd et al.[23] used in calculations.

^{c} Data from Schofield et al.[35]

Summary

Our experience to date in applying cytogenetic techniques in evaluations of persons referred to REAC/TS has confirmed the usefulness of this method in biological dose estimation and in providing information relative to the nature of the radiation exposure. Good agreement between cytogenetic and physical dose estimates has generally been obtained in persons having uniform external exposures to low-LET radiations. In other cases, evaluations of chromosome lesion distribution in lymphocyte metaphases have yielded information relative to non-uniformity of exposure in persons having uneven distributions of dose. Cytogenetic analyses in lymphocytes of individuals internally contaminated with α-emitting radionuclides have demonstrated that the distribution of lesions in their lymphocytes does not conform to a Poisson distribution. Similar observations have been made in human lymphocytes exposed *in vitro* to α radiation from ^{241}Am. These findings verify that cytogenetic evidence of radiation exposure can be obtained by evaluating cultured lymphocytes from persons having measurable body burdens of α-emitting transuranics, and suggest that the induction of multiple lesions is a characteristic finding in human lymphocytes exposed to alpha radiation.

ACKNOWLEDGMENTS
The authors gratefully acknowledge Dr. Bryce Breitenstein, Hanford Environmental Health Foundation, for providing us with blood samples from the Hanford americium 241 accident victim and for valuable discussions and consultations regarding this patient. Likewise we would like to thank Dr. Joseph Ross, University of California at Los Angeles, for providing similar assistance in our evaluations in the recent iridium 192 accident. Within the Medical and Health Sciences Division, we would also like to acknowledge the assistance of Dr. Shirley Fry, REAC/TS, clinician in charge of recent referrals; Ms. Shirley P. Colyer and J. Batson for assistance in cytogenetic analyses in several patients; and E. Frome for statistical analyses of data.
Oak Ridge Associated Universities operate under Contract Number DE-AC05-760R00033 with the U.S. Department of Energy. This article is based on work supported by Department of Energy, Office of Health and Environmental Research and NIH Grant HD08828.

References

1. Bender MA: Chromosome aberrations in irradiated human subjects, *Ann NY Acad Sci,* 114:249–251, 1964.
2. Bender MA: Human radiation cytogenetics, in Augenstien LG, Mason R, Zelle M (eds.): *Advances in Radiation Biology,* Vol. 3. London, Academic Press, 1969, pp. 215–275.

3. Evans HJ: Population cytogenetics and environmental factors, in Jacobs PA, Price WH, Law P, (eds): *Human Population Cytogenetics*. Baltimore, Williams and Wilkins, 1970, pp. 192–216.

4. United Nations Scientific Committee on the Effects of Atomic Radiation. Report. General Assembly Official Records, 24th session, Supplement No. 13, (A/7613). New York, United Nations, 1969, pp. 98–155.

5. Dolphin GW: Biological dosimetry with particular reference to chromosome aberration analysis, in *Handling of Radiation Accidents: Proceedings of a Symposium, Vienna, 1969*. Vienna, International Atomic Energy Agency, 1969, pp. 215–224.

6. Dolphin GW, Lloyd DC: The significance of radiation-induced chromosome abnormalities in radiological protection. *J Med Genet* 11:181–189, 1974.

7. Evans HJ: Use of chromosome aberration frequencies for biological dosimetry in man, in *Advances in Physical and Biological Radiation Detectors, Proceedings of a Symposium on New Developments in Physical and Biological Radiation Detectors, Vienna, 1970*. Vienna, International Atomic Energy Agency, 1971, pp. 593–609.

8. Abbatt JD: Cytogenetic indicators of radiation (and other) damage calibration—present and future practical applications, in *Biochemical Indicators of Radiation Injury in Man, Proceedings of a Scientific Meeting on Biochemical Indicators of Radiation Injury in Man, Paris-Le-Vésinet, France, 1970*. Vienna, International Atomic Energy Agency, 1971, pp. 149–163.

9. Bender MA: *Status of human chromosome aberrations as a biological radiation dosimeter in the nuclear industry*. Brookhaven National Laboratory report BNL-25281, Upton, N.Y., 1978.

10. Lloyd DC, Purrott RJ, Prosser JS, White AD, Dolphin GW, Reeder, EJ, Martin LC, Priseman SJ, Gray SA: Doses in radiation accidents investigated by chromosome aberration analysis. IX. A review of cases investigated, 1978. National Radiological Protection Board, Harwell, England, NRPB-R83, 1979.

11. Lushbaugh, CC, Andrews GA, Hübner KF, Cloutier RJ, Beck WL, Berger JD: "REAC/TS": A pragmatic approach for providing medical care and physician education for radiation emergencies, in *Diagnosis and Treatment of Incorporated Radionuclides, Proceedings of an International Seminar, Vienna, 1975*. Vienna, International Atomic Energy Commission, 1976, pp. 565–577.

12. Littlefield LG, Joiner EE: Cytogenetic follow-up studies in six radiation accident victims—16 and 17 years post-exposure, in *Late Biological Effects of Ionizing Radiation*, Proceedings of the Symposium, Vienna, 1978, Volume 1. Vienna, International Atomic Energy Agency, 1978, pp. 297–308.

13. Perry P, Wolff S: New Giemsa method for the differential staining of sister chromatids. *Nature* 251:156–158, 1974.

14. Littlefield, LG, Colyer, SP, Joiner EE, DuFrain RJ: Sister chromatid exchanges in human lymphocytes exposed to ionizing radiation during G_o. *Radiat Res* 78:514–521, 1979.

15. Crossen PE, Morgan WF: Analysis of human lymphocyte cell cycle time in culture measured by sister chromatid differential staining. *Exp Cell Res* 104:453–457, 1977.

16. Tice R, Schneider EL, Rary JM: The utilization of bromodeoxyuridine incorporation into DNA for the analysis of cellular kinetics. *Exp Cell Res* 102:232–236, 1976.

17. Scott D, Lyons CY: Homogeneous sensitivity of human peripheral blood lymphocytes to radiation-induced chromosome damage. *Nature* 278:756–758, 1979.

18. Buckton KE, Pike MC: Time in culture. An important variable in studying *in vivo* radiation-induced chromosome damage in man. *Int J Radiat Biol* 8:439–452, 1964.

19. Dolphin GW, Purrott RJ: The use of radiation-induced chromosome aberrations in human lymphocytes as a dosimeter, in *Advances in Physical and Biological Radiation Detectors,* Proceedings of a Symposium on New Developments in Physical and Biological Radiation Detectors, Vienna, 1970. Vienna, International Atomic Energy Agency, 1971, pp. 593–609.

20. DuFrain RJ, Littlefield, LG, Joiner EE, Frome EL: Human cytogenetic dosimetry: A dose-response relationship for alpha-particle radiation from [241]Am, *Health Physics* 37:279–289, 1979.

21. DuFrain RJ, Littlefield, LG, Joiner EE, Frome EL: *In vitro* human cytogenetic dose-response systems, in *The Medical Basis for Radiation Accident Preparedness.* New York, Elsevier North Holland, Inc., 1980.

22. Lloyd DC, Purrott RJ, Dolphin GW, Botlon D, Edwards AA, Corp MJ: The relationship between chromosome aberrations and low-LET radiation dose to human lymphocytes. *Int J Radiat Biol* 28:75–90, 1975.

23. Lloyd DC, Purrott RJ, Dolphin GW, Edwards AA: Chromosome aberrations induced in human lymphocytes in neutron irradiation. *Int J Radiat Biol* 29:169–182, 1976.

24. Bauchinger M, Schmid E, Rimpl G, Kühn H: Chromosome aberrations in human lymphocytes after irradiation with 15.0-MeV neutrons *in vitro.* I. Dose-response relation and RBE. *Mutat Res* 27:103–109, 1975.

25. Frome EL, DuFrain RJ: Estimation of the amount of exposure to an environmental clastogen using human cytogenetic dosimetry, in Davis HT, Prairie RR, Truit T (eds.): *1978 DOE Statistical Symposium,* Albuquerque, NM, 1979. U.S. Department of Energy CONF-781108, 1979, pp. 169–172.

26. Ross JF and Holly FE: The 1979 Los Angeles accident: Exposure to an iridium 192 industrial radiographic source, in *The Medical Basis for Radiation Accident Preparedness.* New York, Elsevier North Holland, Inc., 1980.

27. Holly E, Beck WL: Dosimetry studies for an industrial radiography accident, in *The Medical Basis for Radiation Accident Preparedness.* New York, Elsevier North Holland, Inc, 1980.

28. Norman A, Sasaki MS: Chromosome-exchange aberrations in human lymphocytes. *Int J Radiat Biol* 11:321–328, 1966.

28a. Savage JRK: Sites of radiation induced chromosome exchanges. *Curr Top Radiat Res* 6:129–194, 1970.

29. Edwards AA, Lloyd DC, Purrott RJ: Radiation induced chromosome aberrations and the Poisson distribution. *Radiat Environ Biophys* 16:89–100, 1979.

30. Lloyd DC: The problems of interpreting aberration yields induced by *in vivo* irradiation of lymphocytes, in Evans HJ, Lloyd DC, (eds.): *Mutagen-Induced Chromosome Damage in Man.* New Haven, Yale University Press, 1978, pp. 77–88.

31. Schofield GB, Howells H, Ward F, Lynn JC, Dolphin GW: Assessment and management of a plutonium contaminated wound case. *Health Physics* 26:541–554, 1974.

32. Heid KR, Breitenstein BD, Palmer HE, McMurray BJ, Wald N: The 1976 Hanford accident, in *The Medical Basis for Radiation Accident Preparedness.* New York, Elsevier North Holland, Inc., 1980.

Discussion for Section IV

E. KOMAROV: Before closing this session I would like to make a couple of remarks on the last presentations. I'd like to tell you that, of course, we can tell that such techniques could be widely used. I remember our experience in this field. In 1969 we provided to 20 laboratories 100 slides for scoring, and we were astonished. We found complete disagreement between the 20 laboratories in scoring chromosomal aberrations. Of course, since then, we have better accuracy, but still my personal point of view is that it is better to use some central laboratories, which have more expertise and more precise techniques. We do not recommend the widespread use of such methods of biological dosimetry in various establishments. It's better to send a sample of blood to a central laboratory with good techniques, to obtain data from occupationally exposed personnel from throughout the United Kingdom.

M. WILLS: I would like to ask Dr. Littlefield how long do lymphocyte chromosomal changes persist following radiation exposure? Secondly, can you tell if the changes are from a new or old exposure?

L. G. LITTLEFIELD: First, cytogenetic follow-up studies in several groups of irradiated persons, such as A-bomb survivors, Bikini Island fishermen, and patients treated with X-radiation for ankylosing spondylitis, have demonstrated that some lymphocytes bearing radiation-induced chromosome lesions can survive for as long as 15–30 years after exposure. Second, it is not possible to determine if an induced lesion in any single cell resulted from a new or an old exposure. However, a high frequency of so-called "stable aberrations" (i.e., translocations and inversions) relative to rings and dicentrics would indicate that the exposure was not recent.

H. C. ALLEN: Dr. Breitenstein, has the sauna bath (at 200°F) or steam bath been considered for decontaminating skin from "inside out" for radiocontaminated workers?

B. D. BREITENSTEIN: In the americium case presented, a modified sauna bath was used prior to the decontaminating baths during the first month. This was accomplished by putting the patient in a plastic suit and having him sit in a steam filled shower room for 20 minutes. The theory was that the sweating produced would enhance removal of the americium. Sauna baths have been advocated as a means of facilitating decontamination.

K. CARSTAIRS: Would Dr. Littlefield discuss the reasons why dicentric counts are reliable for five weeks. How unreliable are the results after five weeks?

L. G. LITTLEFIELD: Sequential cytogenetic studies in cultured lymphocytes from a person who received a single acute exposure to ^{60}Co radiation demonstrated that the frequency of cells bearing dicentrics remained constant for the first five weeks after exposure, and thereafter began to slowly decline. This is presumably a reflection of the life span of some lymphocytes in the peripheral circulation. It has been estimated from cytogenetic studies by Dr. Buckton of radiotherapy patients that the mean life span of human lymphocytes is approximately 1600 days. Thus, reliable dose estimates can be made after five weeks; but it is necessary to take lymphocyte life span into consideration when making these calculations.

G. L. VOELZ: Dr. Littlefield, you indicated that you could ship samples to the laboratory without any difficulty. I am wondering how you actually ship your samples.

L. G. LITTLEFIELD: We use styrofoam boxes, and we actually send tubes out in most instances to have blood collected. We enclose in the boxes little freezer packs, wrap the blood in insulating material, and just sit the freezer packs around them in order to keep them cool, not frozen, and get them to the lab as quickly as possible.

N. WALD: I think you emphasized the search in the literature for calibration curves for the various nuclides that are of interest because of their involvement in overexposure cases. I'd like to emphasize that for accurate calibration it's probably better for each laboratory that's engaged in studying patients' samples to also run their own calibration curves using their technique rather than relying on the calibration curves in the literature. As a matter of fact, our dose-response curve is not in the literature because we feel that every laboratory should develop its own if it is going to do this kind of radiation cytogenetics.

R.J. DUFRAIN: Publication of the curve in a refereed journal is absolutely essential if it is to be used. If you have your own curve, you should have developed it by the best available techniques, and, therefore, it should be a publishable result. Everybody should have their own curves, or at least be able to show that their technique gives the same result as the published curves.

H. WOLFE: What agents other than those producing ionizing radiation can cause chromosomal abnormalities?

L. G. LITTLEFIELD: Dozens, perhaps hundreds, of agents other than ionizing radiation can cause chromosome damage in mammalian cells. These include numerous chemicals, viruses, chemotherapeutic drugs, etc. Most of these agents induce chromatid-type lesions in exposed cells. I know of only two compounds, streptonigrin and bleomycin, that induce double strand breaks in the DNA of human G_0 lymphocytes that lead to dicentric formation. For this reason dicentric induction in cultured lymphocytes may be considered a reliable indicator of radiation exposure in most instances.

E. KOMAROV: I can add that there are special problems in the identification of chemicals for which we should use the "sister chromatid exchanges (SCE) technique" but not the "chromosome aberration technique." Until now we have been discussing mostly the use of the lymphocytes, but we should not forget that we also have bone marrow cells. We can obtain more recent information because one can use the bone marrow cells for direct scoring without culturing.

M. E. GAULDEN: The peripheral lymphocytes are a very heterogeneous population of cells. There are two types of lymphocytes, the T and the B lymphocytes, which vary greatly in their radiosensitivity. We have recently demonstrated that the PHA, which is used to stimulate these cells at zero dose, gives you from 10 to 18% of the blasts that are the B-lymphocyte cells. As you increase the dose, this percentage of B-cells drops off dramatically. The D zero in our hands for the B cells is 50 rad. So, this is a very heterogeneous population. We also know there are three types of T cells, and they have varying sensitivity. I think it is remarkable that we are getting so much uniformity in this dosimetry business. The point I wanted to make here is that we should not be too complacent about the use of lymphocyte chromosomes.

E. KOMAROV: Yes, of course, all of us are in agreement with this statement.

J. T. BRENNAN: Is there a possibility that sister chromatid exchanges in the second generation lymphocytes could be helpful in cytogenetic dosimetry?

L. G. LITTLEFIELD: No, this method is proving to be a very sensitive indicator of exposure to many chemicals, but not to radiation. Slight increases in sister chromatid exchanges have been reported in human lymphocytes exposed to radiation after incorporation of bromodeoxyuridine, but not in lymphocytes exposed to radiation prior to culture.

L. KREISLER: How accurate for dose estimates is chromosome analysis? Briefly, how and when should the analysis be done?

R. J. DUFRAIN: In cases where short-term medical attention may be necessary (i.e., doses above 50 rem, whole-body), the accuracy of cytogenetic evaluation is precise enough to guide the physician in preparing for treatment. In the cases with low doses (i.e., less than 20 rem, whole-body), routine cytogenetic analysis is much less accurate. Recently Evans and his coworkers estimated it would take 10,000 cells examined for an accurate estimation on individuals receiving 10 rem; this is roughly one year's work for a trained cytogeneticist. From my crude calculations I would estimate 50 to 100,000 cells need to be evaluated for doses below 1 rem, and I am still not sure if this would show a statistically significant elevation above control frequencies. My own feelings are that cytogenetic evaluations are useful medical tools in suspected accidents; however, their uses in legal cases involving low-level exposures must remain questionable. In the case of a Three Mile Island type of incident, I could not consider recommending cytogenetic evaluations.

R. V. DORN, III: Dr. DuFrain, your introduction mentioned deletions, rings, and dicentrics (all with fragments) as possible results of radiation damage. You then gave reasoning for not using deletions and emphasized use of dicentrics for dosimetry. Are the rings not useful, and if not, why not?

R. J. DUFRAIN: The rings are useful; however, there are some problems in distinguishing between small rings and some fragments. Also, the rings occur at much lower frequencies than dicentrics. For example, the cytogenetic studies on the 1979 California accident revealed that only 1 of 49 two-break asymmetric chromosome exchanges was a centric ring.

G. G. CALDWELL: Could the chromosome-analysis method be used to determine radiation exposure in persons present at a nuclear test in 1957 and purportedly exposed to less than 5–10 rem?

R. J. DUFRAIN: In theory chromosome analysis could be applied to this problem. In actual practice the analysis at 20 to 25 years after doses under 10 rem would not be feasible. By that, I mean that the cost could not be justified by the information that would be gained; because to do the study right, it would cost at least $15,000 per individual examined. And after all of this expense, we would probably still not be able to statistically exclude a dose of 0 rem.

K. H. DINGER: In light of the recently published cytogenetic study of shipyard workers in the United Kingdom by Evans, is it feasible, reasonable, and economically justifiable to perform cytogenetic studies in conjunction with current epidemiological studies of populations occupationally exposed to low levels of ionizing radiation?

L. G. LITTLEFIELD: Such studies are feasible. I am not convinced, however, that such evaluations are reasonable or economically justifiable. The results of Evans demonstrated that evidence of radiation exposure could be detected in cultured lymphocytes from groups of persons having cumulative occupational exposures as low as 5–30 rem. However, to demonstrate a statistically significant effect at such low doses, it was necessary to score several thousand metaphases at each dose point. A dose-response relationship was obtained when data from cultures from several persons having similar doses were pooled. However, it was not possible to demonstrate dose-response relationships for individuals within each dose range. These findings suggest that to obtain statistically valid cytogenetic data on specific individuals exposed to doses in the range of occupational limits, it would be necessary to score monumental numbers of metaphases from cultures from each person. In fact, Evans and his associates estimate that one would need to score approximately 10,000 metaphases from a single individual to estimate the cytogenetic consequences of exposure to 10 rem. Since a trained cytogeneticist can score only 50 or so metaphases a day, it would be highly impractical to attempt such a study in large groups of persons having exposures to low doses of ionizing radiation.

A. WOOD: In response to a question from the floor, you (Dr. Littlefield) stated there would be no way of knowing whether dicentrics were caused by a new radiation exposure or perhaps to a recent chest X-ray. Did you intend to imply that the normal clinical chest X-ray procedures cause detectable chromosomal aberrations? What is felt to be the minimal dose of acute, whole-body X-irradiation that will result in measurable cytogenetic changes?

L. G. LITTLEFIELD: I would not expect to routinely detect lymphocyte chromosome aberrations in persons who had received no radiation other than a single chest X-ray. However, cytogenetic lesions are seen in lymphocytes of persons having extensive diagnostic X-ray procedures, such as multiple X-rays, GI series, intravenous pyelograms, etc. Many persons in the general population have had such procedures at some time, and this can be a complicating factor in dosimetry estimates in some individuals. Statistically valid cytogenetic data have been reported following *in vitro* exposures of human lymphocytes to doses of X-irradiation as low as five rads. However these data are obtained at a great investment of time. In this particular report in excess of 6,000 metaphases were scored to obtain data for the five-rad dose point.

J. E. HOLLY: I would like to make a comment on Dr. Gaulden's comment regarding cytogenetic sensitivity. The lower sensitivity is approximately 10 rad, far below even several chest X-rays and below most noncontrast fluoro-exams. The reports of aberrations at doses of 2 R (UCLA) were exams with contrast medium. Later UCLA experiments have proven this to be an effect of contrast-plus-radiation not detectable with radiation or contrast alone.

SECTION V:

Long-term Medical Effects in Populations Occupationally Exposed to Radiation

Published 1980 by Elsevier North Holland, Inc.
K. F. Hübner and S. A. Fry, eds. The Medical Basis for Radiation Accident Preparedness

Introductory Remarks:
Radiation Exposures:
Long-term Effects

W.W. Burr, Jr.

Director, Office of Health and Environment Research, Office of Environment, U.S. Department of Energy.

Several long-term epidemiologic studies now in progress are aimed at evaluating the health effects of occupational exposures to external and internal radiation. In recent years interest has been shown in the lower levels of exposure, especially those within the 1–9 rad range (the lowest dose group in the Japanese atomic bomb survivors studies).

Workers in many industries are potentially exposed to various toxic agents, often at low doses. The atomic industry has been no exception to this general rule. In evaluating occupational exposure to external radiation, the possibility of internal irradiation must also be considered and examined with available data. Several studies described here today continue to provide data relevant to the problem of internal exposure. These studies include uranium workers, plutonium workers (at Hanford, Los Alamos, and other facilities), the classical studies of radium-dial painters, and new studies on thorium workers. Studies of workers in the U.S. and Canada, as well as other countries, will provide data relevant to the acceptability of the occupational standards.

The results of the studies presented here can be compared with findings from other ongoing studies, especially those of the RERF. The assessment of risks associated with radiation exposure at various levels involves the interpretation of findings from all of these epidemiologic studies. This interpretation must involve careful attention to possible confounding factors, to the meaning of statistical tests (which result only in statements of probability), and to the results of experiments on animals. One challenge to the epidemiologists and biostatisticians who conduct these studies is to convey to physicians and to the public the best estimates of risks and the uncertainties involved in such estimation. The risks of low-level radiation must also be placed in perspective with other risks incurred in modern society.

Long-range Studies of Uranium Workers and the Oak Ridge Radiation Worker Population

Anthony P. Polednak

Epidemiology Group, Medical and Health Sciences Division, Oak Ridge Associated Universities, Oak Ridge, Tennessee.

Introduction

With very large external radiation doses, acute effects are of major concern medically. After exposure to radiation at various levels, whether in an accident or in the course of normal work in which radioactive substances are involved, the question of possible long-term health effects arises. It is generally recognized that long periods of time may be required for the manifestation of apparent radiation effects (i.e., certain cancers), as witnessed by recent findings of the Japanese atomic bomb survivors.[1]

The Epidemiology Group at Oak Ridge Associated Universities (ORAU) is concerned mainly with examining associations between occupational radiation exposure and subsequent mortality. Various chemical (especially metal) toxicants are also under investigation mainly as potential confounding variables in studies of the long-term radiation exposure on health. Ongoing studies are concerned with evaluating the mortality experience of past and present workers at Oak Ridge nuclear facilities and of several other occupational cohorts (Table 1).

The facilities have been involved mainly in uranium processing and metal production (National Lead of Ohio, Mallinckrodt Chemical Works in Missouri, and the Y-12 plant under Union Carbide) or uranium enrichment for use in weapons or reactors by an electromagnetic-separation process (Tennessee-Eastman Corporation at the Y-12 plant) or by a gaseous-diffusion process (the K-25 plant at Oak Ridge). The X-10 facility (Oak Ridge National Laboratory) has been concerned with

Table 1. Some Occupational Cohorts Currently Under Study

Facility	Period of operation	Known or estimated total no. of workers
Oak Ridge, Tennessee		
Y-12		
Tennessee-Eastman Corporation	1943-1947	38,000
Union Carbide	1947-present	11,000
Both TEC and Carbide	1943-present	5,000
K-25 (Gaseous Diffusion Plant)	1945-present	40,000
X-10 (Oak Ridge National Laboratory)	1943-present	20,000
Other (two or more of the above)	1943-present	6,000
All Oak Ridge facilities	1943-present	120,000
National Lead of Ohio	1951-present	6,300
Mallinckrodt Chemical Works Uranium Division (Missouri)	1942-1966	4,000

reactor technology, radioisotope production, and research and development of uranium and plutonium fission-product recovery. At each facility, there is (or was) a potential for internal and external radiation exposure.

To facilitate these studies and to aid other DOE epidemiologic studies (such as those of atomic workers at Hanford, Washington, and Los Alamos, New Mexico), the DOE Death Certificate Retrieval Office at ORAU obtains information on the vital status of individual workers through the cooperation of the Social Security Administration (SSA) and state vital-statistics departments. Copies of death certificates are obtained for persons known to have died, and causes of death are coded by a nosologist; presently, all certificates are coded to the eighth revision of the "International Classification of Diseases" (ICD).[2]

Editing and error-correction procedures have been developed for this data base (Table 1), derived from employment records that extend back to the early 1940's. Preliminary analyses have been completed on mortality in two groups of workers at the Y-12 uranium-processing facility, operated by the Tennessee-Eastman Corporation (1943–47) and by Union Carbide Corporation (1947 to the present). The results of these preliminary analyses are outlined here.

Tennessee-Eastman Corporation

The Tennessee-Eastman Corporation (TEC) operated the Y-12 facility from 1943–47 and was engaged in the production of uranium chloride (from uranium oxide) and its enrichment by an electromagnetic separation process. The uranium (enriched in ^{235}U) was sent to Los Alamos for atomic weapons production.

Materials and Methods

A total of about 45,000 persons worked at TEC between 1943 and 1947; analyses have been limited to those who did not remain at the Y-12 plant when Union Carbide assumed operation in 1947 and those who did not work for any other Oak Ridge facility. About 47% of the 38,000 workers were women, but preliminary analyses have focused on male workers because of the method used to ascertain deaths (i.e., searches by the Social Security Administration) produced less complete information on females.

Causes of death were coded from death certificates that were obtained for almost all persons reported dead by the SSA. Expected numbers of deaths were obtained by use of a computer program[3] that applies death rates for U.S. white males, specific for age and calendar year (five-year intervals), to person-years of follow-up (i.e., from year of first employment at TEC until death or the end of 1973).

Uranium Exposure Data

Although film badges were not worn by workers at TEC, exposure levels to penetrating external radiation were low because of the nature of the operation. Air-sampling data are useful in approximating the average exposure of a group of workers performing the same repetitive task or operation.[4] Subgroups of TEC workers have been defined on the basis of reported average levels (μg/m^3) of uranium dust. Briefly, workers in both stages of the electromagnetic separations process (known as "Alpha" and "Beta") were exposed to appreciable average air levels of uranium dust. In the Alpha-stage chemical departments, where UO_3 was converted to UCl_4, average uranium air levels were several times greater than the then current standard (150 μg/m^3), while in the Beta-stage chemical departments average levels were lower (about 50 μg/m^3). Since these processes were carried out in separate buildings and required special security processes for entry, workers in other departments and buildings (e.g., cafeteria, offices, industrial shops) were not exposed to uranium dust.

Uranium levels in the urine of over 1000 chemical workers were also determined at TEC by a fluorescent method, but results are not reported here.

Mortality and Cause of Death

Table 2 shows the mortality experience as of the end of 1973, with observed and expected deaths from selected causes for 4008 males who worked one year or longer at TEC and who worked in departments

Table 2. Tennessee Eastman Corporation:
White Males (N=4008) Employed in Selected Departments for ⩾ 1 Year

Selected Causes of Death	Observed number	Expected number[a]	Obs./Exp.
All causes of death	964	1169.14	0.8l
All infective and parasitic	12	27.05	0.44
All malignant neoplasms	177	211.92	0.84
Buccal cavity and pharynx	8	7.62	1.05
Digestive organs and peritoneum	39	64.06	0.61
Esophagus	6	5.12	1.17
Stomach	4	13.80	0.29
Large intestine	8	18.43	0.43
Rectum	4	7.99	0.50
Liver	3	4.77	0.63
Pancreas	13	12.01	1.08
Respiratory system	68	67.44	1.01
Lung	66	62.56	1.06
Bone	1	1.35	0.74
Skin	1	3.73	0.27
Prostate	10	10.55	0.95
Testis	3	1.57	1.92
Bladder	3	6.12	0.49
Kidney	5	5.51	0.91
Brain, CNS	8	7.45	1.07
Thyroid (1950-73 only)	0	0.50	0.0
Lymphosarcoma and reticulosarcoma (1950-73 only)	5	5.35	0.93
Hodgkin's disease	3	3.52	0.85
Leukemia and aleukemia	9	8.83	1.02
Cancer of other lymphatic tissue (1950-73 only)	3	4.02	0.75
Benign neoplasms	5	3.44	1.45
Diabetis mellitus	11	15.99	0.69
All diseases of blood and blood-forming organs	1	3.11	0.32
All diseases of nervous system and sense organs	10	10.31	0.97
All diseases of circulatory system	454	596.04	0.76
All respiratory diseases	57	61.10	0.93
All diseases of digestive system	50	62.63	0.80
All diseases of genitourinary system	13	18.72	0.69
All diseases of the bones and organs of movement	6	1.86	3.22
Symptoms, senility, and ill-defined conditions	20	11.29	1.77
All external causes of death	105	123.27	0.85
Unknown cause (death certificate not yet obtained)	34		

Total person-years of follow-up	108,592
Mean age at entry	32.3
Mean year of entry	1944.5

[a] Expected numbers are based on mortality rates for U.S. white males, specific for age and calendar years (see text).

indicative of potential exposure to uranium dust. The ratio of observed to expected deaths or standardized mortality ratio (SMR) was less than 1.00 for all causes and for all cancers. Copies of certificates were obtained for 930 of the 964 men (96.5%) reported dead; all deaths were included in the "all causes" category (Table 1), but no correction of cause-specific SMRs was made for deaths from unknown cause.

On the basis of available data on uranium metabolism and toxicity in man and other animals,[5] some diseases of particular interest are cancer of the lung and bone and diseases of the genitourinary tract (because of possible chemical effects of uranium). Tests of statistical significance were applied (the Mantel-Haenszel summary chi-square test[6]), and 95% confidence intervals were calculated for each SMR using either the Poisson assumption or the normal approximation depending upon the number of observed deaths.[7] The 95% confidence interval for the SMR for lung cancer, for example, was 0.83–1.35; that is, in a statistical sense, one could be 95% confident that the "true" mortality ratio was in this range.

The mortality ratio was high for the category, "symptoms, senility, and ill-defined conditions," but this is comprised predominantly of deaths for which the death certificate stated "unknown cause." Also, the death rate for this cause category for Tennessee (1940–60) was about four times the rate for the U.S.[8] The category of "diseases of bones and organs of movement" included four deaths attributed to rheumatoid arthritis; this may be a chance finding, since a large number of comparisons were made. Low SMRs, such as those for diseases of the circulatory system and infectious disease, may represent the "healthy-worker" effect evident in most occupational cohorts.

These mortality ratios (Table 2) should be interpreted with caution. Many of these persons spent most of their lives in Tennessee, and death rates for certain cancer sites are lower in Tennessee than in the U.S. Ratios of age-standardized mortality rates for white males in 1950–69 (i.e., the rate for Tennessee divided by the rate for the U.S.) were 0.67 for cancer of the colon and 0.49 for cancer of the rectum; ratios for lung cancer (0.88) and for all cancers (0.84), however, were closer to 1.00.[9] Corrections should also be made for deaths for which death certificates have not yet been obtained (these are included in the "all causes" category), and incomplete ascertainment of deaths by the Social Security Administration (SSA) system. An estimate of the latter error is being obtained by more intensive follow-up of samples of TEC workers to determine the percentage of deaths among persons not reported as dead by the SSA.

In a group of 720 white males who worked in Alpha chemistry departments, results of a search of all deaths in Tennessee (1949–1974) and in Kentucky (1963–1974) indicated that at least 4–5.5% of all pre-

1974 deaths were not ascertained by the SSA. The SMR for lung cancer was corrected by assuming that: (1) 94% of deaths were ascertained by the SSA, and (2) the percentage of lung cancer decedents among these nonascertained deaths and among the declared dead but lacking a death certificate (Table 2) was the same as the percentage among deaths with certificate. The corrected SMR for lung cancer was 1.16 (72.6 observed ÷ 62.6 expected), with a 95% confidence interval of 0.91–1.47. Thus, a two-fold risk of lung cancer could be excluded, but a risk factor of 1.5 was possible.

These problems will be largely overcome by internal comparisons of mortality (by subgroup) which will be presented in detail in other publications. Table 3 shows that the SMRs for lung cancer and for all cancers were not higher in the group of men who worked in chemical departments than in other groups. Future analyses will consider such factors as age at hire and length of employment in specific departments; a case-control study of lung cancer is also planned.

The mortality experience of TEC workers is being updated to include deaths occurring up to the end of 1978.

Y-12 Plant Under Union Carbide Corporation

Materials and Methods

Preliminary analyses of mortality have been limited to white males who worked at Y-12 (Union Carbide) from 1947 to the present and not at TEC or any other Oak Ridge facility. Men first employed after 1969 have been excluded in order to provide at least four years of follow-up, since

Table 3. Tennessee-Eastman Corporation Cancer Mortality in White Males

	Total no. of men	All cancer		Lung cancer	
Group		Observed no. of deaths	SMR[a]	Observed no. of deaths	SMR
1. Alpha and Beta departments	8,345	335	0.85	116	0.99
(Alpha and Beta chemistry)	(2,051)	(63)	0.78	(23)	0.97
2. Electrical workers	1,172	57	0.91	26	1.42
3. All other (office, etc.)	9,352	494	0.85	182	1.13
4. Total	18,869	886	0.85	324	1.09

[a]Standardized mortality ratio (observed ÷ expected number of deaths), where the expected number is obtained by using mortality rates for U.S. white males.

the analyses were based on the results of a 1974 search for deaths by the Social Security Administration. Methods of analysis of mortality are similar to those outlined above for the Tennessee-Eastman Corporation cohort.

A radiation-monitoring program was initiated in 1950 for radiation film badges and uranium bioassays (urinalysis). Some 4988 men hired before 1970 have been monitored for external radiation. Cumulative occupational radiation (penetrating) doses were low; 1783 men (35.7%) received a cumulative dose of $\geq$ 1 rem, and only 19 men (3.8%) received $\geq$ 10 rem. In 1958 eight workers received estimated total-body doses as high as several hundred rem in a criticality accident (see Dr. K. Hübner's report in this Symposium); these persons were excluded from the present study of the long-term effects of low-level radiation exposure. The 4988 men received a total of 5828 person-rem occupational radiation exposure.

Since internal radiation exposure by inhalation of uranium compounds is the major potential hazard, uranium bioassay and chest-counting data must be examined. Since 1961, about 2200 employees have been monitored by these methods and 49 were restricted from working with uranium for periods of six months or longer because of elevated monitoring results.[10] Data on internal exposures of individual workers will be obtained in the near future.

Mortality and Cause of Death

Table 4 shows observed and expected numbers of deaths from selected causes for the cohort of 4988 men as defined above. Follow-up was from the year of first film-badge record to death or the end of 1973. Copies of death certificates have been obtained for 303 of the 316 persons (95.9%) known to have died.

There was no evidence for statistically significant excesses in numbers of deaths observed over those expected on the basis of death rates for U.S. white males. SMRs for all cancers, cancer of the lung, bone cancer, and leukemia were less than 1.00. The SMR for brain cancer was high (1.97), but not statistically significant (with a 95% confidence interval of 0.79–4.06).

Based on the external radiation exposures in this population and current estimates of excess cancers per 10^6 person-rem, these negative findings are not unexpected. Follow-up of this cohort is continuing, however, and future analyses will involve subgroups based on levels of internal and external radiation exposure.

Other Studies

All of the other cohorts mentioned above (Table 1) are under investigation, and studies are at various levels of completeness. Merged computer files of all Oak Ridge workers are being prepared, including data on

Table 4. Y-12 (Union Carbide) White Males (N = 4,988) First Employed Before 1970, with Film Badge Reading(s)

Selected causes of death	Observed Number	Expected Number	Obs./Exp.
All causes	316	444.43	0.71
All malignant neoplasms	66	82.90	0.80
Cancer of digestive organs	12	22.13	0.54
Cancer of lung	27	26.46	1.02
Cancer of bone	0	0.50	0.00
Cancer of brain and CNS	7	3.56	1.97
Leukemia and aleukemia	3	3.66	0.82
Hodgkin's disease	2	1.82	1.10
Lymphosarcoma	2	2.54	0.79
Other lymphatic tissue	2	1.70	1.18
All diseases of circulatory system	156	211.22	0.74
All respiratory diseases	7	21.76	0.32
Unknown cause (death certificate not yet obtained)	13		
Total person-years (from year of first film-badge reading until death or January 1, 1974)	61,358		
Mean age at entry	34.7		
Mean year of entry	1961.3		

external radiation exposure. These data will be used to test current population estimates of radiation-induced cancers per 10^6 person-rem.

Another study in progress is examining mortality and morbidity among workers exposed to $\geq$ 5 rem external whole-body dose in any year of employment in the Department of Energy or its predecessor agencies (ERDA, AEC, Manhattan Engineering District) from 1943 to the present. Five rem is the currently accepted limit for annual whole-body radiation dose. The purpose of the study is to determine whether adverse health effects are associated with these radiation doses, the majority of which are in the 5–9 rem/year range, and if such effects are greater than those predicted on the basis of current estimates. Presently, about 2300 names are on the roster for this study. Additional persons, at least 1300 in number, will be added from the ranks of shipyard workers in the U.S. Naval Reactor Program.

The results of the studies outlined here can be compared with those from other ongoing studies such as those of Hanford workers,[11] and of Japanese atomic bomb survivors.[1] The assessment of risks associated with radiation exposure at various levels involves the interpretation of findings from all of these epidemiologic studies. Interpretation involves careful attention to possible confounding factors, to the meaning of statistical tests (which result only in statements of probability), and to the results of experiments on animals. One challenge to the epidemiologists and biostatisticians who conduct these studies is to convey to physicians and to the public the best estimates of risks and the uncertainties involved in such estimation. The risks of low-level radiation, to which many thousands of workers have been exposed over the past several decades, must also be placed in perspective with other risks incurred in modern society.

ACKNOWLEDGMENTS
This report is based on work performed under Contract No. DE-AC05-760R00033 between the U.S. Department of Energy, Office of Health and Environmental Research, and Oak Ridge Associated Universities.

Richard R. Monson, M.D., of the Harvard School of Public Health, provided a computer program using abstracted U.S. death rates and person-years tabulation appropriate for cohort studies. Support in computer programming was provided by D. R. Hudson and M. S. Hansard at Oak Ridge Associated Universities, and by the Computer Sciences Division at Union Carbide Corporation, Oak Ridge, Tennessee. Certain data used in this paper was derived from information furnished by the Social Security Administration. The author assumes full responsibility for the analyses and interpretation of the data.

References

1. Beebe GW, Kato H, Land CE: Studies of the mortality of A-bomb survivors. 6. Mortality and radiation dose, 1950–1974. *Radiat Res* 75:138–201, 1978.

2. International Classification of Diseases, Eighth Revision, Adapted for Use in the United States. U.S. Public Health Service Publication No. 1693. Washington, D.C., U.S. Government Printing Office, 1968.

3. Monson RR: Analysis of relative survival and proportional mortality. *Comput Biomed Res* 7:325–332, 1974.

4. Eisenbud M., Quigley JA: Industrial hygiene of uranium processing. *Arch Indust Health* 14:12–22, 1956.

5. Hursh JB, Spoor NL: Data on man, in Hodge HC, Stannard JN, Hursh JB (eds.): *Uranium, Plutonium, Transplutonic Elements*. New York, Springer-Verlag, 1973, pp. 197–239.

6. Mantel N, Haenszel W: Statistical aspects of the analysis of data from retrospective studies of disease. *J Natl Cancer Inst* 22:719–748, 1959.

7. Haenszel W, Loveland DB, Sirken MG: Lung cancer mortality as related to residence and smoking histories. I. White males. *J Natl Cancer Inst* 28:947–1001, 1962.

8. Grove RD, Hetzel AM: Vital statistics rates in the United States 1940–1960. U.S. Public Health Service Publication No. 1677. Washington, D.C., U.S. Government Printing Office, 1968.

9. Mason TJ, McKay FW: U.S. cancer mortality by county. U.S. Department of HEW Publication No. 74–615. Washington, D.C., U.S. Government Printing Office, 1974.

10. West CM, Scott LM, Schultz NB: Sixteen years of uranium personnel monitoring experience—in retrospect. *Health Phys* 36:665–669, 1979.

11. Gilbert ES, Marks S: An analysis of the mortality of workers in a nuclear facility. *Radiat Res* 79:122–148, 1979.

A Continuing Study of Mortality in Hanford Workers

S. Marks and E.S. Gilbert

Pacific Northwest Laboratory, Richland, Washington.

This will consist of an update for those who have heard accounts of our study previously and a recap of the design and essential results for those who have not. The update consists of the addition to the study population of a number of deaths, most of which occurred between 1 April 1974 and 1 May 1977.

For those who are not familiar with the study, I will review briefly the design and methods of analysis. The Hanford plant, which is located in Washington State, started operation in 1944. At first, its mission was the production, chemical separation, and purification of plutonium. Later, a large supporting research effort was developed. More recently, power has been generated in the one remaining active reactor, but additional power reactors are under construction at the site now.

The study of workers at Hanford and certain other sites, such as Oak Ridge, was started in 1964 by Dr. Thomas F. Mancuso of the University of Pittsburg. From that time until now, the Hanford data have been collected by the Hanford Environmental Health Foundation, now headed by Dr. Bryce D. Breitenstein. Until 1976, the data were analyzed by Dr. Barkev S. Sanders. Dr. Sanders' principal analyses were concerned with the measurement of life shortening in the exposed workers.[1] Since 1975, Dr. Ethel Gilbert of our laboratory has conducted independent analyses. The results of her analyses have been presented at various meetings during the past three years and were recently published in depth.[2] Since 1976, Dr. Alice Stewart and Mr. George Kneale have collaborated with Dr. Mancuso in analyzing the data and have published or presented a series of papers containing results that have received widespread distribution.[3,4] Those results and analyses have also occasioned much comment. I will return to this matter briefly before I close.

About 45,000 persons have been employed at the Hanford plant since the start of its operation. The population of radiation workers has been predominantly white and male. The population currently under study by Dr. Gilbert consists of 20,842 white males. The study population does not include workers who died before 1955 or were hired after 1965. These exclusions eliminate virtually no deaths with exposure of interest. The study is limited to mortality, and no attempt has been made to study morbidity. The Social Security Administration (SSA) identifies deaths in the employee population. Oak Ridge Associated Universities (ORAU) has an office that functions in an intermediary role, communicating our personnel rosters in a suitable format to SSA and receiving the results of the search of their files. ORAU also obtains death certificates from the states to establish the cause of death. SSA misses an undetermined number of deaths, which is believed to be about 5% to 8% of the total.

In our study of the role of radiation in health effects, we use the cumulative dose of external, penetrating radiation for each worker. The radiation exposure information available to us is probably as reliable as any in the industry. However, although prior radiation exposure data are obtained routinely now, that information is not available for transfers from other plants that occurred during the early period of plant operation when exposures elsewhere may have been relatively substantial in some poorly monitored installations. It also fails to include any exposure incurred subsequent to the individual's last period of employment at Hanford. The skewed nature of the distribution of cumulative doses in the study population is illustrated in Figure 1.

Dr. Gilbert has used two principal methods of analysis. One involves calculating standardized mortality ratios (SMRs), which compare mortality in the study population with mortality rates for the U.S. population based on vital statistics. The SMR for cause i is defined as follows:

$$SMR_i = 100 \times \frac{O_i}{E_i}$$

where O_i = number of deaths due to cause i observed in the Hanford population; and E_i = number of deaths due to cause I expected in the Hanford population based on age- and calendar year-specific rates for U.S. white males.

Table 1 shows SMRs for broad categories of causes of deaths. In this analysis, Dr. Gilbert divided the population by length of employment into those workers who had periods of employment of less than 2 years and those who were employed for 2 or more years. We see that, among the twenty thousand white male employees who began work before 1965, about two-thirds worked for at least two years. Of the others, only two

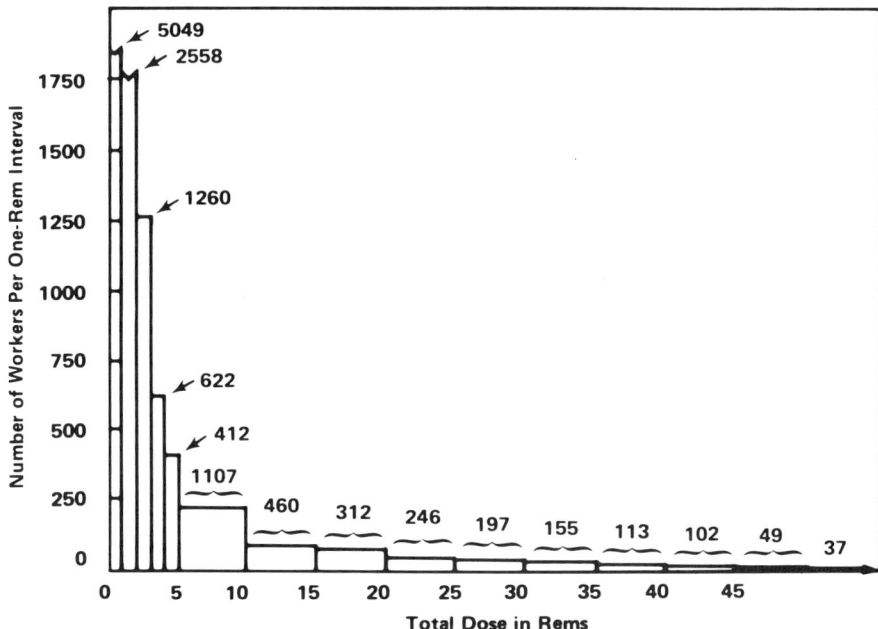

Figure 1. Distribution of cumulative doses for white, male workers employed at least two years.

Table 1. Observed and Expected Deaths and SMRs for White Males

	LENGTH OF EMPLOYMENT					
	<2 YEARS			2+ YEARS		
POPULATION AT RISK	7,767			13,075		
NUMBER WITH 5+ REM CUMULATIVE DOSE	2			2,778		
CAUSE OF DEATH	OBS.	EXP.	SMR	OBS.	EXP.	SMR
ALL CAUSES	1905	2216.6	86	2089	2796.8	75
ALL MALIGNANT NEOPLASMS	319	363.0	88	414	487.7	85
DISEASES OF THE CIRCULATORY SYSTEM	839	965.4	87	955	1254.2	76
ACCIDENTS, POISONINGS AND VIOLENCE	243	222.9	109	216	288.8	75
ALL OTHER CAUSES	423	568.1	74	455	700.8	65

individuals received as much as 5 rem of exposure. This table demonstrates that the "healthy worker effect," which describes the more favorable mortality of workers in clean industries when compared with the general population, is less marked in the short-term than the longer-term worker population. In other words, the mortality experience of the long-term workers is the more favorable. We also observe, as others have done, that the healthy worker effect for cancer is less marked than for other diseases, such as cardiovascular disease. This is not surprising because we would expect cancer to be less influenced than other diseases by favorable working conditions and health programs. The result is that the proportion of cancer cases may be greater among the long-term, more heavily exposed workers than among the short-term, less-exposed workers. This may create the erroneous impression that the long-term, more exposed workers have more cancer when, in fact, the proportion of cancer in those workers may be increased only because they have fewer deaths from other diseases.

The second and more important analytical approach used by Dr. Gilbert involves testing for a relationship between the level of radiation exposure and mortality. In this analysis, she controlled for age, calendar year of death, occupational category, and employment status. Here, we can provide an updated analysis with about a 20% increase in the number of deaths relative to our previous data set. This includes 390 additional deaths of all types, 94 of which are cancer deaths. In this analysis, the worker population is divided into groups according to their cumulative radiation dose, the cutpoints being at 2, 5, and 15 rem. Then, the trend of mortality with increasing exposure is tested. The expected deaths for each category of age, calendar year of death, employment status, and occupation are calculated as if radiation dose were not a factor. If radiation dose were to influence the mortality rates, the observed deaths would significantly exceed the expected in the higher dose groups. The statistical method used here is the Mantel-Haenszel procedure. The statistical test for trend of increasing mortality with dose is called the Mantel test.

Table 2 presents results of the analysis of trend with increasing dose. Here, in order to compress the material into a readable slide, we have pooled the 0 to 2 and 5 rem categories so that the combined groups are displayed as a 0 to 5 rem category. The table shows observed and expected deaths for all causes, for "all cancer" cases, and for several selected cancer types. The p value in the right column gives the level of significance of the one-tailed test. Values below 0.5 indicate an increasingly positive trend at the higher dose levels, whereas values above 0.5 may indicate the opposite, namely, a decreasing trend in higher dose ranges. We see that for all causes the higher dose ranges show fewer deaths than expected. The same is true for all cancer. Corresponding to

Table 2. Observed and Expected Deaths by Exposure Category for White Males

| | EXPOSURE CATEGORY | | | | | | |
| | 0-5 rem | | 5-15 rem | | 15+ rem | | |
CAUSE OF DEATH	OBS	EXP	OBS	EXP	OBS	EXP	VALUE
ALL CAUSES	1982	1969 0	144	147 8	90	99 2	0 88
ALL CANCER	408	400 7	29	32 8	20	23 5	0 81
STOMACH	25	24 8	0	1 9	3	1 3	0 13
LARGE INTESTINE	41	39 6	1	2 1	1	1 3	0 66
PANCREAS	27	27 4	1·	2 9	4	1 8	0 06
OTHER DIGESTIVE ORGANS	33	30 5	0	1 5	0	1 0	0 95
LUNG	115	117 0	16	11 9	7	9 1	0 54
PROSTATE GLAND	32	28 6	2	3 0	0	2 5	0 97
MYELOID LEUKEMIA	7	7 2	1	0 6	0	0 3	0 71
MULTIPLE MYELOMA	4	5 9	0	0 6	3	0 5	0 006

these, we have high p values. Of the specific cancer types, multiple myeloma shows a positive test at the 1% level of significance; the pancreas is not quite significant at the 5% level. Both show correspondingly small p values. At the opposite end of the scale, the prostate gland and the category of "other digestive organs," which includes esophagus, small intestine, liver and gallbladder, show a negative trend with p values greater than 0.95. Myeloid leukemia shows no trend.

The principal difference between our early and current sets of data occurs in cancer of the stomach where we had no cases in the high dose range previously but have three cases now. However, the test for trend is still not significant. In response to suggestions that we attempt to verify the diagnoses, especially for cancer of the pancreas, which is especially likely to be misdiagnosed, we checked back into the medical records of the multiple myeloma and pancreatic cancer cases. We did find that, in one high dose, pancreatic case, there was no autopsy, but the death certificate diagnosis of cancer of the pancreas did not agree with the attending physician's diagnosis, which was cancer of the stomach. We have not changed our formal analysis to reflect this observation because we have not had an opportunity to do a systematic search on all relevant cancer types. However, if that diagnosis were changed, the pancreas would not approach significance while the stomach would have a level of significance somewhere between 5% and 10%. This case illustrates the precarious nature of any conclusions that might be based on the small numbers of cases in each disease category.

We are continuing this study with periodic searches for additional deaths and updates of the analyses. Our most recent submission to SSA includes a group of several thousand workers employed by a construction firm at the plant; many of those workers incurred nontrivial radiation exposure while doing maintenance work. Smoking histories for the plant population are inadequate, but we plan to investigate differences in smoking incidence between different occupational categories in the event that lung cancer becomes a matter of interest in the study. We are also interested in developing an estimate of the percentage of deaths missed in our population by SSA by means of a suitable stratified sampling follow-up study. This would provide the basis for an adjustment of our Standardized Mortality Ratios. Finally, if we can develop a feasible, unbiased system for verification of diagnosis, we will undertake a project directed to that end.

We have recognized for some time that other exposures, principally chemical, could be confounding factors to radiation where trends of increased mortality with radiation exposure are observed. However, obtaining historical information of value about such exposures has proven to be virtually impossible to achieve. At present we are seeking such information about the few high dose myeloma and cancer of the pancreas cases.

I have refrained from commenting on the analyses, results, and conclusions reported by Mancuso, Stewart, and Kneale. If any of you are interested in reading critiques of their studies, I recommend to you reviews by Anderson,[5] Reissland,[6] and the team of Hutchison, MacMahon, Jablon and Land,[7] and our own publications.

To summarize, I have presented an updated analysis of data on the mortality experience of about 12,500 white, male workers who were employed at Hanford for at least two years. The addition of 390 deaths, including 94 cancer deaths, to our data file has not changed our previous results in any important respect. Using a Mantel-Haenszel analysis of trend of mortality with radiation dose, a positive trend of multiple myeloma with increasing dose at the 1% level of significance remains. Cancer of the pancreas shows a doubtful trend with dose. Certain other organs show fewer deaths than expected in the higher dose ranges. All deaths and all cancer deaths display a similar negative trend with dose.

ACKNOWLEDGMENT

This work was supported by the U.S. Department of Energy under Contract EY-76-C-06-1830.

References

1. Sanders B: Low-level radiation and cancer deaths. *Health Physics* 34:521–538, 1978.
2. Gilbert ES, Marks S: An analysis of the mortality of workers in a nuclear facility. *Radiation Research* 79:122–148, 1979.

3. Mancuso TF, Stewart A, Kneale GW: Radiation exposures of Hanford workers dying from cancer and other causes. *Health Physics* 33:369–386, 1977.

4. Kneale, GW, Stewart A, Mancuso TF: Reanalysis of data relating to the Hanford study of the cancer risks of radiation workers, in *The Proceedings of the IAEA Symposium on Late Biological Effects of Ionizing Radiation*, IAEA-SM-224/510, 1978.

5. Anderson TW: Radiation exposures of Hanford workers: A critique of the Mancuso, Stewart, and Kneale report. *Health Physics* 35:743–750, 1978.

6. Reissland JA: An assessment of the Mancuso study. National Radiological Protection Board document NRPB-R79, September 1978.

7. Hutchison GB, MacMahon B, Jablon S, Land CE: Review of report of Mancuso, Stewart, and Kneale of radiation exposure of Hanford workers. *Health Physics* 37:207–220, 1979.

Published 1980 by Elsevier North Holland, Inc.
K. F. Hübner and S. A. Fry, eds. The Medical Basis for Radiation Accident Preparedness

Studies on Health Risks to Persons Exposed to Plutonium

George L. Voelz,* James H. Stebbings, Jr.,* John W. Healy,* and Louis H. Hempelmann+

*Los Alamos Scientific Laboratory, Los Alamos, New Mexico;
+University of Rochester, Rochester, New York.

Man's first opportunity for exposure to potentially harmful amounts of plutomium was during World War II, when industrial scale production began in 1944. Ever since the United States has had an industry employing several thousands of persons who work with this long-lived alpha-radiation emitter that has the important property of producing nuclear energy by fission.

The potential for plutonium to produce adverse health effects, if taken internally, was recognized already in 1944. Thirty years later this subject is vigorously debated with a wider range of subtopics than at any time in its history. One would think as information of health effects has accumulated from studies on animals exposed to plutonium and human follow-up studies, that the areas of controversy would narrow. That has not been the case, at least not in statements designed for public consumption. One of the purposes of this paper is to present data derived from the follow-up on Los Alamos plutonium workers and to evaluate some risk assessments used today to see how well they correlate with these preliminary results.

Studies on persons exposed to plutomium are now beginning to reach an important stage because of the length of time since first exposures. The long physical half-life of ^{239}Pu (24,400 years) and long biological half-time in the body (an estimated 100 years in bone and 40 years in liver)[1] make internal depositions a continuing lifetime exposure. Depositions in humans, now present more than 30 years in the early exposures, already extend well beyond any long-term experiments in animals. Both studies cited here are on persons with long term plutonium depositions, primarily through inhalation exposures.

Plutonium Workers on the Manhattan Project at Los Alamos

In the early 1950s, 26 plutonium workers who had worked on the Manhattan Project at what is now the Los Alamos Scientific Laboratory, Los Alamos, New Mexico, were selected for clinical follow-up studies. These men were judged to have had the highest exposures to ^{239}Pu of any persons at Los Alamos in 1944 and 1945.

The study subjects, whose work histories indicated heavy exposure to plutonium, were selected on the basis of the amount of ^{239}Pu excreted in urine measured by methods available before 1950. The study has been reported in detail.[2,3]

The working conditions in 1944–45 and the circumstances of the plutonium exposures of these men support the notion that inhalation was the primary route of exposure. Eight workers in the group had potentially contaminated wounds and three had chemical burns by plutonium-containing solutions. Most wounds were excised promptly and did not contain plutonium of any significance. The highest quantity of plutonium measured in excised tissues was 2 nanocurie (nCi) in one case. In another person, a known contaminated wound area on a finger is estimated to retain 5 ± 2 nCi of ^{239}Pu.

The 1972 and 1977 examinations, done at Los Alamos, included *in vivo* counting of the chest, liver, and hands; analysis of urine and fecal samples; and comprehensive medical studies. No internally deposited radioactivity significantly above background was found by direct counting *in vivo* methods except for the one wound area described above. Plutonium excretion in urine was used to estimate internal depositions of plutonium by use of the PUQFUA code.[4] The estimated body burdens range from 7 to 230 nCi with an average of 58 nCi and a median value of 33 nCi. Eleven persons in the group exceed the 40 nCi maximum permissible body burden,[5,6] and 21 persons have depositions of 20 nCi or more.

Two individuals in the group have died: one due to a myocardial infarction and the other due to injuries sustained in an automobile–pedestrian accident. The expected numbers of deaths for the group adjusted for age and year of death, based on United States white, male rates, were generated by means of a computer program developed and described by Monson[7] and compared to the observed deaths in Table 1. The low observed mortality is most likely due to positive selection for health status in this group: these men were military

Table 1. Thirty-year Mortality in 26 White, Male Los Alamos Manhattan-District Plutonium Workers

	Observed	Expected	Obs/Exp
All causes of death	2	4.22	0.47
All malignant neoplasms	0	0.77	0.00
All diseases of circulatory system	1	1.80	0.55
All respiratory diseases	0	0.18	0.00
All external causes	1	0.81	1.23
Other	0	0.69	0.00
Average year of entry:		1945.35	
Average age of entry:		24.58	
Total person-years of survival:		782.40	

personnel in 1944–45 and have in general attained a high socioeconomic status.

The medical histories, clinical examination and diagnostic procedures, including blood chemistry profiles, hematology, urinalysis, roentgenograms of chest, teeth, and bones, electrocardiograms, pulmonary exfoliative cytology, and lymphocyte chromosome analysis, revealed findings in these individuals that appear to be within usual expectations of health problems for their ages, average of 56 years in 1976 with a range of 52 to 69 years. The most significant diagnoses were one case each of coronary heart disease, total blindness due to glaucoma, hypertension with possible left ventricular hypertrophy, and bronchitis and early emphysema in a heavy smoker. There are no cases of cancer within the group except for a history of two skin cancers that have been successfully excised.

Mortality Study of Highest Plutonium-Exposed Los Alamos Workers

A mortality study of every Los Alamos worker since the beginning of Los Alamos project who was estimated to have an internal plutonium deposition of 10 nCi or more was begun in 1974.[8] The group is made up of each individual estimated to have that level of exposure based on Los Alamos health physics records as of 1 January 1974. The body burden estimates were calculated with the version of the PUQFUA code[4] then in use. Subsequently a revised PUQFUA code[9] was developed that results in a more accurate estimate of internal depositions. These improved estimates are used in this paper for risk assessment analysis, but the original composition of the group has not been changed.

The group consists of 224 white, male and 17 white, female subjects.

Mortality status was obtained on each individual in the study as of 30 June 1976. The follow-up is 100% complete, despite the 30-year period of follow-up present for most subjects. Thus, there are no missing persons in this mortality study. The data on females is limited by the small numbers and is not discussed further, but is consistent with the mortality data presented here on the males.

The mortality data and some characteristics of the cohort of 224 white, male plutonium workers are presented in Table 2. The average year of entry into the study, 1947, was determined by the time of the subjects' first recorded urine test for plutonium exposure or of the recorded accident resulting in the first presumed exposure. Most subjects would not have received their current or final body burden until some few years after entry into the cohort.

The revised body burden estimates in the group range from < 1 to 215 nCi, with an average of 20 nCi and a median value of 9.5 nCi. Twenty-three persons in the group exceed the 40-nCi maximum permissible body burden and 54 persons have depositions of 20 nCi or more.

Expected mortality rates, age and calendar-year adjusted, are based on United States white male rates and generated by Monson's computer program.[7] The results for broad categories of deaths are shown in Table 2. The expected mortality calculated for this group does not incorporate healthy worker effects.

The standardized mortality ratio (SMR) for total mortality was 54 ($p < 0.001$), malignant neoplasms 64 (not significant), and for diseases of the circulatory system 38 ($p < 0.001$). An SMR of 100 is average. Mortality from malignant neoplasms were one each of the buccal cavity, stomach, large intestine, rectum, lung, bladder, and lymphopoietic system. For the cancer sites of greatest interest following plutonium exposures, liver or bone malignancies did not occur, and only one lung cancer appeared

Table 2. Thirty-year Mortality in 224 White Male Plutonium Workers

	Observed	Expected	Obs/Exp
All causes of death	33	61.3	0.54
All malignant neoplasms	7	10.9	0.64
All diseases of circulatory systems	12	31.8	0.38
All respiratory diseases	3	3.3	0.92
All external causes	8	6.9	1.16
Other	3	8.4	0.36
Average year of entry:	1947.4		
Average age of entry:	30.9		
Total person-years of survival:	6205		

versus an expected 3.2. Tests of statistical significance are not useful for the small numbers of cancer cases present in this study.

The low mortality ratios found in this study are most likely explained by selection biases relative to the general United States population. These include the healthy worker effect for employed populations, plus additional selection for security clearances required for all subjects and military selection for some of the earlier workers. The total influence of such factors is unknown, but healthy worker effects create SMRs between 70 and 90 depending on the precise cause of death and on age. In context our data do not suggest any excess of mortality due to any cause in these workers with the highest plutonium exposures at Los Alamos.

Risk Assessments for Plutonium Exposure

The organs of concern for cancer development following plutonium exposure are primarily the lung, bone, and liver. In these studies, one lung cancer death occurred in the 224 workers, but as noted this is not an unusual finding in light of the three lung cancers expected by adjusted U.S. male statistics. No bone or liver cancers were found in the mortality study. No cancers of internal organs have been diagnosed in the 26 Manhattan District exposed persons who have had their plutonium depositions for over 32 years. Although these studies are limited by the small numbers of subjects studied, they are of interest to determine if the data tends to corroborate or dispute current risk assessment values.

The data on estimated plutonium deposition in the 224 workers are summarized in Table 3. The distribution of individual values of plutonium deposition is given in Figure 1 and nanocurie-years of exposure are distributed as shown in Figure 2. These exposures are predominantly due to ^{239}Pu, but include some cases of ^{238}Pu exposure. The ^{238}Pu depositions in the group represent about 10% of the total activity, but the relative accumulated exposures to ^{238}Pu are less because these

Table 3. Plutonium Exposure on 224 Los Alamos Plutonium Workers

	Living	Dead
Number of workers	191	33
Average deposition	20 nCi	11 nCi
Average nCi-year exposure	461	171
Total nCi-year exposure[a]	88,139	5,652

[a] Summed to 6/30/76 or date of death.

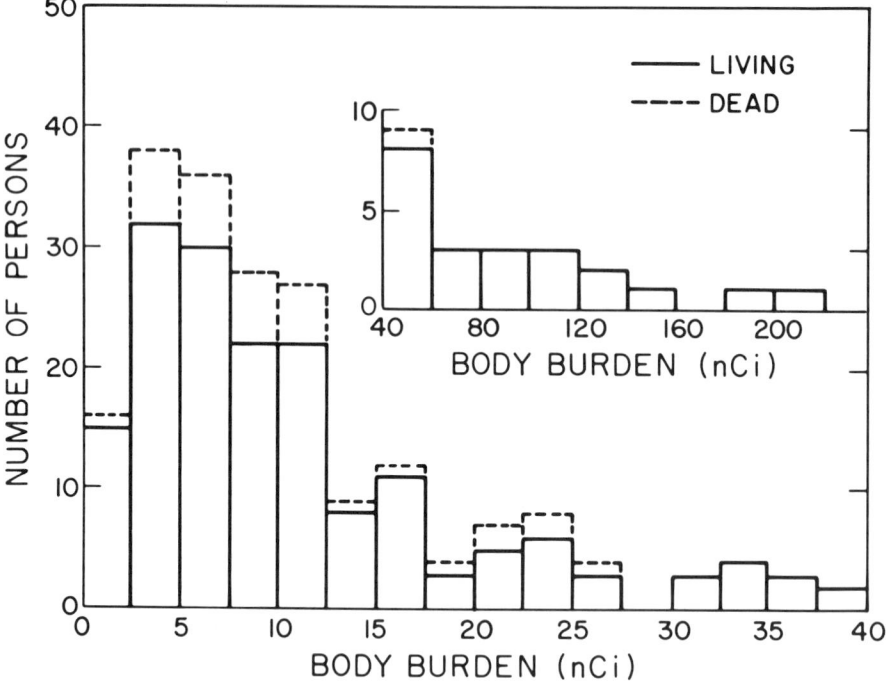

Figure 1. Distribution of body burdens.

exposures are more recent than those to [239]Pu. For the purposes of this discussion, [239]Pu and [238]Pu are combined.

Calculations of the radiation doses to the lung, bone, and liver were done using two different assumptions on the plutonium distribution within the body. The first approach is based on the results of plutonium analyses of tissues from several of the deceased in the group and the plutonium was assumed to distribute as follows for the entire period of exposure: 40% in lung, 30% in bone, 20% in liver, and 10% in other soft tissues, including lymph nodes.

In the second approach, a simplified scheme of the ICRP lung model[1] for the inhalation of an insoluble (class Y) aerosol was used. The measured body burden was assumed to have resulted from an inhalation exposure. The initial lung burden that could have led to this body burden was evaluated from the lung model given in ICRP 19.[1] This lung burden was used to estimate the total lung dose assuming that 40% was eliminated in the first day and the remaining 60% was eliminated with a 500-day half-life. The bone and liver doses were estimated by assuming that 45% of the body burden was in each organ and that the time delays in transferring to these organs from the lung was negligible. This procedure gives high values for the total bone and liver doses because it does not include the 500-day half-life for transfer to the blood or lymph nodes or the 1000-day half-life for transfer from the lymph nodes to the blood.

Dose calculations by these two methods through 1976 are summarized in Table 4. A quality factor of 10 was used throughout, and a dose distribution factor of 5 was used for the bone (5000 g).

Evaluations of the risk of excess cancers developing in this group were made using several contemporary methods. These were made for both the lifetime risk from the exposure received as of 1976 and the excess risk already present by 1976.

Lifetime Excess Cancer Risk

Using the risk coefficients given in the UNSCEAR report,[10] one can calculate an estimate of potential lifetime excess cancers that may occur as a result of the radiation doses delivered to the organs by 1976. These risk coefficients and the potential excess cancers calculated are listed in Table 5. The UNSCEAR risk coefficients are expressed per rad of low-LET radiation. For the purpose of this calculation, a rad of low-LET

Figure 2. Distribution of cumulative exposures.

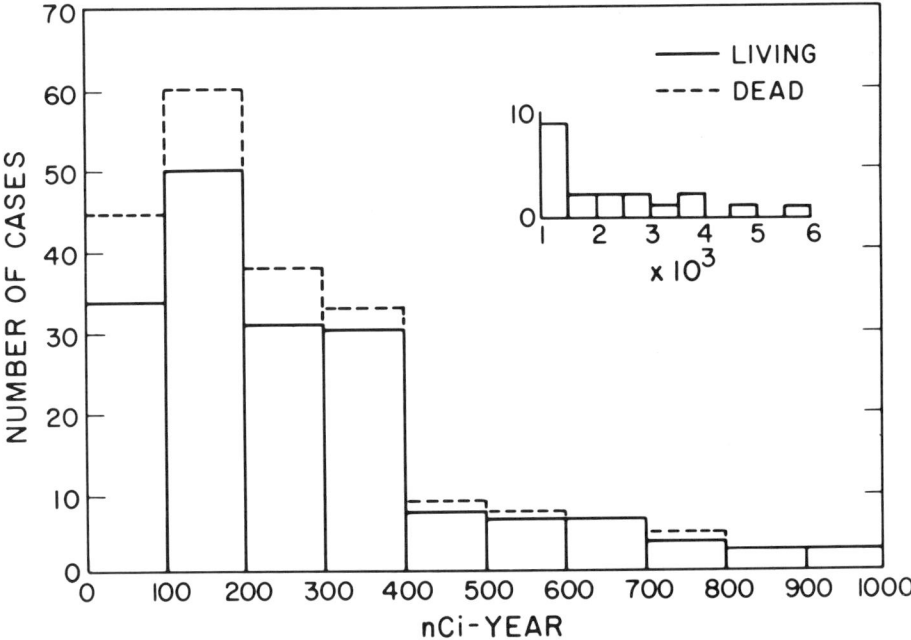

Table 4. Total Estimated Doses in Rems to 224 Los Alamos Plutonium Workers
as of 1976

	Tissue analysis assumptions (rem)	Modified ICRP model (rem)
Lung	35,800	16,800
Bone	26,800	36,400
Liver	10,500	24,000

radiation was considered equivalent to a rem of plutonium alpha radiation.

Lung cancer is the principal risk identified by this calculation and shows a possible lifetime expectancy of one or two excess cases.

A risk hypothesis of Gofman[11] is cited frequently in the press and in expert testimony to assess possible excess lung cancer in persons exposed to plutonium. For weapons-grade plutonium, the material present in the Los Alamos workers, Gofman equates 0.059 μg (3.6 nCi) of plutonium in the lungs of a cigarette smoker to one lung cancer, while 7.56 μg (465 nCi) in lungs of nonsmokers is said to produce one lung cancer. The smoking histories of the 224 plutonium workers is known for over 70% of these subjects. To simplify the problem of complex smoking histories over periods of more than 30 years, subjects were called smokers only if they were current smokers as of 1974 or later, or at the time of death. Past smokers were classified as nonsmokers if they stated they had quit smoking at the time of the last history. Several of these nonsmokers were one to two pack per day smokers for over 30 years, or essentially all the time of their plutonium depositions in the lung. The estimate required an extrapolation from the known percentage

Table 5. Potential Lifetime Excess Cancers in 224 Los Alamos Plutonium
Workers

	UNSCEAR Risk (per rad)	Excess cancers[a]
Lung	50×10^{-6}	0.8 -1.8
Bone	$2\text{-}5 \times 10^{-6}$	0.05-0.18
Liver	$4\text{-}10 \times 10^{-6}$	0.04-0.24
Total		0.89-2.22

[a] Range due to different assumptions used for dose calculations.

of current smokers on a random assignment to the remaining subjects on whom smoking data is not available yet. The error of this procedure is not believed to be significant for this type of estimate.

In calculating the possible excess cancers by this method, an arbitrary 40% of the current total-body deposition was considered to be the lung burden. This is the same assumption of lung distribution used in other estimates above. Although Gofman has indicated that his risk estimate can be based on the plutonium present in the lung initially after exposure, our calculation uses the estimated deposition of plutonium in 1976, nearly 25 years after exposure on the average for the group. The lifetime lung cancer risk by the Gofman method was limited by the authors to no more than one cancer per person although Gofman does not apply such an arbitrary limitation.

This method, using the above criteria, results in an estimate of 52 excess lung cancers in the 224 workers as shown in Table 6. (The estimate would have been 138 excess lung cancers if the lifetime risk per person had not been limited to one cancer per person). Gofman states that the "expected cancer fatalities will occur over about 30 years."[11]

1976 Excess Cancer Risk

Another approach to estimating possible excess cancers due to radiation is described in the BEIR report.[12] Following a latent period, a risk of excess cancers per rem for each year is hypothesized according to the linear, nonthreshold model. Using the average exposure for the group (Table 3) and the average length of exposure, assuming a constant average body burden for this entire period, it is possible to calculate

Table 6. Potential Excess Lung Cancers Predicted by Gofman Hypothesis[a] in 224 Los Alamos Plutonium Workers

Persons at risk	Lung cancer dose[b] (micrograms)	Total lung cancers predicted[c]	Limited lung cancer estimated[d]
Smokers	0.059	135.9	49.6
Nonsmokers	7.56	2.6	2.6
Total		138.5	52.2
Number of first lung cancers calculated to occur by 1976		25	15

[a] Gofman.[11]

[b] The quantity of weapons grade plutonium in the lung that equates to one lung cancer according to Gofman.

[c] Gofman risk estimate used without limitation on number of cancers predicted per person.

[d] Gofman risk estimate arbitrarily limited to a lifetime lung cancer risk not in excess of one lung cancer per person.

possible excess cancers. A latent period of 10 and 15 years was used in separate calculations to estimate a range. The risk coefficients and the results of the calculations for the exposures up to 1976 are shown in Table 7. These estimates suggest that excess cancer in the lung, bone, and liver by 1976 would total less than one-half a cancer for the group.

It is also of interest to consider the number of excess lung cancers that should have appeared by 1976 as predicted by the Gofman risk hypothesis.[11] For this purpose it was assumed that lung cancer at various ages might appear proportionately the same in this worker population as in the general U.S. population. The respiratory cancer mortality was taken from the National Center for Health Statistics, "Vital Statistics of the United States, 1970"[13] and population figures from the 1970 United States census[14] were used to estimate the percentage of cancers that occur by age 60, the average age of these workers in 1976. These data indicate that about 30% of lung cancer mortality occurs by age 60. If one takes 30% of the 52 excess cancers predicted by the Gofman hypothesis, it suggests that about 15 excess lung cancer deaths should have been registered in the group of 224 plutonium workers as of 1976. The possibility that exposure to plutonium accelerates the proportion of lung cancer present at earlier ages or that the higher risk estimate using multiple cancers for some persons is valid would cause the calculated expectation to be even greater than 15 lung cancers by 1976.

Conclusion

The estimation of the risk of cancer development following plutonium exposure is a matter of considerable importance for setting exposure standards and proper protection of workers and the public. A mortality study of 224 Los Alamos white, male workers with the highest exposures to plutonium has shown no excess deaths due to any cause compared to adjusted rates of white males in the United States population. Estimates,

Table 7. Potential Excess Cancers by 1976 in 224 Los Alamos Plutonium Workers

	BEIR risk/yr/rem	Excess cancers[b] by 1976
Lung	1.3×10^{-6}	0.02-0.3
Bone	0.2×10^{-6}	0.02-0.05
Liver[a]	4.0×10^{-7}	0.01-0.06
Total		0.05-0.41

[a] Risk coefficient derived by EPA from thorotrast exposures. No BEIR value available.

[b] Range due to different assumptions used for dose calculations, including latent periods of both 10 and 15 years.

using risk values developed by scientific committees, such as the UN-SCEAR[10] and BEIR,[12] suggest less than one-half a cancer total would be expected in the group by 1976, although lifetime experience may carry a potential of one or two excess cancers in the group. The mortality data in such a small group is not adequate to prove or disprove these estimates, although there is no suggestion of any excess deaths to date.

Other hypotheses suggest the risk due to plutonium is much higher. The Gofman risk hypothesis[11] suggests that 52 out of the 244 persons, or more than one out of five, will develop lung cancer. It is noted that the exposures occurred nearly 25 years ago on the average, so a relatively long latent period has already passed without the development of excess lung cancers in the group. The calculation that 15 excess lung cancer deaths should have been noted by 1976 is believed to be a reasonable, conservative interpretation of the Gofman risk hypothesis. The data in this study suggest that this hypothesis seriously overestimates the risk of lung cancer due to plutonium exposure.

In applying risk estimates, it seems reasonable to expect that predicted and observed excess cancers should correlate. Undoubtedly, risk estimates will be adjusted and refined as more information is compiled. Risk estimates significantly higher than those predicted by the UNSCEAR[11] and BEIR[13] reports are not supported by the human data presented here.

Additional data on workers at major plutonium facilities is now being collected at Los Alamos. It is estimated that nearly 5000 workers in the United States have had positive measurements of internal depositions of plutonium. A larger number of persons with potential exposure, but no evidence of internal deposition, will also be studied. Persons working for the same employer, but with no known potential for plutonium exposure, will be used as control populations. As studies on larger numbers of workers are completed, the human data will improve, and we hope the risk estimates will be modified correspondingly.

References

1. International Commission on Radiological Protection: The metabolism of compounds of plutonium and other actinides. *ICRP Publication No. 19,* Pergamon Press, New York, 1972.

2. Hempelmann LH, Langham WH, Richmond CR, Voelz GL: Manhattan Project Plutonium Workers: A twenty-seven year follow-up study of selected cases. *Health Physics* 25:461–479, 1973.

3. Voelz GL, Hempelmann LH, Lawrence JNP, Moss WD: A thirty-two year medical follow-up of Manhattan Project plutonium workers. *Health Physics* 37:445–485, 1979.

4. Lawrence JNP: A history of PUQFUA. Report *LA-7403-H,* Los Alamos Scientific Laboratory, Los Alamos, NM, 1978.

5. International Commission on Radiological Protection: Report of Committee II on permissible dose for internal radiation. *Health Physics* 3:82, 1960.

6. National Committee on Radiation Protection and Measurements: Maximum permissible body burdens and maximum permissible concentrations of radionuclides in air and in water for occupational exposures. *NCRP Report No. 22,* National Council on Radiation Protection and Measurements, Washington, D.C., 1959.

7. Monson RR: Analysis of relative survival and proportional mortality. *Comput Biomed Res* 7:325, 1974.

8. Voelz GL, Stebbings JH, Hempelmann LH, Haxton LK, York DA: Studies on persons exposed to plutonium, in *Late Biological Effects of Ionizing Radiation,* International Atomic Energy Agency, Vienna, vol. 1, pp. 353–366, 1978.

9. Lawrence JNP: PUQFUA, an IBM 704 code for computing plutonium body burdens. *Health Physics* 8:61, 1962.

10. United Nations Scientific Committee on the Effects of Atomic Radiation: Sources and effects of ionizing radiation. United Nations Publication No. E.77.1X.1, 1977.

11. Gofman JW: The plutonium controversy. *JAMA* 236:286, 1976.

12. Advisory Committee on the Biological Effects of Ionizing Radiations: The effects on populations of exposure to low levels of ionizing radiation. National Academy of Sciences, National Research Council, 1972.

13. National Center for Health Statistics: *Vital Statistics of the United States,* 1970, vol. 2. Mortality, Part A. U.S. Department of Health, Education and Welfare, Public Health Service, Rockville, MD, 1974.

14. U.S. Bureau of the Census: United States Census, 1970. Final Report PC(1)-B1 United States Summary. U.S. Government Printing Office, Washington, DC, 1972.

Long-term Follow-up of Radiation Workers in Canada

D.K. Myers, H.B. Newcombe, and A.M. Marko

Health Sciences Division, Chalk River Nuclear Laboratories Research Company, Atomic Energy of Canada Limited, Chalk River, Ontario, Canada.

Introduction

The principles that have generally been accepted for many years in the field of radiation protection might be summarized as follows: It is highly desirable and indeed essential to prevent exposure to high levels of radiation before any adverse health effects appear, to know what these adverse health effects might be in order that they can be detected if and when they occur, to have some quantitative estimate of the specific risks involved in exposure to any given level of radiation, and to provide compensation when work-related injuries occur.

The long-term follow-up of the health of radiation workers plays a vital role in meeting all four of these goals. Current follow-up studies in Canada range from detailed and elegant prospective studies, which are not expected to yield any evidence of adverse health effects for many decades, if ever, to those retrospective studies of groups of persons exposed to high-radiation doses in the past that will yield data on health risks but where it is often difficult to obtain accurate information either on individual exposures or on identification of the individuals involved.

National Dose Registry

In 1951, the Department of National Health and Welfare established a National Dosimetry service for measuring and recording radiation exposures of medical and industrial radiologists and other related groups of radiation workers. The National Dose Registry has evolved from this particular collection of dose records. Over the past few years, the Registry has been expanded to include, in addition to the National Dosimetry records of occupational exposures of medical radiation technologists and others, those from nuclear power reactor companies (e.g., Ontario Hydro) that carry out their own dosimetry; recently, records from uranium mining companies have also been added to this registry.[1]

The Registry includes records of 250,000 people of which some 70,000 are currently employed as "atomic radiation workers".[1] The rearrangement of the computer records in the National Dose Registry into their final recommended form[2] is expected to be completed in the next few months. By that time, the Registry should cover most occupationally exposed groups in Canada except for airline employees (currently exempt from recording of radiation exposures) and employees of Atomic Energy of Canada Limited. It is expected that these latter records will be included.

The National Dose Registry is used to provide data for routine regulatory control, [2] as required by legislation, in addition to statistics on the average annual exposures of different groups of occupational radiation workers.[3] Because of the centralized nature of the registry and its ability to link records to different types of radiation exposure, the registry can maintain a continuous record of a worker's exposures regardless of the organization or the province in which the person works.

The computer readable data[1,2] comprise two files with information relating to exposures in the current calendar year, plus two permanent files: (a) "lifetime annual history file" with lifetime total dose plus a list of the past yearly contributions to that total for each individual person; (b) a "master identification file" with sufficient personal identifying information to permit recognition of dose histories that have become fragmented and to permit long-term epidemiolgical follow-up of all radiation workers in Canada. The personal identifying information includes: social insurance number, surname, given names, previous surname (if applicable), date of birth, country or province of birth, sex, mother's maiden surname, father's first name, and year of enrollment in the registry. The social insurance number is of course available only for more recent employees, but is not essential for epidemiological follow-up.

Epidemiological follow-up will depend upon computer-assisted matching[4] of the records held in the National Dose Registry[1,2] and those held in the Canadian Morality Data Base,[5] which will be described below. Depending upon pending legislation, a complete national cancer registry for all of Canada may or may not become available in future; data on cancer incidence as well as cancer mortality could be obtained from this cancer registry.

Canadian Mortality Data Base

The Mortality Data Base contains computer readable data on approximately five million deaths recorded in Canada since 1950, together with causes of death as identified by international code numbers.[5] This data base is already being used, and will be used, for a considerable number of follow-up studies,[4] quite apart from the anticipated use in connection with the National Dose Registry. Five such studies to do with irradiated populations will be mentioned later, these being of Ontario uranium miners, fluoroscoped tuberculosis patients, AECL employees, Eldorado Nuclear employees, and INCO-Falconbridge nickel workers.

The special feature of this Mortality Data Base is that it makes use of information that is entered routinely from the death registrations into machine readable form for other purposes, more specifically for the completion of annual death statistics and for the preparation of alphabetic indexes to the bound volumes of death registration forms. The data base is arranged to facilitate rapid computer searching to determine whether members of a study population have died and, if so, the date and cause of death.

The Mortality Data Base is maintained by Statistics Canada, but the records are the property of the provinces. The manner in which it is used is therefore subject to provincial approval. In order to preserve strict confidentiality of the personal information which it contains, all searching must be carried out within Statistics Canada. In general, only bulk statistics are released, although these may under appropriate circumstances be broken down to permit appropriate analyses to be carried out.

This facility is more than a simple death index, since it gives cause of death, and is unique with respect to the accuracy and speed of the computer searching process.

Mortality Studies

Ontario Hydro Workers

The province of Ontario currently derives almost one-third of its electrical power from nuclear power stations. Ontario Hydro is the provincial corporation responsible for electrical supplies to most of the citizens in that province. A long-term follow-up of the mortality of Ontario Hydro employees has been set up and is currently being conducted by T.W. Anderson.[6,7] This mortality study is restricted to pensionable employees.[6] All current pensionable employees, pensioned employees, and deceased employees since 1970 are classified as having been employed at a nuclear power station, at a thermal station (usually coal-fired) or in other jobs (e.g., hydro stations, linemen). The total numbers in each of the three classifications at the end of 1977 were roughly 3400, 2300, and 12,800 respectively.[6] The general results are summarized in Figures 1 and 2, and do not reveal any striking overall differences in mortality from cancer or from all causes; the results to date, like those from Hanford and from Windscale,[8,9] suggest that the predominant difference between nuclear power-station workers and the general population can be attributed to the "healthy-worker" effect. It is anticipated that many decades of further experience would be required before any of the predicted harmful effects of occupational exposures to radiation could be detected.[10,11]

Newfoundland Fluorspar Miners

Fluorspar mining in St. Lawrence, Newfoundland, was carried out from 1933 to 1978. Fluorspar miners are not classified as radiation workers. However, excessive mortality from lung cancer was noted among the

Figure 1. Standard mortality ratios for death from cancer for radiation and other workers at Windscale, U.K., Hanford, U.S.A., and Ontario Hydro, Canada. The incidence of deaths occurring among these workers is compared with that expected for persons in the general population of the same age and the same sex. The numbers in each column represent the total number of deaths observed in each group.[6,8,9]

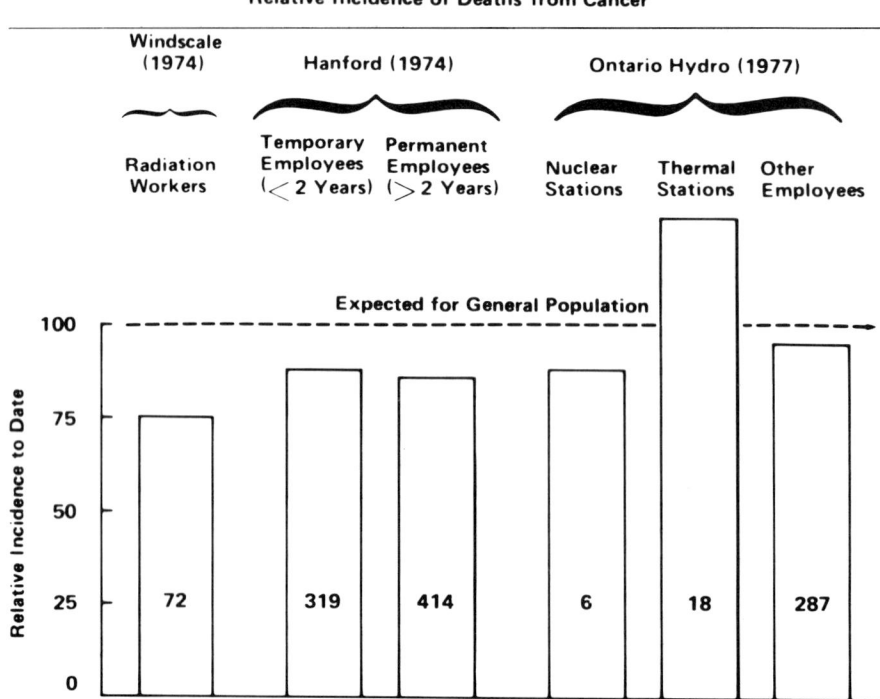

miners and was attributed to accumulation of radon daughters in the fluorspar mine.[12] The first data was published by deVilliers and Windish in 1964.[12] This led to a Royal Commission study,[13] and the data are currently being updated to 1977 by McCullough and coworkers.[1] Some 1900 miners were involved; of these, the majority (1422) had estimated exposures of less than 100 working level months (WLM), while the remaining five hundred had estimated exposures between 100 and 3000 WLM. The data (Figure 3) have been used to calculate risk estimates for induction of lung cancer by exposure to radon daughters;[14,15] there is, however, still considerable uncertainty as to exposure estimates for the pre-1960 period. This study is continuing.[1]

Ontario Uranium Miners

Uranium was mined in the province of Ontario at Bancroft from 1955 to 1964 and at Elliot Lake from 1956 to the present. A nominal roll of some 15,000 persons who worked for one month or more in the uranium mines was compiled by Muller and Wheeler, whose reports (1970–74) indicated an excess of lung cancer deaths among these miners.[16] This finding prompted a Royal Commission study on the health and safety of workers in mines.[17] The excess of lung cancer deaths (Table 1) was attributed to radon-daughter exposures of less than 400 WLM, but no risk estimates were derived from the initial analysis of the data.[17]

Figure 2. Standard mortality ratios for death from all causes for radiation and other workers. Other details as in Figure 1.

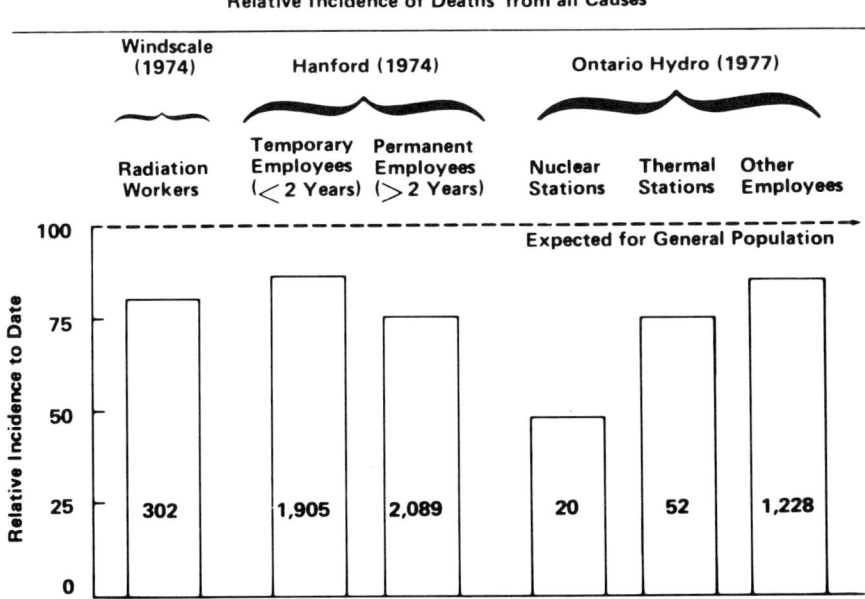

Relative Incidence of Deaths from all Causes

Preliminary risk estimates based on the original data have since been reported,[18,19] but there are some difficulties in the analysis due to, among other things, the lack of age-matched controls.[1,20] There are also the usual difficulties involved in estimation of individual radon-daughter exposures in the absence of personal monitors for each miner, but the available measurements of general levels of radon-daughters in the mines since 1955 are considered to be relatively reliable.

Currently the nominal roll for uranium miners in Ontario is being updated and extended to include, in machine readable format, data on the identity of the miners, their estimated annual exposures in uranium mines and in other hard-rock mines, their work history before and after involvement in uranium mining, as well as medical records.[21] More definitive data from which reliable estimates of risks might be derived are thus anticipated in the near future.

Figure 3. Percent of fluorspar miners in Newfoundland who were known to have developed lung cancer by 1977. The numbers in brackets beside each point represent the total number of miners involved.[1] Radon-daughter exposures are known to be uncertain; this graph is not intended to be used for calculation of risk estimates.

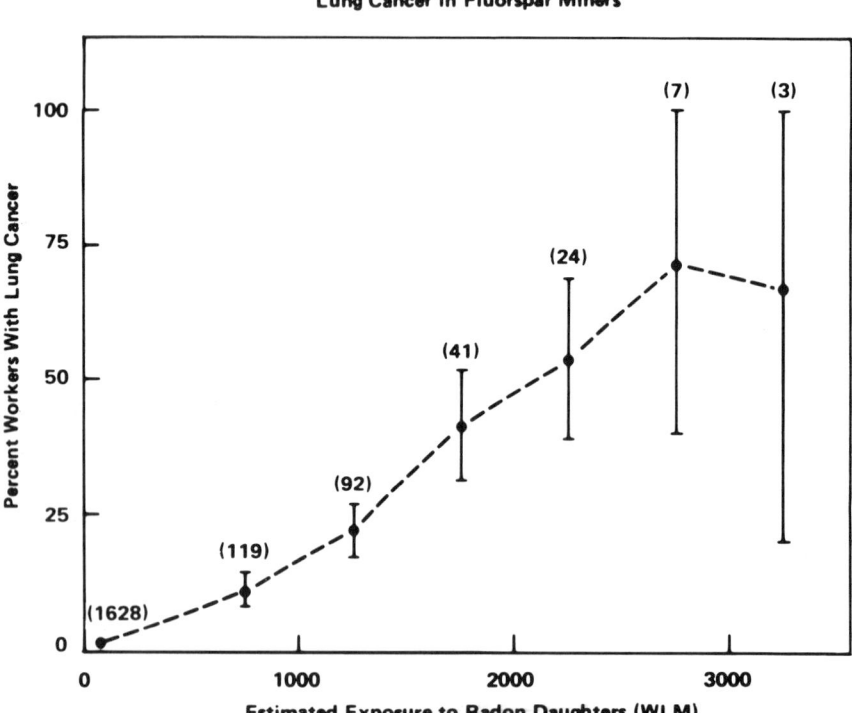

Lung Cancer in Fluorspar Miners

Table 1. Comparison of Actual and Expected Mortality of Ontario Uranium Miners[a]

Cause of death	Observed deaths	Excess deaths compared to	
		all Ontario males	Northern Ontario males
Motor vehicle accidents and suicide	140	13	(-8)
All other violent causes (mainly occupational accidents)	260	174	89
Lung cancer	81	36	33
Other respiratory diseases, arteriosclerotic heart disease, and all other "natural" causes	475	(-162)	(-221)
Total	956	61	(-107)

[a] Data derived from report of the Royal Commission on the Health and Safety of Workers in Mines, Ontario, 1976.

Fluoroscopy Patients

Myrden & Hiltz[22] reported an increase in incidence of fatal breast cancer among women who were repeatedly exposed to fluoroscopic examination of the chest during treatment for tuberculosis in the province of Nova Scotia in the 1930s. The data for this report were obtained by manual searching of relevant files on treatment and on mortality. Newcombe[23] later indicated how these data could be extended by using computers to assist in the linkage of the relevant records. This study is currently being carried out by the National Cancer Institute of Canada in collaboration with Statistics Canada[24] and involves computer-assisted linkage of records of about 100,000 patients who were in the past repeatedly exposed to fluoroscopic examinations. It is not at present anticipated that the final results will provide risk estimates which differ widely from those which are currently accepted.[3,14,15]

Other Long-term Mortality Studies in Progress

Methods by which the health of radiation workers could be followed by studying mortality on a long-term basis were described in detail by H.B. Newcombe in 1976.[11] A program to implement this proposal in order to study the health of workers at Atomic Energy of Canada Limited (AECL) is currently being initiated under the direction of J.L. Weeks.[25] This study, in contrast to that of Ontario Hydro,[6] is not restricted to pensionable employees and will rely heavily on use of the Canadian Mortality Data Base[5] in addition to other sources of information such as pension records.

Personal identifying information, in as far as this is available, will be similar to that used in the National Dose Register.[1,2] Identifying information is frequently incomplete, as it is in many of these studies. Further, exposure records for the period 1945–56 were destroyed in a fire in 1956. Preliminary data from this study are expected to be available within a few years. However, it is anticipated that many decades of additional experience would be required before any of the predicted deleterious effects of occupational exposures could be detected with any degree of certainty.[10,11]

A study similar to those of Ontario uranium miners and of AECL employees is being carried out by J. Abbatt (in collaboration with Statistics Canada and the National Cancer Institute of Canada) for Eldorado Nuclear Ltd.,[26] a crown corporation that has been involved in radium mining at Port Radium in the 1930s and 1940s and later in uranium mining and milling at Beaverlodge in the province of Saskatchewan. Eldorado Nuclear also operates the Port Hope refinery, which was originally built for radium production, but which now handles all uranium refining in Canada. Most of the radium extracted in earlier years was used for medical purposes and for the production of luminous dials. Only about 100 out of 9350 current and recent employees at the Beaverlodge mines had cumulative radiation daughter exposures in excess of 100 WLM. Reconstruction of radiation exposures at the Port Radium mines and the Port Hope refinery during 1930s and 1940s is being attempted[26] but will of necessity be based on fragmentary information.

A related study on the mortality of persons employed by International Nickel Company of Canada (INCO) and Falconbridge Nickel Mines in the Sudbury area in the province of Ontario is also currently in progress.[27] Although this study is not primarily concerned with radiation effects, except in as far as some modest accumulation of radon-daughters seems to be inevitable in all hard-rock mines,[3,21] the results from hard-rock miners are expected to provide vital information for interpretation of the effects of uranium mining on the health of workers. Transfer of miners between the Sudbury area and the Elliot Lake area has been fairly common in the past, and it is to be expected that hard-rock mining experience will have some effect on the health of miners, independent of any exposures to radiation in the uranium mines.[20,21]

Sputum Cytology Surveys

Sputum cytology studies of uranium miners in the U.S.A have shown progressive changes in cellular cytology, similar to those seen in cigarette smokers, that ultimately progressed to development of lung cancer.[28–30] Similar surveys are now being supported both in Saskatchewan and in Ontario by a number of agencies, with P. Band as project coordinator.[31,32] One of the primary purposes of these surveys is to initiate a program for the early detection of lung cancer in uranium miners. To date, the preliminary results available suggest that either radon-daughter exposure or cigarette smoking will increase the chances of finding abnormal cells in the sputum, but that the presence of both risk factors together results in a marked increase in the probability of abnormal cytology.[31] The data agree with previous results indicating that cigarette smoking accelerates dramatically the appearance of lung cancer in uranium miners exposed to high levels of radon-daughters in the past. [33]

References

1. McCullough RS, Stocker H, Makepeace CE: Pilot study of radon-daughter exposures in Canada, in *Conference/Workshop on Lung Cancer Epidemiology and Industrial Applications of Sputum Cytology*. Colorado School of Mines Press, 1979, pp. 183–213.

2. The National Dose Registry of Canada, draft document prepared by National Health and Welfare Group on Dosimetry (D. Grogan, Chairman), 1979.

3. United Nations Scientific Committee on the Effects of Atomic Radiation: Sources and Effects of Ionizing Radiation. United Nations, 1977.

4. Newcombe HB: A method of monitoring nationally for possible delayed effects of various occupational environments. National Research Council of Canada, Report No. NRCC 13686, 1974.

5. Smith ME: The Canadian Mortality Data Base, talk presented to NCIC Workshop on Computerized Record Linkage in Cancer Epidemiology, Ottawa, August 1979.

6. Anderson TW: Ontario Hydro mortality 1970–1977 (4th annual report), September 1978.

7. Anderson TW: The epidemiology of radiation workers, in *Proceedings of Symposium on Research Related to Radiological Safety in the Nuclear Fuel Cycle*. Toronto, Canadian Nuclear Association, 1979.

8. Mark S, Gilbert ES, Breitenstein BS: Cancer mortality in Hanford workers, in *IAEA Symposium on Late Biological Effects of Ionizing Radiation,* vol. 1, 1978, pp. 369–386.

9. Dolphin GW: A comparison of the observed and the expected cancers of the haematopoietic and lymphatic systems among workers at Windscale: a first report. National Radiological Protection Board, Technical Report NRPB-R45, 1976.

10. Reissland JA: The observation and analysis of cancer deaths among classified radiation workers. *Radiological Protection Bulletin* 17:23–27, 1976.

11. Newcombe HB: Plan for a continuing follow-up of persons exposed to radiation in the Canadian nuclear power industry. Atomic Energy of Canada Limited, Report AECL-5538, 1976.

12. deVilliers AJ, Windish JP: Lung cancer in a fluorspar mining community —radiation, dust, and mortality experience. *Brit J Med* 21:94–108, 1964.

13. Report of the (Newfoundland) Royal Commission Respecting Radiation, Compensation and Safety in the Fluorspar Mines, St. Lawrence, Nfld. Queen's Printer, Newfoundland, 1969.

14. The effects on populations of exposure to low levels of ionizing radiation. Report of the Committee on Biological Effects of Ionizing Radiation. U.S. National Academy of Sciences, 1972.

15. Report of the Committee on Biological Effects of Ionizing Radiation (BEIR III). In press.

16. Muller J, Wheeler WC: Causes of death in Ontario uranium miners, in *Proceedings of the International Symposium on Radiation Protection in Mining and Milling of Uranium and Thorium.* Bordeaux, France, 1974.

17. Report of the (Ontario) Royal Commission on the Health and Safety of Workers in Mines (JM Ham, Commissioner). Government of Ontario, 1976.

18. Archer VE, Radford EP, Axelson O: Factors in exposure–response relationships of radon-daughter injury, in *Conference/Workshop on Lung Cancer Epidemiology and Industrial Applications of Sputum Cytology.* Colorado School of Mines Press, 1979, pp. 324–367.

19. Hewitt D: Biostatistical studies on Canadian uranium miners, in *Conference/ Workshop on Lung Cancer Epidemiology and Industrial Applications of Sputum Cytology.* Colorado School of Mines Press, 1979, pp. 264–287.

20. Myers DK, Stewart CG: Some health aspects of Canadian uranium mining. Atomic Energy of Canada Limited, Report AECL-5970, 1979.

21. Wheeler WC, Muller J: Uranium and hard-rock miners study, talk presented to NCIC Workshop on Computerized Record Linkage in Cancer Epidemiology. Ottawa, 1979.

22. Mydren JA, Hiltz JE: Breast cancer following multiple fluoroscopies during artificial pneumothorax treatment of pulmonary tuberculosis. *Can Med Assoc J* 100:1032–1034, 1969.

23. Newcombe HB: Cancer following multiple fluoroscopies. Atomic Energy of Canada Limited, Report AECL-5243, 1975.

24. Miller AB, Lindsay J: Cancer following multiple fluoroscopies, talk presented to NCIC Workshop on Computerized Record Linkage in Cancer Epidemiology. Ottawa, 1979.

25. Weeks JL: A registry for the study of the health of radiation workers employed by Atomic Energy of Canada Limited. Atomic Energy of Canada Limited, Report AECL-6194, 1978.

26. Abbatt J: Follow-up of employees of Eldorado Nuclear, talk presented to NCIC Workshop on Computerized Record Linkage in Cancer Epidemiology. Ottawa, 1979.

27. Roberts R, Shannon H, Julian J: Mortality study of nickel workers, talk presented to NCIC Workshop on Computerized Record Linkage in Cancer Epidemiology. Ottawa, 1979.

28. Saccomanno G, Saunders RP, Archer VE, Auerbach O, Kushner M, Beckler PA: Cancer of the lung: the cytology of sputum prior to the development of carcinoma of the lung. *Acta Cytol* 9:413–423, 1965.

29. Saccomanno G, Archer VE, Auerbach O, Saunders RP, Brennan L: Development of carcinoma of the lung as reflected in exfoliated cells. *Cancer* 33:256–270, 1974.

30. Archer VE: Significance of sputum cytology in relation to radon-daughter injury; and potential uses of sputum cytology in high lung cancer risk groups, in *Conference/ Workshop on Lung Cancer Epidemiology and Industrial Applications of Sputum Cytology.* Colorado School of Mines Press, 1979, pp. 2–9, 469–473.

31. Band P, Feldstein M, Saccomanno G, King G, Watson L: Sputum cytology survey of uranium miners, in *Conference/Workshop on Lung Cancer Epidemiology and Industrial Applications of Sputum Cytology.* Colorado School of Mines Press, 1979, pp. 214–229.

32. Harris R: Give your lungs a break, in *Conference/Workshop on Lung Cancer Epidemiology and Industrial Applications of Sputum Cytology.* Colorado School of Mines Press, 1979, pp. 230–251.

33. Archer VE, Wagoner JK, Lundin FE: Lung cancer among uranium miners in the United States. *Health Physics* 25:351–371, 1973.

Published 1980 by Elsevier North Holland, Inc.
K. F. Hübner and S. A. Fry, eds. The Medical Basis for Radiation Accident Preparedness

The Long-term Follow-up of Radium Dial Painters and Thorium Workers

Austin M. Brues

Center for Human Radiobiology, Argonne National Laboratory, Argonne, Illinois.

The ill effects of ingested radium were first publicized in 1924 when a dentist practicing in the vicinity of Orange, New Jersey, observed cases of jaw necrosis in young women who painted watch and clock dials with radium at a nearby plant.[1] This work had been going on since 1916, and in intervening years several of the dial painters had died with "radium jaw," oral lesions, and progressive anemia that was both aplastic and regenerative in character. Dr. Harrison Martland, the county medical examiner, made a thorough investigation of the situation, reported this as a new occupational disease, demonstrated radioactivity in the breath and bones of the victims,[2] and warned of the hazard of ingestion and injection of radium and mesothorium, and in 1929 published a more detailed report,[3] in which two osteosarcomas were described as occurring in the workers.

Originally, luminous paint had been made with radium 226, but by the time these cases were discovered, mesothorium had been sometimes introduced into the mixture, for economy or for more constant luminosity. Mesothorium 1 is radium 228, the alpha-decay product of natural thorium. This isotope of radium has a very weak beta ray but it begets a chain of radioelements most of which are alpha emitting. One of these is another radium isotope, thorium x or radium 224, whose daughter is thoron, an isotope of radon but with a half-life of only 55 sec, followed by series of three other rather short-lived alpha emitters. Per microcurie, mesothorium appears to be more toxic than radium 226 because of the greater alpha energy in its chain, and it becomes difficult to detect after 40 to 50 years because of its rather short half-life (5.7 years).

A great deal of radium was administered medically, by injection or orally during the 1920s, to an uncounted number of persons, probably a few thousand. Only rarely have such cases been discovered by a radiologist or dentist as having suspicious or characteristic radium lesions. The treatments were given for a variety of indications, particularly hypertension and arthritis, sometimes in attempts to find whether they might be useful in other disorders. A group of schizophrenic patients in a state mental hospital received weekly injections of 10 microcuries each during the period from 1930 to 1932, and a physicist studied the radium retention[4] in the first few months by measuring gamma-ray emission in a calibrated counter and radon loss in expired air. When survivors of this heroic but unsuccessful therapeutic attempt were measured 20 years later, the retention values fit a power function of time with the equation (called the Norris function) $R = 0.54 t^{-0.52}$, where $t =$ time in days.[5] There is some doubt as to the precision of the exponent[6] due to biological variation and some questionable entries in the hospital records, but the model is in general use and appears valid for dosimetric estimates.

In 1925 precautionary rules were introduced in most plants to prevent workers from oral contact with the paint brushes. Although applications of these rules varied somewhat, it is noteworthy that no dial painters who began work after 1925 have been found to have the large or medium radium burdens, which were commonly seen before that time. A large number of dial workers were employed from 1941 to 1947, when luminous airplane instruments were required by the military. This has yielded a large comparison population with low burdens, occupying an important (although largely negative) role in present studies.

Following the war, the new crop of radionuclides posed a considerable health problem in all phases of nuclear business. The radium cases appeared to provide a bridge from animal studies to medications in man; therefore radium studies were strongly encouraged to make full use of the information from this irreplaceable happening, to avoid repetition on a much larger scale, especially since the 0.1 microcurie "safe" level was based on a survey of a relatively small number of early cases.[7]

Both basic and practical questions were raised, similar to those in connection with the Hiroshima–Nagasaki casualties: are any serious unanticipated consequences possible; and what relation exists between exposure level, time, and incidence of malignant tumors? The more practical questions dealt with the human toxicity of bone-seeking fission products and transuramic elements. Animal experiments in abundance yielded much information, but were not adequate to supply numerical toxicity values for man and quite clearly had shown that physical calculations are misleading. Specifically, ^{239}Pu is several times as carcinogenic to bone as radium is because of complex biologic factors of tissue structure and metabolic processes. Therefore, the empirical "permissible burden" of radium was used to derive values for the bone-seekers in general, and the radiobiology laboratories for long-term experiments on beagles were established at Salt Lake City and Davis. These programs were designed to supplement the human studies and have done so on basic as well as empirical levels.

In the mid-1930s, R. D. Evans at the Massachusetts Institute of Technology, who had collaborated with Martland and developed instrumentation for estimating radium content of workers, began to seek out patients for study and therapeutic removal of deposited radium. The procedures developed for removal of lead by Aub and Minot[8] had been suggested by Martland[9] as possibly effective for radium, and parathyroid hormone had been investigated previously.[10] Evans and Aub collaborated in the study of two dial painters, a chemist and an iatrogenic radium case,[11] involving administration of parathormone, thyroid, ammonium chloride, and low-calcium intake; these procedures produced a five- to tenfold increase in the excretion rate, but removed only the most accessible radium, less than 0.01% of the body radium: in lead poisoning the disability is due to soft-tissue and blood lead, while with radium the vulnerable target is bone.

In the ensuing years, the Radioactivity Center at M.I.T. continued to study the radium problems as cases became available. In 1952 a monograph from that laboratory[12] described the findings in 30 cases, some with radium burdens that had been acquired occupationally, others who had received radium as medication. Included were data on measurements of ^{226}Ra and ^{228}Ra *in vivo*, roentgenologic changes in skeletal surveys, and medical observations. Seven of these individuals had developed bone sarcomas or carcinomas of mastoid or paranasal sinuses. A few years later an employment list of dial workers became available, which facilitated the collection of cases for epidemiologic purposes, to a total of over six hundred.[13,14,15] The work of M.I.T. in this period has been discussed at length in these publications.

At Argonne National Laboratory a survey of radium cases was initiated in 1951, following contacts with physicians in the Chicago area, some of whom had identified cases from routine roentgenograms. A few cases were also found among dial workers in an Illinois plant. A summary of the observations was published in 1955.[16] In 1954, C.E. Miller had acquired some group photographs of employees of a dial-painting studio, from patients who had been examined, and by showing them to other patients had learned the names of many others. Eventually in one such photograph taken in 1924, all of the 100 employees have been identified, and almost one-half are living at present.[17] Although no employment records of this plant have been preserved, most of the workers from its inception in 1921 to its dissolution in 1936 have been identified by company photographs and other means, including city directories and common methods of searching names, checked against individual recollections. Reviews of the studies prior to 1968 have been published,[18,19] and a report with abstracts of all cases who were examined was prepared.[20]

A project of the New Jersey State Department of Health was initiated in 1957 and devoted its time to finding and examining persons who had engaged in dial painting in Orange, New Jersey, between 1914 and 1924. Of 978 persons who were identified by name, 328 were found to be living and 269 were known to be dead. A terminal report in 1967[21] summarized the information obtained on those who were examined or on whom outside records were available for study.

A 1974 paper by Sharpe[22] reports the results of 42 autopsies that were performed on persons associated with the New Jersey radium industry and includes much information about the project.

In the late 1960s a majority of the known persons carrying significant radium burdens acquired as a result of occupational exposure, if they were available and cooperative, had probably been under the surveillance of one of the three projects. On the other hand, the number who had received radium internally for medical purposes was unknown; very few of these individuals were to be found on existing lists, and they were not likely to be acquainted with one another (except where whole families had been so treated).

The dial workers are a limited population, large enough to have some statistical usefulness, but small enough to permit detailed longitudinal study, and external physical measurements allow objective, quantitative evidence of the radium intake. The three projects have used rather similar protocols in collecting medical information and the major differences among the population have been (1) geographical, since the three projects were oriented to three local areas where dial painting was one of the small industries, and (2) isotopic, since the midwestern plants used almost pure radium 226, while that used in the northeast was generally spiked with variable amounts of radium 228, the inexpensive daughter of thorium. As mentioned before, this has important implications for radiation dose and for detectability after many years.

In view of the above, a proposal for formation of a Center for Human Radiobiology was made in 1967,[13] and in 1968 it gained approval with the provision that it be established at Argonne National Laboratory. The Center became the repository of the medical and other records of the projects at Argonne, M.I.T., and New Jersey. After a transitional period, clinical studies and whole-body radium measurements were instituted at Argonne in 1971, with assistance from the Radioactivity Center at M.I.T., which is a satellite laboratory of the Center.

Inasmuch as the Center was established to ensure the continuation of the human radium studies that are essential in the formulation of radiation protection standards and procedures for internal emitters in general, a first objective is to determine radium effects in their quantitative relations to dose. It was envisioned that human studies might be broadened to include other internal emitters of radiation and that the population, and data derived from it, would be applicable to study of basic mechanisms, particularly of malignant tumor-induction.[23]

Most of the techniques of study had been developed in the earlier projects. Physical measurements defining the body radium content are made by gamma-ray determinations under standard conditions that relate directly to body content of ^{214}Bi, indicating the radon emanation that has been retained in its physical lifetime. This is then added to the fraction of radon lost, which represents about two-thirds of the original ^{226}Ra and is determined from analysis of expired air. ^{228}Ra is estimated by gamma measurements of its decay products, of which ^{228}Ac is the proximate one. Because of the time-decay of that series (^{228}Ra having a half-life of 5.7 yrs; all of the others are shorter), for *in vivo* measurements at the present time (over 50 years) it has been necessary to assume the original ^{228}Ra intake of previously unmeasured cases from information of the radium isotopic ratios in the early periods, either from analyses of paints or from measurements that were made on contemporary patients. However, radiochemical measurements of autopsy material are sufficiently sensitive to continue to provide direct estimates of radium 228 content.

If one is to estimate the radium content by either gamma or radon measurement alone, an assumption of the total can be made by using stated values of the ratio of emanating to total skeletal radium. Recent studies at the Center have shown, however, that the rate of radon loss by exhalation is dependent on cyclic physiological conditions (probably circulatory) and is significantly higher in the postprandial period,[24] and that in certain modern housing conditions, which include recirculated air conditioning or heating connected with unpaved basement areas, radon concentrations above 10 picocuries/liter may occur, leading to temporary soft-tissue storage of radon that is later exhaled along with that derived from deposited radium.[25]

One of the problems in constructing a total picture of dose-effect relations lies in the number of cases lacking data on radium content. Since these include many of the early cases (as before 1930) a program of exhumation for skeletal measurements and radiographs has been pursued for some time. Besides this, donation of willed bodies, which are available for detailed pathologic study, has been solicited in some cases; it is of interest and reflects well on the personal handling of patients by the staff that some spontaneous offers have been made.

Each patient who comes for medical examination is asked to complete a personal history form and medical questionnaire in advance; a detailed medical history is taken and a thorough routine physical examination with blood samples for hematology and clinical chemistry. Visual examinations by orthorater and audiometry (including bone conduction) are made, an electrocardiogram is taken, and a skeletal X-ray survey is made at least once in persons who consent. (The mean absorbed dose to red bone marrow has been measured by use of an anthropomorphic phantom, and by careful attention to technical details is less than 200 mrad in a person of average build.) Special attention is given to the mastoids and air sinuses and to radiologic changes in the skeleton that might be suggestive of neoplasm, since these are the fully recognized sites of radiogenic neoplasms and fractures, and information in this area is of value to the patient's welfare as well as to the purposes of the study. A full report is sent to the personal physician, a procedure that encourages cooperation.

A release is requested so that outside medical records from hospitals and other sources may be obtained and these are actively being sought. Death certificates are obtained where possible on all deceased cases. Every item of significant clinical importance is coded for computer storage under the SNOP coding system along with date and nature of the source of each item.[26] At the present time, survey of 5400 records has yielded over 140,000 items, an overall average of more than 25, even including a considerable number of records with little useful information. This system provides an excellent index to the records and information can be retrieved in the context of any other data in the computer files.

For epidemiologic purposes, the largest and most satisfactory group is the dial workers. Various unbiased lists (i.e., defined because of recorded exposure) may be separated out from the total, or the unmeasured cases may be eliminated for a dose-effect study. A recent compilation[27] listed 1199 dial workers who had been studied (including radioactivity measurements) and 903 who had not. Most of the recent statistical studies have used the segment of female dial workers who first worked before 1930; this includes all of those who have accumulated over 100 mean skeletal rads, and excludes the World War II painters who had minimal intake.

Because of the fact that the radium burden (which has been widely used in the past as an index) decreases with time, the basic index now being used in the intake dose, which is calculated from available measurements by use of the Norris equation. Previous Argonne investigators[20] have undertaken to calculate maximum burdens by using similar methods and assuming constancy of intake during the working period.

Two mortality studies have been reported from the Center, using death certificate data to distinguish causes; they differed in the segment of the population used, but reached a similar conclusion. One of these studies[27] analyzed the data in a population of 1235 workers and found an excess of 68 deaths as against appropriate life-table values; while by eliminating the risk introduced by the "radiogenic" tumors, the deaths from other causes were approximately the same as in the expected values (excess of five cases). The other study[29] used a segregated cohort of 634 cases, limited to those whose names were obtained from employment and other objective lists. Overall mortality ratios were lower than unity in the groups first employed after 1924 (0.89) and in the group with calculated intake below 50 microcuries (0.86). Cause-specific mortality ratios were elevated at $p < 0.001$ for all malignant neoplasms and for bone and "other and unspecified" malignancy, also at the same significance level. In both of these studies the case records were examined where radiogenic tumor types were involved, and this gave very useful indication of the problems inherent in studies where the only data exist on death certificates.

An examination of the dose-incidence relationship of radiogenic tumors in 759 dial workers whose radium burdens were known[30] disclosed 38 cases of bone sarcoma and 17 of "head" carcinomas (a shorthand term for carcinoma of mastoid and paranasal sinuses). These were fitted by least squares alternately to the commonly used linear-square radiobiologic formula $I = (C + \alpha D + \beta D^2)e^{-\gamma D}$ in which the exponential term indicates cell killing or inactivation, and to combinations of several terms of this formula. The doses were expressed in terms of calculated intake, and ^{228}Ra was assumed to be 2.5 times as effective as ^{226}Ra. The bone tumors best fit the square-exponential model (the search for a linear term yielded a meaningless negative exponent), and the head carcinomas best fit a linear model, although some other formulations could not be rejected. It may not be surprising that these two tumor types are fitted by different models, since there is a growing belief that the sinus epithelium may be primarily irradiated by trapped radon and because of differences in topological distribution of the cells in the target areas. Both of these questions are under examination in the laboratory.

Other studies pursued in the Center include the Marshall-Groer model of bone oncogenesis by alpha radiation which was recently reported.[31] This derives from the application of alternative models to data from the radium study, as well as from animal investigations and other human data. The present model has terms for two initiating events, for growth, cell inactivation and replacement, and a promoting event. Studies by Lloyd on the geometry of the nuclei of cells on the surface of bone and on the dynamics of cell transformation by alpha particles are being continued. Marshall has also developed models of alkaline earth metabolism, as chairman of a task group of the International Commission on Radiological Protection, which will be useful in extending the radium findings to other nuclides.[32]

Continuation of the collection of medical information in the aging radium population is now involving a population of increasing cancer susceptibility. This may entail an increase in soft-tissue neoplasms. A catalog of all of the verified malignancies in the SNOP entry file has been made and is being kept up-to-date: this can be used for any chosen segment of the total recorded cases in the registry.

I should like to deal briefly with the Thorium Study. Although initiated some time ago, it is at present in an active state in gathering information.[33] The Center has been granted access to the employment records of the thorium refining plant in northern Illinois, from the 1930s until recently. A survey of this plant was made by representatives of the Health and Safety Laboratory of the U.S. Atomic Energy Commission in 1953.[34] Apparently the mode of operation has remained much the same. The paper described characteristics of the dusts derived from the monazite sands and of those resulting from the various processes. At that time, two deaths among the workers appeared to have resulted from lung carcinoma, and one lung measurement at postmortem indicated 14 mg thorium per kg. A great deal of information exists on the induction of liver neoplasms by deposited thorotrast (colloidal thorium dioxide). A small amount of alpha-active material is deposited on bone and may be associated with the development of bone tumors.

From the list a selection was made of 558 males who had worked a year or longer; 127 were known dead, 317 of the remainder were located (73%) and 262 of these returned health questionnaires. A random sample of 100 yielded 62 located cases, most of whom have been examined. Additional cases are being selected, and a total of 208 have now been examined and measured. The medical examination scheduled has been similar to that used for radium cases, except that the skeletal survey has been omitted and abdominal radiography substituted. Pulmonary function testing is also done routinely. The physical measurements include gamma-ray spectrometry front and back of chest to determine thorium daughters, especially ^{212}Bi(ThC), and a 50 minute collection of thoron (^{220}Rn) from expired air. Correlations between these measurements are somewhat ambiguous and refinements of technique are being examined. Clearly the ranges of values in individuals are quite wide, through two orders of magnitude in the thoron values. A death certificate survey of the entire population has been undertaken and shows little deviation from expectation except for an apparent increase in accidental deaths compared with white U.S. males.

Film-badge readings have been obtained and the job classifications are being examined. Efforts are being made to secure pathologic material at autopsy or by willed-body arrangements to improve estimates of the body distribution and content of the thorium chain, and its translocations, with reference to the external measurements that are made.

ACKNOWLEDGMENT
Work was performed under the auspices of the United States Department of Energy.

References

2. Blum T: Osteomyelitis of the mandible and maxilla. *J Am Dental Assn* 2:672–674, 1924.

2. Martland HS, Conlon P, Kref JP: Some unrecognized dangers in the handling of radioactive substances. *JAMA* 85:961, 1925.

3. Martland HS: Occupational poisoning in manufacture of luminous watch dials. *JAMA* 92:466–513, 1929.

4. Schlundt H, Nerancy JT, Morris JP: Detection and estimation of radium in living persons. IV. The retention of soluble salts administered intravenously. *Am J Roentgenol Radium Ther* 30, 1933.

5. Norris WP, Speckman TW, Gustafson PF: Studies of the metabolism of radium in man. *Am J Roentgenol Radium Ther Nuclear Med* 73:774–784, 1955.

6. Miller CE, Finkel AJ: Radium Retention in man after multiple injections: the power function re-evaluated. *Am J Roentgenol Radium Ther Nuclear Med* 103:871–880, 1968.

7. Evans RD: Protection of radium dial workers and radiologists from injury by radium. *J Indust Hyg* 25:253–269, 1943.

8. Hunter D, Aub JC: Lead Studies. XV. The effect of the parathyroid hormones on the excretion of lead and of calcium in patients suffering from lead poisoning. *Quart J Med* 20:123–140, 1926.

9. Martland HS: The occurrence of malignancy in radioactive persons. *Am J Cancer* 15:112–193, 1931.

10. Flinn FB, Seidlin SM: Parathormone in the treatment of "radiation poisoning." *Bull Johns Hopkins Hosp* 45:269–275, 1929.

11. Aub JC, Evans RD, Gallagher DM, Tibbetts DM: Effects of treatment on radium and calcium metabolism in the human body. *Ann Int Med* 11, 1938.

12. Aub JC, Evans RD, Hempelmann LH, Martland HS: The late effects of internally deposited materials in man. *Medicine* 31:221–329, 1952.

13. Evans RD, Keane AT, Kolenkow RJ, Neal WR, Shanahan MM: Radiogenic tumors in the radium and mesothorium cases studied at MIT, in Mays CW, Jee WSS, Lloyd RD, Stover BS, Dougherty JH, Taylor GN (eds.): *Delayed Effects of Bone-Seeking Radionuclides,* Univ. of Utah Press, Salt Lake City, 1969, pp. 157–194.

14. Evans RD, Keane AT, Shanahan MM: Radiogenic effects in man of long-term skeletal irradiation, in Stover BJ, Jee WSS (eds.): *Radiobiology of Plutonium,* J.W. Press, Salt Lake City, 1972, pp. 431–468.

15. Evans RD: The effect of skeletally deposited alpha-ray emitters in man. *Brit J Radiol* 39:881–895, 1966.

16. Looney WB, Hasterlik RJ, Brues AM, Skirmont E: A clinical investigation of the chronic effects of radium salts administered therapeutically (1915–1931). *Am J Roentgenol* 73:1006–1037, 1955.

17. Brues AM, Kirsh IE: The fate of individuals containing radium. *Trans Amer Clin Climatological Assn* 88:211–218, 1976.

18. Finkel AJ, Miller CE, Hasterlik RJ: Radium-induced malignant tumors in man, in *Delayed Effects of Bone-Seeking Radionuclides,* 1969, pp. 195–224.

19. Finkel AJ, Miller CE, Hasterlik RJ: Correlation between retrospective estimates of maximum body burden and clinical findings in dial painters 40 years later. *Third Internat. Congress of Radiation Research* (abstract, p. 84) Cortina d'Ampezzo, Italy, 1966.

20. Miller CE, Hasterlik RJ, Finkel AJ: The Argonne radium studies—summary of fundamental data. U.S. Atomic Energy Commission document ANL-7531 and ACRH-106, pp. 596, 1969.

21. New Jersey State Department of Health, Radium Research Project, Epidemiological follow-up of the New Jersey radium cases, November 1957—June 1967, Final report (2 vols.). U.S. Atomic Energy Commission Report NYO-2181-5 (TID4500), 1967.

22. Sharpe WD: Chronic Radium Intoxication: Clinical and autopsy findings in long-term New Jersey survivors. *Environ Res* 8:243–383, 1974.

23. Radiological Physics Division Annual Report. Center for Human Radiobiology, July 1969–June 1970. Argonne National Laboratory Report, ANL-7760. part II, 1970, pp. i–ii.

24. Rundo J, Markun F, Sha JY: Postprandial changes in the exhalation rate of radon produced *in vivo. Science* 199:1211–1212, 1978.

25. Rundo J, Markun F, Plondke NJ: Observation of high concentrations of radon in certain houses. *Health Phys* 36:724–730, 1979.

26. Littman MS, Lucas HF Jr, Sharpe WD, Stehney AF: Radiation epidemiologic surveillance using the systematized nomenclature of pathology. *J Clin Computing* 3:191–197, 1973.

27. Rowland RE, Stehney AF, Brues AM, Littman MS, Keane AT, Patten BC, Shanahan MM: Current status of the study of [226]Ra at the Center for Human Radiobiology. *Health Phys* 35:159–166.

28. Stehney AF, Lucas HF Jr, Rowland RE: Survival times of women radium dial workers first exposed before 1930, in *Late Biological Effects of Ionizing Radiation,* International Atomic Energy Agency IAEA-SM.224/505, Vienna, 1978, pp. 333–351.

29. Polednak AP, Stehney AF, Rowland RE: Mortality among women first employed before 1930 in the U.S. radium dial-painting industry. *Am J Epidemiol* 107:179–195, 1978.

30. Rowland RE, Stehney AF, Lucas HF Jr: Dose-response relationships for female radium-dial workers. *Radiation Res* 76:368–383, 1978.

31. Marshall JH, Groer PG: A theory of the induction of bone cancer by alpha radiation. *Radiation Res* 71:149–192, 1977.

32. Marshall JH, Liniecki J, Lloyd EL, Marotti G, Mays C, Rundo J, Sissons HA, Snyder WS: *Alkaline Earth Metabolism in Adult Man.* New York, Pergamon Press, 1973.

33. Rundo J, Polednak AP, Brues AM, Lucas HF Jr, Patten BC, Rowland RE, Stehney AF: A study of radioactivity and health status of former thorium workers–preliminary report. *Environ Res* 18:94–100, 1979.

34. Albert R, Klevin P, Fresco J, Harris W, Eisenbud M: Industrial hygiene and medical survey of a thorium refinery. *Arch Indust Health-* 11:234–242, 1955.

Published 1980 by Elsevier North Holland, Inc.
K. F. Hübner and S. A. Fry, eds. The Medical Basis for Radiation Accident Preparedness

The United States Radiation Accident and Other Registries of the REAC/TS Registry System:
Their Functions and Current Status

Shirley A. Fry

Medical and Health Sciences Division, Oak Ridge Associated Universities, Oak Ridge, Tennessee.

The REAC/TS Registry System consists of a central comprehensive registry and four satellite registries, named the United States Radiation Accident Registry, the Department of Energy Study (Equal to or Greater than Five Rem Registry), the DTPA Registry, and the Foreign Registry. Each registry is designated to record a specific aspect of the exposure of human beings to ionizing radiation. Using information provided by or drawn from a variety of public and private institutions, the registries record events involving the accidental exposures to radiation in the United States and abroad, the occupational whole body exposure to radiation in excess of current permissible limits of individuals in designated study populations, and individual administrations of diethylenetriaminepentaacetic acid (DTPA) to provide a current tally of such events. The registries are an integral part of the research and educational programs of the REAC/TS group, a subunit of the Medical and Health Sciences Division of Oak Ridge Associated Universities. Instituted in 1974, this system of registries has been restructured in response to the evolution and development of the interests and responsibilities of the medical and scientific communities in general and the REAC/TS group in particular. The registries form the basis for medical follow-up programs designed to be of mutual benefit to exposed individuals and to the studies of the REAC/TS, Epidemiological and Radiopharmaceutical groups of the Medical and Health Sciences Division, and other interested professional groups. Past experience, as documented in the files of the registries, is a useful teacher in courses given throughout the year by REAC/TS staff and invited faculty members for physicians, health physicists, and allied health-care personnel in the management of radiation accidents and persons involved in them.

This paper presents a detailed description of the structure and function of the registry system, together with the current status of the component registries.

Introduction

The registry system developed by the Radiation Emergency Assistance Center/Training Site (REAC/TS) group of the Medical and Health Sciences Division of Oak Ridge Associated Universities records, in one or more of its five registries, events involving exposures of human beings to ionizing radiation that meet certain criteria. In addition to providing a current tally of these events, the U. S. Radiation Accident and the Department of Energy (DOE) Study Registries form a basis for long-term clinical and epidemiological studies by the REAC/TS and Epidemiology groups, which seek to increase knowledge of the health effects of such exposures and improve the therapeutic methods for radiation induced injuries, as shown in Figure 1. The study of the clinical effectiveness and the possible side or adverse effects of chelation therapy with the calcium and zinc ions and diethylenetriaminepentaacetic acid (DTPA), under investigation by the Radiopharmaceutical group, and the educational responsibilities of REAC/TS are also served by the REAC/TS Registry system. REAC/TS role as a responder to requests for emergency and other assistance in radiation accidents and incidents makes the site a logical repository for registries that document these and related events.

The REAC/TS Registry system as it presently exists is the tangible result of the evolution of an avocation of a few physicians into a vocation of national and international proportions, supported by the federal government. Prior to the institution of a national repository for information about radiation accidents at REAC/TS in 1974, information about such events and occupational over-exposures at governmental and contractor facilities and private licensee facilities was recorded and documented ultimately by and for the Atomic Energy Commission (AEC). Descriptions of some accidents and the clinical effects and the management of survivors appeared in literature,[1–54] and the long-term follow-up of the survivors was advocated. However, the actual follow-up was haphazard. Execution of the follow-up depended largely upon the interest and opportunity of individual physicians, generally those who were involved directly in the early care of the survivors of a specific accident. Under these circumstances, continuity of medical follow-up was liable to interruption or abrupt termination by changes in the circumstances of the physicians or the survivors, or both. Consequently, survivors of some serious accidents, notably those at Los Alamos,[2,3] Oak Ridge,[11–15]

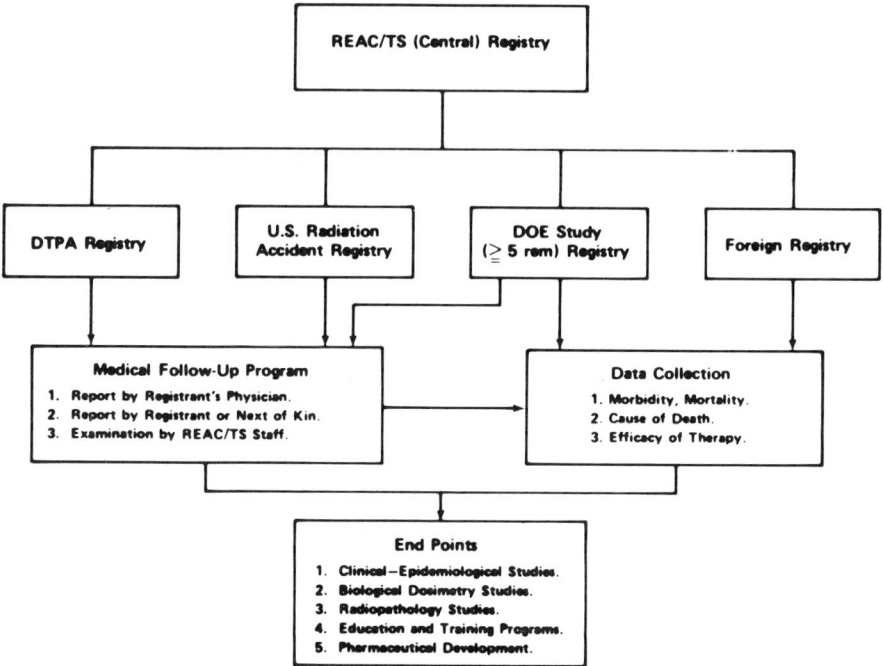

Figure 1. The REAC/TS Registry System as a basis for long-term clinical-epidemiological studies.

Pittsburgh,[43] and the Marshall Islands,[55] were followed consistently at variable intervals; some survivors of other accidents were lost to follow-up after several years as was the case with survivors of the accidents at Eniwetok (1946),[4,5] Argonne (1952),[6] and Lockport (1961).[28] With the exception of the Atomic Bomb survivors, who are not considered here, and the Marshall Islanders and others exposed to radioactive fallout following atmospheric testing of an atomic device at Bikini Atoll in 1954,[55–70] there have been few published reports of the medical follow-up of accidentally irradiated persons.[71,72]

Expansion of the nuclear industry and the growing need for methodical long-term follow-up studies of apparently healthy persons accidentally exposed to acute radiation prompted the development of the U.S. Radiation Accident Registry. In 1974 the Energy Research and Development Administration (ERDA), as successor to the AEC, designated the newly created REAC/TS group[73] to be the custodians of the registry with responsibility for the development and operation of a long-term medical follow-up program.[74] This mandate was supported by an agreement between the recently independent regulatory arm of the nuclear industry, the Nuclear Regulatory Commission (NRC), and the Division of Biological and Environmental Research (DBER) of ERDA to provide for the orderly flow of information about radiation accidents and the persons involved in them, from the NRC to the U.S. Radiation Accident Registry through DBER, as they occurred.

The criteria for events to be included in the U.S. Radiation Accident Registry, with subsequent medical follow-up of persons involved, were developed and adopted by agreement between the directorates of NRC and DBER (ERDA) and the Office of Health and Environmental Research in the Department of Energy (DOE) as successor to DBER (ERDA).[75] Other registries evolved or were developed to meet additional registry needs of REAC/TS. The REAC/TS Case Registry became the repository for cases in which REAC/TS was involved in its role as a Radiation Emergency Assistance Center. Such cases included radiation accident cases, as defined by ERDA (DOE)-NRC (DOE/NRC) selection criteria, and incidents involving persons exposed or suspected of having been exposed to lower doses of ionizing radiation. The Supplemental Registry was developed to record and retain anecdotal information about radiation accidents occurring in the United States and abroad and the medical consequences to the individuals involved.

The Functions and Structure of the REAC/TS Registry System

Because of the increase in the number of personnel and registries, it became necessary to restructure the REAC/TS Registry System in order to facilitate its orderly operation and maintenance. To this end, a central or parent registry has been created to serve four satellite registries as shown in Figure 2. Information flows from the central registry into one or more of the satellite registries according to their selection criteria as shown; if the information provided about an individual event does not meet the criteria of any of the satellite registries, it is retained in the files of the central registry for reference.

Once information about a specific radiation event and the individuals involved in it is registered, files are prepared for the appropriate registries to retain additional information as it becomes available. Information that could identify individuals and other privileged information is kept separate and physically secure in correspondingly numbered medical files. Any relevant information contained in these files is made available to the files of the registries in abstract form without identification. In this way appropriate files of the registries can be made available to students of radiation accidents and other professional groups while maintaining the privacy of the individuals involved. The characteristics of the individual registries will be described.

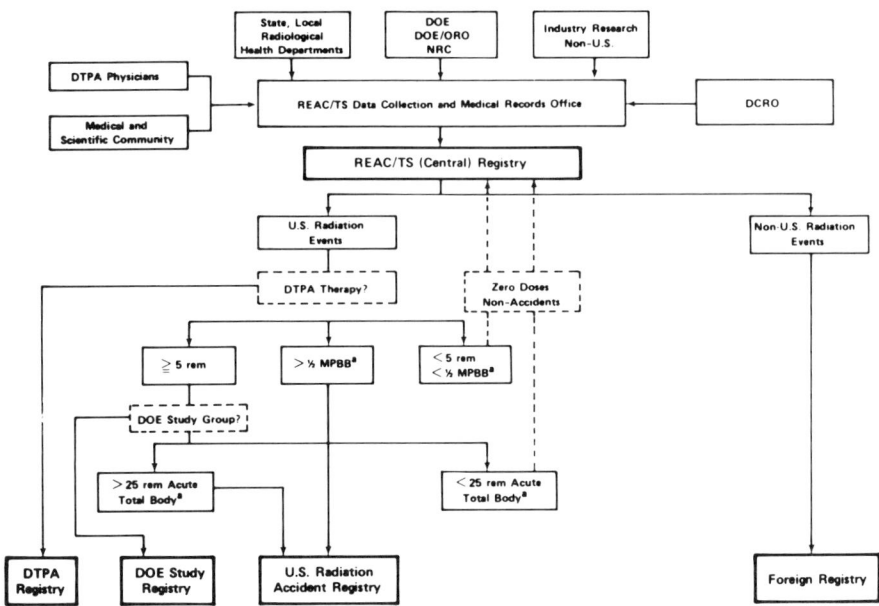

Figure 2. The REAC/TS Registry System. A diagrammatic representation of the flow of information into and from the REAC/TS (Central) Registry.

The REAC/TS (Central) Registry

This registry provides for the registration of all events that come to the attention of REAC/TS directly or indirectly (shown in Figure 2) and all events that involve the known or suspected exposure of human beings to ionizing radiation. Pertinent information about such events is recorded irrespective of the known or suspected exposure dose, the type or location of the accident, or the source of the information. Comprehensive registration of events is undertaken in this manner to prevent information "slipping through the cracks."

When REAC/TS is notified of a known or suspected radiation exposure the event is recorded in the REAC/TS Registry log book and is assigned a sequential four digit registration number. Individuals involved in the event are identified by an additional four digit number only, beginning with 0001 for each event. The key to the system and data bank rests in a single, secured working notebook in which the names of events and individuals involved in them are linked to registry numbers. Characteristic lack of accurate biological and exposure data early in the post-exposure stage frequently delays the evaluation of a radiation event against the selection criteria of the satellite registries. Meanwhile, registration of the event in the REAC/TS (Central) Registry ensures retention of the information in the Registry files until such time as accurate data become available and a critical evaluation of the event can be made. When an evaluation has been made, the event may be found to qualify for inclusion in one or more of the satellite registries; the registration is made accordingly with information about the event being entered into the files of the appropriate registry or registries. The central registry file for a specific event indicates the satellite registry or registries to which the event has been designated; if the event does not qualify for inclusion in any of the satellite registries, the information is retained in the central registry file for reference only. Subsequently, information about the exposure and the biological and clinical effects on the persons involved is extracted from the records, encoded, and entered into a data bank together with information about the extent and type of assistance provided by REAC/TS.

At the present time 238 events involving approximately 3880[1] individuals are included in this registry.

The DTPA Registry

The DTPA Registry is one of the more recently developed satellite registries in the REAC/TS Registry System. In it are recorded administrations of DTPA to individuals known to have been or suspected of being contaminated internally with one or more actinides. Authorization to administer the drug is given by the Medical and Health Sciences Division of ORAU, managers of the Food and Drug Administration's (FDA) Investigational and New Drug (IND) protocol. Each site at which there is a physician so authorized has been given a sequential, low-digit registry number. Registration of individuals to whom DTPA is administered at each site is recorded by the second four-digit sequential number. Individual administrations of DTPA, their efficacy, and any side or adverse effects are reported by ORAU to the FDA annually, a system that makes REAC/TS a logical repository for this registry. At this time administrations of DTPA to 390 individuals at 12 sites have been recorded in the registry. Some of the radiation events in which these individuals were involved, which necessitated their treatment with DTPA, also qualify for registration in the U.S. Accident Registry; consequently individuals may be registered in more than one of the REAC/TS satellite registries in addition to the REAC/TS (Central) Registry. Registration of these and other events into other satellite registries proceeds as shown in Figure 1. An example of dual registration is the case of the individual

---

[1]Uncertainties in the numbers of persons involved in some radiation accidents outside the U.S. make this an approximate total.

involved in the accident at Hanford in 1976, who as the result of the accident required DTPA therapy and is therefore registered in the DTPA Registry. He was contaminated internally in excess of one half of a maximum permissible body burden. The event qualified for registration in the U.S. Radiation Accident Registry where the individual and others involved in the accident are also registered.

The Department of Energy (DOE)-Study Registry

The DOE-Study Registry, known colloquially as "The Equal to or Greater than Five Rem" Study Registry, is being developed to provide a basis for epidemiological evaluation of the health and mortality of persons who, over the past thirty or more years, have exceeded "permissible" exposure limits in their employment with DOE and its predecessors. Populations being studied currently for the Department of Energy include persons exposed to ionizing and neutron radiation in excess of the current occupational limits of whole body exposure to or greater than 5 rem per annum, or 3 rem per quarter, and who are past or present employees at the facilities of the Manhattan Project, the Atomic Energy Commission, the Energy Research and Development Administration, Department of Energy, or United States Navy Reactor Program (civilian employees). Rosters of these persons have been submitted to the Registry through the Epidemiological group of the Medical and Health Sciences Division of ORAU. Individuals have been registered according to site. Preliminary studies of mortality in these populations are in progress using information from death certificates collected by the DOE Death Certificate Retrieval Office operated by ORAU.

Some persons qualifying for registration in the DOE-Study Registry also qualify for registration in the U.S. Accident Registry because their exposure was acute and in excess of the dose criteria of the U.S. Radiation Accident Registry. Examples of dual registration of this type are the individuals involved in radiation accidents at Argonne National Laboratory in 1952 and at the Oak Ridge Y-12 Plant in 1958. While employed at these AEC facilities, they received whole-body exposure in excess of 5 rem in a calendar year, thus qualifying for registration in the DOE-Study Registry. The same exposure was also acute and, in some cases, in excess of the selection dose criteria for the U.S. Radiation Accident Registry where, as a consequence, they are registered. Thus far 18 persons have been found to qualify for registration in both registries.

Currently the DOE-Study Registry includes approximately 2400 persons from 22 sites. It is anticipated that approximately 1800 present or former civil employees of the U.S. Navy's Reactor Program will be added to this Registry in the near future.

The United States Radiation Accident Registry

The United States Radiation Accident Registry was developed under the guidance of the USAEC, its activities were formalized by ERDA and continued by DOE. It records those events occurring in the United States and its territories in which one or more persons accidentally received doses of ionizing radiation equal to or in excess of the criteria agreed to by ERDA and the NRC in 1974. The persons meeting these criteria qualify for long-term medical follow-up programs; the criteria are shown in Table 1.

In the early years of the nuclear industry, the most frequently registered type of radiation injury was due to acute whole-body irradiation, which was usually the result of an accidental critical excursion. The first of this type of accident, in which human beings received doses of radiation to the whole body in excess of 25 rem, occurred in June 1945 at the Los Alamos Scientific Laboratory (Los Alamos 0).[1] There have been no radiation accidents involving accidental critical excursions in the United States since 1964,[37,38,39] largely due to the benefit of experience and to the development of automated operating processes at remote sites. The type of radiation-induced injury registered most frequently in recent years has been the result of high dose local exposure, commonly to the hands.[10,41,46,48,76] Injuries of this type are frequently associated with unshielded industrial radiographic sources. In these cases any concomi-

Table 1. Radiation Dose Criteria for Selection of Cases for Long-Term Medical Follow-up[a]

Condition	Criteria
1. Dose to Whole Body, Active Blood-Forming Organs or Gonads	25 rem
2. Dose to Skin of Whole Body or Extremities	600 rem
3. Dose to Other Tissues or Organs From External Source	75 rem
4. Internal Burdens	½ NCRP Maximum Organ Burden[74]
5. Medical Misadministration	All misadministrations, provided they also result in a dose (if a radiation source) or a burden (if a radiopharmaceutical), equal to or greater than the criteria for conditions 1, 2, 3, or 4 above.

[a] Agreement between directorate of Regulatory Operations (NRC) and Division of Biomedical and Environmental Research (ERDA) regarding long-term medical follow-up of significant exposures.

tant total body dose tends to be low and of less biomedical consequence than the local exposure.

The 88 accidents recorded in the United States Radiation Registry have involved a total of 596 persons, of whom 267 were exposed to radioactive fallout on the Marshall Islands following a nuclear test at Bikini Atoll in 1954. The seemingly large number of persons involved in radiation accidents, although small in comparison to the numbers of persons involved in other types of accidents,[77,78] reflects the scope of registration of individuals in this registry. If the exposure dose of one person involved in a radiation event meets the one or more of the ERDA (DOE)/NRC selection criteria given in Table 1, all other persons involved in the same event are also registered whether or not their doses meet the same criteria. This procedure is designed to increase the data base in order to allow comparison of morbidity and mortality in groups of persons who received high exposure doses with those who received little or none of the same type of radiation exposure. The numbers of persons who received doses (rads) resulting in clinically significant effects are shown in Table 2. Of these, approximately forty persons sustained serious injuries in the form of severe bone marrow depression and/or

Table 2. Registrants in the U.S. Radiation Accident Registry Grouped According to Dose (1945 — September 1979)

Accidents According to DOE/NRC Criteria	88
Persons Involved	596[a]
Persons With $\geqslant$ Dose Criteria.	295[b]
Persons, Acute Total Body Irradiation $\geqslant$ 25 rem	54[c]
Persons, $\geqslant$ 100 r Acute Total Body Irradiation	35
Persons, Acute TBI Plus Local $\geqslant$ Dose Criteria	22
Persons, $\geqslant$ r, Acute TBI Plus Local	5
Persons, Acute Local Irradiation Only, $\geqslant$ 600 rem	45
Persons, Significant Local Lesions Only	31[d]
Persons, Contaminated Internally $\geqslant$ ½ MPBB	19
Medical Misadventures	7
Persons Involved in Medical Misadventures	49[e]
Fatalities.	7[f]

[a] Includes 239 Marshall Islanders plus 28 U.S. Servicemen exposed to fallout in 1954.

[b] Includes 82 Marshall Islanders plus 28 U.S. Servicemen exposed to fallout in 1954.

[c] Marshall Islanders and U.S. Servicemen exposed to fallout in 1954 are not included in this or subsequent totals.

[d] Lesions requiring surgical repair or necessitating amputation.

[e] Includes 42 persons from larger group overexposed to therapeutic source due to calibration error and seven persons involved in six medical misadministrations involving isotopes.

[f] Includes three victims of blast injuries in SLI accident, and four fatalities as a direct result of radiation.

local lesions that required amputation of portions of digits or limbs. There has been no fatality in the United States directly attributable to the acute effects of accidental exposure to radiation since 1964.[39,40]

Except for the interagency agreement [ERDA(DOE)/NRC 1974] there is no provision for the mandatory registration of radiation accidents in the private domain. The NRC is responsible only for those materials and facilities for which it issues licenses and abrogates its control of these in "agreement states."[2] Thus there exists a large crack through which falls information about radiation accidents occurring in areas in which the NRC has no responsibility. In addition X-ray defraction units and non-isotopic sources are the responsibility of the individual states. In these situations much of the early information about an accident or suspected accident comes from physicians and others seeking medical assistance from REAC/TS in dealing with their problem. This system has resulted in the less than complete registration of all radiation accidents. Nevertheless, as the result of Holmesian investigational methods and information provided to us by colleagues and former students, we believe the registry has recorded most of the acute whole-body exposures of equal to or in excess of 25 rem and a majority of the local exposures in excess of 600 rem that have occurred in the United States. The reporting and registration of medical misadventures is believed to be far less complete. In order to improve upon this registration record, an appreciation of the registry program and its purposes is needed. It has been our experience that there is willing cooperation from informed physicians and others at the location of a radiation accident. Such cooperation may include acting on behalf of REAC/TS physicians to recruit the accident survivor(s) into the long-term medical follow-up program.

Because of the selection criteria of the other satellite registries, it is theoretically possible for an individual to be registered in the DOE-Study Registry and the DTPA Registry in addition to the U.S. Radiation Accident Registry; such a situation has not yet arisen.

The Foreign Registry

Although there has been involvement of a few members of the REAC/TS staff in the management of survivors of radiation accidents occurring outside the United States, most of the information leading to the registration of events in the Foreign Registry is largely secondhand and anecdotal. The most common sources of this type of information are the open literature, personal communications, and the news media. Attempts

---

[2]Agreement States (25): Alabama, Arizona, Arkansas, California, Colorado, Florida, Georgia, Idaho, Kansas, Kentucky, Louisiana, Maryland, Mississippi, Nebraska, North Carolina, North Dakota, Nevada, New Hampshire, New Mexico, New York, Oregon, South Carolina, Tennessee, Texas, Washington.

are made subsequently to learn of the circumstances of the accidents from the physicians and scientists directly involved, but with varying degrees of success. No efforts have been made to identify or follow directly the individuals involved and anecdotal information on their progress is recorded as it becomes available. This registry provides a frame of reference for the comparison of the radiation accident experience in the United States with that in other countries and also increases educational resources.

Twenty-eight radiation events involving approximately one hundred ninety-five persons are recorded in this registry; of these, twenty-four events (c. 77 persons) are believed to involve doses (rads) in excess of the ERDA(DOE)/NRC criteria for serious exposures.[3] There is information about 10 fatalities that can be related directly to the acute effects of exposure to ionizing radiation.

Follow-up Programs

Designs for the long-term follow-up of survivors of radiation accidents (registrants in the U.S. Radiation Accident Registry), and persons whose doses were less than the DOE/NRC criteria but in whose evaluation and/ or management REAC/TS was involved, have been described by Hübner et al.[74]

Ideally, recruitment of persons involved in radiation accidents or suspected accidents into such a program begins at, or soon after the time of the accident. The scope, purposes, and benefits of the program are explained by REAC/TS physicians or their surrogate. Although the benefits of participation in the program are largely societal, the participant and his physician do have access to and the support of experts in radiation medicine. There is no remuneration for participation in the program. The decision to participate can be made by the individual at any time, and he/she is equally free to withdraw from the program. Participation begins when the individual provides written permission for the release to REAC/TS of medical records, including those from hospitals and clinical laboratories and relevant exposure data from his/her employers; permission is sought for the data obtained from these records to be used for the purposes of the REAC/TS programs. The participant is also asked to agree to allow annual contact, direct or indirect, for the purposes of updating his/her health status. A complete medical history including personal, family, and occupational histories is obtained at the time of enrollment in the follow-up program. Experience has taught the value of obtaining conditional permission to participate from persons

[3]This is an approximate total; it does not include persons believed to have been involved in an accident in 1958 in the U.S.S.R.

involved in incidents in which accurate dosimetry is not immediately available. Their participation is confirmed if the dose estimates for one or more persons in the group are later found to be in excess of the DOE/NRC dose criteria, in which case the incident qualifies to be registered as an accident.

The process of recruitment is relatively simple if REAC/TS physicians are involved directly in the evaluation and management of the irradiated person(s). If their involvement is indirect, or if notification is anecdotal only, it may be necessary to enlist the cooperation of the attending physician to explain the purposes and benefits of participation in the follow-up program. It is our experience that both informed attending physicians and potential participants are interested and willing to cooperate with REAC/TS in the follow-up program.

For obvious logistical reasons it is more difficult to recruit the person who was involved in a radiation accident years earlier, who may or may not be identified, and who was never followed for the Registry or has been lost to follow-up. Ironically it has been easier to identify and search for persons involved in radiation accidents that occurred in the private sector than it is to trace persons involved in radiation accidents that occurred in the public sector. Even if an individual is located, there is some risk of a negative, even hostile, response to the initial contact. For this reason we prefer to make the initial contact through a physician or other suitable official known to the individual, although this is possible only in a few cases. However, we have been fortunate in eliciting positive responses to direct initial contacts in the majority of cases.

In the past year some follow-up information about 71 persons involved in 30 radiation accidents in the U.S. prior to 1978 has been obtained from a variety of sources; of these, 42 persons had been previously lost to follow-up by the Registry. Survivors of accidents in Oak Ridge in 1958 and 1971 were examined at REAC/TS; survivors of other accidents were followed through their physicians, or directly by mail or telephone. The results of the follow-up of some of these persons have been reported to the conference by the physicians involved. The report of the twenty-four-year follow-up of the Marshall Islanders is expected to be released in the near future. Anecdotal information is available about an additional 110 radiation accident survivors. The NRC and others continue to help our efforts to locate survivors of other accidents and to recruit them into the program.

A follow-up program for registrants in the DTPA is being developed. It is anticipated that the follow-up of the majority of these persons will be achieved with the cooperation of the physician who administered the DTPA, or other plant or personal physicians for persons who have changed jobs or retired.

Medical surveillance of registrants in the DOE-Study Registry is under consideration. A program conducted similarly to that for DTPA Registry registrants can be implemented for the entire study population or for subpopulations within the study group.

As the late effects of radiation are generally nonspecific, medical follow-up should be based on a good medical history, with special reference to past medical, personal habits, family, and occupational histories, and physical examination. Updating of the medical history— including changes in personal habits, occupational environment, exposures to chemicals, and diagnostic and therapeutic radiological exposures—should continue on a regular basis. A regular physical examination and evaluation should include a CBC with differential leukocyte count and routine urinalysis. The results of quantitation analysis of serum immunoglobulins may be useful indicators of early but nonspecific malignant changes (A. Soloman, personal communication). Special attention should be given to the examination of those organs or systems in which specific histological changes or an increased incidence of neoplasms have been recognized to occur in persons exposed acutely to some levels of ionizing radiation, for example, the lens, the hematopoietic and reticuloendothelial systems, the thyroid gland, the lungs, and skin.[79]

Conclusion

There have been ample demonstrations of the delayed effects, notably the carcinogenic effect, of ionizing and neutron irradiation. Data have been obtained from many well-designed animal studies and extensive epidemiological studies of human populations exposed to radioactive fallout[54-69,79] or therapeutically exposed to radiation as reported in UNSCEAR 1977.[80] Results of these studies have indicated that animal data cannot be extrapolated to humans under all conditions. This suggests that studies of the effects of radiation in humans are essential for the proper estimation of dose–response and risk in human populations. Most studies in exposed human populations have been confounded by pre-existing disease, stress, and/or malnutrition. It is, therefore, important to have available the data that describe radiation effects in "healthy" or "normal" populations. Some of these populations are identified in one or other of the REAC/TS registries. Because these populations are relatively small, it is important that the registration of them should be as complete and current as possible. This may be achieved for populations drawn from employment and other rosters, but is more difficult when the events (e.g., radiation accidents) occur infrequently at widely separated and possibly unrelated locations, which are served by a variety of regulatory bodies. To register this latter type of event for the ultimate purposes described in this paper requires the cooperation of some individuals and organizations in a spirit of altruism. We hope that a request for cooperation in these endeavors would not be an undue imposition. This, and earlier conferences, have been instrumental in providing current information on a number of accidents and study populations, and, it is hoped, in publicizing the need and mechanisms for the reporting of radiation incidents and accidents both in the United States and abroad. We hope similar conferences will be convened periodically. In the interim, we would welcome and encourage the exchange of information about accidental radiation exposures wherever possible, while hoping that the incidence of new exposures is minimized by education and technical advances.

ACKNOWLEDGMENTS
The author wishes to thank Clarence C. Lushbaugh, M.D., and Karl F. Hübner, M.D., for their helpful critical evaluation of the text.

Oak Ridge Associated Universities operates under Contract Number DE-AC05-760R00033 with the U.S. Department of Energy.

References

1. Aebersold P, Hempelmann LH, Slotin L: Report of accident of August 21, 1945, at Omega Site LAMD 120, September 21, 1948.

2. Hempelmann LH, Lisco H, Hoffman JG: The acute radiation syndrome. A review of nine cases. *Annals of Internal Medicine* 36(2):279–510, 1952.

3. Hempelmann LH: The assessment of acute radiation injury, in *Proceedings of a Scientific Meeting on Diagnosis and Treatment of Acute Radiation Injury*. Geneva, WHO, 1961, pp. 49–66.

4. Knowlton NP, Leifer E, Hogness JR, Hempelmann L, Blaney LF, Gill DC, Oakes WR, Schafer CL: Beta ray burns of human skin. *JAMA* 141(4):239–246, 1949.

5. Brown JB, McDowell F, Fryer MP: Surgical treatment of radiation burns, in *Surgery, Gynecology, and Obstetrics*. 88:609–622, 1949.

6. Hasterlik RJ, Marinelli LD: Physical dosimetry and clinical observations on four human beings involved in an accidental critical assembly excursion, in *Proceedings of International Conference on the Peaceful Uses of Atomic Energy*. Geneva, United Nations, 11:25–34, 1956.

7. Cronkite EP, Bond VP, Dunham CL (eds.): Some effects of ionizing radiation on human beings: A report on the Marshallese and Americans accidentally exposed to radiation from fallout and a discussion of radiation injury in the human being, Washington, D.C., TID 5358, U.S. Government Printing Office, 1956.

8. Tsuzuki M: Radiation injury due to radioactive fallout, in *Proceedings of International Conference on Peaceful Uses of Atomic Energy*. Geneva, United Nations, 11:132–133, 1956.

9. Miyoski K, Kumatori T: Characteristics of hematological findings of the Japanese fisherman exposed to radioactive ashes in the Bikini area, in *Proceedings of VII International Congress of Hematology*. Tokyo, Pan Pacific Press, 1962, pp. 29–35.

10. Allen WR: Ignorance, experimentation and tragedy: Radiation injury to the hand. *Journal of the Kansas Medical Society* September:447–453, 1966.

11. *Accidental Radiation Excursion at the Y-12 Plant June 16, 1958.* Unclassified report, United States Atomic Energy Commission Report Y-1234, Union Carbide Nuclear Company, Y-12 Plant, 1958.

12. Brucer M: *The Acute Radiation Syndrome: A Medical Report on the Y-12 Accident June 16, 1958.* Unclassified report, United States Atomic Energy Commission ORINS-12. 25, Oak Ridge Institute of Nuclear Studies, 1959.

13. Hurst GS, Ritchie RH, Emerson LC: Accidental radiation excursion at the Oak Ridge Y-12 Plant. III. Determination of radiation doses. *Health Physics* 2:121–133, 1959.

14. Andrews GA, Sitterson BW, Kretchmar AL, Brucer M: Accidental radiation excursions at the Oak Ridge Y-12 Plant. IV. Preliminary report on clinical and laboratory effects in the irradiated employees. *Health Physics* 2:134–138, 1959.

15. Andrews GA, Sitterson BW, Kretchmar AL, Brucer M: Criticality accident at the Y-12 plant, in *Proceedings of a Scientific Meeting on the Diagnosis and Treatment of Acute Radiation Injury.* Geneva, WHO, 1960.

16. Stratton WR: Review of criticality accidents: Technology, engineering, and safety, in *Progress in Nuclear Energy Series IV.* New York, Pergamon Press, 1960, pp. 163–205.

17. Jammet H, Mathé G, Pendiĉ B, Duplan JF, Maupin B, Laterjet R, Kalic D, Schwarzenberg L, Djukic Z, Vigne J: Etudes de six cas d'irradiation totale accidentele. *Revue Francaise d'Etudes Cliniques et Biologiques* 4:210–225, 1959.

18. Radojicic B, Hajdukovic S, Antic M: Follow-up studies of exposed persons in the zero-energy reactor accident at Vinca, in *Proceedings of IAEA Scientific Meeting on the Diagnosis and Treatment of Acute Radiation Injury.* WHO, Geneva, 17–20 October, 1960. International Document Service, Division of Columbia U. Press. 1961, pp. 105–111.

19. Jammet HP: Treatment of victims of the zero-energy reactor accident at Vinca, in *Proceedings of IAEA Scientific Meeting on the Diagnosis and Treatment of Acute Radiation Injury.* WHO, Geneva, 17–20 October 1960. International Document Service, Division of Columbia University Press, 1961, pp. 83–103.

20. Pendiĉ B: The zero-energy reactor accident at Vinca, in *Proceedings of a Scientific Meeting on Diagnosis and Treatment of Acute Radiation Injury.* WHO, Geneva, 17–20 October, 1960. International Document Service, Division of Columbia University Press, 1961, pp. 67–81.

21. Institute of Nuclear Sciences "Boris Kidrich" Yugoslavia criticality accident, October 15, 1958. *Nucleonics* 17(4):106, 154–156, 1959.

22. Paxton HC, Baker RD, Maraman WJ, Reider R: Los Alamos criticality accident December 30, 1958. *Nucleonics* 17(4):107–108, 151, 1959.

23. Shipman TL: A radiation fatality resulting from massive overexposure to neutrons and gamma rays, in *Proceedings of a Scientific Meeting on Diagnosis and Treatment of Acute Radiation Injury.* WHO, Geneva, 17–20 October, 1960.

24. Shipman TL (ed.): Acute radiation death resulting from accidental nuclear critical excursion. *Journal of Occupational Medicine.* Special Supplement 3(2):146–192, 1961.

25. Lushbaugh CC, Grier RS, Benson JS, Peterson DF: Clinical cause of case K in acute radiation death resulting from an accidental nuclear critical excursion. *Journal of Occupational Medicine.* Special Supplement 3(2):150–154, 1961.

26. Petersen DF: Clinical pathology and biochemistry in acute radiation death resulting from an accidental nuclear critical excursion. *Journal of Occupational Medicine.* Special Supplement 3(2):155–159, 1961.

27. Kurshakov NA (ed.): Sluchay ostroy luchevoy bolezni u cheloveka (A case of acute radiation sickness in man). *Gosudarstvennoe Izdatel'stvo Meditsinskoy Literatury,* (Moskva), 150, 1962.

28. Howland JW, Ingram M, Mermagen H, Hansen CL: The Lockport incident: Accidental partial body exposure of humans to large doses of X-irradiation, in *Proceedings of a Scientific Meeting on Diagnosis and Treatment of Acute Radiation Injury.* WHO, Geneva 17–20 October 1960. International Document Service, Division of Columbia University Press, 1961, pp. 11–26.

29. Holfield C: SL-1 accident. Atomic Energy Commission Investigation Board Report. Joint Commission on Atomic Energy. Congress of the United States, June, 1961.

30. Horan JR, Gammil WP: Health physics aspects of the SL-1 accident. *Health Physics* 9:177–186, 1963.

31. Petersen DF: Neutron dose estimates in SL-1 accident. *Health Physics* 9:231–232, 1963.

32. Rossi EC, Thorngate AA, Larson FC: Acute radiation syndrome caused by accidental exposure to cobalt 60. *Journal of Laboratory and Clinical Medicine* 59(4):655–666, 1962.

33. Bliss SP: Medical aspects of an accidental exposure to Van de Graaff generator, in *Premier Collague International sur la Protection Aupres des Grands Accelerateurs,* 18–20 January 1962. Paris, Presses Universitaires de France, 1962, pp. 35–36.

34. Andrews GA: Mexican ^{60}Co radiation accident. *Isotopes and Radiation Technology* 1:200–201, 1963–64.

35. Fuqua PA, Norwood WD, Marks S: Biological effects of human radiation exposure. Report of a criticality accident. *Journal of Occupational Medicine* 7(3):85–93, 1965.

36. McCandless JB: Accidental acute whole-body gamma irradiation of seven clinically well persons. *JAMA* 192(3):185–188, 1965.

37. Industry's first radiation accident, studied by AEC, firms. *Nucleonics* 22(9):21, 1964.

38. Auxier JA: Nuclear accident at Wood River Junction. *Nuclear Safety* 6(3):298–300, 1965.

39. Karas JS, Stanbury JB: Fatal radiation syndrome from accidental nuclear excursion. *New England Journal of Medicine* 262(15):755–761, 1965.

40. Fanger H, Lushbaugh CC: Radiation death from cardiovascular shock following a criticality accident. *Arch of Pathology* 83:446–460, 1967.

41. Maxfield WS, Porter GH: Accidental radiation exposure from iridium 192 camera, in *Proceedings of IAEA Symposium on Handling Radiation Accidents.* Vienna, International Atomic Energy Agency, 1969.

42. Lanzl HL, Rozenfeld ML, Tarlow AR: Injury due to accidental high-dose exposure to 10 MeV electrons. *Health Physics* 13:241–251, 1967.

43. Schenk RS, Gilberti MV: Four extremity radiation necrosis. *Archives of Surgery* 100:729–734, 1970.

44. Baron JM, Yachin S, Polcyn R, Fitch FW, Sturner W: Accidental radiogold ([198]Au) liver scan overdose with fatal outcome, in *Proceedings of IAEA Symposium on the Handling of Radiation Accidents.* Vienna, International Atomic Energy Agency, 1969.

45. Beninson D, Placer A, Vander Elst E: Estudio de un caso de irradiacion humana accidental, in *Proceedings of an IAEA Symposium on the Handling of Radiation Accidents.* Vienna, International Atomic Energy Agency, 1969.

46. Krizek TJ, Ariyan S: Severe acute radiation injuries of the hands. *Plastic and Reconstruction Surgery* 51(1):14–22, 1978.

47. Vodopick H, Andrews GA: Accidental radiation exposure. *Archives of Environmental Health* 28:53–56. 1974.

48. Kumatori T, Hirashima K, Ishihara T, Kurisu A Sugiyama, Hashizume T: Radiation accident caused by an iridium 192 radiographic source, in *Proceedings of IAEA Symposium, Handling Radiation Accidents.* Vienna, International Atomic Energy Agency, 1977, pp. 35–42.

49. Accidental exposure involving X-ray spectrometer unit. *Serious Accidents.* United States Atomic Energy Commission. Issue 338, December 6, 1974.

50. Hot-cell operator received an estimated 400 rad dose. *Nuclear Safety* 17(4):495–496, 1976.

51. Steidley DK, Zenk GS, Ouellette R: Another ⁶⁰Co hot cell accident. *Health Physics* 36:437–441, 1979.

52. Jacobson A, Wilson BM, Banks TE, Scott RM: Iridium 192 overexposure in industrial radiography. *Health Physics* 32:291–293, 1977.

53. Ruber LS: The Riverside radiation tragedy. *Columbus Monthly* April:52–66, 1978.

54. Steidley DK, Zenk GS, Ouellette R: Another ⁶⁰Co hot-cell accident. *Health Physics* 36:437–441, 1979.

55. Bond VP, Conrad RA, Robertson JS, and Weden EA Jr: Medical examination of Rongelap people six months after exposure to fallout, WT-937. Operation Castle Addendum Report 4.1A, April 1955.

56. Cronkite EP, Dunham CL, Griffin D, McPherson SD, Woodward KT: Twelve-month postexposure survey on Marshallese exposed to fallout radiation, BNL 384, August 1955.

57. Conrad RA, Huggins CE, Cannon B, Lowrey A: Medical survey of Marshallese two years after exposure to fallout radiation. *JAMA* 164:1192, 1957.

58. Conrad RA: March 1957 medical survey of Rongelap and Utirik people three years after exposure to radioactive fallout, BNL 501, June 1958.

59. Conrad RA: Medical survey of Rongelap people, March 1958, four years after exposure to fallout, BNL 534, May 1959.

60. Conrad RA: Medical survey of Rongelap people five and six years after exposure to fallout, BNL 609, September 1960.

61. Conrad RA: Medical survey of Rongelap people seven years after exposure to fallout, BNL 727, May 1962.

62. Conrad RA: Medical survey of Rongelap people eight years after exposure to fallout, BNL 780, January 1963.

63. Conrad RA: Medical survey of the people of Rongelap and Utirik Islands nine and ten years after exposure to fallout radiation (March 1963 and March 1964), BNL 908, May 1965.

64. Conrad RA: Medical survey of the people of Rongelap and Utirik Islands eleven and twelve years after exposure to fallout radiation (March 1965 and March 1966), BNL 50029, April 1967.

65. Conrad RA: Medical survey of the people of Rongelap and Utirik Islands thirteen, fourteen, and fifteen years after exposure to fallout radiation (March 1967, March 1968, March 1969), BNL 50220, June 1970.

66. Conrad RA: Medical survey of Marshallese people five years after exposure to fallout radiation. *Int J Radiat Biol* Suppl 1:269–281, 1960.

67. Conrad RA, Hicking A: Medical findings in Marshallese people exposed to fallout radiation: Results from a ten-year study. *JAMA* 192:457–459, 1965.

68. Conrad RA: A twenty-year review of medical findings in a Marshallese population accidentally exposed to radioactive fallout. BNL 50424, Brookhaven, New York, 1974.
69. Conrad RA: Acute myelogenous leukemia following fallout radiation exposure. *JAMA* 232(13):1356–1357, 1975.
70. Kumatori T, Ishihara T, Ueda T, Miyoshi K: Medical survey of Japanese exposed to fallout radiation in 1954 (A report after 10 years). NP-15891, National Institute of Radiological Sciences, Chiba, Japan, 1965.
71. Ingram M, Howland JW, Hansen CL, Angel CR: Continuing clinical observations on dose estimates one year after a radiation accident. *Health Physics* 8:519–522, 1962.
72. Pendič B, Djordjevič O: Chromosome aberrations in human subjects five years after whole-body irradiation. *Yugoslav Physiol Pharmacol ACTA* 4(3):231–237, 1968.
73. Lushbaugh CC, Andrews GA, Hübner KF, Cloutier RJ, Beck WL, Berger JD: "REACTS" A pragmatic approach for providing medical care and physician education for radiation emergencies, in *Proceedings of IAEA Seminar on the Diagnosis and Treatment of Incorporated Radionuclides*. Vienna, International Atomic Energy Agency, 1976, pp. 565–577.
74. Hübner KF, Andrews GA, Lushbaugh CC, Tompkins E: A follow-up study program for persons irradiated in radiation accidents, in *Proceedings of IAEA Symposium Handling Radiation Accidents*. Vienna, International Atomic Energy Agency, 1977, pp:57–69.
75. Maximum permissible body burdens and maximum permissible concentrations of radionuclides in air and in the water for occupational exposure; recommendations of the National Committee on Radiation Exposure. NCRP report No. 22, National Bureau of Standards Handbook 69, 1959.
76. Saenger EL, Kereiakes JG, Wald N, Thoma GE: Clinical course and dosimetry of acute hand injuries to industrial radiographers from multicurie sealed gamma sources, in *Proceedings of the Third International Congress of International Radiation Protection Association*. United States Atomic Energy Commission, Office of Information Services (Tech. Div.). Part 1, pp. 773–782, 1974.
77. Kelsey CA: Comparison of relative risk from radiation exposure and other common hazards. *Health Physics*. 35(2):428–429, 1978.
78. Statistical Abstract of The United States, 1979. 99th Annual Edition. U.S. Department of Commerce, Bureau of the Census, p. 78.
79. Beebe GW, Kato H, Lard CE: Studies of the mortality of A-Bomb survivors. 6. Mortality and radiation dose, 1950–1974. *Radiation Research* 75:138–201, 1978.
80. United Nations Scientific Committee on the Effects of Atomic Radiation 1977: Sources and effects of ionizing radiation. Annex G, pp. 361–423, 1977.

Discussion for Section V

T. A. LINCOLN: The expected rate on malignant neoplasms of brain and CNS is based on data of what time period? Several studies being performed in several locations for workers with widely differing occupational exposures have revealed elevated SMRs for these diseases. Is it possible that some other factor besides exposure could be changing the observed rates faster than the expected rate?

A. P. POLEDNAK: The method of analysis takes into account changes in brain cancer rates that have occurred over time. That is, expected numbers of deaths from brain cancer are calculated by multiplying person-years of follow-up (in five-year age and calendar-year intervals from 1940–44 through 1970–74) for U.S. white males. The 1970–74 rates, however, are based on rates to 1971 only, so that any recent increases in 1972 and 1973 (when follow-up was terminated in these analyses) could have a very slight effect.

It should be noted that brain cancer death rates for white males in Tennessee are not lower than rates for U.S. white males. The ratio of age-standardized death rates for brain cancer in Tennessee (vs. U.S.) white males for 1950–69 is 1.12. Although the SMR for brain cancer was high (1.97) in the Y-12 (Union Carbide Corporation) population, the 95% confidence interval was wide (0.79–4.06); and, thus, the SMR was not statistically significant at the 0.05 level. Also noteworthy is the SMR of 1.07 in the Y-12 (Tennessee-Eastman Corporation) cohort.

Interpretation of the results of such statistical tests is always difficult. If the excess is real and not due to chance, it is unlikely to be related to radiation exposure. The possibility of an effect of occupational exposure to some toxic agent should be considered, perhaps in a case-control study of all brain cancers in Oak Ridge nuclear workers. This study would also need to consider other factors, such as alcohol consumption, which has been associated with brain cancer in a recent study. Finally, it is possible that bias in assessment of brain cancers has occurred in other studies of occupational groups using morbidity and mortality data. Another possibility is that certain brain cells are highly sensitive to a variety of chemical agents, as manifested in brain cancers. Obviously, further studies are needed in the emerging field of neurotoxicology.

J. TAYLOR: It would seem that a relatively large, well-documented population of persons exposed to low-level external exposure exists in past and present members of the U. S. Navy Nuclear Propulsion Program. Are epidemiological studies other than the ongoing ship-yard worker studies on this group contemplated?

A. P. POLEDNAK: Occupational radiation exposures in the U.S. Naval Reactor Program have been summarized recently by M. E. Miles. As Miles observes, the total lifetime radiation exposure from work associated with naval nuclear propulsion plants for all personnel monitored since 1954 has averaged only about 1 rem per person, and very few persons have received ≥ 5 rem in any year. Radiation exposures in shipyard personnel have been somewhat higher, with about 1,300 recorded exposures of ≥ 5 rem in any year. The shipyard workers, mostly civilians, are under study by the Department of Epidemiology at Johns Hopkins University; the results of that study, which will require years of effort, will be relevant to the assessment of health effects of occupational radiation exposures in other groups (such as the naval nuclear propulsion personnel). To my knowledge, a study of naval propulsion personnel has not been undertaken. In view of the time and expense involved in epidemiologic studies, it may be prudent to focus on groups such as the shipyard workers with enough cumulative exposure (person-rem) to allow assessment of health risks that are more meaningful statistically.

K. C. CARSTAIRS: Can the "healthy-worker effect" be quantified? If so, how would the interpretations of this afternoon's data be affected?

A. P. POLEDNAK: It is difficult to quantify the "healthy-worker effect," partly because the magnitude will vary from one cohort to another due to differences in self-selection for employment, in medical criteria for acceptance for employment, and quality of medical follow-up and treatment during and after employment. There has been little evidence for a "healthy-worker effect" for cancer mortality, however, and cancers are of major interest in long-term studies of radiation affects. Interestingly, an effect could be produced if workers were selected by employers on the basis of cigarette smoking habits (since this variable is correlated with risk of several types of cancer), but this has apparently not occurred. The problem is overcome, at least in part, by using internal "controls" or comparison groups derived from the same working population but differing in radiation (or other) exposure level under study as has been done by Drs. S. Marks and E. Gilbert. Such factors as length of employment were also considered by these investigators. Similar methods of analysis will be used for the Oak Ridge nuclear worker population.

L. B. SZTANYIK: Dr. Brues, have you any data on leukemia incidence among radium-dial painters, and on the possible dose absorbed in bone marrow from gamma rays of radium?

A. M. BRUES: Leukemia incidence is not impressive among the dial painters, and there is no significant increase; the early deaths from "pernicious" anemia might have been leukemia cases, but we have no evidence of this. Estimates of the marrow dose from radium in bone have been forwarded, but I do not have them at hand.

W. K. SINCLAIR: Dr. Fry, may I clarify a question with respect to the registries? The DOE $\geqslant 5$ rem Registry is presumably derived from occupational exposures reported from within DOE operations and laboratories to DOE Headquarters. Are these registered solely at REAC/TS?

S. A. FRY: Yes.

W. K. SINCLAIR: Does NRC maintain a similar Registry for occupational workers among their licensees?

S. A. FRY: NRC reports accidents to the REAC/TS Accidents Registry above the 25-rem-limit whole-body exposure, etc. The question about NRC licensee occupational exposures was answered by Dr. Roy Parker who said yes.

J. F. ROSS: I should like to ask Dr. Fry about persons who have been seen over a period of time. If I started, I could probably reconstruct data without too much trouble. I can think of 25–30 exposures that have never been reported to you and probably never been reported to the State of California (OSHA). Are you interested in this type? If this data is to be presented to you, what would be the liability that would accrue to the employers of these people who had been exposed?

s. a. fry: I do not have the legal background to answer this question so I will refer it to Dr. Collins.

v. p. collins: This question has come up before, of course. The adversary system results in both sides climbing upon the docket until the court is convinced by one side or the other. At this time I think opinion agrees that the employer, who is entitled to his case, might at least resent the free provision of information on an accident.

j. f. ross: I should like to amplify this a little bit as a physician. I would like to keep the government off my back and out of my pocket. What my question really comes down to is what is the security of the data that is provided to REAC/TS? What is its availability to other government agencies, employers, and bureaucrats? What do you do, supposing somebody says "we're going to raise hell with these people all around the country."? Can they get the data, or is it not going to be available to them?

s. a. fry: The medical and other identifiable data is kept securely as privileged information and is not available to other agencies. Relevant information from this source is made available to the registries only in abstract form, without identification, and would be available together with information from the open literature, such as official accident reports.

m. e. gaulden: In view of the fact that your lower limit for a radiation accident is 25 rem, are you interested in reports on human embryos and fetuses that receive that dose and do not undergo therapeutic abortion and go to term? And if so, you again want to be very concerned about the confidentiality of the information.

s. a. fry: We are interested in reports of this type of exposure. We already have reports of one or two such cases in the Registry. Again, any medical or identifiable information will be kept securely and treated as any other privileged information.

m. e. gaulden: I have one more question about the legal aspects. Is anyone keeping any sort of registry on the legal aspects of these accidents? The number of questions I get from the public about legal aspects really makes one exceedingly nervous about the whole business.

v. p. collins: I doubt that there is a legal registry *per se*, but those interested could use the law libraries, which do something called "shepherdizing," which is running down all aspects of a case. I'm sure all these attorneys representing a plaintiff have been kept very busy at it. There is within the past few months a book "Cancer" published by Matthew Bender which addresses this problem.

R. PARKER: I'd like to say something about NRC. Current regulatory system requires all licensees to file an immediate report of whole-body exposure in excess of 25 rem, extremity exposure in excess of 325 rem, and skin doses of 150 rem. A 24-hour report should be filed for exposures in excess of 5 rem, extremity doses in excess of 75 rem, and skin doses of 30 rem and a 30-day report of all exposures that are in excess of the applicable 3 rem rule or 1.25 rem/quarter. These reports should be filed, according to the regulations, with the NRC in a report in such a way that the identification (name, Social Security number, and date of birth of that individual) is maintained separately and does not appear on the document.

SECTION VI:

Reactor Incidents: Medical Preparedness and Planning

Medical Planning for Situations Involving Large Populations

Victor P. Bond

Brookhaven National Laboratory, Associated Universities, Inc., Upton, New York.

Medical preparedness of the range of nonwarfare nuclear incidents and accidents involving large populations should be concentrated primarily on public health considerations, as opposed to the additional measures that would be appropriate for the usual gamut of medical emergencies. Although industrial accidents in a nuclear facility could conceivably involve up to a dozen workers requiring treatment for traumatic or burn injuries, with or without radiological complications, the "large population" situation affecting the general public is likely to be devoid of traumatic or burn injury related directly to the incident.[1] The highest exposures from external gamma radiation, and these to a relatively small fraction of the population, are unlikely to exceed a few tens of rem. Exposure to internal emitters are also likely to be in the relatively low-dose range that will not result in detectable early effects,[2] although prophylactic measures may be considered, for example, to reduce the uptake of radioiodine. Hence, it is unlikely that there will be any requirement for patient treatment associated with direct effects of the incident, radiation-related or otherwise, and hospitalization will not be required. Realistic planning must emphasize an educational program to familiarize medical and paramedical personnel, and decision makers, with the special conceptual and practical problems associated with radiation exposure and radioactive contamination.

Even though only "low-level" exposure with no immediate clinical consequences will be involved, adequate familiarization with potential consequences must include consideration of the effects of exposure over the entire dose range and an appreciation of the potential and real effects as a function of dose. Special attention should be paid to the probabilities of late carcinogenic (and mutagenic) effects. Armed with such knowledge, the public health physician can then deal effectively and realistically with the primary and basic public health problem faced, namely one of "optimization," or cost–benefit balancing. The problem is to balance the benefit of any reduction in the risk of potential radiation effects in the population (achievable by taking specific measures to reduce the radiation dose) against the real and immediate harmful effects of the measures required to reduce the radiation dose.

A number of real, practical, and difficult questions involving optimization must not only be addressed but acted on without delay: should the entire population be evacuated? Should evacuation of subgroups of that population (e.g., pregnant women, children, the elderly) be accomplished? Should hospitalized and bed-ridden patients be translocated? As a corollary, should medical and paramedical personnel be asked to remain to care for the sick, if the population is evacuated? Should health physics and other emergency personnel be asked to remain in the area? Should prophylactic measures such as nonradioactive iodine be used in the general population or for special subgroups? To repeat, for each of the above, the benefit of further reducation in the (already small) risk of potential late effects, must be balanced against the costs and the real, immediate, and probably serious, if not lethal, consequences of instituting the measures to reduce the radiation dose.

An equally important and related problem involves the concerns and questions of those in the involved population during and subsequent to the actual incident. The physician in a community is and must be the principal direct source of information on possible radiation effects, and an informed medical community can do much to allay unnecessary fears in the population. Thus the physician must be informed adequately to allow him to deal with probabilistic questions, and thus to respond authoritatively and objectively to the real concerns about potential radiation effects of various kinds. As an additional benefit the well-informed physician will be immeasurably better equipped to handle similar questions relating to exposure associated with diagnostic X-ray and nuclear-medicine procedures.

The problems involved in optimization are not trivial on any scale and must not be underrated. Only extensive familiarization with the many and complex facets on the overall radiological problems will provide one with the confidence to act rationally and effectively under such circumstances.

References

1. WASH-1400, An assessment of accident risks in U.S. commercial nuclear power plants, in *Reactor Safety Study*, Appendix VI. United States Nuclear Regulatory Commission, October 1975.

2. *Manual of Protective Action Guides and Protective Actions for Nuclear Incidents*. Environmental Protection Agency, Office of Radiation Programs, Environmental Analysis Division, September 1975.

Environmental Health and the Windscale Incident

Geoffrey Brealey Schofield

British Nuclear Fuels Limited, Sellafield Seascale, Cumbria CA20 1 PG, England.

The Windscale Establishment of British Nuclear Fuels Limited is located on the northwest coast of England, near Whitehaven, on a plain three miles wide between the sea and the foothills of the Cumbrian mountains. The site was developed by the government during the 1939–1945 war as an Ordnance Factory under the name of Sellafield. When, after the war, military work on nuclear energy in the U.K. was started, the Sellafield site was acquired by the Ministry of Supply, Department of Atomic Energy, as the location for the plutonium producing "piles," and for the plutonium separation plant. Work started on site in September 1947, and the first "pile" reached criticality in October 1950, the second in June 1951. In parallel with construction of the reactors, a chemical plant was built to treat the fuel rods after irradiation. The reprocessing complex was commissioned in 1951 and received its first irradiated fuel in January 1952, and fuel reprocessing on the site has therefore been in progress for just over 27 years.

In 1957, the first Windscale Piles were closed down following the much publicized "Windscale Incident"—a fire in No. 1 Pile.

The nature and cause of the nuclear reactor accident at Windscale in October 1957 have been described in the summary report of the Committee of Inquiry set up by the Atomic Energy Authority and published in a Command Paper (Atomic Energy Office, 1957).[1] The environmental aspects have been discussed in the second report by the Medical Research Council on the Hazards to Man of Nuclear and Allied Radiations.[2] The events leading up to the accident occurred on 8 October, during a routine release of the energy that had become stored in the graphite moderator as a result of the normal operation of the reactor. The Committee concluded that the accident had been caused by local overheating of the uranium fuel elements, the canning of which had failed, exposing the uranium and allowing it to oxidize. The temperatures in the affected channels continued to rise, leading to the combustion of the graphite. By the evening of Thursday, 10 October, the fire had spread and was affecting about 150 channels, permitting the release of substantial amounts of the radioactive fission products from the reactor.

Radioactivity Released

The amount of radioactivity released during the accident is not known precisely, but approximate estimates were made from the measurements of the radioactive iodine deposited on the ground in this country, and from measurements on air filters obtained both in the United Kingdom and on the continent of Europe. The following list shows an assessment of the amounts of various isotopes released:

iodine 131	20,000 curies
tellurium 132	12,000 curies
caesium 137	600 curies
strontium 89	80 curies
strontium 90	2 curies

Exposure to External Radiation

Before the accident, routine gamma-radiation surveys in West Cumbria made with ionization chambers fixed in survey vehicles had shown that the natural gamma background varied according to position over a range of 4–10 μR per hour, with a mean value of 7 μR per hour. As a result of the accident the principal sources of external radiation to which the public were exposed were the deposited iodine 131, tellurium 132, and iodine 132. Dunster et al.[3] estimated the integrated gamma dose to people living in the area of maximum deposition as 30–50 mR. Integration of the results of Chamberlain [4] gives a total gamma dose of 75 mR, no allowance being made for the shielding effect of houses. There would also be small additional external doses from the passing cloud of radioactive material and from deposited, long-lived fission products, but it can be concluded from the investigations made that these were less than that from deposited radioiodine. Apart from the problems relating to the exposure of affected personnel on the site, concern also arose as to the possible danger to the general public arising from external irradiation and from inhalation and ingestion of radioactive material. It was possible at an early stage to exclude the necessity for any emergency measures in regard to inhalation or external irradiation, but early measurements of deposition showed that it would be necessary to consider prohibiting the consumption of milk, particularly by children.

Radiation Doses Incurred in Human Thyroids

The main risk to members of the public arose from the contamination of milk, and control measures were introduced to take account of this hazard. In a few instances, however, there was reason to suspect that the control of milk had not been fully effective, and in these instances individuals were invited to the laboratories at Windscale and measurements were made of the activity of iodine 131 in their thyroids. In addition, some members of the public who were more representative of those in the down-wind area were similarly invited for measurement. The results of these thyroid measurements are given in Table 1. Details of the method of calculation of the thyroid doses shown in this table have been published.[3]

The highest dose to a child's thyroid was estimated as 16 rads and the corresponding figure for an adult's thyroid was 4 rads. In addition to the measurements given in the table for persons in the down-wind sector, approximately 113 other thyroid measurements were made on members of the public living in other places in the vicinity. Of these, 107 showed a dose of zero, and the highest dose was 1.2 rads.

Since the control of milk was based on large numbers of assays, there was every reason to believe that the members of the public were satisfactorily protected against excessive doses of internal radiation, and the measurements made on thyroid glands gave confirmation to this view.

Table 1.   Radiation Doses in Human Thyroids [a]

Place	Range (miles)	Average dose (rads)		Maximum dose (rads)	
		Adults	Children	Adults	Children
Seascale	2	0.5(18)[b]	0.8 (9)	1.4	3.9
Drigg	4	1.4 (8)	3.9 (3)	2.8	7.3
Holmrook	4.5	1.4 (7)		2.7	
Ravenglass	6	1.8 (8)	12.2 (3)	4.0	16.1
Bootle	11	1.4(12)	6.0(11)	3.4	9.8
Millom	19.5	0.4(29)		1.8	
Ulverston	23	0.5 (5)	4.4 (3)	1.4	11.4
Barrow	24	0.3 (9)		1.1	

[a] Persons who lived in the down-wind sector (130-160 degrees from Windscale, but who were not in the Windscale Works at the time of the accident, are represented.

[b] The number of persons examined is shown in brackets.

Alternative supplies of milk for certain areas had been brought in, and at no time was there any shortage. Of the other possible sources of internal contamination—vegetables, eggs, meat, and water—none was found to require restriction.

The use of contaminated milk for human consumption in any form was prohibited when its content of iodine 131 exceeded a level that might have been injurious to infants. It is important to recognize, however, that none of the milk would have led to an unacceptable irradiation of the thyroid if it had been used for the preparation of cheese, butter, or other manufactured produce.

Effluent Discharges from Windscale

In assessing the environmental health aspects of activities at Windscale, the possible results of effluent discharges to the sea and the atmosphere must also be taken into account, as well as those from the 1957 accident described above. The liquid effluents from Windscale are discharged to sea under specified conditions, provided that the government authorizing ministries are satisfied of the need to discharge the waste and that its environmental impact accords with the U.K. policy.

The authorization permitting discharge of gases, mists, and dusts into the atmosphere requires the company to use the best practicable means to minimize the radioactivity of the waste discharged. No quantitative limits for the wastes discharged are specified at present, but the company is required to measure the amount of radioactivity in samples taken from the different outlets, and to keep records of the discharges. For the major plants, the effluents are released to the environment via tall stacks, in order to achieve good dispersion and dilution before they reach ground level.

In the marine environment two important pathways of potential radiation exposure are currently identified: external radiation exposure of an individual who works over estuarine sediments while netting salmon at the estuary of the River Esk at Ravenglass, and the consumption of fish and shellfish caught in the north Irish sea. Discharge of radioactive effluent into the sea causes some uptake of radioactivity in marine animals such as fish. In particular, the radioisotopes caesium 134 and caesium 137 are readily absorbed in the soft tissue of fish and shellfish and man. In recent years there have been increased discharges of these caesium isotopes from the fuel element storage ponds at Windscale and the levels of radiocaesium in fish and shellfish have increased in the same number. Therefore members of the public who eat such fish will receive some additional radiation exposure due to their ingestion of caesium. For most of the period concerned, the estimated radiation doses to the critical groups as defined by ICRP[5] have been less than 10% of the ICRP

Dose Limits, and for the general public a much smaller amount (about a tenth of that of the critical group, i.e., 5 mrem/year). There has been an increase in the exposure of the critical group of fish eaters during the last three years, but still within ICRP dose limits, because of the exceptional discharges of caesium 137 from the magnox fuel storage ponds. The caesium discharges to sea are being reduced by special measures being taken in the plant to deal with this problem and a steady reduction in the environmental impact of these discharges can be expected.

Environmental Health

In any discussion on the health impact[6] of the Windscale facilities, two populations may be identified: those who are occupationally exposed by virtue of their work on the site, amounting to about 5000 persons between the ages of 18 and 64; and the general population of the West Cumbria area, which numbers about 135,000 people of all ages. This latter area also contains an administrative district called "Copeland," which has a population of about 70,000 and which is immediately adjacent to the Windscale site. The health of the work force on the site has been constantly monitored since 1949 and the figures for the mortality experience of this population from 1962 to 1975 are included in Table 2. The proportion of females in the work force is extremely small, and therefore these figures apply only to males. The actual number of deaths is compared with the number of deaths that would have been expected on the basis of the statistics for the whole of England and Wales (with

Table 2. Ratio of Actual to Expected Deaths by Cause for Windscale Male Employees and Pensioners, 1962-1975

Cause of death	Employees aged <65		Pensioners aged >65		All employees and pensioners		A:E
	Actual	Expected	Actual	Expected	Actual	Expected	
All causes	296	360	150	184	446	544	0.8
All neoplasms ICD 140-239	72	97	33	43	105	140	0.8
Respiratory neoplasms ICD 162-163	25	41	11	17	36	58	0.6
Leukemia ICD 204-207	2	2	1	0.8	3	3.5	0.9
Ischemic heart disease ICD 410-414	138	113	60	54	198	167	1.2

appropriate adjustments for age structure of the populations).[7] A more comprehensive exercise is currently being undertaken, which will provide the mortality experience pertaining to all those who have ever been employed at the Windscale Establishment.[8] It is intended to relate the mortality figures not only to radiation, but also to other environmental and social factors.

The collection of health statistics for the West Cumbria is a somewhat complicated procedure, dependent on the assembly of information from a number of smaller administrative districts. A further complication arises because the boundaries of the various health authorities and health districts in the U.K. do not necessarily coincide with those of the administrative districts already referred to. Further difficulties have arisen in the collection of health information due to the fact that a complete revision of the Area Health Authority boundaries took place in 1972, and allowances have had to be made in order to attempt to compare data obtained prior to this date with that which is being currently received. However, on the positive side, the geographical location of West Cumbria is such that the total population has only shown slight variations over the past 30 years, and the population turnover is relatively small compared with most other regions in the U.K. As stated above the population of the West Cumbria Health District is about 135,000, and Table 3 sets out the mortality experience for certain defined conditions in the area from 1971 to 1977.[9] In order to allow a comparison to be made with the occupational health statistics, the figures have again been expressed as a function of the national data. An attempt has also been made to examine the incidence of other more specific mortality data which it has been suggested may be relevant to radiation exposure. Table 4 is concerned with the leukemia incidence in the Copeland Administrative District, which has a population of about 70,000. Table 5 compares the incidence of congenital birth malformations and stillbirths with the national figures.

With due regard to the ^{131}I release at Windscale in 1957, the death rate from carcinoma of thyroid in West Cumbria has been examined for the years 1963 to 1977. The average incidence of thyroid carcinoma in the U.K. is about 0.85/100,000 of the population, and during the years under consideration the average incidence of this disease in the Copeland area (population 70,000) of West Cumbria is 0.73/100,000, with a random spread of cases. Therefore there is no specific indication of an increase in this particular cancer in the context of the 1957 Windscale Incident.

Preparedness and Planning

The Windscale Incident of 1957 resulted in a great deal of work being carried out in order to establish a better technical basis for decision taking in emergency situations. Moreover, following the wide range of

Table 3. Ratio of Actual to Expected Deaths by Cause and Sex for All Ages in the West Cumbria Health District (Pop. 135,000), 1970-1977

Cause of death	Sex	1970	1971	1972	1973	1974	1975	1976	1977	Average Actual:Expected
All causes	M	1.07	1.10	1.11	1.14	1.30	1.26	1.09	1.04	1.14
	F	0.96	0.93	1.01	1.07	1.27	1.22	1.05	0.94	1.06
All neoplasms ICD 140-239	M	1.02	0.97	0.97	1.04	1.05	1.07	0.92	0.89	0.99
	F	0.85	0.81	0.99	1.07	1.13	1.18	0.96	0.98	1.00
Respiratory neoplasms ICD 160-163	M	0.87	0.81	0.89	1.00	0.87	0.81	0.83	0.87	0.87
	F	0.47	0.79	0.63	0.58	0.84	0.89	0.79	0.74	0.72
Neoplasms of breast ICD 174	F	0.58	0.77	0.84	0.87	0.87	1.03	0.84	1.19	0.87
Leukemia ICD 204-207	M	0.40	0.80	0.80	0.60	1.20	1.20	0.20	0.20	0.68
	F	0.75	1.50	1.00	2.00	1.50	–	1.00	1.25	1.13
Ischemic heart disease ICD 410-414	M	1.23	1.32	1.34	1.27	1.57	1.43	1.26	1.19	1.33
	F	1.03	1.14	1.15	1.24	1.40	1.57	1.21	1.06	1.23

Table 4. Leukemia Deaths 1963-1976 for All Ages

Year	England and Wales		Copeland Borough Council		Copeland C.M.R.
	Deaths	Rates/m Population	Deaths	Rates/m Population	
1963	2830	60.2	3	40.3	
1964	2867	60.5	2	26.8	
1965	2860	59.9	8	107.5	
1966	2896	60.2	4	53.9	
1967	2904	60.0	4	54.0	
1968	3132	64.5	6	81.0	
1969	3051	62.5	4	54.2	
1970	2984	60.9	3	40.9	
1971	3019	61.8	7	97.5	
1972	3124	63.7	1	14.0	
1973	3045	61.9	6	84.6	
1974	3101	63.0	7	98.6	
1975	3194	64.9	2	28.3	
1976	3192	64.9	2	28.7	
Total	42,199	Avg. 62.1	59	Avg. 57.9	Avg. 93

Table 5. Notification of Congenital Malformations, 1964-1977

	West Cumbria Health District		Copeland Borough Council	
Year	No.	Rate per 1000 live and still births	No.	Rate per 1000 live and still births
1964	43	16.0	12	7.9
1965	44	17.1	12	8.6
1966	30	12.6	11	8.8
1967	49	20.5[a]	30	23.4
1968	46	21.0[a]	30	25.3[a]
1969	23	10.6	10	8.4
1970	19	9.2	10	9.1
1971	23	10.8	12	10.5
1972	24	12.9	14	14.3
1973	18	9.9	14	13.9
1974	21	12.1	16	16.5
1975	16	9.7	10	11.0
1976	30	18.3	20	22.6
1977	17	10.6	7	8.6
Total 1964-1977	403	Avg. 13.7[b]	209	Avg. 13.5

[a] Thalidomide effect.

[b] Average in England and Wales = 20.0.

investigations carried out on all aspects of the environment (e.g., milk and other food stuffs), it became possible to establish criteria such as emergency reference levels which could be related to such environmental measurements.

Another highly important outcome of the Windscale Incident was the establishment of a Local Liaison Committee whose original terms of references were as follows:

To define responsibilities and action to be taken by all interested parties in the event of a district hazard arising from a site incident at Windscale and Calder Works, to reassure local opinion of the hazards involved, and to create an administrative machinery for the protection of the population in the event of a serious incident.

The Local Liaison Committee acts as a formal interface with the site management and various public bodies, such as police, local and district councils, public health authorities, the emergency planning units, trade unions, and representatives from the public utilities and organizations having responsibility for the public environment. It should be emphasized that the Local Liaison Committee is an active body, which has always met regularly, annually or more often.

The Windscale management, in consultation with relevant external bodies, has produced a comprehensive District Emergency Scheme, which is approved by the Government Nuclear Installations Inspectorate. An outline of this scheme has then been made available to the local population by incorporating the document in the various public libraries. From the medical standpoint, the provisions of the District Emergency Scheme relate to activities such as personal monitoring procedures and the distribution of potassium iodate tablets. Although not specifically mentioned in the text, the provision of close liaison between the BNFL Medical Departments and the National Health Service Organizations.

Finally, it should be emphasized that close surveillance is, and always has been, undertaken of the health of the local population and of the work force at Windscale by public health authorities and the BNFL Medical Departments respectively.

References

1. Atomic Energy Office. *Accident at Windscale No. 1 Pile on 10 October 1957.* HM Stationery Office, Cmnd. 302, 1957.

2. Medical Research Council. *Hazards to Man of Nuclear and Allied Radiations,* 2nd report. HM Stationery Office, Cmnd. 1225, 1960.

3. Dunster HJ, Howells H, Templeton WL: District surveys following the Windscale incident in October 1957, in *Proceedings II International Conference Peaceful Uses Atomic Energy,* vol. 18, pp. 296, 1959.

4. Chamberlain AC: *Relation between measurements of deposited activity after the Windscale Accident of October 1957.* AERE. HP/R. 2606.

5. Annals of the ICRP, ICRP Publication No. 26, 1977.

6. Schofield GB: Environmental health aspects of nuclear energy, Seminar on environmental health impact assessment. Copenhagen, World Health Organization, 1978.

7. Office of Population Censuses and Surveys Mortality Statistics. DH2. No 1., 1974.

8. Clough EA, Schofield GB, Ward FA: Mortality Rates among Windscale and Calder Workers. International Symposium on Biological Implications of Radionuclides released from Nuclear Industries. Vienna 1979. IAEA.

9. Office of Population Censuses and Surveys Mortality Statistics, West Cumbria Health District. SD 25, 1970–1977.

The Three Mile Island Incident in 1979: The State Response

Niel Wald

*Department of Radiation Health, Graduate School of Public Health,
University of Pittsburgh, Pittsburgh, Pennsylvania.*

In response to the request that I review the TMI incident which began on 28 March 1979 at the Three Mile Island (TMI) Nuclear Power Station from the point of view of the State of Pennsylvania, I have been trying to decide what information would be most useful. The TMI incident was a unique experience in the literal sense, and we should certainly try to derive the maximum benefit from it in improving our capability to deal with such a problem. On the other hand, it is a bit too early to have developed a final analysis in adequate depth and perspective of this very complex event.

One of the unusual features that has to be recognized in discussing the incident is that there is not really a very clearly discernible end-point. There are continuing concerns as there are continuing operations at the plant, and even though we are six months down stream there are still problems and uncertainties. Another unusual consideration is that there are many on-going studies on the TMI incident; at least six formally constituted groups are looking into the matter of what happened at TMI and the investigations are not complete. Indeed the report of the President's Commission on the Accident at Three Mile Island is due in about five days. Therefore I don't think it would be useful to give you all of the complicated details of what went wrong and the suggested reasons for what happened in specific terms.

What might be useful is the format that many other speakers at this symposium have followed in discussing the various radiation accident cases. This is, to share our observations of these radiation-related occurrences that hopefully are limited in their frequency and therefore are not likely to be part of the personal experience of many individuals, with emphasis on the health impact and its management. I shall therefore describe what the TMI incident looked like through the eyes of the health team at Harrisburg, Pennsylvania, in the period from the beginning of the incident through the first week to ten days, or what the clinicians among you might call the acute stage. I do so not as a state employee, but primarily on the basis of having been called in as a consultant by the Pennsylvania State Health Department, which in turn had the responsibility to advise the governor concerning appropriate measures to take for the health and safety of the people of the state. I also have served for a number of years as a member and chairman of the Governor's Advisory Committee on Atomic Energy Development and Radiation Control, and since the TMI incident, as a member of the Governor's Commission to Study and Evaluate the Consequences of the Incident at Three Mile Island. I will discuss the state response during the incident and then give you some idea of the continuing state response and of what has been done in the six months that followed the acute stage.

The Three Mile Island Nuclear Power Station is located in Pennsylvania at the location shown in Figure 1. Because of its proximity to the state capital in Harrisburg, the incident may have received more prompt state-level attention that it might have elsewhere in the state.

Regarding the mechanics of the incident, since this has already been widely published, all I will note is the fact that there was a problem with a steam generator that shut down the reactor. The basic difficulty was one of a heat build-up in the reactor core because the cooling systems were not functioning as they were supposed to. The other point that should be noted is that contaminated water from the primary cooling system went from the reactor containment vessel to the auxiliary building, which was not fitted to contain gases and vapors. This led to the release of xenon 133 and a small amount of iodine 131 into the off-site area.

We are interested in the health aspects of the problem, what the state was faced with, and what it did. The State of Pennsylvania is like about half of the 50 states in that during the 1960s, when environmental issues were emphasized, the legislature separated some activities that had previously been considered health responsibilities and put them under a new Department of Environmental Resources. Among these was the sole focus of radiation protection competences in the state, the Bureau of Radiological Health, now called the Bureau of Radiation Protection (BRP), where the first impact was felt.

The utility had the responsibility, which it carried out, of notifying the Office of Inspection and Enforcement of the Nuclear Regulatory Commission (NRC) in Region I, in which the plant is located, about the abnormal occurrence. It also notified the Pennsylvania Emergency Man-

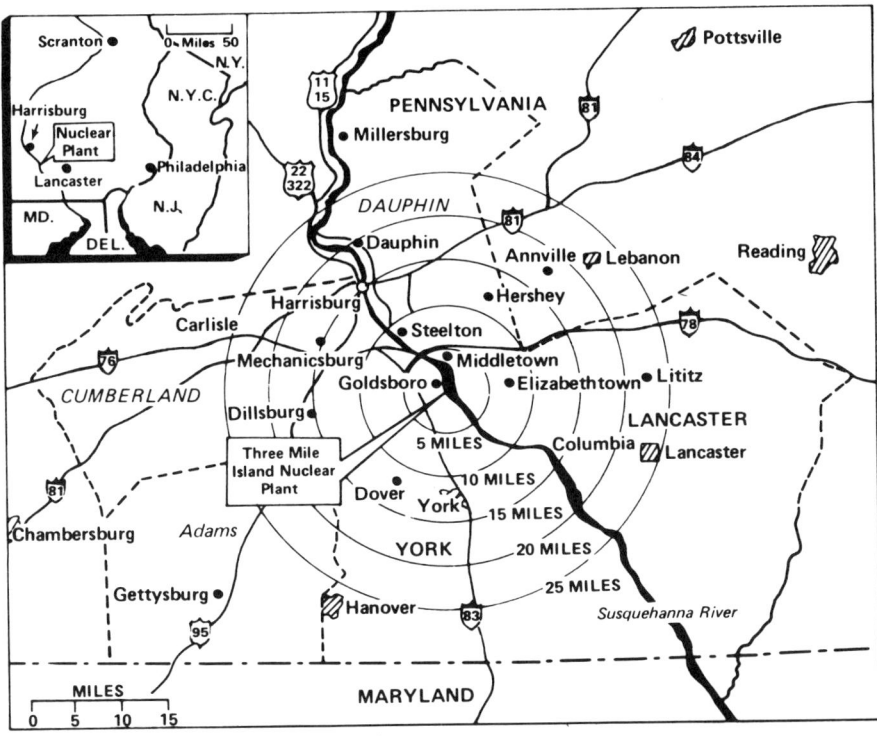

Figure 1. Geographic location of the Three Mile Island Power Station. From the *New York Times*, 2 April 1979.

agement Agency (PEMA), about the problem. The Department of Environmental Resources was then contacted by PEMA. The notification was made about 7:00 A.M. on March 28 although the problem began about 4:00 A.M.

The sequence went as follows: the BRP duty officer, a nuclear engineer, received the call from PEMA. He determined the nature of the problem by telephone and then notified the key state officials in the executive department about the fact that some radioisotope releases were coming from an unknown location at the TMI plant, which turned out to be the auxiliary building previously mentioned. The levels were low, and therefore, there was no great alarm initially and the information seemed to be useful in planning purposes. Further measurements were made, and information was transmitted to the NRC in Washington.

There were increased communications back and forth between government officials in Washington and Harrisburg, the utility personnel, the media, and the public. Over the next two days a certain amount of confusion and lack of coordination developed. A number of federal agencies, including the Department of Energy (DOE), the Department of Health, Education, and Welfare (HEW), the Communicable Disease Center (CDC), the Food and Drug Administration (FDA), and the Environmental Protection Agency (EPA), had been called in by then at the behest of both the NRC and the state BRP to help with a major requirement. This was the continuing assessment of the amount of radioactivity being released from the plant and the off-site dose commitment, i.e., the amount of radiation exposure of the off-site population. BRP quickly found itself in the situation of giving its entire effort first to making measurements and then, when the above-mentioned help arrived, to collating and assessing the information from the various sources as well, for administrative use. The relatively small group performed very well, but after several days, the round-the-clock crisis tempo began to interfere with performance. The monitoring data collection and coordination was organized ultimately under the DOE personnel at a separate location from BRP to reduce the tremendous amount of confusion and communication difficulties that were building up. They then sent the information back to BRP and, in turn, the state executive personnel received their information that way.

A brief summary of the already published dosimetry effort[1] may help to give you a feeling for the nature of the measurements. Thermoluminescent dosimeters were used by the utility, or its radiation monitoring group, plus additional ones subsequently put in the field by NRC. There were also a few BRP dosimeters in the area. A hypothetical cumulative maximum dose of approximately 83 mrem is based on continuous exposure at a point half a mile north of the plant where no one lives. Based on the TLD measurements, the person-rem exposure of the population from March 28 through April 7 adds up to about 3300 person-rem. That is simply the average dose times the number of people. Using about 2,000,000 people in a 50 mile area around the TMI plant one comes up with this kind of number. The average dose to a typical individual within 50 miles was 1.5 mrem, and for one within 10 miles, 8 mrem.

Another estimate of the off-site exposure was based on plume measurements based on over 200 DOE aircraft measurements tracking plumes with specially equipped helicopters. The result of this was to give an isodose plot of the dose out-of-doors for any particular time period. Figure 2 gives as an example, a ten-mile plot that represents the first weeks' exposure. One can then get a feeling for the geographic distribution of the exposure in millirem. The total population exposure estimated by this method at the end of the first week was about 2000 person-rem in the 50 mile area with an average of 0.9 mrem. The major escape of radioactivity was in the first week, the second week adding only about 50 person-rem.

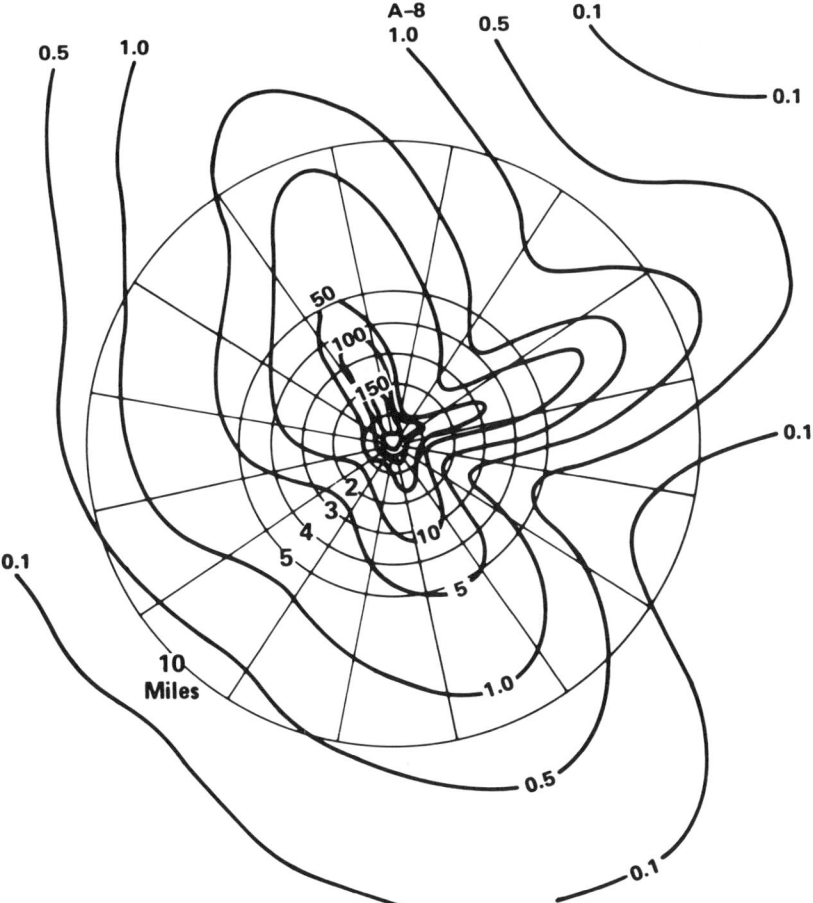

Figure 2. Department of Energy 10-mile exposure profile (mR) for the period 28 March through 3 April 1979.[1]

It was important to measure the radioisotopic release of ^{131}I to the environment. Airborne activity was measured and levels were very much lower than we received from a Chinese nuclear-weapons test, which produced fallout in Pennsylvania a couple of years earlier. The thyroid dose estimate based on these air releases came to about 3 mrem for the first week, a vanishingly small exposure.

What about intake from ingestion? In the surface sampling area, hundreds of samples were taken of air, soil, water, milk, and food. A very thorough search for activity was made in the environment, including the raw milk from the dairy farms in the area. The highest milk reading was 40 picocurie/l of ^{131}I and that was in a very transient and localized distribution. Most of the samples were near or below the detection limit of the measurement system at about 10 or 11 picocurie/l.

For the population itself, urinalyses were done at NIH in 39 people and whole-body counts by an NRC contractor in 721 individuals who volunteered for this, particularly in the town of Middletown. No activity was found other than what one would expect from the general population except for a few instances of radon exposure unrelated to the TMI incident.

As can be seen from the foregoing, the radioactivity resulted in very low exposure estimates. The real health stress had to do with the perception of what was going on. The psychological impact of perceived hazard was indeed a health problem that had to be dealt with. On the one hand, the state officials and the public were getting the impression that the early reassuring information from the utilities was not as credible as one would like. On the other hand, they were getting the perception that perhaps some technical and administrative federal government people were over-reacting. In fact, an NRC order to evacuate, which was not followed, came through on the third day on the basis of one reading that was misinterpreted and later found not to be valid.

There was a lot of confusion in information gathering and communication. Telephone communication was virtually impossible at the BRP, although it was the only resource at the state level for radiation protection information. It was very difficult to get a call through to find out what the Bureau of Radiation Protection was learning about radiation exposures reported to it by the large support team of federal agency technical personnel that had been mobilized and subsequently organized under DOE. Concordant official information was badly needed and the NRC's Division of Reactor Regulation headed by Howard Denton took over at that point by White House designation to serve as the sole source to transmit federal information to the utilities, the State of Pennsylvania, and the public. At the same time, Governor Thornburg became the sole source of state information to the public. In addition to making use of the more usual media communications, one of the most helpful steps he took was to set up and publicize a hot-line telephone number manned by his staff, which anyone in the area could call to get current factual information about their TMI-related concerns.

One of the major needs was for interpretation of the health impact of that information to get through to the decision makers at the state level where the public health and safety responsibility lay. What was the State Health Department role in all this? In Pennsylvania it is important to realize that although we have 67 counties, only 6 of them have County Health Departments so the State Health Department plays a very large role at the county level as well as the state level. What happened in March 1979 was that the Secretary of Health had been in office for approximately two weeks. The Deputy Secretary of Administration had come on board that day. The Secretary of Health, Dr. Gordon MacLeod said, "Upon hearing of the accident on the morning of 28 March 1979, I asked immediately for the person responsible for radiation health within the Department and found that there was no unit. I then asked for the liaison person with the Department of Environmental Resources and its Bureau of Radiation Protection, and found that there was a person who had had that responsibility and he left the department six months previously. I further asked for library references, the technical resources in terms of literature and journal articles and found that the library of the Department had been dismantled some two years previously for budgetary purposes."[2] That's when I got a phone call in Pittsburgh from Dr. MacLeod asking for my assistance.

I think it is important to recognize that when emergency plans delegate the management of the off-site problems related to reactor accidents to the state, even in a relatively sophisticated and up-to-date state like Pennsylvania, that this is currently what is likely to happen. However, the health problems were addressed, and I did go to Harrisburg to try to help out.

The first need was to develop a good communications link between the Health Department and BRP so that information about actual and potential radiation exposure was getting to the Secretary of Health, who was being called on daily by the governor to advise him on various problems. This was arranged with the help of medical personnel on loan from HEW's CDC, and the FDA's Bureau of Radiological Health (BRH), as well as dedicated additional phone lines and DOE's daily dosimetry briefings.

The next problem was the question of the desirability of evacuation or a recommendation that pregnant women and preschool children leave the area. On that issue, by the third day of the incident, the governor received information both from NRC and HEW recommending this. He also had information from the State Department of Health, and did make the precautionary recommendation. A similar decision was made independently by many of the people living in the area who saw a beautiful view of the TMI cooling towers out of the windows of their homes. The advisory was terminated in about 10 days.

The next problem was the issue of prophylactic action beyond the recommended departure of pregnant women and preschool children. This was stimulated by an observation emerging from technical information being developed by NRC. There was major concern about a possible "hydrogen bubble" in the reactor vessel, which could interfere with the mode of core cooling being used and even possibly result in an explosion and venting of radioactive gases and water from the containment. Although hindsight has indicated that this was not a real possibility, the technical view at the time was given to the state officials and the public, all of whom were very concerned about the possibility of explosion and wide release of radioactivity for several days. The heads of a number of state agencies, some cabinet members, and I participated in a number of meetings over those days to discuss and advise the Governor and Lt. Governor about possible responses to the potential health problems.

I will defer to Dr. Rasmussen to explain why the "bubble" concern emerged and why it turned out later not to be the problem that it initially appeared to be. The perception of the hazard, nonetheless, was real and suggested a possible need for evacuation of a population. The state plan was based on a 10-mile evacuation zone. Some federal sources, including the chairman of the NRC in an interview with the press, pushed it up to 20 miles, which meant the planners at PEMA had to redo their standing evacuation plan because many of the evacuation reception areas were within 20 miles. This caused three days and nights of 24-hour duty on the part of the civil defense people in the surrounding counties that were involved. It was a very major and stressful use of resources that was triggered by what was later, regretfully, indicated to be not a studied decision but simply a casual informal statement.

The next issue was the question of prophylactic use of potassium iodide (KI). The prophylactic use of KI has been recommended particularly by NCRP Report 55,[3] by a task group chaired by Dr. Eugene Saenger. It said that effective protection of the thyroid gland is attainable by taking 100 mgm daily doses of KI, and that it should be administered to nuclear facility workers immediately in the event of releases of radioiodine whose projected absorbed dose to the thyroid gland is 10–30 rad or more. It also said that KI should be considered for the public if estimates of the total thyroid absorbed dose exceed 10 rad. The governor received an impressive memorandum through the White House from HEW prescribing this kind of therapy on 3 April. It recommended that the workers in the plant and others on TMI "begin taking blocking doses now." It also recommended making KI "now personally available" to people in an area of perhaps up to 10 miles from the plant.

By 3 April the concern about a hydrogen explosion from that "bubble" had been dissipated by further technical thinking. The ^{131}I levels in milk had shown their first rise as the analyses of samples collected earlier had been completed and reported. If one had followed through on HEW's first recommendation, one would have been ignoring the action guide in NCRP Report 55, i.e., the indication of expectation of 10 rem to the thyroid, since nobody at TMI anticipated 10 rem to the thyroid nor did they get it.

To carry out HEW's secon recommendation, to have KI then made personally available to people up to 10 miles, meant distribution of KI bottles to almost 200,000 people. We had received KI from FDA by this time, but since the public was then being informed that there was no likelihood of a major explosive release from containment, and that milk levels were well below action levels, people could well have interpreted KI distribution as another round of conflicting official statements and actions. Further psychological stress and a total breakdown of an authority credibility could have resulted. In view of the source and route of the recommendations, we ended up having to spend considerable thought, time, and effort in a nonproductive manner in justifying our decision not to follow them.

Let us now consider very briefly the follow-up since the end of the acute stage of the TMI incident. A number of studies subsequently have been initiated by the state, particularly the Departments of Health and of Welfare. Already concluded is a census of the five-mile population, which is some 27,000 people. This was a voluntary census with about 95% participation that gives information about the population including where they were, how long they were there, where they worked, as well as where they lived, and whether they stayed or left the area on any of the first ten days. There is a study of pregnancy outcomes in the area, which is part of a study in progress for three years before the incident but which now will allow a pre- and postaccident comparison. There was also a pre-existing state program for a monitoring of the incidence of congenital hypothyroidism that will allow similar comparisons.

Assessment of health has been included despite the very low radiation exposure estimates because other stresses, including the psychological trauma of this event in particular, could well have had an impact on health. A study of health impact by utilization studies of in- and out-patient medical and psychiatric facilities is in progress.

There will be an individual estimation of the dose for the people living within 5 miles of TMI as a refinement on lumping 2,000,000 people into a person-rem estimate. This is to be based on the census information on each individual's location plus the dose distribution patterns described earlier, made sector by sector, to arrive at each individual's dose estimate. The feasibility of some cytogenetic evaluation is under consideration. Long-term disease frequency surveillance, the kind of follow-up Dr. Schofield discussed, is planned for this population as well. We should have a very well-defined population base because of the census that has already been carried out.

Other groups have also been responding to the problems raised by the TMI incident at a federal level, as well as a state level. For example, there is now a NRC publication NUREG 0610,[4] which was distributed for comment two weeks ago. It lists classes of accidents and instructions in a tabular format, indicating what the licensee and what the state or local off-site authority should do in incidents of four classes of severity.

Finally, a booklet has been prepared by PEMA[5] for distribution by electric utilities using nuclear power to people in the area of their nuclear reactors. It describes the alarm systems and how the public will get information in an emergency. It also discusses the ameliorative options of sheltering, as well as thyroid blocking and evacuation.

The state has also revised its emergency plans. The Commonwealth of Pennsylvania Disaster Plan gives much more detail about the local level and the chain of command, and who will do what than we ever had before. The State Department of Health had completed a draft of its first Radiological Emergency Response Plan, which also goes into detail of who does what, the composition of various teams for response to this kind of emergency, and where the facilities and resources are for such things as evacuation and the medical care of people who are evacuated.

A lot has happened in the past six months since the TMI incident began. I hope to leave you with a clearer idea of the kind of problems one faces if all the detailed planning for off-site radiation emergency management is not in place, as it was not when we had to deal with the problems. I have also reviewed some of the corrective steps that have been taken since. If we don't have final answers on what should be done, and I haven't indicated that we do, at least we are attempting to learn from the experience and to start addressing the problems that will have to be studied further for proper state management of the health impact of such incidents.

References

1. Ad Hoc Population Dose Assessment Group: Population dose and health impact of the accident at the Three Mile Island Nuclear Station. Stock No. 017-001-00408-1, Superintendent of Documents, Washington, D.C., May 10, 1979.

2. MacLeod GK: Oral deposition to the President's Commission on the Accident at Three Mile Island. 23 July 1979, p. 5.

3. National Council on Radiation Protection: Report 55, Protection of the thyroid gland in the event of release of radioiodine. Washington, D.C., 1 August 1977.

4. Nuclear Regulatory Commission: NUREG 0610, Draft emergency action level guidelines for nuclear power plants. U.S. Nuclear Regulatory Commission, September 1979.

5. Pennsylvania Emergency Management Agency: What you should know about nuclear radiation incidents. Commonwealth of Pennsylvania, Harrisburg, PA, September 1979.

The Three Mile Island Incident in 1979:
The Utility Response

Roger E. Linnemann

Radiation Management Corporation, Philadelphia, Pennsylvania.

Introduction

With the balance provided by some distance in time and space from the accident that occurred at Three Mile Island in March 1979, it is now possible to sort out what did and did not happen, to reflect on the medical implications of possible large-scale radiation release, and to offer some suggestions on handling any possible future mishaps.

The drama at Three Mile Island (TMI) was underscored by the fact that all professionals at the site—medical, industrial, governmental—were presented with a new and unique situation. None of us had ever handled a potentially serious reactor accident because in the twenty-five year history of commercial nuclear power generation in this country there has never been a medically significant radiation injury. Moreover, all the traumatic injuries and radiation overexposure cases associated with reactors would be limited in number to the several plant workers who might be present at the time of a minor mishap.

This should not be interpreted to mean, however, that medical measures for the care of radiation injuries in the event of large-scale radiation release were not in place. The fact is that detailed emergency medical plans were operational at TMI, as they are at every nuclear reactor, from its first day of on-line power generating operation. The reasons for this lie, of course, in the rigorous standards placed on all nuclear utility operators by the Nuclear Regulatory Commission (NRC). NRC regulations require that plant operators submit detailed informational schedules outlining their plans for the medical management of on-site accidents as part of the lengthy pre-licensing procedures that must be concluded before construction of the plant is even begun.

These schedules focus on medical preparedness for on-site accidents (e.g., extensive first aid in the plant to treat worker injury) and go on to include plans for the safety of people living in the area and for environmental protection measures. NRC regulations require that plant operators demonstrate a sound medical capability to handle radiation injuries before being given a license to operate.

These detailed NRC guidelines do not normally extend to off-site injuries. Although this practice might have to be reconsidered in light of TMI, disaster planning for the general population is left largely to the state and federal agencies. The rationale underlying this decision relates to the extreme rarity of serious radiation accidents. Because not one had occurred in the twenty-five years of nuclear power generation in this country, plans for handling large numbers of area residents are spelled out in general terms only.

Another important consideration generally overlooked in the rush of events at TMI is the fact that utilities have no authority to order people to take any action whatsoever. They are charged with the accurate reporting of the situation but have no powers beyond that. This creates a grey area where responsibilities are not clearly defined and immediate measures are perhaps inappropriately left to the judgment of those in charge at the site of an accident.

At TMI this had unfortunate consequences. Although no injuries occurred and no lives were lost in what has been termed this country's worst nuclear accident, the possible sequelae demand our careful attention. For the danger here is one of over-reaction; that is, government officials sensitized by media claims of widespread mishandling may respond with measures that will prove ineffective and unworkable. In my view there is an overriding danger that regulations promulgated in the immediate aftermath of TMI may go too far.

Regional Medical Planning

Although the NRC guidelines are rigorous and demanding, each plant must adapt its planning to the medical facilities available in its area. Among the utilities served by Radiation Management Corporation of Philadelphia, a three-tier plan has been developed for the management of on-site injury. Because radiation injuries are an extremely rare occurrence, we have cooperated with the Department of Radiology at the Hospital of the University of Pennsylvania to develop a regional approach for Three Mile Island that has proved effective in reducing the cost and enhancing the effectiveness of treatment.

In this hierarchy, the first level of care is the first aid available on-site in the plant itself. Equipment and trained personnel are prepared at all times to provide immediate care to an injured worker and to prepare him for evacuation if necessary. At Three Mile Island, the in-plant medical resource consists of a first aid team and a radiation technician team, supervised by the plant's health physics officers. A first aid room is equipped to render life-saving measures and decontamination is supported by an in-plant radioisotopic laboratory that evaluates exposures and does routine analyses. Other plant personnel are also trained, and their training is updated on an annual basis in a continuing effort to provide competent first aid at the site.

To augment the first immediate level of care, each nuclear reactor plant is associated with a nearby support hospital. At TMI the support hospital is the Hershey Medical Center, located just ten miles away from the plant. The primary objectives at this level are to support life, decontaminate the patient, and begin the initial evaluation of the patient's radiation injury. Any seriously injured patient is transported to the hospital by the Middletown Ambulance Service, which is also equipped and trained to handle a radioactively contaminated individual. Hershey Medical Center has a Radiation Emergency Area (REA) that is well equipped to provide emergency treatment and to decontaminate the patient while limiting the spread of contamination and radiation hazard to the attendants.

Supporting the regional medical care in the event of a major nuclear accident is the Radiation Medicine Center at the Hospital of the University of Pennsylvania. This tertiary-care facility provides the trained personnel and costly equipment needed for definitive evaluation and treatment; it coordinates all three levels of care, provides back-up support, and maintains the preparedness of each of the other units with a continuing program of scheduled visits, audits, and training/exercises. The president of Radiation Management Corporation is Associate Professor of Clinical Radiology at the University of Pennsylvania Medical School and serves as coordinator of their radiation medicine facilities.

This regional approach to emergency planning has an added advantage in that it concentrates the equipment, facilities and trained personnel needed for the immediate evaluation and treatment of radiation injuries at or near the site of a reactor. Therefore, we are confident that the units involved in the Emergency Medical Assistance Program at TMI could readily have expanded their capabilities to handle almost any number of on-site injuries resulting from a serious accident at the plant. Our experience indicates that most injuries of this kind require emergency handling for trauma or illness; radiation exposure was below the levels where anything more than simple decontamination and follow-up were needed.

Three Mile Island

At Three Mile Island there is no question that the medical plans in place were adequate to handle the actual dimensions of the accident, as is documented by the chronology of events.

Radiation Management Corporation (RMC) received its first call through its 24-hour emergency communications network at 7:15 on the morning of 28 March 1979. Dr. Brennan, who took the call, was informed that no injuries had occurred but that an on-site emergency had been declared. He immediately set into motion the often-tested, but never-before-used, plans to deal with a situation of this kind: the Radiation Emergency Medical Team (REM-Team)—a physician, health physicists, and technicians—was dispatched to TMI. Radiation Emergency Coordinating Committee members at the Hospital of the University of Pennsylvania were briefed on the situation, and the Radiation Surgery Suite was made ready for any possible use. These measures were implemented within minutes of the initial phone call and remained in place throughout the period of crisis. Dr. Brennan also notified key medical and health physics personnel around the country to stand by in case consultation was required.

From the start, constant contact was maintained between the plant and RMC officers in Philadelphia. Dr. Linnemann returned from Germany (where he had been testifying in behalf of the Gorleben Project), and both he and Dr. Brennan remained at the site until April 6, when the crisis period was considered ended.

It was soon apparent that the most immediate need at TMI was for laboratory support. Sample-taking supplies at the plant were augmented as soon as possible, and qualified personnel were dispatched to the site to begin the process of data gathering. Because of the highly charged atmosphere, even minimal overexposures were attended to at once with the added decontamination supplies that had been shipped in from Philadelphia.

The psychological reassurance needed by workers and their families was supplied by RMC physicians during a series of "house calls"; one worker whose slight overexposure had been magnified by the attention of the media was seen several times at home.

Meanwhile, at Hershey Medical Center, the nearby support hospital, the Radiation Emergency Plan long in place was being reviewed along with community plans to handle a general disaster. The problem was twofold: first, they had to handle more than the usual few contaminated and injured employees from the plant; and second, they needed to plan for any large number of off-site area residents who might appear with real or imagined contamination and overexposures. Taking the most probable need first, plans were made to expand the Radiation Emergency

Area to handle and triage almost any number of employee injuries. Actually, this should not have proved difficult; any hospital prepared to accept one contaminated and injured patient could easily expand its techniques to handle more than one. This is especially so because traumatic injury always takes precedence over radiation injury. Radiation injury seldom, if ever, constitutes a life-threatening event. Therefore, a hospital could implement its normal disaster triage plan by categorizing each patient for treatment according to the severity of his traumatic injury. The only salient difference would be to do so while limiting the contamination to one easily isolated part of the hospital. During the crisis at TMI, augmented decontamination supplies were immediately in place to handle any expanded operations of this kind.

In order to cope with the other possibility of large numbers of people with real or imagined injury, Hershey Medical Center adapted its disaster plans in a number of ingenious ways. Plans were made to route people to a large area adjacent to the REA. Multiple shower facilities were set up, and an auditorium was prepared where people could gather for briefings and basic informational services. In this way the overwhelming psychological needs of frightened, anxious people could be attended to by professional staff while plans were made to begin the selective laboratory testing needed to determine the actual extent of exposure. Had substantial iodine releases actually occurred, potassium iodide would probably have been administered in this setting.

It should be emphasized that the levels of radiation released at TMI were actually very low. The maximum level, measured at a site 0.5 miles distant from the plant was 87 mrem. Therefore, there was never any real reason to consider treating large numbers of people for radiation overexposure, and there was certainly never any real need for large numbers of hospital beds.

After the Emergency Medical Assistance Program had been implemented at TMI and the small number of actual medical problems attended to, we found that our role altered. As the tense shutdown got underway, RMC's major and continuing involvement became one of extensive support in significant nonmedical areas. For example, soon after the onset of the accident it was apparent that the on-site laboratory—important as a source of ongoing analyses of samples—had been rendered useless by the high levels of background radiation in the building. RMC's laboratories in Philadelphia were immediately placed on 24-hour operation. Large numbers of in-plant and off-site samples were transported to these central labs, and results were reported immediately to on-site officials at TMI by telephone. RMC's mobile laboratory was also dispatched to the site to assess ongoing radiation exposures.

Food processors in the area sent samples for analysis, as did private citizens living within twenty miles of the plant who requested that we check everything from candy bars to dead chickens. As would be expected, there was a concomitant need for added quantities of survey instruments, respirators, and chemicals. Three respirator testing units were also dispatched to the site to aid in respirator fittings for the huge influx of workers to assist in control of the reactor.

As the events at TMI unfolded, reliable data concerning environmental levels of radiation became an overriding consideration. NRC officials requested that RMC supplement the in-place environmental monitoring systems with 47 thermoluminescent dosimeter (TLD) stations. Since our equipment was nearby and operational, we were able to respond to this request without delay. Information gathered from these stations was being supplied by late Saturday afternoon, three days after the accident. Daily readings at these stations indicated that environmental levels were never more than slightly above background.

There was additional evidence that background radiation levels at Three Mile Island were low. As it happened, the RMC mobile whole-body counter was at TMI as part of the routine procedure surrounding the scheduled refueling of the Unit 1 reactor. An extremely sensitive instrument used primarily to measure the normal levels of radiation present in human beings at all times, RMC's counter can detect internal contamination on the order of 1 mrem. Although it was no more than a few yards from the damaged reactor at the time of the accident, the counter was in perfect operating condition as soon as it had been decontaminated by a hosing down with water. The whole-body counter is so sensitive that any important radiation release greater than 20 mR/hour would have rendered it inoperable. For some time, however, the significance of its immediate routine operation was somehow overlooked and this valuable information was not emphasized in our public information efforts.

The whole-body counter remained on site throughout the emergency, acting as a continuing source of valuable information. For example, of the 150 whole-body counts performed on workers, only one showed activity barely exceeding investigative levels. That is one-twentieth of the annual permissible dose for a specific isotope and organ, in this case ^{131}I and the thyroid.

These continuing requests to RMC for additional equipment and supplies suggest several important modifications in emergency medical planning for radiation accidents. In the event of any future mishap a number of whole-body counters should be available as soon as possible. Other supplies and equipment urgently needed at the site of any radiation release should also be stored in a central location accessible and easily transportable to the site of an accident.

The accident at TMI underscored the fact that the most serious defect in planning for radiation accidents may lie in the vital area of public information. Any rational response to the danger of possible radiation overexposure depends on the public's perception of the dimensions and possible effects of the accident; at TMI there is no question that the information needed for sound public judgment had not been adequately assimilated by the people and their elected officials. Moreover, a considerable amount of the confusion concerning the actual effects of radiation extended to the medical community as well, suggesting that radiation medicine has not done an adequate job in communicating its tenets and findings to other professionals.

At TMI, however, this had significant consequences. For example, patients unable to obtain the sound information they desired from their usual source of medical reassurance, their physician, compounded the panic and confusion of the event. Some poorly informed medical personnel left the area, seriously compromising the care of patients already in hospitals and long-term care facilities. Had any large-scale accident occurred, this lack of trained personnel would have had very serious consequences. The events of TMI underscore our belief that better information must be supplied to both lay and professional audiences.

With the perfect vision of hindsight, we now know that adequate information of this kind cannot be disseminated against the background of an ongoing crisis. That is, if we want people living in the area of a nuclear reactor to respond sensibly in the event of a mishap, we must supply easily comprehended guidelines concerning the effects of radiation long before any untoward event has occurred. For example, people should know that it takes about 75,000 mrem delivered over a short period (hours) before symptoms of acute radiation sickness (nausea and vomiting) would occur. Physicians should know that under large scale emergency conditions, patients would not be hospitalized for doses less than 150,000 to 200,000 mrem.

If this information had been available and well understood prior to the accident, it would have been quite clear that there was no need either for large numbers of hospital beds or for the hasty evacuation of the area. As a matter of fact, the only excess emergency room load would have been that resulting from automobile accidents as overwrought drivers left the area in an ill-planned evacuation.

Even if radiation levels many times higher than those measured at TMI had occurred, rational steps could have been taken to effectively reduce any biological effects. Civil defense measures, for example, could reduce exposure by 60% to 90%, if residents were advised to remain indoors with the air conditioning off or to take shelter in prepared areas. In the event of extensive radiation release, civil defense officers could have effected an orderly organized evacuation of the area.

But rational responses of this kind depend on a high level of informed public awareness, and this should be based on environmental dosimetry of a similarly high level. In any future event it would be wise to ask selected citizens to wear dosimeters and place others inside and outside of homes. I feel that information of this kind can be expressed graphically and meaningfully to people living in the area of a nuclear reactor; moreover, it demonstrates a quality of candor that has been lacking in our earlier relations with the people among whom we operate. It is clear, however, that the relationship between radiation dose levels and biological effects must be understood long before any accident occurs. Community leaders should be identified and their assistance engaged in these ongoing efforts.

In the event of any future large scale off-site release of radiation from a nuclear power plant, plans should be in place to gather people at a central REA; following showers, decontamination, and a change of clothing, selective bioassays—white blood cell counts, whole body counts, fecal and urine analysis, and somewhat more selectively, chromosome analysis—should be performed to determine the extent of radiation release.

Any pre-existing educational plan must also emphasize the importance of the administration of potassium iodide. At TMI, as rumors ran rampant, public confusion compounded the difficulty of treating large numbers of people with a little known drug. In March of 1979, it should be remembered that the problem was exacerbated by the recent events of Jonestown; to many people potassium iodide sounded suspiciously like potassium cyanide. Since even drinking a solution out of a small paper cup might have triggered an unpleasant response, officials judged that the administration of potassium iodide would have been difficult, if not impossible, had it actually been needed. But if a more serious radiation release should occur, potassium iodide is an effective rational treatment method with few side effects. For this reason efforts must be made prior to any accident to prepare people living in the area of nuclear plants for this important preventive public health measure.

Conclusions

The impact of the events at TMI will be discussed and debated for years to come. In my view the important immediate findings are positive ones. First, of course, the system worked. The plant designed to contain radioactivity in the event of an accident did exactly that; the threat of meltdown was remote and the need for emergency evacuation or for large numbers of hospital beds was never real. Secondly, from RMC's point of view, our system worked too. The regional medical approach to radiation accidents was tested and found to be quite sound. In addition, we were able to respond to unanticipated needs in a timely and effective fashion.

This does not mean, however, that there are no important lessons to be learned at TMI. Greatly improved public information efforts are clearly needed. Films, booklets, brochures, television instruction units— every modern means should be employed to accurately define the dose-effect relationship of radiation. Normally occurring levels of radiation should be quantified, for example, so that people living in the area of a nuclear plant will be able to assess the negligible effect of the reactor on their daily lives. I believe that we should also step up our informational efforts to the medical profession, supplying them with the data needed to impart accurate information in response to the needs of patients.

Another easily taken measure involved the stock-piling and mainte-nance of large amounts of supplies and equipment. Since the quantities needed far exceed those available at any one nuclear facility, central storage plans must be developed. Mobile laboratories, respirators, chem-icals, and survey meters could be maintained, truck-mounted, and ready for immediate dispatch to the site of a radiation accident. In this way the proven effectiveness of the regional approach can be extended from medical to nonmedical areas. Expanded and improved public information efforts can also be organized along regional lines to reduce the costs and improve the effectiveness of the materials needed to convey these vital measures.

In conclusion, I wish to state my belief in the inherently rational behavior of most people. An informed individual can live quite comfort-ably in the area of a reactor if he can appraise and evaluate possible consequences. Fear and terror can be eliminated by information and education. With any reasonable Civil Defense plan and good dissemina-tion of information, there should be no excuse for any off-site person in any type of reactor accident to receive even a symptomatic dose of radiation (75,000 mrem).

Medical Preparedness on Radiation Accidents at the Ringhals Power Plant

William Jessen

Ringhals Thermal Power Production, S-430 22 Väröbacka, Sweden.

The Ringhals plant started in 1973. Since then we have had no radiation accidents worth mentioning. Of course, we have had injuries, but almost all were without contamination. The Ringhals plant, with two reactors at work and two others waiting for government permission to start, employs about 900 persons.

In the plant area three nurses and one doctor work in a modern clinic. About 35 persons are educated and employed in radiation protection and radiation survey, and also have some training in first aid. We have an ambulance of our own and specially trained ambulance drivers. When accidents occur a radiation protector has to follow the ambulance and assist the hospital staff when necessary. There are also recently built decontamination facilities and, depending on the character of the injuries, we can take care of decontamination of most of the injuries by ourselves.

Although we don't have actual experience in handling these cases, we have learned a great deal from the U.S.A. and from West Germany. We appreciated especially Dr. Linnemann's lectures in November 1978 in Gothenburg, where he spoke to Swedish technicians and physicians.

I am pleased about the cooperation with the local hospital in Varberg. We have trained for handling accidents with the staff there. We have placed special equipment for radiation detecting, for blood tests, and other necessary instruments at the hospital. We've decided on a plan for action, made an educational film, and continue to train together at least once a year. We also have contacts with regional hospiials to handle extra patients with severe injuries, such as great damage in the blood-building system or extensive burns.

We started investigations about lymphocyte aberrations together with the NRPB in England. We found three cases. It is rather unusual that everything has been done without any support or instructions by government authorities.

We are aware that we still have very much to learn, but we also hope that we never shall use this knowledge.

K. F. Hübner and S. A. Fry, eds. The Medical Basis for Radiation Accident Preparedness

Specialized Medical Sections for the Treatment of Radiation Injuries from Accidents in Nuclear Power Plants

Živan Deanović, Milivoj Boranić, and Branko Vitale

"Rudjer Bosšković" Institute, Department of Experimental Biology and Medicine, Zegreb, Yugoslavia.

We shall describe preparations of a small, developing country for the care and treatment of radiation casualties that may occur in connection with the installation of nuclear power plants. Our premise was that small countries, in proportion to their possibilities, should solve these problems as rationally and economically as possible.

Precautions against a possible radiation or nuclear accident should start with the transport of the nuclear fuel and mounting of the fuel bundles. Emergency situations may also arise on the occasion of starting up the plant, during its exploitation, or at its decommissioning. In spite of considerable technological perfection and obligatory coefficients of safety, some factors still remain beyond satisfactory control (fatigue of materials, "human factor," elementary disasters, etc.). Consequently, the Public Health Service must be prepared to respond through its network of medical institutions to specific needs that may arise with the introduction of nuclear power exploitation.

Without neglecting the importance of the first aid performed after an accident immediately in the plant itself, nor the importance of the first medical care and general therapy extended by physicians in a local hospital, this presentation is limited to the organization of the final, highly specialized treatment (diagnostic and therapeutic) of the persons that have been severely injured in a radiation or nuclear accident. Such casualties include persons that have been irradiated from an external source, contaminated superficially (over the skin), or both, as well as the persons that have incorporated a radionuclide, and/or at the same time suffered burning or wounding.

In the organization scheme proposed by us, the leading idea was to group and establish suitable medical (or surgical) sections for the acceptance, diagnostic work-up, and treatment of various radiation casualties, around a strong clincical center in which the different specialists, as well as most of the needed equipment, would already be available. Such a center, with ongoing efforts aimed at introducing highly specialized diagnostic and therapeutic methods in the field of transplantation, nuclear medicine, and clinical toxicology, offers the best opportunity for creating a nucleus of experts of various branches. Specialized sections would be developed around this nucleus, and the inter- and intra-disciplinary collaboration inaugurated. For economical reasons and for the educational purposes, these sections should operate during the accident-free period, accepting and treating appropriate types of patients (Table 1).

Section for Intensive Care under Sterile Conditions

Persons that have received less than 4 Sv (<400 rem) over a major part of the body are directed to this section, which normally belongs to the Department of Hematology and accommodates patients with acute leukemia who are receiving aggressive chemotherapy. The care in sterile conditions allows free regeneration of the hemopoietic tissues, i.e., a safe and relatively quick recovery without comprehensive therapeutic intervention. Satisfactory function of this section requires an adequate education of the personnel and strict implementation of the specific operative regimen. Aseptic conditions must be achieved at least by means of light plastic isolation tents with a pressurized air-filtration system. In addition to the facilities and means for the prevention of infection (including fungus), the section should also be able to cope with the hemorrhagic syndrome.

Section for the Transplantation of Bone Marrow

Persons that have received 4 Sv or more (>400 rem) over a major part of the body are transported to the transplantation section, which is also affiliated with the Department of Hematology. Here the patients are accommodated in sterile units ("modules"). They are made of Perspex, provided with gloves for handling the patient, and supplied with pressurized, sterile air. In incident-free period, these units normally accommodate patients with severe aplasia of bone marrow (of any etiology) awaiting the bone marrow transplant, or recovering after it. Tissue typing of the prospective donor and the host is a prerequisite before the procedure. Aspiration of the marrow for the transplantation is done under general anesthesia of the donor in a surgical room by means of multiple (several hundred) punctures of the iliac crest. The marrow,

Table 1. Specialized Medical Sections for the Treatment of Radiation Injuries

During the accident-free period: Radiation accident management training courses	In the case of a radiation accident: Type of injury	Radiation accident medical response staff
1. Department of Hematology Leukemia center Section for intensive care under sterile conditions	Irradiated < 4 Sv	Section for intensive care under sterile conditions
2. Department of Hematology Center for bone-marrow aplasia Section for transplantation of bone marrow	Irradiated > 4 Sv	Section for transplantation of bone maroow (with sterile units)
3. Department of Nuclear Medicine	All contaminated and combined casualties	Triage station (identification and body distribution of the contaminants/facilities for urgent decontamination)
4. Department of Industrial Toxicology Section for heavy metals decorporation	Persons with incorporated radionuclides of high toxicity	Section for decorporation of radionuclides (alkaline and rare earths, transuranium elements)
5. Department of Traumatology Section for bone transplantation and implantation of artificial joints	Persons with contaminated wounds	Section for surgery of contaminated wounds
6. Department of Plastic Surgery Section for treatment of burns	Heavy burned and contaminated casualties	Section for treatment of contaminated burns

collected into a plastic bag, is then infused intravenously into the recipient. Intensive care in the sterile (or at least aseptic) environment helps the patient survive aplasia until the transplant "takes" and begins to function. It is important to eradicate all endogenous foci of infection before the transplantation. In addition to the control of the hemorrhagic syndrome, these patients would also require a continuous care of the water and electrolyte balance, since severe diarrhea may occur after higher doses of radiation, which damage the gastrointestinal mucosa.

In case of considerable external or internal contamination, especially with highly radiotoxic substances, an urgent intervention is indicated, particularly so if the contamination is combined with mechanical or thermal trauma (wounds or burns). For all casualties with such a contamination, Department of Nuclear Medicine forms a detached triage station.

Triage Station

This station must have a separate entrance, and should be provided with equipment for detection and identification of the contaminants, as well as the facilities for decontamination of the skin and accessible mucosal surfaces. If the radionuclides have been incorporated, the person is checked by a whole-body counter in order to determine the type, amount, and distribution of contaminants. Some measures for preventing the resorption and deeper penetration of highly radiotoxic elements (such as the long-living "bone seekers") are so urgent that they should be undertaken immediately in the triage station, if not performed earlier. For this purpose, the station should be provided with several holding rooms, as well as with a separate sewage draining into a special collector for radioactive liquid waste.

If a protracted internal decontamination is necessary—as in the case of transuranic alpha emitters—the victim should be transferred to the next section.

Section for Decorporation of Radionuclides

This section would be organized by the Department of Industrial Toxicology. The staff of this department includes clinicians experienced in the application of chelating agents to patients intoxicated with heavy metals. Victims needing such a decontamination treatment should be accommodated separately, and their excrements should drain into a sewage system connected with the special collector for the radioactive material (waste). A pulmonogical team should be at hand in order to carry out the pulmonary lavage in cases of inhalation of compounds such as $^{239}PuO_2$. Of course, excrements, as well as all washing fluids, must go through an accurate measurement of radioactivity before disposal.

If a person has been contaminated and wounded or burned, the triage station should only carry out an ordinary decontamination of the unin-jured skin, and the casualty would be directed to the corresponding surgical section. It is obvious that emergency treatment of the injury takes precedence over emergency treatment of the contamination.

Section for the Surgery of Contaminated Wounds

This surgical area should be furnished with laminar air-flow facilities and organized in the manner to avoid any possibility of secondary infection, since contaminated wounds heal slowly and are very susceptible to infection. The surgical room must be large enough to accommodate the monitoring and measuring equipment as well as the health-physics staff. Operation instruments should be available in triplicate sets, as they have to be measured and changed during the surgery of the contaminated wound to avoid propagation of radioactivity. In the accident-free period this highly sterile surgical area, affiliated to the Department of Trauma-tology, would be used for bone transplantation and implantation of artificial joints. However, periodic training and perfection courses would be necessary to maintain the teams. A postoperative intensive-care unit and several double-bedded rooms belong in this section.

Some incidents, particularly in a pressurized water reactor (PWR), may cause combined injuries, such as burns and irradiation or contami-nation. Heavy casualties of this kind should be transferred to a special section of the Plastic Surgery Department for the contaminated burns.

Section for Contaminated Burns

Treatment of heavily burned victims is the preoccupation of plastic surgeons. After general preparations that include decontamination by washing or rinsing and excision of necrotic parts in a "septic" surgical room, the surgeons would in a second step cover the skin defect with an auto- or heterotransplant. A highly sterile treatment of such patients is required, since the burned surfaces are an excellent medium for the growth of bacteria. In case of a concomitant serious radioactive contamination, a fast propagation of the contaminant must be taken into consideration, because it has free entrance to the blood and lymph vessels. Specialists for dosimetry and radiotoxicology might advise the surgeon to extirpate even the regional lymph nodes, and suggest the appropriate timing of such an operation—if indicated at all.

Finally, a dead person that has been heavily contaminated should be sent to the Unit of Pathology, which must be furnished with a shielded and cooled storage vault. The autopsy in this case, as well as the burial, would require special precautions.

From these statements it is obvious that beside special premises and facilities, the care and treatment of radiation casualties require extensive collaboration of multidisciplinary teams. Education of adequate specialists, both medical and paramedical, for this purpose is a problem of high priority. For this reason, permanent international exchange of experience in this field would be of great benefit for all countries, but particularly for countries starting their own nuclear power programs.

A Review of the Reactor Safety Study

Norman C. Rasmussen

Department of Nuclear Engineering, Massachusetts Institute of Technology, Cambridge, Massachusetts.

Introduction

This paper reviews the methods used by the Reactor Safety Study (WASH 1400)[1] in assessing the risk to the public from nuclear power plant operation. In addition to the methods, the paper will discuss the results of the study and their relation to the accident at Three Mile Island. The goal of the Reactor Safety Study was to assess the risk to the public from accidents in nuclear power plants of the type we build and operate in the United States today. The study did not consider risk from other parts of the nuclear fuel cycle and did not attempt to assess the risk resulting from deliberate human acts such as sabotage. It included risks to the public but did not attempt to estimate the risk to the plant work force or losses to the operating utilities. The study was started in 1972, and a draft report was issued in 1974. The comments from organizations and individuals on the draft report were considered in preparing the final report, which was issued in October of 1975. The study involved about 70 people plus consultants and cost about $4 million to complete.

The Study Methodology

The work in the study was divided into seven basic tasks, illustrated in Figure 1. Task 1 was to identify those events that could lead to the release of serious amounts of radioactivity that could affect the public health or damage public property. Task 2 was to determine the probability

Basic Seven Tasks in Reactor Safety Study

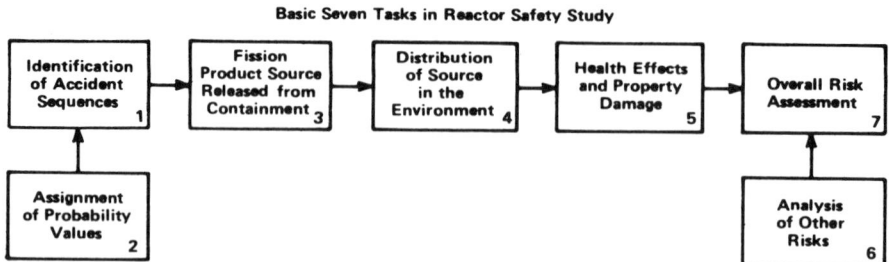

Figure 1. Basic seven tasks in reactor safety study.

of these various plant failures called accident sequences. Task 3 was an analysis to estimate the amount of radioactivity leaked from the containment under the conditions defined by the accidents identified in Task 1. Task 4 was to calculate how any released radioactivity would be distributed in the environment. Task 5 was to estimate the health effects and property damage caused by the released radioactivity. Task 7 was to sum up the risk from all the individual accident sequences identified to determine an overall risk for six consequences whose risk the study estimated. The remaining task, identified as Task 6 in the figure, was to make similar analyses of other risks that society now is exposed to for the purpose of comparing them to the nuclear risks.

The task was simplified by an analysis that showed that the public risk would be dominated by those accidents that involved the release of radioactivity from the fuel itself. This was concluded because by far the largest inventory of radioactivity is trapped inside the fuel during normal operations. The fuel effectively contains the radioactive fission products in the uranium-dioxide matrix unless it is severely overheated, essentially to its melting point of 5000°F. Thus the study focussed its attention on those plant failures that could lead to serious overheating or melting of the fuel. Although there are other failures in the plant that could release some radioactivity, the amounts of radioactivity in these other parts of the plant are quite small compared to the inventory in the fuel, and the probability of release is no greater than for fuel melt. For this reason the study group concluded that such events would contribute negligibly to the overall risk.

In order to identify those failures that could produce serious overheating or melting of the fuel, the study group noted that such overheating could only occur for conditions that produced a serious heat imbalance in the plant, that is, conditions that undercooled the fuel by failing to remove the heat generated, either because the heating rate was in excess of the cooling system capacity, or because the cooling system was not removing heat at the rate it was designed to. These were identified as the overpower case and the undercooling case. Analysis led us to conclude that although certain conditions that could lead to the chain reaction rate in excess of the normal power level were possible, their likelihood was relatively small as compared to failures that could lead to improper cooling of the fuel. Thus in the study we found that the major contribution to the risk of release of radioactivity was caused by failure of the cooling system to perform properly in one of two ways. The first condition, called loss of cooling accident (LOCA), are those failures that lead to the loss of the primary coolant itself. This can come about by ruptures in the primary system or by safety valves that remain open when they should not. The second mode of failure are failures in the heat removal system in which the coolant is present, but various functions required to move the heat from the fuel to its ultimate heat sink fail.

To identify the accident sequences in an organized, logical way, the study used a technique called event trees for the initial analysis. Figure 2 shows a simplified version of an event tree to illustrate the method. The event tree starts with an initiating event, in this case a pipe break, which is a form of loss of coolant accident (LOCA). The analyst must then, through his knowledge of the system, identify various plant func-

Figure 2. Simplified event tree for a loca in a typical nuclear power plant.

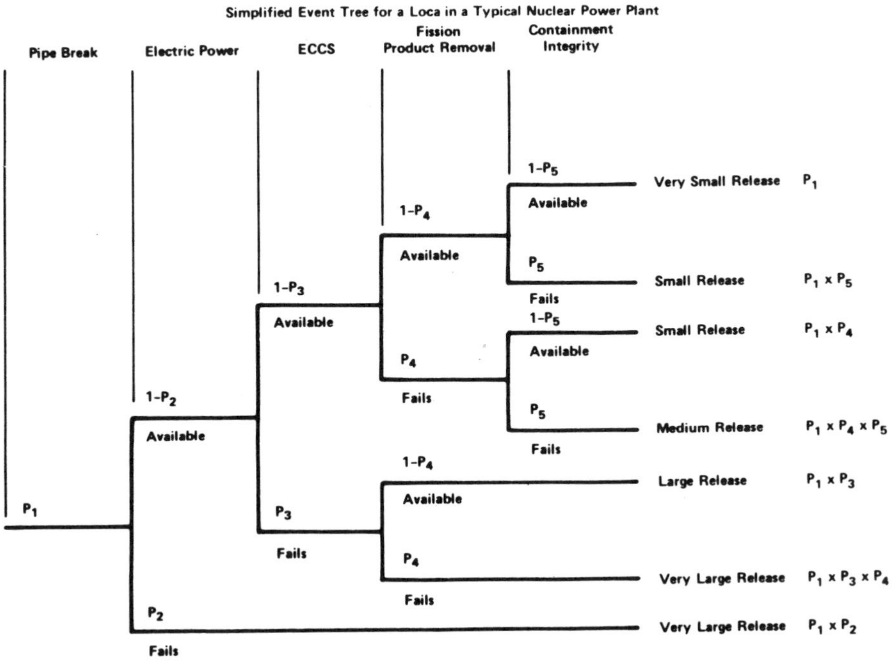

Simplified Event Tree for a Loca in a Typical Nuclear Power Plant

tions that will affect the outcome of this initiating event. In this case the functions identified are: availability of electric power, the availability of the emergency core cooling system (ECCS), the fission product removal system, which is a system that washes radioactive aerosols out of the containment, and finally the integrity of the containment itself. In Figure 2, at each branch point the path that goes up represents successful function or availability of the system that provides this function. When the path goes down at the branch point, it represents failure of this system to perform its design function. Thus we see a variety of possible paths through the tree, each of which represents a possible state of the plant following the initial event pipe break. Not all possible branches are shown because, for example, if electric power fails, the emergency core cooling system (ECCS) cannot operate, so there is no choice shown on that line. In addition, the fission product removal system cannot operate, and if these two systems fail the core will melt and rupture the containment, so containment integrity is not available either. Thus we see the bottom line on this tree has one step, failure of electric power, and leads directly to a very large release of radioactivity.

The Ps on the figure are meant to indicate the probability of that particular path at any particular branch point. Thus any one path's total probability can be obtained by multiplying the probabilities at the various branches together. The final column on the chart shows this. It should be noted that, in general, these probabilities, the values of P, are quite small, so that a good approximation is to assume that (1-P) is essentially one. That approximation has been made in determining the probability shown in the final column. Clearly, there may be dependences between the various probabilities. That is, the value of the probability of ECCS function failure P_3 may depend upon, in some way, the conditions created by the pipe break itself P_1. Thus, in the analysis one must be careful to assess any dependences that may exist between the probabilities. This analysis is often called the common cause or common mode failure analysis of the system. Thus, if done with care, the event tree allows the analyst to define all the possible final states that might result from the initial event, in this case a pipe break, and indicates what the probability of the various outcomes might be if a method is available to determine the values of the Ps in the chart. In this study, six different event trees were developed to cover the spectrum of initiating events that could lead to core melt.

To determine the values of the probability, another logic method was used. This method is called fault tree analysis, and is indicated in a very simplified way in Figure 3. In the figure we have shown a simplified fault for the failure of the electric power system to provide power to the emergency safety features (ESF) of the plant. You will note that the logic is somewhat the reverse of the event tree logic. In the fault tree we start

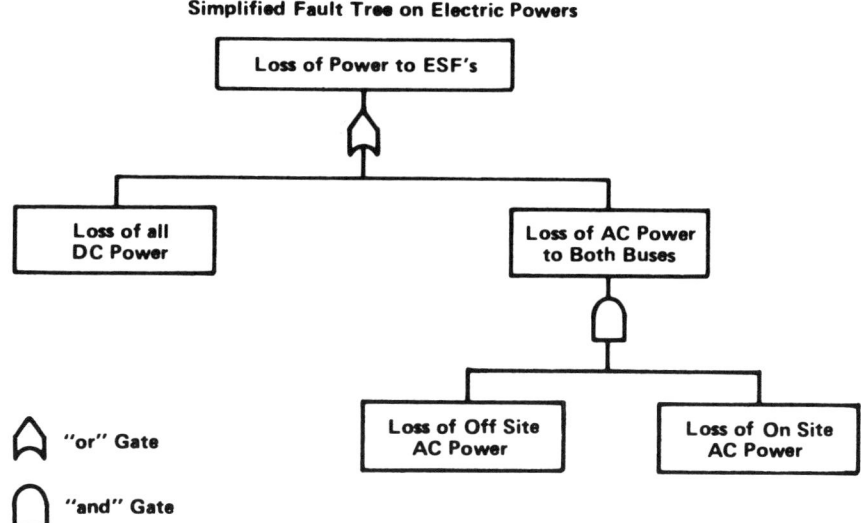

Figure 3. Simplified fault tree on electric powers.

with some undesired outcome and ask how it might have happened. In the event tree we start with some initial event and ask what are all the possible outcomes. Referring to Figure 3, we see that loss of power to the emergency safety features can be caused by loss of DC power or loss of AC power. This is so because there is a direct current system that activates the controllers to the various electrical equipment, and there is an alternate current system that provides the power to operate the equipment. Thus loss of either means loss of ability for those systems to function properly, and on the chart it is indicated by the symbol called an OR gate, which simply means that the top event will occur if either one or the other of the two lower events happens.

To illustrate another type of logic that occurs in the tree we further analyze loss of AC power. AC power is provided by two different sources, each of which is capable of operating the emergency safety features. These are the off-site power, that is the connection of the utility grid, and the on-site power, the station diesel generator. To lose all AC power, both sources must be lost, so they are related to the box loss of AC power through a symbol called an AND gate, which indicates that both must occur for the event above to happen. The analyst knows that the probability of the top event in this case is the product of the probability of the two lower events, whereas in the case of the OR gate the probability of the event above is, to a first approximation, the sum of the probabilities of the two lower events. If the tree is developed to lower and lower levels, that is, to smaller and smaller parts of the plant, one finally obtains a series of failures—failure of the operator to throw the switch, failure of the switch to work properly, the solenoid sticks, the valve sticks, the pump fails, and so on. From experience with equipment of this type in a variety of operations under similar conditions, we can obtain an estimate of how likely these events are to occur. With the probabilities of these bottom events, called primary events, and the relationships that indicate how their probabilities are related to each other, one can propagate the probabilities upward through the tree and determine the probability of the top event.

Fault trees based on these principles were drawn for some twenty different plant systems. These were systems identified by the event trees as affecting the outcome of various initiating events. Thus the fault trees were used to obtain the probabilities and the probabilities were combined, as indicated, by the event trees to determine the probability of various failure states of the plant. Careful analysis of these conditions was required to determine whether serious fuel overheating would result or not. The application of fault trees and event trees thus provided a method for carrying out Tasks 1 and 2, indicated in Figure 1.

Task 3 was carried out by an analysis of the conditions created by the failures identified in Task 1. These analyses allowed the group to determine whether fuel melting had occurred or not. And, given that fuel melting had occurred, further analysis was done to estimate how much radioactivity would be released. The release of radioactivity could come about by various kinds of failures of the containment itself. The group assumed that if the core melted, the containment would surely fail. However, there were different ways in which the containment might fail, and these different ways could release different amounts of radioactivity. The result of step 3 was to generate a histogram of the magnitude of release of radioactivity versus the likelihood of release of radioactivity.

The final result of this analysis was a histogram of the type shown in Figure 4. This figure was the result obtained for a PWR in the study (of course a similar histogram was developed for a BWR). The ordinate gives the probability per year of a release. The abscissa gives the release magnitude as one of nine different categories. Category nine represents quite small releases up to category one which is the largest release. In Table 1 the fraction of the core inventory of various fission products released in each category are tabulated.

In the analysis all identified accidents are assigned to one of the nine categories according to the calculated release of radioactivity. The probabilities of all accident sequences assigned to that category are then summed to get the final histogram shown in Figure 4.

The next step was to develop a model for calculating the consequences of the release of radioactivity. This computer code calculated five

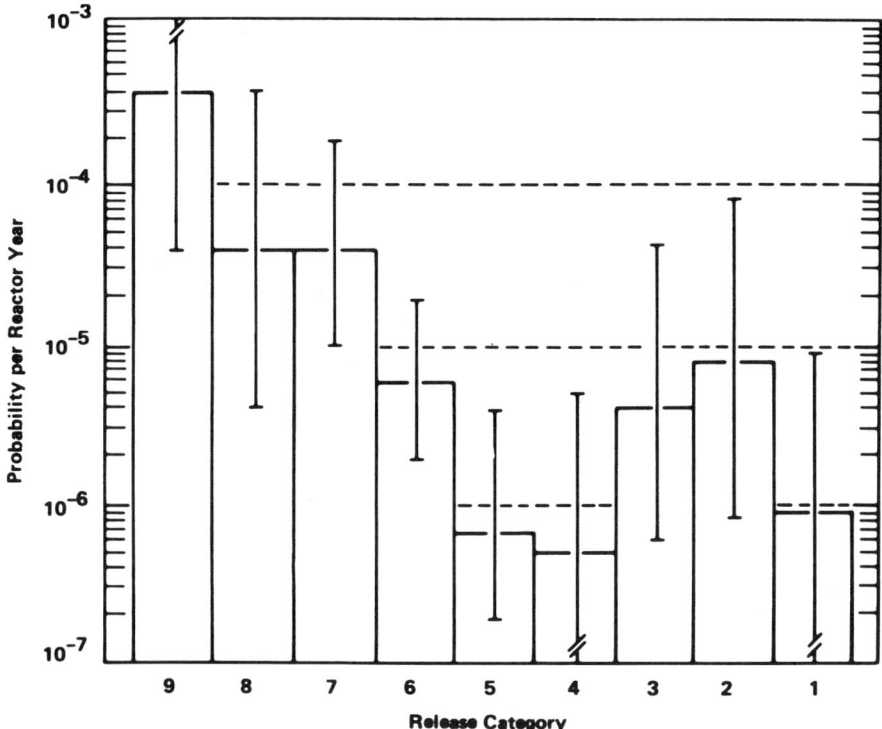

Figure 4. Histogram of PWR radioactive release probabilities.

different health effects, plus the economic loss in dollars due to property damage, clean-up costs, and cost of relocating people. The five health effects considered were early fatalities (fatalities within one year); early injuries (nonfatal injuries requiring medical care); cancer fatalities (cancer deaths that might be expected in a ten to forty year period after the accident); thyroid injury (latent nonfatal effects of the thyroid gland that would require medical care); and genetic effects.

The consequence code, called CRAC, used a Gaussian Plume model to predict how radioactivity was dispersed under prevailing weather conditions. The input data required was the release histogram, demographic data from the Census Bureau out to 500 miles from the site, and a year's worth of weather data from the site. Using a Monte Carlo method the code calculated the magnitude of a large number of possible accident consequences and the probability of these various consequences. The reader interested in more details about the model is referred to Appendix 6 of the Reactor Safety Study.[1]

Table 1. Summary of Accidents Involving Core

Release category	Probability (yr⁻¹)	Time of release (hr)	Duration of release (hr)	Warning time for evacuation (hr)	Elevation of release (m)	Fraction of core inventory releases[a]							
						Xe-Kr	Org-I	I-Br	Cs-Rb	Te	Ba-Sr	Ru[b]	La[c]
PWR 1	7×10^{-7}	1.5	0.5	1.5	25	0.8	6×10^{-3}	0.6	0.4	0.4	0.05	0.4	3×10^{-3}
PWR 2	5×10^{-6}	2.5	0.5	1.5	0	0.9	7×10^{-3}	0.7	0.5	0.3	0.06	0.02	4×10^{-3}
PWR 3	5×10^{-6}	2.0	1.0	1.5	0	0.8	6×10^{-3}	0.2	0.2	0.3	0.02	0.02	3×10^{-3}
PWR 4	5×10^{-7}	2.5	3.0	1.5	0	0.5	2×10^{-3}	0.09	0.04	0.03	5×10^{-3}	3×10^{-3}	4×10^{-4}
PWR 5	1×10^{-6}	2.5	4.0	1.5	0	0.2	2×10^{-3}	0.03	9×10^{-3}	5×10^{-3}	1×10^{-3}	6×10^{-4}	7×10^{-5}
PWR 6	1×10^{-5}	12.0	10.0	1.5	0	0.2	2×10^{-3}	8×10^{-4}	7×10^{-4}	1×10^{-3}	9×10^{-5}	7×10^{-5}	1×10^{-5}
PWR 7	6×10^{-5}	10.0	10.0	1.5	0	5×10^{-3}	2×10^{-5}	2×10^{-5}	1×10^{-5}	2×10^{-5}	1×10^{-6}	1×10^{-6}	2×10^{-7}
PWR 8	4×10^{-5}	0.5	0.5	N/A	0	2×10^{-3}	5×10^{-6}	1×10^{-4}	5×10^{-4}	1×10^{-6}	1×10^{-8}	0	0
PWR 9	4×10^{-4}	0.5	0.5	N/A	0	3×10^{-6}	7×10^{-9}	1×10^{-7}	6×10^{-7}	1×10^{-9}	1×10^{-11}	0	0
BWR 1	9×10^{-7}	3.0	2.0	2.5	25	1.0	7×10^{-3}	0.50	0.40	0.70	0.05	0.5	5×10^{-3}
BWR 2	2×10^{-6}	3.0	0.5	2.5	0	1.0	7×10^{-3}	0.60	0.30	0.10	0.04	0.07	2×10^{-3}
BWR 3	1×10^{-5}	28.0	5.0	2.5	0	1.0	7×10^{-3}	0.08	0.05	0.20	0.03	0.06	3×10^{-3}
BWR 4	3×10^{-5}	9.0	0.5	2.5	0	1.0	7×10^{-3}	0.10	0.07	0.07	9×10^{-3}	6×10^{-3}	9×10^{-4}
BWR 5	1×10^{-5}	5.0	2.0	2.5	0	0.6	3×10^{-3}	0.05	0.02	0.05	2×10^{-3}	3×10^{-3}	6×10^{-4}
BWR 6	1×10^{-4}	30.0	5.0	N/A	0	4×10^{-4}	3×10^{-8}	6×10^{-12}	4×10^{-11}	8×10^{-14}	8×10^{-16}	0	0

[a] A discussion of the isotopes used in the study is found in Appendix VI of Reference 1. Background on the isotope groups and release mechanisms is found in Appendix VII of Reference 1.

[b] Includes Mo, Rh, Tc.

[c] Includes Nd, Y, Ce, Pr, Pm, Np, Pu, Zr.

Results

The results of the analysis were presented in three different ways often used for expressing risk. The societal risk was defined as the average annual impact of a 100-reactor industry of the type of reactors analyzed in the report. The individual risk was the average probability that any particular individual would suffer a given health effect as a result of a nuclear-plant accident. The results for these two types of risks are given in Table 2.[1]

The third method of presentation was complementary, cumulative probability distributions that expressed the probability of an accident of any given size or larger. Such plots were prepared for each of the consequences. Figure 5 gives such a plot for the consequence of early fatalities. The results of the curves for the three latent health effects are summarized in Table 3. The numbers in the table are the expected annual rate of incidence of these three effects over a 30-year period, starting about ten years after the accident. For comparison, the normal incidence rate experienced by the exposed population is also given. From Table 2 it can be seen that the latent cancer fatalities are on average about 700 times greater than the early fatalities. This is because in a large fraction of accidents exposure levels are so low that no early fatalities are expected, but the relatively low doses to a fairly large population do lead to some expected latent cancer fatalities. In the largest accident identified at a probability of one in 10,000,000 per 100 plants per year, the ratio of latent fatalities to early fatalities is 45,000/3300 = 13.6.

Table 2. Approximate Average Societal and Individual Risk Probabilities per Year from Potential Nuclear Plant Accidents[a]

Consequence	Societal	Individual
Early fatalities[b]	3×10^{-3}	2×10^{-10}
Early illness[b]	2×10^{-1}	1×10^{-8}
Latent cancer fatalities[c]	7×10^{-2}/yr	3×10^{-10}/yr
Thyroid nodules[c]	7×10^{-1}/yr	3×10^{-9}/yr
Genetic effects[d]	1×10^{-2}/yr	7×10^{-11}/yr
Property damage ($)	2×10^{6}	–

[a] Based on 100 reactors at 68 current sites.[1]

[b] The individual risk value is based on the 15 million people living in the general vicinity of the first 100 nuclear power plants.

[c] This value is the rate of occurrence per year for about a 30-year period following a potential accident. The individual rate is based on the total U.S. population.

[d] This value is the rate of occurrence per year for the first generation born after a potential accident; subsequent generations would experience effects at a lower rate. The individual rate is based on the total U.S. population.

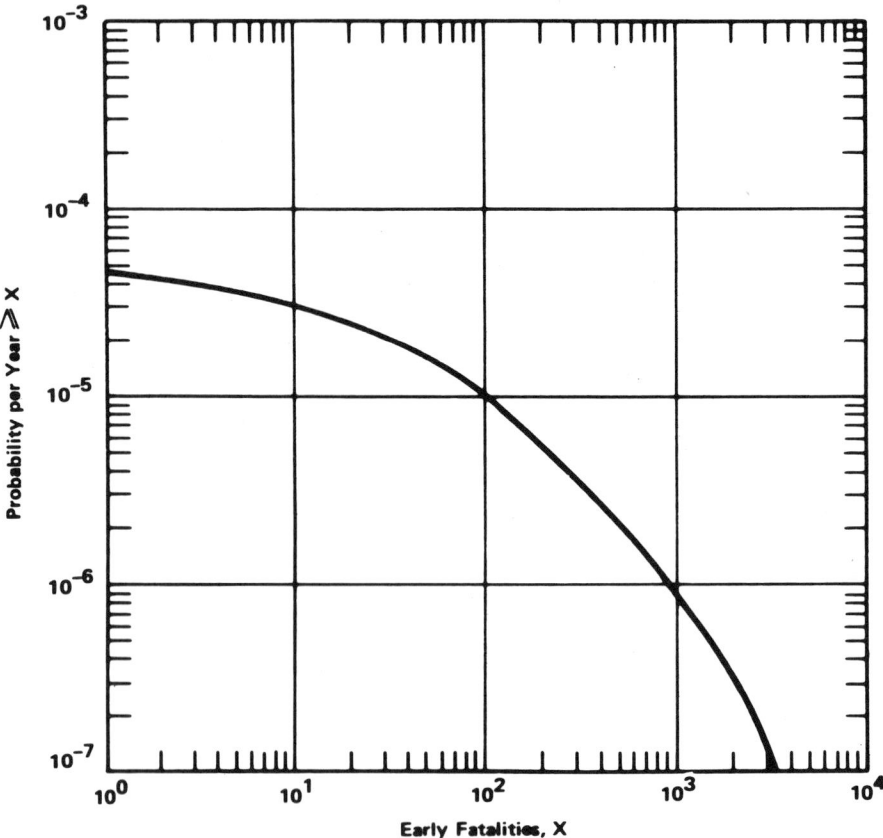

Figure 5. Probability distribution for early fatalities per year for 100 reactors.[1] Approximate uncertainties are estimated to be represented by factors of 1/4 and 4 on consequence magnitudes and by factors of 1/5 and 5 on probabilities.

The Reactor Safety Study and Three Mile Island (TMI)

Many people have asked how well the Reactor Safety Study (RSS) identified a failure of the type that occurred at TMI. There are several levels at which this question may be addressed.

The first approach is to ask just how well the RSS identified the likelihood of a release of radioactivity of the type that occurred at TMI. Although the actual release at TMI does not exactly fit one of the nine categories, it comes close to a category-nine release. From Figure 4 we see such a release has a median probability of release of 4×10^{-4}, or one in 2500 per reactor per year; the uncertainty is $\pm$ a factor of ten. Thus the study predicts that the frequency of such events should lie between one in 250 and one in 25,000 per plant per year. At the time of the event there were about 400 plant years of PWR experience. Thus,

Table 3. Consequences of Reactor Accidents for Various Probabilities for 100 Reactors

Chance per year	Consequences		
	Latent cancer[b] fatalities (per year)	Thyroid nodules[b] (per year)	Genetic effects[c] (per year)
One in 200[a]	<1.0	<1.0	<1.0
One in 10,000	170	1400	25
One in 100,000	460	3500	60
One in 1,000,000	860	6000	110
One in 10,000,000	1500	8000	170
Normal Incidence	17,000	8000	8000

[a] This is the predicted chance per year of core melt for 100 reactors.[1]

[b] This rate would occur approximately in the 10 to 40 year period after a potential accident.

[c] This rate would apply to the first generation born after the accident. Subsequent generations would experience effects at decreasing rates.

using the study results, one concludes that such an event had a significant probability of occurring in the first 400 plant years of experience. To this extent such an event is consistent with the predictions of the study. Clearly, however, the event would have also been consistent with a much higher predicted probability.

The second approach is to ask how well the RSS identified the specific events at TMI as a possible source of trouble. The initiating event at TMI was a loss of feedwater to the steam generator. This was followed by a pressure rise in the primary system, which opened the safety relief valve (SR). The auxiliary feedwater system (AFWS) was turned on but it failed to work for the first eight minutes. The reactor protection system (RPS) was automatically initiated to shut down the plant, and it functioned properly. After the pressure surge the safety relief valve should have closed; it failed to do so, leading to a small LOCA.

Events such as this should appear in the transient event tree for the PWR. Figure 6 from the RSS shows this tree. The initial event in the figure, designated T, was caused by the loss of feedwater. Event K, the reactor protection system, functioned properly; thus one follows the line upward. The secondary system relief valve (SSR) worked, but the power conversion system (PCS) failed because of loss of feedwater, so function M failed; thus we go down at this branch point. The auxiliary feedwater failed, so function L is a failure. The safety relief valve opened, so function P is a success. The safety relief valve failed to reseat, so function Q is a failure. The chemical volume control system (CVCS) was not needed, nor was the residual heat removal system (RHRS), so they

TE	RPS	SSR& PCS	SSR& AFWS	SR/ VO	SR/ VR	CVCS	RHRS	No.	Sequence
T	K	M	L	P	Q	U	W		

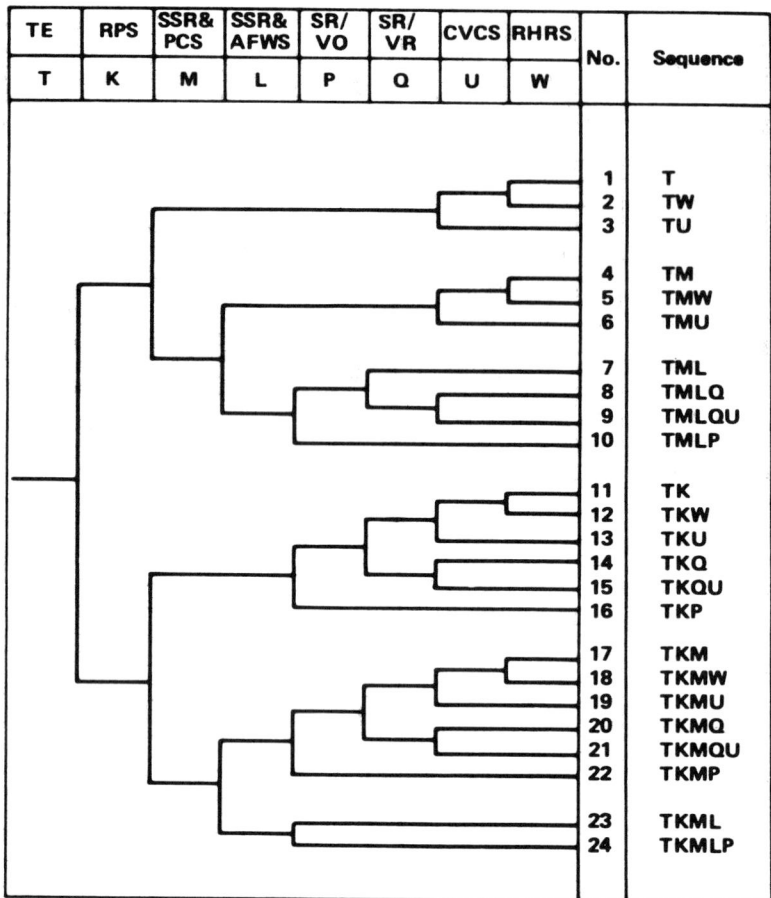

No.	Sequence
1	T
2	TW
3	TU
4	TM
5	TMW
6	TMU
7	TML
8	TMLQ
9	TMLQU
10	TMLP
11	TK
12	TKW
13	TKU
14	TKQ
15	TKQU
16	TKP
17	TKM
18	TKMW
19	TKMU
20	TKMQ
21	TKMQU
22	TKMP
23	TKML
24	TKMLP

Figure 6. PWR transient event tree.

need not be considered. Basically what happened initially was event TMLQ.

The event TMLQ was predicted to lead to core melt, except that a footnote suggests that this event leads to a small LOCA, and under some conditions core melt may not occur. Clearly the RSS analysis identified the status of the plant for the first few minutes of the accident as a serious condition that might lead to core melt. However, within eight minutes the AFWS was recovered, so event L became a success and later the open relief valve was isolated so that Q became a success. In the end core melt was averted, but not until very serious overheating of the fuel had occurred. Thus the analysis did identify in a general sense the possibility of an accident of the type that occurred, and further that it was potentially a very serious accident. It, of course, did not predict in precise detail the actual events.

I believe there were two main shortcomings of the RSS analysis of this event. The first concerned the generation of large volumes of noncondensable gas, mainly hydrogen. The study did consider that large amounts of hydrogen would be generated by a core melt, and the burning of this hydrogen might compromise the containment. However, the study conservatively assumed that if conditions serious enough to produce large amounts of hydrogen existed that the core would melt and it would melt through the pressure vessel, so consideration was never given to the fact that this hydrogen might be trapped in the primary system. Thus there was no analysis of the possibility that hydrogen collecting in the primary system could possibly interfere with proper cooling of the fuel. This possibility turned out to be a serious concern during the first few days of the TMI event.

The second shortcoming was that the study implicitly concluded that a category-nine release, because it would have a minimal health impact, was a trivial accident. Even though TMI will clearly have a minimal health impact, no one can conclude it was a trivial accident in terms of its psychological impact on the public or its impact on the nuclear industry. Thus I conclude that these small accidents in terms of health impacts must be considered in more detail in future analyses of overall reactor safety.

Conclusions

It is clear that in light of all the added information that has accumulated since the RSS was issued in 1975, a number of the aspects of the study can now be updated and improved. The Nuclear Regulatory Commission has carried out or now has underway many of these improvements and changes. To date none of this work has altered the results of the RSS significantly compared to the uncertainty of plus or minus a factor of 5 assigned in the original report. Therefore the basic conclusion of the report that the risks to public health from reactor accidents are small compared to other risks that are currently accepted remains valid. In my opinion this statement remains valid even in light of the accident at Three Mile Island. It does seem clear, however, that intermediate-sized accidents (less than core melt, but greater than design basis accidents) warrant more careful consideration than they have received to date.

Reference

1. Reactor safety study: An assessment of accident risks in U.S. commercial nuclear power plants, United States Nuclear Regulatory Commission, WASH-1400 (NUREG-75/014), October 1975.

Discussion for Section VI

V. P. BOND: Dr. Rasmussen, may I ask a question, which you have already addressed in part, concerning "human engineering." Aircraft and other complicated machines, including large nuclear reactors, have become quite complex. In a serious emergency, even the informed and competent individual can perhaps be overwhelmed by the rapid receipt of large amounts of information. It is said that under such circumstances there is a tendency to form a hypothesis early as to what is happening, and to favor selectively thereafter information that tends to confirm this initial impression, even if available information indicates strongly that the impression is wrong. What is your view of the seriousness of these possibilities?

N. C. RASMUSSEN: The tendency you refer to has certainly been observed in the operation of many large machines. To improve the situation I feel we must take more advantage of the ability of large computers to handle large amounts of information and to process it accurately. Certainly the accident at Three Mile Island clearly showed there is room for considerable improvement in this area.

J. T. BRENNAN: Unofficial reports noted that at TMI two important valves were in the wrong position many hours before the accident. Does this kind of error require special evaluation?

N. C. RASMUSSEN: Yes, it certainly does. We must develop procedures to prevent the occurrence of such an event. There are several procedures or changes in design that could accomplish this.

D. J. SIGMAR: There is presently a large amount of radioactive liquid in the TMI reactor building. What is a reasonable perspective on its significance, and what should one do to get rid of the problem?

N. C. RASMUSSEN: This water must be processed by ion exchange to remove the radioactivity. By this process the levels of activity can be lowered to very safe standards, and then the water can be released.

W. K. SINCLAIR: You described the initial event at TMI as TMLQ and you also said there was no possibility of a hydrogen-oxygen explosion in the vessel. What was the situation as it would be described by the Wash 1400 procedure at the time of the critical period between March 30 and April 2?

N. C. RASMUSSEN: Wash 1400 concluded that TMLQ would level to core melt in most circumstances. However, it noted that the stuck open valve might provide enough water flow to prevent core melt. At TMI, after 8 minutes, failure L (auxillary feed water system) was recovered.

S. MILLER: In the event of a worst-case accident, as outlined in Wash 1400, what would the nature of the cloud shine and ground-deposition fallout from the plume be? And how long would it last?

N. C. RASMUSSEN: As you must realize this depends upon the weather conditions and the distance from the plant. I can not give a specific answer to your question, but the Wash 1400 computer code will calculate the quantities you desire for any given set of weather conditions.

Index